Measuring Well-Being

Measuring Well-Being

Interdisciplinary Perspectives from the Social Sciences and the Humanities

Edited by

MATTHEW T. LEE, LAURA D. KUBZANSKY, AND
TYLER J. VANDERWEELE

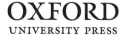

OXFORD
UNIVERSITY PRESS

OXFORD
UNIVERSITY PRESS

Oxford University Press is a department of the University of Oxford. It furthers
the University's objective of excellence in research, scholarship, and education
by publishing worldwide. Oxford is a registered trade mark of Oxford University
Press in the UK and certain other countries.

Published in the United States of America by Oxford University Press
198 Madison Avenue, New York, NY 10016, United States of America.

© Oxford University Press 2021

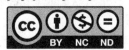
Library of Congress Cataloging-in-Publication Data
Names: Lee, Matthew T., 1972– editor. | Kubzansky, Laura D., editor. |
VanderWeele, Tyler J., editor.
Title: Measuring well-being : interdisciplinary perspectives from
the social sciences and the humanities / edited by
Matthew T. Lee, Laura D. Kubzansky, and Tyler J. VanderWeele.
Description: New York, NY : Oxford University Press, [2021] |
Includes bibliographical references and index.
Identifiers: LCCN 2020039398 (print) | LCCN 2020039399 (ebook) |
ISBN 9780197512531 (hardback) | ISBN 9780197512555 (epub) |
ISBN 9780197512562
Subjects: LCSH: Well-being—Research—Methodology. |
Quality of life—Research—Methodology. | Social indicators. | Economic indicators.
Classification: LCC HN25.M4195 2021 (print) | LCC HN25 (ebook) | DDC 306—dc23
LC record available at https://lccn.loc.gov/2020039398
LC ebook record available at https://lccn.loc.gov/2020039399

DOI: 10.1093/oso/9780197512531.001.0001

1 3 5 7 9 8 6 4 2

Printed by Integrated Books International, United States of America

Contents

PART 3 ADVANCING THE CONVERSATION ABOUT MEASUREMENT

PART 4 SCHOLARLY DIALOGUE ON THE SCIENCE OF WELL-BEING

Contributors

Paul V. Allin, CStat, FRSA
Visiting Professor
Department of Mathematics
Imperial College London
London, UK

Michael J. Balboni, PhD, ThM, Mdiv
Instructor
Department of Psychiatry
Harvard Medical School
Boston, MA, USA

Anne Baril, PhD
Lecturer
Department of Philosophy
Washington University in St. Louis
St. Louis, MO, USA

Jennifer Morozink Boylan, PhD
Assistant Professor
Health and Behavioral Sciences
University of Colorado Denver
Denver, CO, USA

Colin Farrelly, PhD
Professor
Department of Political Studies
Queen's University
Kingston, ON, Canada

Guy Fletcher, PhD
Senior Lecturer
Department of Philosophy
University of Edinburgh
Edinburgh, UK

Donald E. Frederick, PhD
Research Affiliate
Human Flourishing Program
The Institute for Quantitative Social
Science
Cambridge, MA, USA

Jon Hall, MSc
Policy Specialist
United Nations Development
Programme
New York, NY, USA

Jeffrey A. Hanson, PhD
Senior Philosopher
Human Flourishing Program
Harvard University
Cambridge, MA, USA

John F. Helliwell, PhD
Professor Emeritus
Vancouver School of Economics
University of British Columbia
Vancouver, BC, Canada

Andrew T. Jebb, PhD
Scientist
Institute for the Study of Human
Flourishing
University of Oklahoma
Norman, OK, USA

Eric S. Kim, PhD
Assistant Professor
Department of Psychology
University of British Columbia
Vancouver, BC, Canada

Julie A. Kirsch, PhD
Postdoctoral Fellow
Department of Family Medicine and
Community Health
University of Wisconsin—Madison
Madison, WI, USA

Laura D. Kubzansky, PhD, MPH
Lee Kum Kee Professor
Department of Social and
Behavioral Sciences
Harvard T. H. Chan School of
Public Health
Boston, MA, USA

William A. Lauinger, PhD
Associate Professor of Philosophy
Religious Studies and Philosophy
Chestnut Hill College
Philadelphia, PA, USA

Matthew T. Lee, PhD
Director of Empirical
Research
Human Flourishing Program
Harvard University
Cambridge, MA, USA

Katelyn N. G. Long, MSc, DrPH
Postdoctoral Fellow
Human Flourishing Program
Harvard University
Cambridge, MA, USA

Sonja Lyubomirsky, PhD
Distinguished Professor
Department of Psychology
University of California,
Riverside
Riverside, CA, USA

Seth Margolis, PhD
Graduate Student
Department of Psychology
University of California, Riverside
Riverside, CA, USA

Eileen McNeely, PhD, MS, RN
Executive Director
Sustainability and Health Initiative for
NetPositive Enterprise
Department of Environmental Health
Harvard T. H. Chan School of
Public Health
Boston, MA, USA

Neil G. Messer, BSc, MA, PhD
Professor
Department of Theology, Religion, and
Philosophy
University of Winchester
Winchester, UK

Daniel J. Ozer, PhD
Professor
Department of Psychology
University of California, Riverside
Riverside, CA, USA

Carol D. Ryff, PhD
Director, Institute on Aging
Hilldale Professor of Psychology
University of Wisconsin—Madison
Madison, WI, USA

Eric Schwitzgebel, PhD
Professor
Department of Philosophy
University of California, Riverside
Riverside, CA, USA

Victoria S. Scotney, BA
Graduate Student
Psychological Sciences
Purdue University
West Lafayette, IN, USA

Louis Tay, PhD
William C. Byham Associate Professor
Industrial-Organizational Psychology
Department of Psychological Sciences
Purdue University
West Lafayette, IN, USA

Claudia Trudel-Fitzgerald, PhD
Research Scientist
Department of Social and Behavioral
Sciences
Harvard T. H. Chan School of
Public Health
Boston, MA, USA

Tyler J. VanderWeele, PhD
John L. Loeb and Frances Lehman Loeb
Professor of Epidemiology
Departments of Epidemiology and
Biostatistics
Harvard T. H. Chan School of
Public Health
Boston, MA, USA

K. Vish Viswanath, PhD
Lee Kum Kee Professor
Department of Social and Behavioral
Sciences
Harvard University and Dana-Farber
Cancer Institute
Cambridge, MA, USA

Dorota Węziak-Białowolska, PhD, dr hab
Research Scientist
Department of Environmental Health
Harvard T. H. Chan School of
Public Health
Boston, MA, USA

Mark R. Wynn, BA, DPhil
Nolloth Professor of the Philosophy of
the Christian Religion
Faculty of Theology and Religion
University of Oxford
Oxford, UK

Juan Xi, PhD
Associate Professor
Department of Sociology
University of Akron
Akron, OH, USA

Introduction

Matthew T. Lee, Laura D. Kubzansky, and Tyler J. VanderWeele

Policy-makers, researchers, employers, and governments are expressing growing interest in well-being (Diener et al., 2017; see also Chapter 1 by Helliwell, and Chapter 2 by Allin, both in this volume). Scholarly and popular works on the topic are also finding a broad audience (e.g., Gaffney, 2011; Seligman, 2012; Volf, 2015). According to the US Centers for Disease Control and Prevention (CDC, 2020) there is "no consensus around a single definition of well-being," but the CDC claims that it generally refers to "judging life positively," "feeling good," and the experience of good physical health. Thus, a sense of well-being is informed by both how individuals feel psychologically as well as by their actual state of physical health and their feelings about that. Religious people also include theological elements in their appraisal of overall well-being. As might be expected, the study and measurement of a concept as broad as well-being remains challenging. This has complicated efforts to track the trends in well-being over time and across cultures, which also affects our ability to understand the antecedents and consequents of well-being. Large national surveys routinely measure health and economic circumstances, but people attach just as much importance to other aspects of their life, including being happy and having a sense of purpose, living well, having good relationships and being connected, and numerous other facets of well-being (VanderWeele, 2017; VanderWeele, McNeely, & Koh, 2019; Lee et al., 2020). Beyond individuals, it is necessary to consider the well-being of groups of people, including organizations, communities, and nations. Antecedents and consequences of well-being at a societal level might differ from those at the individual level and could include such domains as the positive contribution of a group to its members or to flourishing more broadly, the extent to which a climate of mutuality prevails within a group, and a shared sense of collective vision and mission (Phillips & Wong, 2017; VanderWeele, 2019).

Matthew T. Lee, Laura D. Kubzansky, and Tyler J. VanderWeele, *Introduction* In: *Measuring Well-Being*. Edited by: Matthew T. Lee, Laura D. Kubzansky, and Tyler J. VanderWeele, Oxford University Press (2021).
© Oxford University Press. DOI: 10.1093/oso/9780197512531.003.0001

This edited volume, *Measuring Well-Being: Interdisciplinary Perspectives from the Social Sciences and the Humanities,* focuses on both conceptual and practical challenges in measuring well-being in the hope of moving the field in the direction of greater integration and perhaps even synthesis while also recognizing that hegemony is undesirable and that diverse voices and perspectives are always valuable. Given such diverse interests related to well-being, it is not surprising that well-being measures—both objective and subjective—have proliferated in recent years. *Subjective well-being* refers to a person's self-reported "global assessment of all aspects" of their life (Diener, 1984), whereas *objective well-being* refers to a set of societal circumstances generally captured by material, tangible, and quantitative indicators. Even when considering just one facet of well-being, subjective well-being, numerous domains have been identified along with related measures, including life satisfaction, positive affect, absence of negative affect, sense of purpose, positive relationships, personal growth, optimism, engagement, mastery, and autonomy. The abundance of subjective well-being measures may arise in part from attempts to capture more specific dimensions or because conceptual definitions also vary widely. In addition, many of these measures focus only on psychological experiences of well-being and do not include other important dimensions of well-being (e.g., physical health) that are also constitutive of well-being broadly defined (CDC, 2020). Another complexity is that an individual might self-report a low level of subjective well-being even in the absence of significant mental health problems such as anxiety or depression. Further complicating this picture, researchers have also identified people who express a high level of subjective well-being but also experience an elevated level of psychopathology (Suldo, 2016).

Some definitions of well-being include material conditions such as income, political conditions like having a voice in governance, and environmental conditions such as the degree of physical safety or the presence of pollution (Stiglitz, Sen, & Fitoussi, 2009). These objective circumstances—sometimes labeled as aspects of "quality of life"—are certainly "fundamental to well-being" (CDC, 2020), but treating them as domains of well-being per se might contribute to conceptual confusion due to the conflation of predictors and outcomes. After all, the overall well-being of some individuals is more sensitive to a reduction in income, while others may be more affected by a diminishment of political voice. This is why the CDC and others advocate the assessment of living conditions separately from psychological appraisals of life satisfaction, happiness, and other aspects of subjective well-being. This confusion of well-being predictors and outcomes is evident in the definition of well-being used by the Commission on the Measurement of Economic Performance and Social Progress. On the one hand, a variety of objective measures are included in a "multi-dimensional definition" of well-being, but the Report also states that "these dimensions *shape* people's well-being" (Stiglitz et al., 2009, pp. 14–15, emphasis added), implying that they are separate from well-being. Well-being per se is not defined, although the term is frequently used, and the language in the Report sometimes shifts to "quality of life" (p. 15). In another place, "happiness" and "well-being" (p. 10) are mentioned separately, whereas most discussions of subjective well-being would include happiness. As these examples demonstrate, one of the challenges in taking stock of the field of well-being is sorting through the variability in how the concept "well-being" is defined. In sum, with a bewildering array of measures available and ambiguity regarding when and how to measure particular aspects of well-being, knowledge in the field is in danger of becoming scattered, inconsistent, and difficult to reconcile (Hone, Jarden, Schofield, & Duncan, 2014).

Some of the chapters in this volume engage with philosophical and theological traditions on happiness, well-being, and the good life, while others evaluate recent empirical research on well-being and its measurement and consider how measurement requirements may vary by context and purpose. Some chapters draw on the practices and perspectives of the author's home discipline for the purpose of contributing to a conversation across multiple disciplines. Other chapters are truly interdisciplinary as they integrate methods and synthesize knowledge across disciplines. By leveraging insights shared across diverse disciplines, the various chapters explore how research to date can help make sense of the proliferation of different measures and concepts within the field, and also propose new ideas to advance the field (see the exchange in Part 4 of this volume between VanderWeele, Trudel-Fitzgerald, Allin, Farrelly, et al. [Chapter 17, as well as Chapter 19 by VanderWeele, Trudel-Fitzgerald, & Kubzansky] and Ryff, Boylan, & Kirsch [Chapters 18 and 20]).

Contributors represent numerous disciplines including psychology, economics, sociology, statistics, public health, theology, and philosophy. This collected work may be useful not only for researchers primarily focused on well-being, but also for scholars across a range of disciplines who may be considering how well-being interacts with or touches on other problems of interest, including educational reform, the strengthening of democratic institutions, and economic empowerment. Furthermore, our chapters may provide some practical guidance for public policy, public health, or social science or for clinical practitioners and researchers seeking to measure, monitor, and study well-being or who are interested in well-being but may need an introduction to the conceptual and measurement issues in the field (see especially Part 4 of this volume).

The Goals of the Volume and Its Origins

This volume developed out of the Interdisciplinary Workshop on Happiness, Well-Being, and Measurement held at Harvard University on April 5–6, 2018. With funding from the John Templeton Foundation and the Lee Kum Sheung Center for Health and Happiness, this gathering of active scholars of well-being in the social sciences and humanities was co-organized by Tyler VanderWeele, Laura Kubzansky, and Vish Viswanath and hosted by the Human Flourishing Program at Harvard University, in conjunction with the Lee Kum Sheung Center for Health and Happiness, at the Harvard T. H. Chan School of Public Health. Moving beyond the eudaimonic versus hedonic measurement debates of the past, workshop participants focused principally on how to make progress in knowledge despite the uncoordinated proliferation of measures across relatively siloed disciplines. This aspiration is consistent with the trend in many scientific fields toward "convergence research," which "entails integrating knowledge, methods, and expertise from different disciplines and forming novel frameworks to catalyze scientific discovery and innovation" (National Science Foundation, 2019).

We hope that the workshop—and our volume—contributes to the development of a *well-ordered science of well-being*. As Chapter 6 (by Farrelly; p. 195) in this volume puts it, the "ultimate goal" of well-ordered science is its "ability to enable us to flourish." In other words, we aim to provide tools for addressing key questions about well-being that can be used by scholars whose empirical studies inform public policy and public understanding. These tools may prove useful for informing the social and political processes that aim to promote the greatest amount of complete well-being, or flourishing, for the greatest number of people. The theologians and philosophers who contributed to this volume might hasten to point out that this end is not necessarily as universally valued or as utilitarian as this phrasing might make it seem.

The Harvard workshop launched a discussion of these issues and provided a space for participants from a variety of disciplines to share their perspectives on well-being, take stock of the field as a whole, and co-create recommendations to guide future research. The workshop was organized around five questions.

1. What aspects of well-being should governments measure?
2. What aspects of well-being should large multiuse public health and social science cohort studies measure?
3. What should researchers conducting well-being studies measure as a predictor or as an outcome?
4. To what extent is it possible to attain consensus on how to define and measure well-being? To what extent is it necessary?
5. How can knowledge about the distribution, effects, and determinants of well-being expand when we are using so many different measures?

Starting from their own vantage point as scholars who have each made significant contributions within their own disciplines, these psychologists, philosophers, epidemiologists, sociologists, theologians, and others shared their insights and challenged each other to explore possibilities for interdisciplinary integration and synthesis.

The workshop convened both senior and junior scholars across multiple disciplines. It is rare for scholars generally used to speaking to others within their own discipline to open their cherished ideas to cross-examination by representatives from other disciplines, especially those that operate from different epistemic, metaphysical, and ontological foundations. But both the conference and the volume aimed for "hospitality" (Hampson & Boyd-MacMillan, 2008, p. 98; Lee & Yong, 2012) across disciplinary lines, the debate about intractable "epistemic crises" in interdisciplinary communication notwithstanding (MacIntyre, 1984, 1988, 1990). Dissonance was welcome, but a spirit of "the pursuit of truth in the company of friends" prevailed (Palmer, 1998, p. 90). That spirit continues in the volume, which concludes with a convergent set of recommendations offered by nineteen co-authors, a dissenting response by several other workshop participants, a response to the dissent, and a rejoinder. We believe such dialogue is essential to a healthy and well-ordered science.

It is our hope that this volume will strengthen the potential for further interdisciplinary conversation within the research community and in the domain of public policy and that it will bring together the best insights from this lively discussion. In the first section of our volume, chapters identify key questions about well-being that have been explored by empirical social science. In later chapters, contributors provide discussion of some of the underpinnings of our understanding of well-being from the perspectives of theology and philosophy, as well as discussing the extent to which these views inform social scientific conceptualizations and investigations.

Philosophical and Theological Underpinnings of Well-Being: Toward a Rapprochement with Social Science

A great deal of valuable scholarship has been conducted within a single disciplinary silo, and moreover, we are not suggesting that interdisciplinary synthesis is always possible or desirable. However, there is also enormous insight to be gained by the process of convergence or consilience. Bringing together scholars from diverse disciplinary backgrounds for a two-day workshop is no guarantee that they will be influenced in a meaningful way by ideas from each other's disciplines. Perhaps the most challenging aspect of any attempt to integrate the social sciences and the humanities is that social science research on well-being often begins with materialist assumptions about human life. On the other hand, scholarship in the humanities often discusses nonmaterialist matters that are difficult, and in some cases impossible, to measure with the methods of empirical science (see also Hood, 2012; Porpora, 2006).

From the vantage point of disciplines in the humanities such as philosophy and theology, complete well-being may be understood as having both *penultimate* and *ultimate* ends (Chapter 10, by Messer, and Chapter 11, by Wynn, both in this volume). Ultimate ends are considered most important, whereas penultimate ends are subordinate. For example, an ultimate end connects well-being in the deepest sense to an "eschatological hope" (Chapter 10, p. 287) in salvation, transcendence, eternal life, or communion with God or Nature, depending on the religious or spiritual tradition. Whereas nonspiritual appraisals of happiness and life satisfaction may constitute ultimate ends from a secular perspective, these ends are considered subordinate from a theological perspective. For example, one empirical study found that people engaged in religiously empowered benevolent service frequently defined well-being "in terms of doing God's will," even if this meant giving up some amount of the more commonly cited well-being outcomes, including physical health, financial stability, "material success, prestige, or the adoration of other people" (Lee, Poloma, & Post, 2013, p. 97). This is one example of a social science study that focused on an ultimate end, although it is somewhat atypical in the field well-being.

The debate about ultimate and penultimate ends does not simply reflect a disagreement between social science and the humanities. Within a single discipline in the humanities, Kant's (1785/2005) distinction between *perfect* and *imperfect* duties mirrors the ultimate–penultimate end dichotomy and further demonstrates the role that worldviews play in defining the ultimate ends of human life. Kant (1785/2005, p. 40), a disciplined thinker renowned for his steadfast commitment to a routine of long work days, disparaged the idyllic life of the "South Sea islanders," which he saw as devoted "merely to idleness, amusement, and propagation of the species." In Kant's view, fulfillment of such imperfect duties, however competently discharged and conducive to a deep subjective sense of happiness and life satisfaction, represented a neglect of the gifts of reason and self-development consistent with the inherent dignity of a rational being. Such a life of pleasure could not be the appropriate fulfillment of the perfect duty, or the attainment of the ultimate end, of a properly human life. Kant's argument is grounded in reason, not theology, and certainly not in the self-reports that provide the foundation for much empirical research on well-being. This is one of the challenges of interdisciplinary dialogue about well-being: some humanities scholars may focus on what reason or theology suggests to them that people *ought* to value, rather than what social science findings reveal about what people *say* they value. A well-ordered science of well-being might benefit from more consideration of such incommensurate epistemological and conceptual commitments.

Social scientists have also attempted to understand the role of penultimate and ultimate concerns in relation to different experiences of well-being. Maslow (1971, p. 271), for example, understood the former as related to "Deficiency-needs" (D-needs like hunger for food or craving for social status, which derive from a sense of not having enough) and the latter as related to the "realm of Being" (B-needs, which include the classic philosophical staples of truth, goodness, and beauty and understood as originating in wholeness rather than a sense of deficit). People could to some extent realize their potential in relation to D-needs and be described, in Maslow's (1971, p. 271) famous phrase, as "self-actualizers." But this self-actualization was at a relatively low level of human development because it was not rooted in ultimate ends. Such individuals might not be aware of the limitations of their growth, a claim that is also made by philosophers such as Kierkegaard, as we will discuss.

Something greater than self-actualization is required. For Maslow, what is needed is *self-transcendence*, in the sense of commitment to a Platonic form or a cause greater than the self. This may involve a religious awakening or conversion, or a perception of "the sacred within the secular" (Maslow, 1971, p. 273) that signifies a nonreligious ultimate end in alignment with a secular worldview. Those who orient their lives toward Being-needs like truth and goodness and away from Deficiency-needs such as material comfort and social status "have transcended self-actualization" (Maslow, 1971, p. 272).

From the standpoint of research on well-being, individuals who are "transcenders" according to this definition may actually present as less "happy" or "satisfied" in a conventional sense and more prone to "cosmic sadness" (or "B-sadness," Maslow, 1971, p. 279) over the inherent suffering in the world and the sense that much of this suffering is the preventable result of human ignorance. Transcenders may be more aware of the reality of the suffering of others and their duty to work toward solutions, rather than employing escapist coping mechanisms, than the "'merely-healthy' self-actualizers" featured in Maslow's (1971, pp. 271) much more widely cited early writings (Koltko-Rivera, 2006). Numerous philosophers and scholars in other traditions affirm this position. Maslow and Kant share a similar sense that our understanding of well-being should align with the kind of being that humans are. Reason was an ultimate value for Kant, Maslow promoted B-values, Aristotle emphasized eudaimonia, and theologians have prioritized salvation or doing God's will.

Penultimate ends include hedonic happiness, job satisfaction, physical health, financial stability, satisfying interpersonal relationships, and the like. These ends, which may be considered ingredients of a flourishing life, often drive large-scale patterns of human migration (Clark et al., 2019). Unless constrained by legal or social factors, people tend to "vote with their feet" by moving to communities that offer greater opportunities for these kinds of well-being. More eudaimonic or spiritual goals, such as achieving a meaningful life or responding to a religious calling, can also drive human behavior, even when attaining these goals may mean sacrificing other aspects of well-being, at least for a time (Lee et al., 2013). The 105 Puritans who landed in Plymouth in 1620, to take a classic example, suffered predictably great material hardships as a result of following their religious aspirations. Nearly half of this group died the first winter (Philbrick, 2006).

In Western societies today, people less frequently have to choose paths that allow them to satisfy penultimate but not ultimate well-being or vice versa. For example, seeking places where religious freedom is possible does not necessarily impose a high cost on other domains of well-being. And, in fact, these different ends are often complementary. For example, increased religious service attendance and spiritual practices predict a variety of other well-being outcomes, including greater happiness, along with lower depression and illegal drug use (Chen & VanderWeele, 2018). Furthermore, social science research has shed light on the types of religious practices that may be most beneficial for well-being (i.e., public religious activity), as well as identifying important group differences in this overall pattern (Maselko & Kubzansky, 2006). But it is also true that well-being for the early Puritan settlers of the United States, as well as for various religious groups today, is grounded in theological presuppositions that may not resonate with dominant trends in the contemporary United States, Canada, and nations of Western Europe. In fact, with regard to defining well-being and scholarly activities around understanding and studying well-being, the general emphasis in these societies since at least the twentieth century has been on material comfort and the self-actualization of the rights-bearing individual—"happiness" as an individual's personal project and disciplined responsibility—rather than on fidelity to religious interdicts or collectivistic norms (Binkley, 2014; Rieff, 2007). Similarly, constructs such as "character" and "virtue," which are highly valued in theological and philosophic perspectives on well-being and considered as important markers of a flourishing life (VanderWeele, 2017; Lee et al., 2020), are instead contested and even sometimes disparaged in some social science perspectives on well-being, particularly within sociology (Sayer, 2019). These disparate underpinnings of how we understand well-being are difficult to reconcile. In the lay population, the contemporary quest for well-being also involves "adaptive preferences" (Elster, 1983/2016) in social systems that more readily encourage the attainment of penultimate rather than ultimate ends (Lee, 2019).

Serious engagement with scholars in the humanities may encourage reevaluating some of the presuppositions of the social scientific study of well-being (see Chapter 19, by Messer, and Chapter 11, by Wynn, both in this volume). For example, although theologians find much value in the work of a psychologist like William James, they also note that "the aesthetic goods that arise in [religious] conversion cannot be adequately identified using a purely secular vocabulary, since the beauty that is disclosed in such experiences has inherently, from the vantage point of the experiencer, a theological structure" (p. 327). In addressing this issue, Wynn (p. 330) further notes that, at least for James, religious states of being can only serve as an "enablers of well-being," not "constituents" of it. In other words, a conversion experience might promote happiness and life satisfaction (penultimate ends), but, conceived in this reductionistic manner, conversion per se cannot constitute well-being itself. Wynn does point out that psychology and theology are not always in competition; they may in fact work together to promote some aspects of well-being, as we have already seen (e.g., Chen & VanderWeele, 2018). So some degree of rapprochement is possible. In this regard, Wynn's chapter exemplifies interdisciplinary hospitality. And yet more dialogue is needed to sort out the extent to which religious and nonreligious domains of well-being are in fact "diverse and not fully commensurable" (Chapter 10, by Messer, p. 293, in this volume).

Several streams of thought in humanities disciplines and some branches of psychology recognize the need to distinguish experiences of well-being that are truly markers of flourishing from those that might partly derive from self-alienation and unhealthy psychological defense mechanisms (Chapter 15, by Xi & Lee, in this volume). One example is the abuse of drugs to gain temporary pleasure at the expense of long-term well-being, although the subtler forms of maladaptive coping identified by philosophers like Kierkegaard will likely be more contested. In the Western tradition, the fundamental issue is highlighted by the Biblical verse about gaining the whole world but losing one's soul (Matthew 16:25–26). *Self-alienation*, or not understanding what is truly good for the self and acting from this ignorance in ways that are harmful in the long run, often involves fixation on socially sanctioned penultimate ends rather than ultimate ends. Socialization processes may condition people to desire apparent goods that are not in their best interests or that produce unintended consequences, as when the unskillful search for material comfort and security for one's in-group leads to conflict and war with an out-group and eventually ends up harming the self/in-group. In addition to philosophical and theological arguments, as an empirical matter, a deep sense of inner peace may not be consistent with the patterns of excessive striving and material acquisition that characterize some aspects of contemporary Western culture. Socrates recognized this tension more than 2,400 years ago—long before the advent of the media-saturated consumer

society—when he promoted a simple, rather austere society as an ideal setting for peaceful flourishing. His interlocutor in a Platonic dialogue labeled
this the "city of pigs" because it was lacking in most of the refinements that
we now take for granted as a birthright. Socrates agreed "that many will not
be satisfied with the simpler way of life," which would lead them to take "a
slice of our neighbor's land. . . . And so we shall go to war" (Plato, 275/2012,
pp. 318–319).

For Socrates, this social dynamic produces a city "in the grip of a fever,"
but it was unlikely that residents would be aware of their fevered strivings
and the great suffering such insatiable ambitions inevitably produce. "Fever"
implies a kind of delirium that generates compulsive behaviors that appear
irrational from a spiritual perspective but quite reasonable to the one in the
grip of the fever. Writing from a very different vantage point than Socrates
more than two millennia later, the Christian philosopher Kierkegaard (1849/
1980, p. 25) also hinted at this fever with these provocative words: "in the
most secret hiding place of happiness there dwells also anxiety, which is despair . . . because for despair the most cherished and desirable place to live is
in the heart of happiness." Also writing from a Christian perspective, though
much earlier than Kierkegaard, Augustine (1950/413–426) argued that a fevered city would not be a place of deepest well-being because it is not "rightly
ordered" with regard to penultimate and ultimate ends.

Kierkegaard (1849/1980, p. 43) demonstrated that a happiness that is
"completely dominated by the sensate" is not a secure happiness, although
a situation of complacency might prevail among people who are not fully
aware of their hidden despair or its source in spiritual malaise. A comparative sociological analysis provides support for Kierkegaard's contention by
showing that societies in a sensate rather than spiritual phase of development
tend to emphasize technological development and shallow, often decadent,
forms of happiness rather than ultimate ends (Sorokin, 1937–1941). Jewish
philosopher and mystic Martin Buber's (1923/2000, p. 97) classic work *I and
Thou* affirms Kierkegaard's notion of "happy" despair by way of a memorable
description of privileged people who offer "a superior smile, but death lurks
in their hearts." According to Buber, we realize our full humanity in I–Thou
relations, in which each person treats the other as a sacred subject and as an
end in themselves. In his view, the experience of the "Divine" arises not only
in the individual, but in the relation "between the I and Thou," and "love" is
properly understood to be "the responsibility of an I for a Thou" (Pfuetze,
1973, pp. 155, 201; see also Buber, 1923/2000, p. 66).

In a mass society characterized by many impersonal, transactional relationships, people may be conditioned to enact the I–It relational form of treating others as objects, merely as means to ends. This pervasive feature of contemporary life may not be at the forefront of consciousness for most people—including many social scientists—which is why it is helpful to distinguish both conceptually and empirically between short-term, superficial types of well-being and more healthy and enduring forms. Interdisciplinary research might help correct inaccurate perceptions of well-being and foster deeper individual and collective experiences or flourishing. The analysis offered by Buber (1923/2000, p. 97), who referred to the central dynamic in sensate societies as the "despotism of the proliferating It," provides an impetus for social science and the humanities to co-develop an enhanced understanding of well-being. From this perspective, despite a level of creature comfort unsurpassed in human history, the complete well-being of people in I–It relations is limited by the depersonalized and desacralized quality of their awareness and interactions: "What has become an It is then taken as an It, experienced and used as an It, employed along with other things for the project of finding one's way in the world, and eventually for the project of 'conquering' the world" (p. 91). In such contexts, Buber argued that love tends to be experienced as a sentimental emotion, which is a pale substitute for the sacred responsibility of an I for a Thou. And absent this sense of sacred stewardship for the world-as-Thou, environmental degradation and pervasive human conflict may coexist with relatively high levels of individual, penultimate, subjective well-being. In some cases, such well-being may take the form of Kierkegaard's despair-hiding-in-happiness.

This raises important questions regarding additional forms of well-being, such as peace, communal well-being, and spiritual well-being, that are explored in this book. We believe future research exploring the associations between current measures of well-being and the new measures presented in our volume, such as the comprehensive measure of meaning (Hanson & VanderWeele, Chapter 12), inner peace (Xi & Lee, Chapter 15), and Christian spiritual well-being (VanderWeele, Long, & Balboni, Chapter 16), will be informative and create a deeper understanding of well-being as discussed earlier. Negative correlations across some of these measures, or at least some domains captured by these measures, are certainly possible. For example, is hedonic happiness positively or negatively related to inner peace or the domains of Christian spiritual well-being? How do such measures relate to "rich and sexy well-being" (Margolis et al., Chapter 13), or community well-being (VanderWeele, Chapter 14)? How might a consideration of the balance of I–It and I–Thou relationships in an individual's social network, or in a society more broadly, affect these associations across measures? Do the associations hold for both penultimate and ultimate ends? For both Maslow's merely healthy actualizers and his self-transcenders? These are just a few of the fresh questions that arise when an interdisciplinary approach is used.

We have argued in this section that it is helpful if both social scientists and laypersons draw on the humanities to more fully consider the philosophical and theological underpinnings of well-being, and we have highlighted Maslow's later work as an example of moving in this direction, at least to a greater degree than his earlier work. But social science offers something of great value to the humanities as well, as many of the chapters in our volume illustrate. Consider the voluminous humanistic writing across the centuries extolling empathy, altruism, and various forms of selfless benevolence. Psychologist Adam Grant's (2013) empirical work is just one example of an emerging body of social science literature showing that unbridled empathy and altruism can be harmful and unsustainable (see also Bloom, 2016; Oakley, Knafo, Madhavan, & Wilson, 2011). It is much more effective to be an "otherish" giver and express skillful concern for both one's own *and* others' interests, rather than being a selfless (self-sacrificing) giver (Grant, 2013, p. 158). The implications of this empirical work for well-being are clear: "when concern for others is coupled with a healthy dose of concern for the self, givers are less prone to burning out and getting burned—and they're better positioned to flourish" (Grant, 2013, p. 158). This is not to suggest that the humanities were blind to this kind of insight. Indeed, the latest research findings confirm at least some ancient wisdom (Bloom, 2016). The research substantially adds to our understanding of how philosophical or theological ideals are lived out by real people in different social settings (see also Lee et al., 2013). And Grant's research findings are potentially more persuasive in shifting large-scale organizational practices than humanistic scholarship because organizational leaders seek to justify decisions in terms of scientific evidence and validated "best practices." In other words, the social sciences and the humanities are mutually enriching.

And yet, despite the rise of positive psychology; the proliferation of well-being interventions and "wellness" programs in the workplace; and increased scholarly, popular, and policy attention to well-being, social science research has documented that happiness has been consistently falling in the United States (Helliwell, Layard, & Sachs, 2019)—a country that has recently been described as a "mass addiction society" (Sachs, 2019, p. 124)—and "deaths of despair" are on the rise in both the United States and the United Kingdom (Case & Deaton, 2017; Dwyer-Lindgren et al., 2018; Joyce & Xu, 2019). We may gain a more complete understanding of the challenges to well-being, and possible solutions to these challenges, from integrating the enormous power of the social sciences to document and understand patterns and causal relationships with the deep wisdom of the humanities. In some cases, this synthesis may encourage scholars to focus attention on a smaller number of essential well-being measures in order to make comparisons across populations (see Chapter 17), while in other instances such integration may encourage the development of new measures of neglected aspects of well-being (see Chapters 12 through 16).

One helpful path forward is to draw on the humanities to guide the development of tradition-specific measures of spiritual well-being. A useful example is provided by VanderWeele, Long, and Balboni (Chapter 16 in this volume). Informed by a rich understanding of the theology of a specific group—the authors offer a Christian measure as a template for the development of measures in other traditions—researchers will be better able to use such measures in combination with other measures of well-being to gauge the associations between penultimate and ultimate ends and the common pathways that shape both (VanderWeele, 2017). As noted in Chapter 13, it is instructive that the correlation between a rather superficial measure of well-being ("the Rich and Sexy Well-Being Scale, which measures 'low-brow' lifestyle goods: wealth, sex, beauty, and social status") and eudaimonic well-being is quite high (r = 0.56; see Chapter 13, by Margolis, Schwitzgebel, Ozer, & Lyubomirsky, p. 381, in this volume). But this correlation also suggests a large amount of unexplained variance, similar to the empirical association of a happy life and a meaningful life (Baumeister, Vohs, Aaker, & Garbinsky, 2013). As these findings illustrate, more dialogue between social scientists and scholars in the humanities is warranted.

Overview of the Chapters

We have organized the volume into three parts. The first part, "Empirical Research and Reflections on Well-Being Measurement," contains five chapters written by social scientists. This section begins with "Measuring and Using Happiness to Support Public Policies" by John F. Helliwell, an economist and the lead author of the World Happiness Report. It engages philosophical and empirical arguments in favor using people's evaluations of the quality of their lives in order to guide public policies in support of well-being. Helliwell (Chapter 1, p. 30) argues in favor of using the "data from everyday life, not to isolate different theories of well-being, but to see how these theories cohere or compete in supporting people's judgments about how their lives are going." Armed with this understanding, policy-makers should be better able to promote flourishing. In Chapter 2, Paul Allin offers "Reflections on the Introduction and Use of Official Measures of Subjective Well-Being in the UK" from his vantage point as former Director of the Measuring National Wellbeing Programme in the UK Office for National Statistics. He makes the case for using four subjective well-being questions in the UK's Annual Population Survey in terms of practical utility, and he argues that this criterion should be used to determine how to assess other topics as well. After noting the limited uptake of survey findings beyond academia, he then argues that statisticians must do more to engage with politics, public opinion, and other domains of broader impact in order to make a meaningful difference in the quality and quantity of well-being in the world. Psychologists Louis Tay, Andrew T. Jebb, and Victoria S. Scotney contributed Chapter 3, "Assessments of Societal Subjective Well-Being: Ten Methodological Issues for Consideration." They discuss the appropriate units of analysis, concerns about translation across cultural contexts (e.g., measurement equivalence), domain-specific versus general measures of well-being, and other important methodological issues which have not been given adequate attention in previous research. If followed, their well-reasoned recommendations—including the use of curvilinear methods when appropriate—might lead to more consistent and valid empirical findings.

Psychologists Carol D. Ryff, Jennifer Morozink Boylan, and Julie A. Kirsch provided Chapter 4: "Linking Eudaimonic and Hedonic Well-Being to Health: An Integrative Approach." They offer a detailed review of these two types of well-being, including reflections on ancient Greek philosophy and more recent psychological understandings. They explore how these well-being types are related to various aspects of physical health and call for an integrative approach to research on well-being. Their review further discusses "challenged thriving" (p. 97), or experiencing well-being in the midst of illness and life challenges. As a follow-up to the review of multiple aspects of health presented in Chapter 4, the next chapter, Chapter 5, offers a more specific focus on whether and how psychological well-being influences longevity and selects the most rigorous studies as a means to advance the field. Titled, "A Review of Psychological Well-Being and Mortality Risk: Are All Dimensions of Psychological Well-Being Equal?" this chapter was written by Claudia Trudel-Fitzgerald, Laura D. Kubzansky, and Tyler J. VanderWeele, with collective expertise in epidemiology, health psychology, social psychology, statistics, and related fields. Their review reveals how distinct dimensions of psychological well-being may differentially impact mortality as well as the biobehavioral pathways involved. Purpose in life and optimism appear to have the strongest associations with mortality, while happiness appears less strongly related, and research on other aspects of well-being is currently inconclusive. They offer twelve recommendations for further research, including the incorporation of more than one psychological well-being dimension in research designs, administering repeated measures of these dimensions, and evaluating if these relationships vary by sociodemographic characteristics.

The second section of the volume, "Conceptual Reflections on Well-Being Measurement," contains six chapters written primarily from the perspective of the humanities, especially philosophy and theology, along with an interdisciplinary chapter grounded in biology. The first chapter in this section is Chapter 6, by Colin Farrelly, a political scientist/philosopher: "'Positive Biology' and Well-Ordered Science." Synthesizing across philosophy, geroscience, and positive psychology, the author builds a strong case for a "positive biology" that focuses on successful aging and promotion of happiness. He argues that including "the positive" in our scholarly endeavors, rather than simply focusing on disease and deficits contributes to a well-ordered science. Whereas a disordered science is characterized by epistemic vices that make it more difficult to "secure the desired aims of health, peace and economic prosperity" (p. 195), a well-ordered science facilitates these desired aims, thereby promoting the ability to flourish. He notes the imbalance between lavish research funding to support the study of disease (negative biology) compared to much more limited support for research on exceptional health and flourishing. A positive biology would "celebrate a curiosity-driven mindset" (p. 213) as a basis for improved scientific investigation that would assist the attainment of desired outcomes rather than just the avoidance of negative ones.

Chapter 7, "Philosophy of Well-Being for the Social Sciences: A Primer," was contributed by the philosopher Guy Fletcher. As a primer, this chapter is especially helpful for social scientists interested in an overview of how philosophers approach the study of well-being, especially how they "preserve a common subject matter for debate, even in the presence of radical disagreement," how they understand theories that make use of the crucial distinction between intrinsic and instrumental goods, the methods they employ (e.g., thought experiments), and some current disagreements between psychology and philosophy. The chapter notes that a "rapprochement" between social science and the humanities is problematized by current philosophical thinking about "genuine conceptual pluralism," a "radical kind of pluralism" in which words like "well-being" refer to incommensurate underlying constructs (p. 225). One constructive pathway out of this situation might be for philosophers to develop theories of specific types of well-being (penultimate vs. ultimate types, for example) and then, in light of this conceptual clarity, social scientists might proceed with appropriately delimited empirical study.

Chapter 8, by William A. Lauinger, also a philosopher, is "Defending a Hybrid of Objective-List and Desire Theories of Well-Being." Lauinger (p. 230) proceeds from the premise that there are two primary and distinct "visions of what human beings are." The first is Aristotelian and conceives of humans as having capacities that both enhance functioning and reflect the "kinds of things they are, that is, as human beings" (p. 230). "Objective-list" theories of well-being proceed from this perspective and include such "basic goods" as friendship, accomplishment, and knowledge (p. 232). The other vision, informed by Jacques Lacan, views human beings "as unique individuals with different sets of intrinsic desires" and advances a more subjective theory of well-being built around sets of desires that vary across people. The author defends a hybrid of these two theories to build a more coherent account of well-being. Next in order is Chapter 9, "The Challenge of Measuring Well-Being as Philosophers Conceive of It," by philosopher Anne Baril. This interdisciplinary chapter explores the congruence between philosophical understandings of well-being and a psychological measure of well-being developed by Carol Ryff and used in more than 750 empirical studies. Baril argues that there is some congruence with regard to the measurement of friendship, although less so for the other domains of the psychological well-being scale. And yet, despite the congruence on even this single domain, she argues that the measure will not "enable us to identify, with perfect accuracy, who among respondents has realized the basic good of friendship and who has not" (p. 277). Still, she concludes by promoting "interdisciplinary deference" and ends on an optimistic note that "meaningful collaboration" is indeed possible (pp. 278–279).

The final two chapters in this section were written by theologians. Chapter 10, by Neil G. Messer, is titled, "Human Flourishing: A Christian Theological Perspective." This chapter develops an understanding of flourishing in terms of the ultimate ends of human beings as created by God: "the fulfilment of God's good purposes" (p. 285). These purposes include relationship with God and with others, living an integrated life (in which mental and physical aspects combine into a well-functioning whole), and living out a vocation. This vision of well-being contrasts with the focus of many social scientific studies, which Messer (p. 299) argues should "encourage a critical self-awareness" among researchers. Furthermore, this theological account of well-being could serve as an alternative model to the two dominant approaches of social science research: the hedonic and eudaimonic accounts. A measure related to the theological account is provided in Chapter 16 by VanderWeele, Long, and Balboni. The final chapter in this section (Chapter 11) is "Comparing Empirical and Theological Perspectives on the Relationship Between Hope and Aesthetic Experience: An Approach to the Nature of Spiritual Well-Being" by Mark Wynn. This chapter offers reflections on the relationships between hope, beauty, and spiritual experience (which involves "a sense of oneness, or being united with the universe, or a love of the entire world," as well as "a conception of the fundamental nature of things") and spiritual well-being. In Wynn's (p. 306) understanding, spiritual well-being refers to "living successfully" in terms of this fundamental nature. To explore more concretely what this might mean, he brings the psychological work of William James into conversation with the theology of Thomas Aquinas. He notes some fundamental differences but also some possible points of convergence, including the possibility of a more "hopeful engagement with the world" (p. 333). As with the previous chapter, this theological account of well-being aims at ultimate ends.

The third section of the volume, "Advancing the Conversation about Measurement," continues the interdisciplinary approach of the book. These five chapters introduce new measures of selected aspects of well-being, with initial psychometric testing provided in two of them. One of these chapters also explores empirical relationships among different types of well-being. In the section's first chapter (Chapter 12), philosopher Jeffrey Hanson and epidemiologist Tyler J. VanderWeele contribute "The Comprehensive Measure of Meaning: Psychological and Philosophical Foundations." The authors rely on philosophical scholarship to enrich "an emerging consensus" in psychology with regard to a tripartite structure of meaning consisting of "cognitive coherence, affective significance, and motivational direction" (p. 339). This enables the elaboration of dimensions within this three-part framework and ultimately to the selection of twenty-one survey items to form a comprehensive measure of meaning. They suggest that their measure may overcome significant conceptual limitations in other measures and demonstrate the value of bringing social science and the humanities into dialogue. Further work will be needed in terms of psychometric evaluation of the measure.

The psychologists Seth Margolis, Eric Schwitzgebel, Daniel J. Ozer, and Sonja Lyubomirsky co-authored Chapter 13, titled, "Empirical Relationships Among Five Types of Well-Being." This chapter explores the relationships among the five main conceptualizations of well-being found in the literature—hedonic well-being, life satisfaction, desire fulfillment, eudaimonia, and non-eudaimonic objective-list well-being—along with other measures of well-being, including a new measure of "desire fulfillment." The associations are moderately strong and suggest some overlap, but the authors ultimately conclude that that "empirical findings based on one type of well-being measure may not generalize to all types of well-being" (p. 377). In addition, associations with Big Five personality traits varied across types of well-being. Consistent with a theme that runs throughout the volume, they argue for greater attention to the "philosophical value commitments" (p. 403) and, we would suggest, to the philosophical/theological underpinnings that are involved in the selection of some measures of well-being and not others.

The next two chapters propose new measures of well-being concepts that have not been previously subjected to empirical study. Chapter 14, "Measures of Community Well-Being: A Template," by Tyler J. VanderWeele, offers a new measure of community well-being with six domains: flourishing individuals, good relationships, proficient leadership, healthy practices, satisfying community, and strong mission. The measure can be adapted to accommodate different units of analysis from families, to schools, to religious communities, to neighborhoods, and to nations. This is important because well-being at the community level is distinct from, but is also inclusive of, the well-being of individuals. Integrating the well-being of individuals and communities leads to a more complete assessment of flourishing. Psychometric evaluation is still needed. In Chapter 15, sociologists Juan Xi and Matthew T. Lee offer "Inner Peace as a Contribution to Human Flourishing: A New Scale Developed from Ancient Wisdom." Here the authors develop a new measure of inner peace and provide an initial psychometric evaluation based on five empirical studies. Results suggest that inner peace is comprised of three dimensions: acceptance of loss, transcendence of hedonism and materialism, and inner balance and calmness. Given that philosophers and theologians have emphasized the centrality of inner peace for the good life, the authors hope that their three-dimensional construct will inform future research on human flourishing.

Chapter 16 is "Tradition-Specific Measures of Spiritual Well-Being," by Tyler J. VanderWeele, public health researcher Katelyn N. Long, and theologian and clinical researcher Michael J. Balboni. Although the overwhelming majority of the world's population identifies with a religious tradition, research on well-being often overlooks religious or spiritual components of complete flourishing. The authors argue in favor of tradition-specific measures of spiritual well-being rather than a generic measure, and they propose a new measure of Christian spiritual well-being as a template for the development of measures for other traditions. This measure contains thirty items across six domains: beliefs, practices, service, communion with God, Christian character, and relationships. By integrating feedback provided by Protestant, Catholic, and Orthodox theologians, pastors, priests, spiritual directors, and laity, the authors sought to develop a measure that would be appropriate for all three of these foundational traditions within Christianity. However, the measure still requires psychometric testing.

Finally, we conclude the fourth and final part of the volume ("Scholarly Dialogue on the Science of Well-Being"), with a lively dialogue starting with "Current Recommendations on the Selection of Measures for Well-Being," Chapter 17, co-authored by nineteen of the scholars invited to the Harvard well-being conference that launched this book. Led by Tyler J. VanderWeele, Claudia Trudel-Fitzgerald, and Laura D. Kubzansky, this group attempted to bring coherence to the measurement arena, partly in response to a common concern expressed by other investigators that clear guidance regarding measurement is lacking, in part due to the proliferation of measures and inconsistent conceptualization. In developing provisional guidance, they considered the number of items that might be included in different kinds of surveys, as well as the distinct purposes of the research, as this might differ for government, multiuse cohort, or psychological well-being surveys. The recommendations were intended to provide guidance about practical decisions that must be made under certain constraints. Carol D. Ryff, Jennifer Morozink Boylan, and Julie A. Kirsch advanced this dialogue by offering a critique of these recommendations in their Chapter 18, "Advancing the Science of Well-Being: A Dissenting View on Measurement Recommendations." The three principal authors of the recommendations chapter, Tyler J. VanderWeele, Claudia Trudel-Fitzgerald, and Laura D. Kubzansky, offered their "Response to 'Advancing the Science of Well-Being: A Dissenting View on Measurement Recommendations'" (Chapter 19). To close the conversation (at least for now), Carol D. Ryff, Jennifer Morozink Boylan, and Julie A. Kirsch provided a rejoinder (titled "Response to Response: Growing the Field of Well-Being," Chapter 20). We then offer a short concluding chapter that draws together the central themes of the entire volume.

Conclusion

The twenty chapters offered in this volume reflect the perspectives of leading representatives of a variety of social science and humanities disciplines. Some of the insights offered by the contributors are more readily assimilated than others. The consideration of both objective and subjective aspects of well-being, representing a hybrid model of their interrelationships, seems rather uncontroversial. Some of the theological interests in ultimate ends are less likely to be wholly represented in the work of social scientists who may be more grounded in materialist presuppositions. But we believe the field will advance if scholars begin to acknowledge that subjective well-being is not complete well-being and that it may be valuable to also consider spiritual well-being, for example, in relation to other forms of well-being, given its importance for so much of the world's population. With a broader spectrum of measures to consider, it may be possible to assess how these different forms of well-being relate to each other.

There are some limitations to the work presented in this book. First, many of the new measures that have been proposed have not been subjected to psychometric testing. Some of this testing is now in progress, but results were not available when the volume went to press. Second, the engagement with non-Western cultures was quite limited as most of the discussion of well-being related to Western contexts and philosophical and theological traditions. But many of the contributions could inform research on non-Western traditions; the new measure of tradition-specific Christian spiritual well-being was offered as an example with the hope of encouraging the development of other tradition-specific measures by content experts. Finally, not all of the chapters involved deep interdisciplinary engagement, and, when this did occur, it generally involved two disciplines, often philosophy and psychology. But for many contributors, the interdisciplinary dialogue enriched the discussion notably. We hope bringing these different perspectives together in a single volume will both provide useful tools for future research and scholarship and inspire further hospitality across disciplines.

About the Authors

Matthew T. Lee is Director of Empirical Research at the Human Flourishing Program in the Institute for Quantitative Social Science at Harvard University and coauthor of The Heart of Religion (Oxford University Press, 2013). He is also Distinguished Visiting Scholar of Health, Flourishing, and Positive Psychology at Stony Brook University's Center for Medical Humanities, Compassionate Care, and Bioethics, and he previously served as Chair of the American Sociological Association's Section on Altruism, Morality, and Social Solidarity. His research explores pathways to human flourishing, benevolent service to others, and the integration of social science and the humanities.

Laura D. Kubzansky is Lee Kum Kee Professor of Social and Behavioral Sciences and co-Director of the Lee Kum Sheung Center for Health and Happiness at the Harvard T. H. Chan School of Public Health. Dr. Kubzansky has published extensively on the role of psychological and social factors in health. Ongoing research includes studying biobehavioral mechanisms linking emotions, social relationships, and health; defining, measuring, and modifying aspects of well-being; and workplace conditions in relation to well-being. She has served on the leadership team for multiple training programs for junior scholars and is primary investigator or co-investigator on numerous grants.

Tyler J. VanderWeele is the John L. Loeb and Frances Lehman Loeb Professor of Epidemiology in the Departments of Epidemiology and Biostatistics at the Harvard T. H. Chan School of Public Health, Director of the Human Flourishing Program, and Co-Director of the Initiative on Health, Religion, and Spirituality at Harvard University. His research concerns methodology for distinguishing between association and causation in observational studies, and his empirical research spans psychiatric, perinatal, and social epidemiology; the science of happiness and flourishing; and the study of religion and health, including both religion and population health and the role of religion and spirituality in end-of-life care. He has published more than 300 papers in peer-reviewed journals and is author of the book Explanation in Causal Inference (Oxford University Press, 2015).

Author Note

This work was supported in part by a grant from the John Templeton Foundation, by the Lee Kum Sheung Center for Health and Happiness, and by the Human Flourishing

Program at Harvard University. The views expressed in this chapter represent the perspectives of the authors and do not reflect the opinions or endorsement of any organization. We have no known conflict of interest to disclose. Correspondence concerning this chapter should be directed to Matthew T. Lee, Human Flourishing Program, Harvard University, 129 Mt. Auburn St., Cambridge, MA, 02138 (matthew_lee@fas.harvard.edu).

References

Augustine. (413–426/1959). *The city of God.* New York: Modern Library.

Baumeister, R. F., Vohs, K. D., Aaker J. L., & Garbinsky. E. N. (2013). Some key differences between a happy life and a meaningful life. *Journal of Positive Psychology, 8,* 505–516.

Binkley, S. (2014). *Happiness as enterprise: An essay on neoliberal life.* Albany: State University of New York.

Bloom, P. (2016). *Against empathy: The case for rational compassion.* New York: HarperCollins.

Buber, M. (1923/1970). *I and thou.* New York: Scribners.

Case, A., & Deaton, A. (2017). Mortality and morbidity in the 21st century. *Brookings Papers on Economic Activity,* 397–476.

Centers for Disease Control and Prevention (CDC). (2020). *Health-Related Quality of Life (HRQOL): Well-being concepts.* Centers for Disease Control and Prevention. Retrieved from https://www.cdc.gov/hrqol/wellbeing.htm

Chen, Y., & VanderWeele, T. J. (2018). Associations of religious upbringing with subsequent health and well-being from adolescence to young adulthood: An outcome-wide analysis. *American Journal of Epidemiology, 187*(11), 2355–2364.

Clark, C. M. A., Buoye, A., Keiningham, T., Kandampully, J., Rosenbaum, M., & Juraidini A. (2019). Some foundational factors for promoting human flourishing. *Humanistic Management Journal,* 4, 219–233.

Diener, E. (1984). Subjective well-being. *Psychological Bulletin, 95*(3), 542–575.

Diener, E., Heintzelman, S. J., Kushlev, K., Tay, L., Wirtz, D., Lutes, L. D., & Oishi, S. (2017). Findings all psychologists should know from the new science on subjective well-being. *Canadian Psychology, 58*(2), 87–104.

Dwyer-Lindgren, L., Bertozzi-Villa, A., Stubbs, R. W., Morozoff, C., Shirude, S., Unützer, J., . . . Murray, C. J. L. (2018). Trends and patterns of geographic variation in mortality from substance use disorders and intentional injuries among US counties, 1980–2014. *JAMA, 319,* 1013–1023.

Elster, J. (1983/2016). *Sour grapes: Studies in the subversion of rationality.* Cambridge: Cambridge University Press.

Gaffney, M. (2011). *Flourishing.* London: Penguin UK.

Grant, A. (2013). *Give and take: A revolutionary approach to success.* New York: Viking.

Hampson, P. J., & Boyd-MacMillan, E. (2008). Turning the telescope round: Reciprocity in psychology-theology dialogue. *Archive for the Psychology of Religion, 30,* 93–113.

Helliwell, J. F., Layard, R., & Sachs, J. D. (2019). *World happiness report 2019.* New York: Sustainable Development Solutions Network.

Hone, L. C., Jarden, A., Schofield, G. M., & Duncan, S. (2014). Measuring flourishing: The impact of operational definitions on the prevalence of high levels of wellbeing. *International Journal of Wellbeing, 4*(1), 62–90.

Hood, R. (2012). Methodological agnosticism for the social sciences? Lessons from Sorokin's and James's allusions to psychoanalysis, mysticism, and Godly love. In M. T. Lee & A. Yong (Eds.), *The science and theology of godly love* (pp. 121–140). DeKalb: Northern Illinois University.

Joyce, R., & Xu, X. (2019). *Are the inequalities seen today a sign of a broken system? Launch of the IFS Deaton review of inequalities.* London: Institute for Fiscal Studies. Retrieved from https://www.ifs.org.uk/publications/14109

Kant, I. (1785/2005). *Fundamental principles of the metaphysics of morals.* Mineola, NY: Dover.

Kierkegaard, S. (1849/1980). *The sickness unto death.* Princeton, NJ: Princeton University.

Koltko-Rivera, M. E. (2006). Rediscovering the later version of Maslow's hierarchy of needs: Self-transcendence and opportunities for theory, research, and unification. *Review of General Psychology, 10*(4), 302–317.

Lee, M. T. (2019). Promoting human flourishing beyond foundational concerns. *Humanistic Management Journal, 4,* 235–237.

Lee, M. T., Poloma, M. M., & Post, S. G. (2013). *The heart of religion: Spiritual empowerment, benevolence, and the experience of God's love.* New York: Oxford University.

Lee, M. T., Weziak-Bialowolska, D., Mooney, K. D., Lerner, P. J., McNeely, E., & VanderWeele, T. J. (2020). Self-assessed importance of domains of flourishing: Demographics and correlations with well-being. *Journal of Positive Psychology,* in press.

Lee, M. T., & A. Yong. (2012). *The science and theology of Godly love.* DeKalb: Northern Illinois University.

MacIntyre, A. (1984). *After virtue: A study in moral theory (2/e).* Notre Dame, IN: University of Notre Dame.

MacIntyre, A. (1988). *Whose justice? Which rationality?* Notre Dame, IN: University of Notre Dame.

MacIntyre, A. (1990). *Three rival versions of moral enquiry: The Gifford lectures.* Notre Dame, IN: University of Notre Dame.

Maselko, J., & Kubzansky, L. D. (2006). Gender differences in religious practices, spiritual experiences and health: Results from the US General Social Survey. *Social Science and Medicine, 62,* 2848–2860.

Maslow, A. H. (1971). *The farther reaches of human nature.* New York: Viking.

National Science Foundation. (2019). *Convergence research at NSF.* National Science Foundation. Retrieved from https://www.nsf.gov/od/oia/convergence/index.jsp

Oakley, B., Knafo, A., Madhavan, G., & Wilson, D. S. (Eds.). (2011). *Pathological altruism.* New York: Oxford University.

Palmer, P. J. (1998). *The courage to teach: Exploring the inner landscape of a teacher's life.* San Francisco, CA: Jossey-Bass.

Pfuetze, P. (1973). *Self, society, existence: Human nature and dialogue in the thought of George Herbert Mead and Martin Buber.* Westport, CT: Greenwood.

Philbrick, N. (2006). *Mayflower: A story of courage, community, and war.* New York: Penguin.

Phillips, R., & Wong, C. (2017). *Handbook of community well-being research.* Dordrecht: Springer.

Plato. (275 BCE/2012). *The republic.* London: Penguin.

Porpora, D. V. (2006). Methodological atheism, methodological agnosticism and religious experience. *Journal for the Theory of Social Behavior, 36,* 57–75

Rieff, P. (2007). *Charisma: The gift of grace, and how it has been taken away from us.* New York: Vintage.

Sachs, J. D. (2019). Addiction and unhappiness in America. In J. F. Helliwell, R. Layard, & J. D. Sachs (Eds.), *World happiness report 2019* (pp. 123–131), New York: Sustainable Development Solutions Network.

Sayer, A. (2019). Critiquing–and rescuing–character. *Sociology.* doi.org/10.1177/0038038519892532.

Seligman, M. E. (2012). *Flourish: A visionary new understanding of happiness and well-being.* New York: Simon and Schuster.

Stiglitz, J., Sen, A., & Fitoussi. (2009). *Report by the commission on the measurement of economic performance and social progress.* Paris: Commission on the Measurement of Economic Performance and Social Progress.

Sorokin, P. (1937–1941). *Social and cultural dynamics (4 Volumes).* Cincinnati, OH: American Book.

Suldo, S. (2016). *Promoting student happiness: Positive psychology interventions in schools.* New York: Guilford.

VanderWeele, T. J. (2017). On the promotion of human flourishing. *Proceedings of the National Academy of Sciences, 114,* 8148–8156.

VanderWeele, T. J. (2019). Measures of community well-being: A template. *International Journal of Community Well-Being.* Retrieved from https://doi.org/10.1007/s42413-019-00036-8.

VanderWeele, T. J., McNeely, E., & Koh, H. K. (2019). Reimagining health: Flourishing. *JAMA, 17,* 1667–1668.

Volf, M. (2015). *Flourishing: Why we need religion in a globalized world.* New Haven, CT: Yale University.

PART 1

EMPIRICAL RESEARCH AND REFLECTIONS ON WELL-BEING MEASUREMENT

1

Measuring and Using Happiness
to Support Public Policies

John F. Helliwell

Abstract

This chapter summarizes the philosophical and empirical grounds for
giving a primary role to the evaluations that people make of the quality
of their lives. These evaluations permit comparisons among communities, regions, nations, and population subgroups; enable the estimation
of the relative importance of various sources of happiness; and provide
a well-being lens to aid the choice of public policies to support well-
being. Available results expose the primacy of social determinants of
happiness and especially the power of generosity and other positive social connections to improve the levels, distribution, and sustainability of
well-being.

Over the past half century, and especially over the past twenty-five years, research and widespread public interest have combined to create possibilities
for using happiness data to broaden the methods and content of public policies. Happiness data offer the possibility to restore to economics the breadth
of purpose and methods it had two centuries ago, when happiness was considered the appropriate goal for private actions and public policies. They can
also help guide health sciences as they move beyond the treatment of illness
to the creation and maintenance of good health. More generally, happiness
data can enable ethics and welfare economics to be driven by evidence rather
than assumptions. What types of data and research are most likely to support
these changes?

John F. Helliwell, *Measuring and Using Happiness to Support Public Policies* In: *Measuring Well-Being.*
Edited by: Matthew T. Lee, Laura D. Kubzansky, and Tyler J. VanderWeele, Oxford University Press (2021).
© Oxford University Press. DOI: 10.1093/oso/9780197512531.003.0002

The Importance of Measuring the Quality of Life

Among the many ways of defining and measuring happiness, the most central, from both philosophical and policy perspectives, are the evaluations that individuals make of the quality of their own lives. From a philosophical standpoint, it has been argued that ancient ethical philosophy "gets its grip on the individual at this point of reflection: am I satisfied with my life as a whole, and the way it has developed and promises to develop?" (Annas, 1993, p. 28). There are ancient and modern philosophical arguments about which aspects of thought and experience are most central to a good life. Ryan and Deci (2001) distinguish two opposing approaches, one hedonic and the other eudaimonic, with the former emphasizing a balance of pleasures over pain, thereby echoing the ancient Epicurean view, and the other emphasizing the development of human potential in a virtuous form, echoing the ancient Stoic philosophers. Ryff et al. (Chapter 4, this volume) make use of the hedonic versus eudaimonic division proposed by Ryan and Deci and emphasize Aristotle's contributions to the latter branch. For both Aristotle and Epicurus, happiness (eudaimonia) was the objective, and a life of virtue a likely route to get there (Annas, 1987).

In my view, Aristotle's most important contributions to the modern reframing of applied ethics lie not in his emphasis on excellence and purpose, but on two other fronts: first, hypothesizing that a good life is likely to combine elements of the viewpoints later identified as Epicurean and Stoic[1] and, second, that the right answers require evidence as much as introspection. "We must therefore survey what we have already said, bringing it to the test of the facts of life, and if it harmonises with the facts we must accept it, but if it clashes with them we must suppose it to be mere theory" (Nicomachean Ethics, book 10, 1179, 20–23, from Helliwell, 2003, p. 333).[2] I therein see Aristotle advocating the use of data from everyday life, not to isolate different theories of well-being, but to see how these theories cohere or compete in supporting people's judgments about how their lives are going.[3] I agree with Owen Flanagan's (2007) proposal that this line of necessarily interdisciplinary inquiry should be called *eudaimonics*.

Therefore I would argue that life evaluations are not just part of a measurement strategy for a philosophy based on the achievement of a favorable balance of pleasure over pain, as would be implied by classing them as hedonic variables. They are much more than that. They provide a central mediating device that can be used to establish the relative importance of various values and experiences, to measure the quality of life, and to support policy choices likely to improve human flourishing. What are the specific characteristics of life evaluations that enable them to do all this?

Because they are overall assessments, they provide an umbrella measure of the quality of life. If they are collected in sufficient numbers from representative samples, they can be used to measure the quality of life in communities of all sizes, from the neighborhood to the nation and beyond. Because they are umbrella measures, they can be used to power research into the relative importance of various aspects of life and hence to inform policy judgments requiring choices among alternative ways to design and deliver public services. Because they are umbrella measures that can nonetheless be collected with any desired degree of granularity, they are able not just to measure differences in the quality of life in different locations and population subgroups, but also to explore the reasons for those differences. Another advantage of direct measurement is that the distributions of responses can be used to estimate the statistical significance of differences over time and among population subgroups.

Life evaluations ask how well life is going rather than what is going wrong. As such, they have more resonance with emerging trends within a number of disciplines to focus on understanding and improving the positive features of life rather than on identifying and repairing what has gone wrong (Chapter 6, this volume). The underlying presumption is that such a shift in focus will broaden the range of scientific understanding in important directions and thereby offer better ways to sustainably improve lives in organizations and communities large and small.

In summary, life evaluations provide umbrella measures that grasp life at its central point. They can be used not just to measure but also to explain why people differ in their life evaluations, thereby providing a focus of attention for the general public and policy-makers alike as they search for something that is able to encompass and reconcile otherwise competing measures of welfare. This centrality of life evaluations as an empirical construct capable of deep meaning was recognized by ancient philosophers and has, in modern times, made them the most relied-upon measure of subjective well-being. Are they also measures of happiness? Here it is crucial to distinguish two quite separate uses of the term "happiness," one relating to a felt emotion and the other to a cognitive judgment about the extent to which one is happy about something.[4] People quite clearly know whether they are being asked about the emotion or, alternatively, about how they value something. Hence answers to questions about happiness yesterday are quite different from answers to life evaluation questions asking people about how happy they are with their lives as a whole. In the latter case, the answers are structurally similar to answers about life satisfaction or other life evaluations. In the former case, the answers clearly relate to the current emotional context. Thus those who are asked both types of question are quick to see the context in which they are asked about happiness and answer appropriately in both cases, reflecting their ability to see the logic of the conversational context (Grice, 1975). This should help dispel fears that the abundance of terms necessarily creates a confusion of results. Indeed, the fact that the answers differ in just the ways that theory would suggest should increase confidence in both types of measure.

How Does This Approach Differ from Alternative Ways of Measuring Human Progress?

This approach differs fundamentally from three other ways of assessing human progress.

Gross Domestic Product and Similar Measures

National accounts of income and expenditure provide a well-established measure of market-based economic activity. To use gross domestic product (GDP) or gross national product (GNP) as measures of national welfare has long been recognized as mistaken. Almost fifty years ago, Nordhaus and Tobin (1972) proposed an experimental *measure of economic welfare* (MEW) that attempted to correct for many of the recognized short-comings of GNP accounting. They realized that their measure was still far too narrow to represent welfare more broadly construed but felt that "the 'social indicators' movement of recent years still lacks a coherent, integrative conceptual and statistical framework" (Nordhaus & Tobin, 1972, p. 9). Life evaluations are now seen by many as providing a plausible way to fill that gap.

Healthy Life Expectancy

Healthy life expectancy involves an adjustment to reduce life expectancy by an amount reflecting some estimate of the welfare costs of morbidity. As welfare accounting moves toward a broader use of subjective well-being to assess the welfare costs of ill health (Peasgood, Foster, & Dolan, 2019), the measure of healthy life expectancy is likely to be further adjusted to reflect the value that individuals place on good health when reporting their life satisfaction. Even the current data have been found to have a strong role in explaining international differences in life satisfaction (e.g., see table 2.1 in the World Happiness Report [WHR] 2019).[5]

Indexes of Economic and Social Progress

Composite social indicators constructed by experts based on their own conceptions of what a good life comprises have been used for more than fifty years—as documented in a special issue of *Social Indicators Research*[6] celebrating fifty years of social indicators research—to supplement or perhaps replace GDP as means of gauging social progress. Within the social indicators movement there has long been a tension between those who value having multiple social indicators, with each being seen as important in its own light and right, and those who see the importance of having a single composite measure that could provide a way beyond relying on GDP per capita as the default proxy measure of progress. The essential difficulty with such indexes is their reliance on somebody's decisions about which aspects of life to consider, how to empirically represent their quality, and, most importantly, how to weight the different sectoral measures to provide a single overall indicator. Such indicators differ according to the policy preferences and theoretical presumptions of their designers. In the absence of some overall primary measure of well-being, there is no empirical way to choose among competing indexes. Their constructed nature means that they cannot be used to estimate the relative importance people place on various aspects of their lives since those weights have already been built into the index itself.

Thus, for example, the Human Development Index (HDI) prepared by the United Nations Development Programme is an equally weighted average of three indicators, one for GDP per capita, one for healthy life expectancy, and one for average education levels (Anand & Sen, 1994). By its very nature, it cannot provide information about the relative importance of these different aspects of development nor about what may be missing from the picture. The choice of items included owes much to Sen's capabilities approach (Sen, 1994), although none would argue that the coverage is comprehensive or that the relative importance of the components is as assumed by the equal weighting. The Organisation for Economic Co-operation and Development's (OECD) Better Life Index (Durand, 2015) finesses the weighting question by presenting a dashboard of indicators and inviting individual users to choose their own weights to develop an overall indicator. That procedure leaves equal weighting as the default option for the media and most users.

A better way of making use of the diverse measures used in indexes of human progress is to treat them as variables that can be used to explain variations over time or among communities and countries in a primary umbrella measure. The primary measures are interesting in themselves, but their real value to public understanding and policy only appears when it becomes possible to uncover some plausible reasons for their effects on well-being over time and among population subgroups. The various social and economic indicators included in composite measures are often ideal candidates for explanatory roles since they reflect topics and aspects of life long thought to be important to human progress. They can then be used, in combination with often-ignored social context variables, to help explain life evaluations, with the results being used to estimate the relative importance of the various factors. Measures of domain satisfaction can likewise be used to help unravel the relative importance of different aspects of life, while multi-item measures of subjective well-being, such as the ten questions in five domains of flourishing proposed by VanderWeele (2017), can be used to help unpack the movements in overall life evaluations or, alternatively, as independent items to be linked to different aspects of life. Understanding the interplay among alternative ways of measuring well-being deserves to remain a central focus for research.

Specific Measurement Issues

One Question or Many?

If and when there is agreement to use life evaluations as a primary measure, there will remain issues about how they should be measured. There are four questions or groups of questions that have been widely used. These include

- the Diener et al. (1985) five-question Satisfaction with Life Scale (SWLS),
- the Cantril ladder question used in the Gallup World Poll,

- a satisfaction with life as a whole (these days, now, or nowadays) question, as recommended by the OECD (2013) and used by the European Union (EU) and many national statistical offices, and
- a question asking respondents how happy they are with their lives (one of the two life evaluation questions used in the European Social Survey).

There is a general research case to be made for surveys to include some redundancy in life evaluations, first, to build understanding of how these alternatives are related and, second, because there is evidence in favor of the presumption that multiple measures can help to increase the signal-to-noise ratio. There is, however, always a tradeoff to consider between asking more questions of the same respondents versus increasing the overall sample coverage. In the case of the five-question SWLS, it has been found that most of the overall information comes from answers to the life satisfaction question. This suggests that to use a single life satisfaction question in large population-based samples might represent the best use of survey resources. Research comparing the SWLS and a single-item SWL question in three large surveys finds that the two measures provide essentially the same information (Cheung & Lucas, 2014) thereby justifying single-item measures as a preferred choice in large-scale surveys where survey space needs to be rationed.

Where two different life evaluation questions have been used in the same survey, they have been found to attach similar relative importance to the chosen sets of explanatory variables and to produce slightly tighter fits if their average value is used. This was first shown for the Gallup World Poll, when the Cantril ladder and the life satisfaction question were both asked of the same respondents, on the same 0–10 scale, in one survey wave (Helliwell, Barrington-Leigh, Harris, & Huang, 2010, table 10.1). The same was found using data from the European Social Survey, which regularly asks two life evaluation questions, one on life satisfaction and the other on happiness with life as a whole, each on the same 0–10 scale. Once again, although the means and distribution shapes were slightly different, the coefficient estimates were very similar, and tighter estimates were obtained by averaging responses to the two questions (Helliwell, Huang, & Wang, 2018). One of the advantages of having different questions asked in the same survey is that it allows one to discern with greater assurance whether surveys that use different question forms are thereby getting answers that are materially different. For example, before there was life satisfaction data from the Gallup World Poll, it was hypothesized that the larger income effects being found in the Gallup World Poll than from earlier work using World Values Survey data were due to the particular ladder framing used for the Cantril ladder. This hypothesis was rejected by the data because the results based on the life satisfaction answers were essentially the same as those from the Cantril ladder. Without having both questions asked in the same survey, this would not have been discovered.

What About Emotions and Purpose?

Much earlier research has shown that positive and negative affect have different correlates and structures from each other (Diener & Emmons, 1984) and from life evaluations. This led the UK Office for National Statistics (ONS) in 2011 to introduce a set of four key questions, on a 0–10 scale, in their Annual Population survey: one life satisfaction question, one on positive emotion (happiness yesterday), one on negative emotion (anxiety yesterday), and one asking whether overall respondents feel that the things they do in their lives are worthwhile. These questions were chosen, as documented in Allin (Chapter 2, in this volume), on the basis of prevalence in previous surveys and public consultations. Should these four questions be seen as alternatives or complements? Within the framework proposed in this chapter and also adopted in the WHR, the life evaluation question provides the central evidence recommended by Aristotle, while positive and negative emotions, and a sense of life purpose, are all to be expected to play a role in explaining life evaluations. The affect measures, because of their short-term focus, are ideally suited to laboratory experimental contexts in which the interventions considered are so small in magnitude or duration that changes in overall life evaluations would not be expected. When asked in general surveys, affective measures can also help to disentangle the channels through which changes in life circumstances come to influence life evaluations. The aggregate results in successive editions of the WHR have suggested a strong positive role for positive affect in explaining life evaluations, with little or no effect coming from the indicators of negative affect, all of which are also less prevalent and less influential than the positive emotions in the Gallup World Poll data. The social variables that are so strong in the WHR findings are mediated to an important extent through positive affect.[7] There is a presumptive role for a sense of life purpose (Chapter 4, in this volume), but this question has not been widely enough asked in large-scale surveys for general conclusions to be reached. There is also need for more comparisons among a wider variety of measures of psychological well-being (Chapter 13, in this volume).

How Many Response Options?

Life evaluations are now generally asked on an 11-point scale anchored by 0 and 10. All of the available evidence suggests that longer scales carry more information than shorter ones. The UK ONS asks its affect questions on the same 0–10 scale. The Gallup World Poll asks its affect questions on a binary yes/no scale. There are two advantages in using the same 0–10 scale for all subjective well-being questions. First, it enables easier comparison of the information provided by life evaluations and affect measures. Second, the longer scale permits the distribution of well-being to be measured and its consequences analyzed. By contrast, from the binary answers one can only learn what fraction of the population has the attribute in question. The binary nature of such data means that they cannot provide a meaningful measure of inequality.

Method Effects

Survey methods are in flux as face-to-face interviews are being replaced by cheaper methods, land line phones are being supplanted by cell phones, and various online completion methods are coming into greater use. Online methods are more easily adapted for increasing the longitudinal component of repeated population-based surveys at modest cost, but at some risk of misrepresentation. Given the persistence of a digital divide, online methods require cross-validation by other methods since some recent evidence (Arim & Schellenberg, 2019) shows that selection effects may lead to online panels delivering life satisfaction estimates that differ seriously from population-based life evaluations. There is also some evidence of method effects, with one analysis of the ONS life evaluations finding higher life evaluations for telephone than for face-to-face interviews (Dolan & Kavetsos, 2016).

Survey Context Effects

It is to be expected that survey answers may depend on the context in which they are asked. Thus US survey respondents who were asked the Cantril ladder question gave on average lower responses if, immediately prior to that question, they were asked a question about national politics, with the negative effect being concentrated among respondents who held unfavorable views about the current political context (Deaton & Stone, 2016). In a similar vein, it has been found that life satisfaction answers in different rounds of the Canadian General Social Survey (GSS) differ according to the overall topic of the survey (e.g., being lower in the time-use cycle) (Bonikowska, Helliwell, Hou, & Schellenberg, 2014). These findings have been seen by some as a caution against reliance on survey responses. The ease with which framing effects can be delivered in laboratory settings more or less guarantees that similar issues would arise in a survey context. What is encouraging is how these effects are of a direction and size indicating that people take the questions seriously and answer them appropriately. For example, middle-aged respondents reporting themselves to be having trouble juggling competing demands for their time are those whose life satisfaction is lower in the time-use waves of the Canadian GSS. This makes any such effects easier to guard against and easier to allow for when samples are being pooled. In the case of the Canadian GSS, the coefficients on all the key variables of interest are very similar for each of the GSS waves. Therefore a fixed-effects adjustment for each survey wave permits the data to be efficiently pooled. In general, there is a case to be made for including life evaluations in a demographic block, with a similar structure for each survey, and at sufficient remove from questions or contexts that have been found (or might be expected) to influence responses. For example, in the Canadian Community Health Survey (CCHS), which asks the life satisfaction question as part of the demographic block and has a similar content from wave to wave, there are no differences in the years where differences appeared among GSS waves with a different subject focus. In summary, survey context matters, but its effects can be minimized and adjustments can be made where context differences remain.

What Do Life Evaluations Reveal About the Sources of a Happy Life?

Possibilities for learning about the sources of happier lives depend crucially on what data are available and used in research. Much of the earliest individual-level research relied mainly on age, gender, education, and income since those were among the relatively few variables available in experimental and survey studies. This led to corresponding conclusions that only a small proportion of the individual-level happiness differences could be explained and the analogous inferences that most of the variance was due to idiosyncratic personality differences, including individual set-points with a potentially large genetic component. This conclusion illustrates the importance of measuring what matters to people.

It is not sufficient to know how satisfied people are with their lives since nothing can be done with this information without an informed view of what makes for better lives. To know more about what features of life are conducive to health and happiness requires that all the relevant aspects of life need to be measured and considered. This is difficult to achieve in the large-scale surveys required to benchmark happiness for a variety of geographic and demographic groupings. Providing a full range of explanatory variables requires a mix of variety and coverage that is achieved by including at least a core set of subjective well-being questions in all of a nation's population-based surveys. These include especially the whole range of social surveys, whether their focus is on health, employment, education, aging, neighborhoods, or the social context. To help unpack causal directions and isolate the effects of confounding factors, it is also essential to monitor subjective well-being before, during, and after any significant policy changes. This also applies to experimental studies, regardless of whether their well-being consequences are the driving force in the policy design process. Measuring several dimensions of psychological well-being also permits a clearer understanding of the multiple possible pathways from higher psychological well-being to improved physical health (Chapter 5, in this volume).

In the absence of much larger samples of survey and experimental data, it is impossible to draw definitive conclusions about the relevant importance of various aspects of life, especially in the presence of complicated feedbacks and many confounding factors. But emerging evidence suggests that the social sources of well-being, especially those delivered in person, are of even greater importance than previously thought (Helliwell & Putnam, 2014). In recent World Happiness Reports, six factors have been found to explain three-quarters of the differences in average life evaluations among countries and over time. Two of these factors have already been mentioned: GDP per capita and healthy life expectancy. The other four factors, all reflecting some aspect of the social fabric widely construed, are having someone to count on in times of trouble, a sense of freedom to make life choices, generosity, and a trustworthy environment, as proxied by the absence of corruption in business and government. Calculations in WHR 2017 (Helliwell, Huang, & Wang, 2017, p. 37) show that to move those in the countries with the lowest values of each of the four social variables up to the world average would raise life evaluations by almost 2 points (1.97) on the 0–10 scale. Such a change is about half as great as the entire range of national average life evaluations and is more than that associated with similar changes in both income per capita and healthy life expectancy (from the bottom to world average). The largest gains come from the measure of social support (having someone to count on in times of trouble [1.19 points]). This difference is about equal to the gains from the 16-fold increase in per capita incomes required to shift the three poorest countries up to world average income levels. The importance of the social variables does not disappear, even at higher happiness levels. If countries with world average levels of the four social variables could raise them to the average of the three top countries for each of the four social variables, life evaluations would be higher by an additional 1.29 points. These calculations, being based on correlations rather than more directly causal evidence, are intended mainly to reveal the relative size of the likely effects of social factors in comparison to the more established measures of income and good health.[8]

Research based on surveys with a larger range of potential driving variables shows even greater primacy of the social and, within the social, the dominance of the local.[9] To feel a sense of belonging in an atmosphere of mutual support and trust is of first-order importance. This goes far beyond being free from the risk of attack by others (e.g., as measured by fear of walking the streets at night, with remedies promised by the gated community); it is the capacity to feel embedded in a community where trust, belonging, and mutual support are the accepted norms.

Among the social variables, the one that has received the least previous research and policy attention is generosity. Generosity, and prosocial behavior in general, is much more prevalent and has greater links to subjective well-being than people and policy-makers think (Aknin, Whillans, Norton, & Dunn, 2019). The fact that people enjoy being engaged in social activities that help others opens the door to a wide range of win-win policy choices (e.g., where schoolchildren and those in elder care get the chance to care for and teach each other, thus creating valuable resources while enriching lives).[10] The fact that benevolent acts make the benefactor happier increases their chances of being repeated. But the related fact that people underestimate their own happiness rewards from benevolence should perhaps be ignored because much of the happiness gain from benevolent acts arises if and when they are done unselfishly (Helliwell & Aknin, 2018). This information gap is perhaps best filled by the Golden Rule, with its central role in all religious doctrines and moral philosophies, thereby providing a norms-based incentive to act in ways that increase happiness for givers and receivers of generous thoughts and actions.

To expand the opportunities for making positive social connections will, however, require reversing some of the increasingly risk-averse professionalism of recent decades in the social services and will require flatter and more open administrative structures for decision and action. To harness pro-social actions most effectively requires that people be offered more chances to engage with others in joint searches for better lives. This will involve changes not only in the content of policies, but also in the ways they are designed and delivered.[11]

Measuring the Distribution of Well-Being, and Why It Matters

If life evaluations provide an umbrella measure of the quality of life, it would seem theoretically obvious that well-being inequality would provide a broader measure of inequality than could be derived from the separate measures of inequality in income and wealth, health, education, and friendship. Most previous studies of inequality have relied on income inequality when studying the effects of inequality on health (Pickett & Wilkinson, 2015) and happiness (Alesina, Di Tella, & MacCullough, 2004). But recent research (Goff, Helliwell, & Mayraz, 2018; Nichols & Reinhart, 2019) has shown that inequality in the distribution of life evaluations is more powerful than income inequality in several explanatory roles where inequality is thought to be a factor. This is an important finding. If average life evaluations are an appropriate measure of community welfare, then the effect of happiness inequality on life evaluations provides an empirical measure of a society's aversion to inequality (Helliwell, 2020). In the absence of this evidence, moral philosophers and policy-makers alike have had to assume the weights needed to construct a social welfare function. The distribution of costs and benefits among the population must always be a central aspect of policy evaluation. The evidence suggests that people significantly prefer less inequality in the distribution of well-being, and these estimates provide the basis for comparing policies with differing impacts on the distribution of well-being. This in turn suggests, but does not necessarily require, a policy framework that explicitly targets those most in misery because there is also evidence that policies which generally improve the social context (e.g., increasing social trust or community belonging) may provide their largest benefits to those in circumstances least likely to make them happy—in particular ill-health, unemployment, and discrimination.[12]

Measuring and Understanding Community and National Well-Being

Does the average level of life evaluations in a community provide the best measure of well-being in that community? That is certainly what is assumed when national averages are measured and taken to represent quality of life within a nation. At the national level, there are qualms and qualifications based on possible linguistic and cultural differences in response styles that might raise problems of comparability. Although response style differences have been shown to exist, they do not appear to be large enough to disturb the general finding that life evaluations are comparable across countries since they are found to depend on the same factors, to roughly the same extent, throughout the world (Helliwell, Huang, & Harris, 2009). This conclusion is also supported by evidence showing that immigrants have life valuations similar to those born locally despite coming from countries with very different institutions, histories, and cultures (Helliwell, Shiplett, & Bonikowska, 2020).

What about comparisons among communities within a country? At this level there is more uniformity of language and culture, but also greater potential for selection effects that cause happy and unhappy people to end up in different neighborhoods based on their tastes, education, ethnicity, and incomes. Also, for a variety of reasons, communities can come to have their own characteristics, partly shaped by their histories and driven by the quality of the interactions among those who live there. Various features of a neighborhood have been found to have important effects on the subsequent life experiences of those who move there (Chetty & Hendren, 2018). Such studies that track individuals as they move are relatively rare. In the larger range of studies that find correlations between neighborhood characteristics and average individual happiness, there is a prevailing difficulty in accounting for selection effects and, more generally, in unpacking the expected two-way causal linkages between individual happiness and various measures of community characteristics, especially ones that track the social context.

Returning to the central question of measuring community-level happiness, how should we answer the frequent suggestion that community-level well-being somehow lies above and beyond the average subjective well-being of the people who live there? If we are interested in assessing the quality of what is added by the community to the happiness of its residents (and its visitors and nonresident workers—two important categories often ignored), then it is clearly necessary to adjust for differences between communities in respect of the characteristics of the individuals who live there. There are two methods for doing this. One is to obtain independent measures of community-level factors that have been assumed or found to improve resident happiness and combine these into an index of community well-being.[13] The problems with such indexes are the same as those outlined earlier for national indexes: how to choose, and then weight, the components, and how to tell whether the resulting differences between communities are significantly large. The second method is to collect information about the characteristics of a community as a whole and of the individuals in that community, and then use empirical work and available natural and controlled experiments to explain the life evaluations of residents. This can help to establish the relative importance of different aspects of community life. As noted by VanderWeele (Chapter 14, in this volume), the communities of interest may include not just those defined by geographical boundaries, but also by common interests, activities, beliefs, and friendships that span geographic boundaries.

In my view, the most appropriate measure of the quality of life in a community (and in a country or region) is the average reported life satisfaction of its residents. To help unpack the role played by qualities specific to a community, rather than by qualities brought to the table by those living there, is and will always remain a difficult research question.[14] Answering that question is aided greatly by the collection and use of variables of the sort proposed as candidate components of a community well-being index.

Using Happiness Data and Research to Support Public Policies

Happiness data and research require widespread measurement if they are to have any impact on public policies. But will the availability of data be enough to trigger public policies based on well-being? Paul Allin (Chapter 2, in this volume) notes that the translation of UK subjective well-being data into research and policy applications has been relatively slow. What is needed to encourage the process? Successful transition is likely to require several further steps once the data are available and in easy reach. First, policy interest will be greater when there is widespread public interest in and acceptance of happiness data. This can be initiated by widespread distribution and preliminary analysis by national statistical agencies.

At the global level, the availability of internationally comparable life evaluations from the Gallup World Poll has spurred widespread interest in how happiness compares across countries, which in turn has led to many books and articles and even new research institutions examining the lives and policies of the happiest countries, most particularly the Nordic countries.

Once data are made readily available to outside users, along with matching data on a variety of those features of life likely to support better lives, this should spur academic and institutional research covering a wide range of national and sectoral policy issues. This research base can in turn support the reform of benefit-cost analysis so that it compares policies on the basis of how much they improve the levels and distribution of life satisfaction. This is perhaps the most important step in the transition since it can be done piecemeal and without fanfare, not requiring any high-profile political precommitments to a new policy focus. It gives policy analysts a better set of tools and the capacity to bring a broader view of life into policy discussions and decisions.[15] For new policy evaluation methods to be effectively designed and widely accepted will require, over the longer run, training new generations and retraining older ones within academic disciplines and public policy schools to rethink the assumptions and methods ingrained in established texts and curricula. A corresponding process has been under way for a few years longer in the study of global warming and other environmental issues. The shift toward subjective well-being as a practical focus for public attention and policy design will take longer. It permeates a range of disciplines, and requires similar transdisciplinary approaches if it is to succeed. If it does succeed, then it should foster more appropriate and sustainable solutions to all policy problems, including those facing the social, political, and physical environments, at all levels, from the neighborhood to the globe.

Notes

1. "Aristotle argues that all our actions are, in some way, for the sake of a single end. Obviously, people are not all aiming at the same determinate end; the final end is a highly unspecific end that nonetheless unifies our actions. The only halfway specific

thing we can say about it is that everyone agrees that it is eudaimonia. This doesn't help much, because people disagree as to what eudaimonia is, some thinking that it is pleasure, others virtue, others virtue exercised in favorable conditions. Epicurus will defend the first option, the Stoics the second, Aristotle himself the third: this sets the framework of ancient ethical debate that continues to this day" (Annas, 1993). As quoted by Keyes and Annas (2009, pp. 197–198).

2. This has modern echoes in the "pragmatic subjectivism" of Haybron and Tiberius (2015).

3. This led me to appoint myself as Aristotle's research assistant, a position made possible through the increasingly widespread availability of answers to the central question he proposed. I similarly expect that ethical philosophy will develop an empirical aspect. This may be slow in coming, as Fletcher (Chapter 7, this volume) reports that modern philosophers still think that empirical work based on data from ordinary lives cannot help to mediate or resolve philosophical debates about the relative importance of different theories of the sources of happiness.

4. Amartya Sen utilized linguistic philosophy to make this distinction in his keynote address to the January 2013 Rome Science Congress. His primary reference was to the later Wittgenstein (1953), with roots attributed to Gramsci via Sraffa, as described in Sen (2003). Gramsci's view of "spontaneous philosophy," whereby meaning is derived from everyday linguistic usage, was also central to English linguistic philosophy, partly through Wittgenstein (1953), wherein meaning is based on the logic of the conversations in which words are used (e.g., Grice, 1975).

5. Richard Layard has suggested (2020, p. 205) that, for valuing health policies and perhaps more broadly, healthy life expectancy should be given even more weight by multiplying average life satisfaction by health life expectancy (or Health Adjusted Life Years [HALYs]). If the current measures of life satisfaction already embody the full value that individuals attach to healthy life expectancy, then to multiply life satisfaction by the number of healthy years would exaggerate their relevance to average national happiness.

6. The overview paper by Land and Michalos (2018) is followed by a series of invited comments.

7. Cohn et al. (2009) additionally find increased resilience to be a pathway from positive affect to life satisfaction.

8. Because the social factor answers come from the same surveys as the life evaluations, there is a risk that they might be correlated, even at the aggregate level, because of idiosyncratic happiness differences that might affect life evaluations and the answers to the social questions. This risk was tested for by dividing the national samples randomly in two and then using the average social variable responses from one half of the sample to explain the average life evaluations of the other half. The results were almost completely unaffected, as shown in table 10 of online statistical appendix 1 of WHR 2018.

9. For example, the Canadian General Social Survey has asked separately about a sense of belonging to one's local community, province, and to Canada as a whole. All are significantly positive, but the power of the local belonging is significantly the largest, more

than three-quarters of a point on the 0–10 life satisfaction scale even holding constant the significant effects from trust in co-workers and trust in neighbors (Helliwell and Wang, 2011, table 4–1).

10. For examples and references, see Helliwell (2019).

11. The "how" aspects are sometimes referred to as "procedural utility" (Stutzer and Frey, 2006). For more examples, see Helliwell (2019) and part III of Helliwell, Huang, Grover, and Wang (2014).

12. See Helliwell, Aknin et al. (2018, figure 4) for evidence from the European Social Survey that people living in a high-trust environment are more resilient in the face of each of these negative circumstances, while Daley, Phipps, and Branscombe (2018) show that a sense of community belonging protects youth with disabilities from the negative well-being effects of perceived discrimination.

13. See VanderWeele (Chapter 14, this volume) and the references therein.

14. For reviews of open issues, see Sampson, Morenoff, and Gannon-Rowley (2002) and Van Ham and Manley (2012).

15. On this point, see also Durand and Exton (2019).

About the Author

John F. Helliwell is a Distinguished Fellow of the Canadian Institute for Advanced Research. He is also Professor Emeritus of Economics at the University of British Columbia and a Research Associate of the National Bureau of Economic Research. He was previously a member of the National Statistics Council 2001–2015. His books include *Globalization and Well-Being* (University of British Columbia Press), *The Science of Well-Being* (Oxford University Press), *Well-Being for Public Policy* (Oxford University Press), *International Differences in Well-Being* (Oxford University Press), and the WHR. His current research is mainly on the sources and consequences of subjective well-being, with a special focus on the social determinants of well-being and the policy applications of well-being research.

Author Note

In revising the draft I have been greatly aided by suggestions from Paul Allin, Ed Diener, Jon Hall, Dan Haybron, Laura Kubzansky, Richard Layard, Matthew Lee, Steve Mulhall, Max Norton, Grant Schellenberg, Louis Tay, and Tyler VanderWeele. I also thank the John Templeton Foundation for supporting open access publication of this and all chapters in the volume. The views expressed in this chapter represent the perspective of the author and do not reflect the opinions or endorsement of any organization. I have no known conflict of interest to disclose. Correspondence concerning this chapter should be directed to John F. Helliwell, Vancouver School of Economics, University of British Columbia, 6000 Iona Drive, Vancouver BC Canada V6T1L4 (john.helliwell@ubc.ca).

References

Aknin, L. B., Whillans, A. V., Norton, M. I., & Dunn, E. W. (2019). Happiness and pro-social behavior: An evaluation of the evidence. In J. F. Helliwell, R. Layard, & J. Sachs (Eds.), *World happiness report 2019* (pp. 67–86). New York: Sustainable Development Solutions Network.

Alesina, A., Di Tella, R., & MacCulloch, R. (2004). Inequality and happiness: Are Europeans and Americans different? *Journal of Public Economics, 88*(9–10), 2009–2042.

Anand, S., & Sen, A. (1994). *Human development index: Methodology and measurement.* World Development Report Occasional Paper. New York: United Nations Development Program.

Annas, J. (1987). Epicurus on pleasure and happiness. *The Society for Ancient Greek Philosophy Newsletter.* 146. https://orb.binghamton.edu/sagp/146

Annas, J. (1993). *The morality of happiness.* Oxford University Press, Oxford.

Arim, R., & Schellenberg, G. (2019, June 4). An assessment of non-probabilistic online survey data: Comparing the carrot rewards mobile app survey to the Canadian community health survey. *Statistics Canada Analytic Studies: Methods and References, 21.* https://www150.statcan.gc.ca/n1/pub/11-633-x/11-633-x2019002-eng.htm

Bonikowska, A., Helliwell, J. F., Hou, F., & Schellenberg, G. (2014). An assessment of life satisfaction responses on recent statistics Canada surveys. *Social Indicators Research, 118*(2), 617–643.

Chetty, R., & Hendren, N. (2018). The impacts of neighborhoods on intergenerational mobility I: Childhood exposure effects. *The Quarterly Journal of Economics, 133*(3), 1107–1162.

Cheung, F., & Lucas, R. E. (2014). Assessing the validity of single-item life satisfaction measures: Results from three large samples. *Quality of Life Research, 23*(10), 2809–2818.

Cohn, M. A., Fredrickson, B. L., Brown, S. L., Mikels, J. A., & Conway, A. M. (2009). Happiness unpacked: Positive emotions increase life satisfaction by building resilience. *Emotion, 9*(3), 361.

Daley, A., Phipps, S., & Branscombe, N. R. (2018). The social complexities of disability: Discrimination, belonging and life satisfaction among Canadian youth. *SSM-Population Health, 5,* 55–63.

Deaton, A., & Stone, A. A. (2016). Understanding context effects for a measure of life evaluation: How responses matter. *Oxford Economic Papers, 68*(4), 861–870.

Diener, E., & Emmons, R. A. (1984). The independence of positive and negative affect. *Journal of Personality and Social Psychology, 47*(5), 1105.

Diener, E. D., Emmons, R. A., Larsen, R. J., & Griffin, S. (1985). The satisfaction with life scale. *Journal of Personality Assessment, 49*(1), 71–75.

Dolan, P., & Kavetsos, G. (2016). Happy talk: Mode of administration effects on subjective well-being. *Journal of Happiness Studies, 17*(3), 1273–1291.

Durand, M. (2015). The OECD Better Life Initiative: How's life? and the measurement of well-being. *Review of Income and Wealth, 61*(1), 4–17.

Durand, M., & Exton, C. (2019). Adopting a well-being approach in central government: Policy mechanisms and practical tools. In Global Happiness Council (Eds.), *Global happiness and wellbeing policy report 2019* (pp. 140–162). http://www.happinesscouncil.org

Flanagan, O. (2007). *The really hard problem: Meaning in a material world.* Cambridge, MA: MIT Press.

Goff, L., Helliwell, J., & Mayraz, G. (2018). Inequality of subjective well-being as a comprehensive measure of inequality. *Economic Inquiry, 56*(4), 2177–2194.

Grice, H. P. (1975). Logic and conversation. In P. Cole and J. L. Morgan (Eds.), *Syntax and semantic (Vol. 3, speech acts)* (pp. 41–58). New York: Academic Press.

Haybron, D. M., & Tiberius, V. (2015). Well-being policy: What standard of well-being? *Journal of the American Philosophical Association, 1*(4), 712–733.

Helliwell, J. F. (2003). How's life? Combining individual and national variables to explain subjective well-being. *Economic Modelling, 20*(2), 331–360.

Helliwell, J. F. (2019). How to open doors to happiness. In Global Happiness Council (Eds.), *Global happiness and wellbeing policy report 2019* (pp. 9–26). http://www.happinesscouncil.org

Helliwell, J. F. (2020). Three questions about happiness. *Behavioural Public Policy, 4*(Special Issue 2), 177–187.

Helliwell, J. F., & Aknin, L. B. (2018). Expanding the social science of happiness. *Nature Human Behaviour, 2*(4), 248.

Helliwell, J. F., Aknin, L. B., Shiplett, H., Huang, H., & Wang, S. (2018). Social capital and prosocial behavior as sources of well-being. In E. Diener, S. Oishi, & L. Tay (Eds.), *Handbook of well-being*. Salt Lake City, UT: DEF Publishers. doi:nobascholar.com

Helliwell, J. F., Barrington-Leigh, C. P., Harris. A., & Huang, H. (2010). International evidence on the social context of well-being. In E. Diener, J. F. Helliwell, & D. Kahneman (Eds.), *International Differences in Well-Being*, (pp. 291–325.) New York: Oxford University Press.

Helliwell, J. F., Huang, H., & Harris, A. (2009). International differences in the determinants of life satisfaction. In B. Dutta, R. Tridip, & E. Somanathan (Eds.), *New and enduring themes in development economics* (vol. 5, pp. 3–40). New Delhi: World Scientific.

Helliwell, J. F., Huang, H., Grover, S., & Wang, S. (2014). *Good governance and national well-being: What are the linkages?* OECD Working Papers on Public Governance No. 25. doi:10–1787/5jxv9f651hvj-en

Helliwell, J. F., Huang, H., & Wang, S. (2017). The social foundations of world happiness. *World happiness report 2017* (pp. 8–47). New York: Sustainable Development Solutions Network.

Helliwell, J. F., Huang, H., & Wang, S. (2018). New evidence on trust and well-being. In Uslaner, R. (Ed.), *The Oxford handbook of social and political trust* (pp. 409–446). New York: Oxford University Press.

Helliwell, J. F., & Putnam, R. D. (2004). The social context of well-being. *Philosophical Transactions of the Royal Society B, 359*(1449), 1435–1446.

Helliwell, J. F., & Wang, S. (2011). Trust and wellbeing. *International Journal of Wellbeing, 1*(1), 42–78.

Keyes, C. L., & Annas, J. (2009). Feeling good and functioning well: Distinctive concepts in ancient philosophy and contemporary science. *Journal of Positive Psychology, 4*(3), 197–201.

Land, K. C., & Michalos, A. C. (2018). Fifty years after the social indicators movement: Has the promise been fulfilled? *Social Indicators Research, 135*(3), 835–868.

Layard, R., with Ward, G. (2020). *Can we be happier? Evidence and ethics.* New York: Penguin.

Nichols, S., & Reinhart, R. J. (2019). Well-being inequality may tell us more about life than income. https://news.gallup.com/opinion/gallup/247754/wellbeing-inequality-may-tell-life-income.aspx

Nordhaus, W. D., & Tobin, J. (1972). Is growth obsolete? In *Economic Research: Retrospect and prospect (Vol. 5, Economic growth)* (pp. 1–80). Cambridge, MA: National Bureau of Economic Research.

OECD. (2013). *OECD Guidelines on Measuring Subjective Well-being.* Paris: OECD Publishing. http://www.oecd.org/statistics/Guidelines%20on%20Measuring%20Subjective%20Well-being.pdf

Peasgood, T., Foster, D., & Dolan, P. (2019). Priority setting in healthcare through the lens of happiness. In Global Happiness Council (Eds.), *Global happiness and wellbeing policy report* 2019 (pp. 27–52). http://www.happinesscouncil.org

Pickett, K. E., & Wilkinson, R. G. (2015). Income inequality and health: A causal review. *Social Science and Medicine, 128,* 316–326.

Ryan, R. M., & Deci, E. L. (2001). On happiness and human potentials: A review of research on hedonic and eudaimonic well-being. *Annual Review of Psychology, 52*(1), 141–166.

Sampson, R. J., Morenoff, J. D., & Gannon-Rowley, T. (2002). Assessing "neighborhood effects": Social processes and new directions in research. *Annual Review of Sociology, 28*(1), 443–478.

Sen, A. K. (1994). Well-being, capability and public policy. *Giornale Degli Economisti e Annali di Economia, 53*(7/9), 333–347.

Sen, A. K. (2003). Sraffa, Wittgenstein, and Gramsci. *Journal of Economic Literature, 43*(4), 1240–1255.

Stutzer, A., & Frey, B. S. (2006). Political participation and procedural utility: An empirical study. *European Journal of Political Research, 45*(3), 391–418.

VanderWeele, T. J. (2017). On the promotion of human flourishing. *Proceedings of the National Academy of Sciences, 114*(31), 8148–8156.

Van Ham, M., & Manley, D. (2012). Neighbourhood effects research at a crossroads. Ten challenges for future research Introduction. *Environment and Planning A, 44*(12), 2787–2793.

Wittgenstein, L. (1953). *Philosophical investigations.* Oxford: Blackwell.

2

Reflections on the Introduction of Official Measures of Subjective Well-Being in the United Kingdom

Moving from Measurement to Use

Paul V. Allin

Abstract

From 2011 onward, the United Kingdom's national statistics office has included four subjective well-being questions in its continuous Annual Population Survey. The specific motivation for this was so that summary statistics about subjective well-being would inform a new, broader assessment of national well-being, along with a selection of other, largely objective measures. There was also a perceived policy need for subjective well-being data, and the questions have also been added to other official surveys. This chapter reviews how and why the four questions were chosen. In particular, I focus on the "practical utility" of the subjective well-being statistics because this concept is at the heart of the case for having official statistics on this or any other topic. I report some progress in policy take-up of well-being statistics, though little media coverage, and a lack of evidence about whether people are thinking differently about their goals and their well-being based on well-being measures. I suggest that more should be done to encourage decisions and actions to be taken, informed by these measures. The work undertaken by the UK's national statistics office is essentially supply-side, helping to develop and maintain a robust, national data infrastructure. This is necessary but not sufficient. Official statisticians must engage more with politics, policy, businesses, academia, and public opinion, thereby helping to stimulate demand for all of their outputs, including well-being measures. I also pose a question: Are

Paul V. Allin, *Reflections on the Introduction of Official Measures of Subjective Well-Being in the United Kingdom* In: *Measuring Well-Being*. Edited by: Matthew T. Lee, Laura D. Kubzansky, and Tyler J. VanderWeele, Oxford University Press (2021). © Oxford University Press. DOI: 10.1093/oso/9780197512531.003.0003 developments of national well-being measures something to be left to each nation to consider, or are there benefits in encouraging international cooperation and exchange of good practice, which is generally valued in the fundamental principles for official statistics?

From 2011, the UK's national statistics office has added four subjective well-being questions to its continuous household survey covering the UK, the Annual Population Survey (APS). The purpose of the APS is to provide information on important social and socioeconomic variables at local levels: in addition to well-being, topics covered include employment and unemployment, housing, ethnicity, religion, health, and education. The survey is a structured random sample covering the whole of the UK household population using either face-to-face or telephone interviews for data collection. Young people under the age of 16 are excluded. The survey also does not cover adults living in communal establishments, such as nursing and care homes, homeless hostels, or prisons. The target sample is of the order of 350,000 adults each year and, with an overall response rate of currently around 45%, the Office for National Statistics (ONS) has achieved sample sizes of more than 150,000 adults each year. Survey estimates are weighted before publication so that they are representative of the UK adult population.

The decision to collect and publish official subjective well-being data in the United Kingdom came at the confluence of two increasing streams of interest in such data. One of these is the "Beyond GDP" agenda (e.g., Fioramonti, 2013) seeking to widen the definition of progress beyond just the economic performance of a country as measured by its gross domestic product (GDP), a prominent official statistic. The report by the Commission on the Measurement of Economic Performance and Social Progress (Stiglitz, Sen, & Fitoussi, 2010) had made a number of recommendations, including that "Statistical offices should incorporate questions to capture people's life-evaluations, hedonic experiences and priorities in their own survey" (p. 18). Although strictly a report commissioned by the then President of France, the recommendations were clearly aimed at a global audience, not least through the support of the Organisation for Economic Cooperation and Development (OECD). The ONS saw all the Commission's recommendations as adding substantially to evidence of the need for wider measures of national well-being, including subjective well-being.

The second motivating factor was cognizance of a desire for a "better politics" (Dorling, 2016), in which people's well-being is seen as the goal of government and of public policy. While Clark (2018, p. 245) has more re- cently noted a "remarkable rise in the interest shown by economists in subjective variables in general and in particular measures of subjective well- being," I suggest that his assessment that this change in economics has taken place over the past 40 years should be read as referring to academic research rather than to public policy. Nevertheless, by the time of a change of govern- ment in the United Kingdom in 2010, the appetite for well-being in public policy had reached the highest levels of government. The ONS gained gov- ernment funding for a Measuring National Well-Being Program.

The ONS Program had two interlinked strands. The first strand was to add questions on subjective well-being to household surveys. The second strand was to consult widely about what matters to the British public before devel- oping a set of indicators to publish as an assessment of national well-being that would be broader than GDP (Allin & Hand, 2014, chapter 7). ONS con- tinues to publish both summary statistics about the subjective well-being data (which it now describes as personal well-being) and a full set of more than 40 national well-being indicators. The first four indicators in the na- tional well-being set each relate to one of the four questions. Around two in five of the other indicators draw on other subjective data, and the others are objective indicators. The ONS four subjective well-being questions have been added to other UK official surveys, and all these data are being ana- lyzed, for example to understand how subjective well-being varies between areas and how different factors might influence well-being.

In this chapter, I review how and why the four questions were chosen. I place the questions in their context as official statistics: these are statistics envisioned as "an indispensable element in the information system of a democratic society, serving the government, the economy and the public with data about the ec- onomic, demographic, social and environmental situation," according to the United Nations fundamental principles for official statistics. In particular, we focus on the "practical utility" of the subjective well-being statistics because this is at the heart of the case for having official statistics on any topic (UN, 2014).

The Office for National Statistics Four Subjective Well-Being Questions

Since April 2011, the UK's ONS has been asking the following four subjective well-being questions as part of its continuous APS (ONS, 2018a):

Overall, how satisfied are you with your life nowadays?

Overall, to what extent do you feel the things you do in your life are worthwhile?

Overall, how happy did you feel yesterday?

Overall, how anxious did you feel yesterday?

(All on a 0–10 scale, where 0 is "not at all" and 10 is "completely")

These are all broad-brush questions about well-being. The questions are subjective, in the sense that they capture what the respondent reports as their perception of their well-being when asked about it. They are not objective measures, such as height or weight, which could be independently verified and which are mainly the kind of questions asked in official surveys. However, subjective questions have a long history of beneficial use in social and medical research, with a theoretical underpinning. There is also the point that apparently objective questions may have an element of subjectivity in how the respondent interprets what information is meant to be supplied.

The four questions are drawn from different approaches to well-being (see Allin & Hand, 2014, chapter 4, for an overview of subjective well-being measures). The first of the ONS questions is a summary, evaluative measure, in effect inviting the respondent to step back and reflect on how their life is going overall and their satisfaction with their life. This and variants of it have been widely used over many years (Pavot & Diener, 1993). One version is the *Cantril ladder*, on which respondents are shown a picture of a ladder with 10 rungs, numbered from 0 (worst possible life) to 10 (best possible life) and invited to say on which rung they feel they are standing. This is used in the Gallup World Poll, from which data on life satisfaction country by country are presented in the series of World Happiness Reports (Helliwell, Layard, & Sachs, 2019).

The second of the ONS questions is from the eudemonic tradition, sometimes referred to as the psychological, functioning, or flourishing approach to well-being. It draws on self-determination theory and taps into such things as the respondent's sense of meaning and purpose in life, connections with family and friends, a sense of control, and whether they feel part of something bigger than themselves. Although all of this is to be captured in a single question, we should acknowledge the complex nature of flourishing and that there is not a standard definition of it. Two authoritative summaries are "a combination of feeling good and functioning effectively, and the experience that life is going well" (Huppert & So, 2013) and "a state in which all aspects of a person's life are good" (VanderWeele, 2017).

The third and fourth of the ONS questions are a pair in which the respondent is asked about their experience of the previous day, specifically how happy and also how anxious they were then. These two questions are focusing on the respondent's positive and negative emotional experiences (or affect) over a short, recent timeframe to measure personal well-being on a day-to-day basis. Kahneman and Ris (2005) discuss how life experience/affect differs from life evaluation.

Question testing was undertaken, including by mode and to check that there would be no impact on response rates for the APS (see ONS, 2018b, for more details). All four questions appear to solicit thoughtful and consistent responses, although there is always scope for more cognitive research into how respondents come up with their replies.

As we will see later, the potential policy and academic research users of the new ONS data on subjective well-being tended to have rather general requirements. The four questions were judged to be the best way of meeting the requirements of potential users. The precise questions were chosen by the ONS with academic support and stakeholder review. There has been some ongoing engagement with potential policy users and with internal and external organizations inside and outside of government who support and encourage policy development informed by evidence, including an independent What Works Centre for Wellbeing.

The ONS decided to opt for subjective well-being questions already proved through use elsewhere, primarily to reduce the time taken to confirm questions to be added to its existing survey. There were other benefits to this (e.g., so that policy-makers and academic researchers would be able to compare the new ONS data with existing academic results). ONS also chose to use questions for which there was already an archive of results to help set the data collected by ONS in context, if possible. The data collection strategy was selected to meet what appeared to be the prevailing needs of potential policy and academic users, which was for a broad assessment of subjective well-being that could be analyzed by many dimensions and for local areas. This was provided by asking a few questions of many people in a survey in which many other variables were also collected. There were emerging policy requirements for more in-depth assessments of subjective well-being, but it was envisaged that these should be met in other surveys, where the ONS four questions could be used as the starting point for a more detailed set of questions.

Before embarking on this work to initiate subjective well-being questions in its survey, the ONS investigated if it could leverage experience from other countries that were already tracking subjective well-being. It found interest but no experience of asking subjective well-being questions in surveys conducted by other European national statistical offices prior to 2010. The French national statistical office (INSEE) was preparing to include such questions in two, one-off surveys on time-use and quality of life, and planning was under way to include well-being questions in the survey of income and living conditions conducted in each European Union country in a harmonized way (known as EU Survey on Income and Living Conditions [EU-SILC]), which resulted in a well-being module in the EU-SILC of 2013. The module included a life satisfaction question that was almost the same as the ONS version (with "these days" rather than "nowadays") and the same "worthwhile" question. The module also asked about satisfaction with eight aspects of life, such as commuting time, and included five self-rated questions about affects and emotions over the 4 weeks prior to interview (Eurostat, 2013, pp. 384–385).

In terms of official surveys in countries outside the European Union, the exemplar was Canada, where there is a track record of research on well-being using the personal well-being data collected in Statistics Canada's General Social Survey (GSS) annually since 1985, although this did not appear to have strong traction with policy-makers. There was some political interest in well-being measurement across Europe, particularly stimulated by French support of the Commission on the Measurement of Economic Performance and Social Progress and its commitment to take debate on the Commission's findings to international gatherings and meetings. What stands out about the United Kingdom is that the Prime Minister spoke at the launch of the ONS measurement program and, on several other occasions, in support of the measures and confirming that government had a role in improving well-being (see later discussion).

The Vision for Official Statistics

According to United Nations' fundamental principles for national *official statistics* (known as *federal statistics* in the United States), "Official statistics provide an indispensable element in the information system of a democratic society, serving the government, the economy and the public with data about the economic, demographic, social and environmental situation. To this end, official statistics that meet the test of practical utility are to be compiled and made available on an impartial basis by official statistical agencies to honour citizens' entitlement to public information" (UN, 2014, p. 1).

In practice, official statistics are driven by the needs of government, and much of the data is derived from administrative sources. Government also provides resources for surveys and censuses that are a significant source for official statistics. It funds data processing, dissemination, and development of new sources, such as the growing use of data science and the big data generated by operational and transactional systems.

The UN principles are designed to ensure that official statistics are also an essential public asset. The established position is that statistics such as these "enable journalists, citizens and politicians to discuss society as a whole, not on the basis of anecdote, sentiment or prejudice, but in ways that can be validated" (Davies, 2017, para. 6). But as Davies (2017, para. 6) also points out, this position is not held by everyone, and "attitudes towards quantitative expertise have become increasingly divided. From one perspective, grounding politics in statistics is elitist, undemocratic and oblivious to people's emotional investments in their community and nation."

The challenge for official statisticians in the contemporary information space is to recognize that they are competing with other providers of statistics who may be using official data, research outputs from academia and think tanks, commentators, and a plethora of opinions on social media who may be promoting alternative facts. Official statisticians therefore need to provide trustworthy and trusted statistics. They need to operate in ways that build confidence in the people and organizations that produce official statistics and data. They need to use data and methods that produce quality-assured and trusted statistics. These efforts are enhanced by recognizing and meeting society's needs for information (UK Statistics Authority, 2018).

The Case for UK Official Statistics on Personal Well-Being

The United Kingdom has a statutory regulator of official statistics, called the Office for Statistics Regulation, which assessed the ONS's statistics about subjective well-being against its code of practice in 2014, concluding that these statistics do meet the code and so merit National Statistics status. The code sets out 14 principles, grouped under the three pillars of trustworthiness, quality, and value. Trustworthiness, for example, includes looking to find professional capability and independent decision-making and leadership within the organization producing the statistics under scrutiny, while value is about finding evidence that the statistics support society's needs for information (UK Statistics Authority, 2018, pp. 14–15). The Authority noted that the ONS had reported that the statistics "are used in the policy making process by Government and for the monitoring, evaluation and measurement of policy. In addition, ONS identified that the statistics are used for international comparison purposes and to provide evidence which enables a broader understanding of the nation's progress and inform decision making by individuals and groups" (UK Statistics Authority, 2014, p. 5).

This is a rather general description of the need for official statistics on subjective well-being, and there were no specific details of the policy uses. Elsewhere in the Authority's report there is recognition that the case was made on the convergence of two requirements, which are those we noted in the Introduction as the twin stimuli for the ONS measurement program. They are still only described in broad terms. One of these was an emerging focus on individual well-being as an objective of public policy and that government should seek to improve well-being (also called social welfare or social value) through its policy priorities and implementation— and be held to account by demonstrating that well-being had improved. For example, this might lead politicians and policy officials to consider how to increase the personal agency of individuals—their sense of having more control in their life—if this can be shown to increase well-being. Similarly, it is about providing services that meet the population's needs in well-being terms.

The second requirement was the "Beyond GDP" agenda, especially the report by the Commission on the Measurement of Economic Performance and Social Progress (Stiglitz et al., 2010). This was a clarion call for wider measures of societal progress. The Commission recommended including indicators of quality of life, the state of the environment, and the sustainability of development, as well as improvements and enhancements to existing measures of economic performance. It was a significant staging post in the increasing realization that there is more to national well-being than economic growth. A proper understanding of well-being and progress can only be gleaned from a range of statistics—including the subjective assessment of personal well-being—beyond the more economically oriented measures traditionally defined in national economic accounts. It is these wider metrics that should inform not only national government policy but also the decisions made by civil society, business, and the public.

There is much to commend in the system of national accounts. They are based on internationally agreed concepts, definitions, and measures, of which GDP is but one headline measure. However, the critique of GDP set out by the Commission and elsewhere (e.g., Fioramonti, 2017) has three main strands. First, there are some weaknesses in how well GDP performs in what it is meant to do (i.e., measure all the economic activity in the country over a given period). Second, there is a demand for what GDP is not: the requirement here is for a measure, or measures, of national well-being, broadly defined, from which a better assessment of progress can be made than by using GDP alone. This wider measure of well-being provides particularly important information needed to assess the long-term sustainability of current economic growth. Third, the dominance of GDP statistics is seen by some as supporting the hegemony of GDP growth, defining or even driving how we live our lives to the exclusion and possible detriment of other things. Hence, critics of GDP argue that more subjective measures might broaden and improve the national discussion of how to define what it means to be doing well.

In a speech at the launch of the ONS Measuring National Well-Being Program, the Prime Minister said that, from April 2011 "we will start measuring our progress as a country not just by how our economy is growing, but by how our lives are improving; not just by our standard of living, but by our quality of life (Cameron, 2010, para. 1). However, it was a measurement program that was being launched, not any specific policy action. The Prime Minister stated his belief that "government has the power to help improve wellbeing" and that, in time, measuring well-being "will lead to government policy that is more focused not just on the bottom line, but on all those things that make life worthwhile" (Cameron, 2010, paras. 9 and 13). But one cannot but help seeing this as another example of what Bryson (2015, p. 428) observed, that Britain is "outstanding at counting what it has, but not so good at holding on to it."

Official Statistics as Tools for Social Change

If we are to move from measurement to action, and if the vision of official statistics having practical utility is to be realized, then we should consider how official statistics can be used in effecting social change. We have a reasonable understanding of the public policy process. Policymakers in UK central government follow a policy cycle known as ROAMEF, an acronym taken from its stages: determining the Rationale for policy; Objectives; Appraisal of options; Monitoring of implementation; Evaluation; and Feedback. Well-being data could be used in a number of these stages, for example to set the context in the rationale phase and in evaluating the impact of the policy as implemented (Allin, 2014, p. 448).

A recent working paper from the OECD, drawing on emerging use of well-being indicators in policy, suggests a number of benefits. For example, such indicators provide "a more complete and coherent picture—and in particular drawing attention to outcomes that matter to people's living conditions and quality of life, but that are often not currently considered in routine policy analysis" as well as supporting "the strategic alignment of outcomes across government" and tackling the silos within government agencies can operate (Exton & Shinwell, 2018, p. 17).

The OECD working paper also suggests that incorporating well-being statistics into policy might need behavior change among policy-makers, which could be brought about through both soft and firm processes (Exton & Shinwell, 2018, p. 19). *Firm processes* are akin to changing (and enforcing) the rules, for example on how policy options are defined and compared, and putting in place a well-being framework for government spending. *Soft measures* include raising awareness of well-being evidence among policy professionals, especially through training, and increasing access to well-being evidence.

Policy products such as legislation and regulation are not the only factors that influence behavior in society, even when policy implementation extends to the use of insights from behavioral economics to nudge people to do things differently. Human behavior may also respond to market incentives, as well as being rooted in ethical and cultural values and attitudes. (One useful source on the latter set of influences is the World Values Survey [www.worldvaluessurvey.org/wvs.jsp], which is not part of official statistics but which includes long-term data on well-being for more than 50 countries, along with many other variables.) All of these drivers of behavior change interact in ways we do not fully understand. There would seem to be multiple opportunities to draw on official statistics in building an evidence base for decision-making, action, and evaluation, except that we do not have a clear map of the whole process from which we can identify points and nodes where official statistics might be most useful.

This lack of understanding is apparent from the many descriptions of the use of specific sets of official statistics, which invariably contain only a list of rather generic categories of user or usage (an example of this was given at the beginning of the previous section). It is not easy to ascertain how public goods, free at the point of delivery, are used. Nevertheless, there must be scope to build a better picture of users and potential users of official statistics. Techniques of marketing and customer engagement widely used in the commercial sector could be adapted for application to official statistics (e.g., Statistics User Forum, 2019, annex 1, paras. 12–17).

The official statistics on well-being that are the focus here were introduced in response to a call for a potentially huge social change, nothing less than to reposition economic growth (especially year-on-year increase in GDP) as a means to an end, not as the end in itself. The big picture of "Beyond GDP," which reaches out to related concerns about our impact on the environment and on climate change, also needs to allow for the assessment of the sustainability of development. Stiglitz et al. (2010, pp. 19–21) recommended a well-identified dashboard of indicators, interpretable as variations in stocks, plus indicators of proximity to dangerous levels of environmental damage.

The rationale for the new measures was the belief that "We will not change our behaviour unless we change the ways we measure our economic performance" (Stiglitz et al., 2010, p. vii). This, it turns out, is only half of the picture. New measures are necessary but they are not sufficient. Governments, businesses, households, and individuals need to take action informed, either directly or indirectly, by the wider measures. One of the ways this is being tackled in the United Kingdom is through a What Works Centre for Wellbeing (https://whatworkswellbeing.org/), an organization that aims to put high-quality evidence on well-being into the hands of decision-makers in government, communities, businesses, and other organizations. This is one of a number of centers for evidence-informed policy and practice in the United Kingdom, elsewhere in the European Union, and in the United States and Australia.

One of the drivers for these kinds of centers is that the producers of evidence are often working in supply-side mode. That is, they concentrate on the pursuit of knowledge and data, rather on its usefulness and its applicability. The ONS Measuring National Well-being Program started with public consultation and with interaction with policy makers. However, there is a danger that delivery of statistical and data outputs will be just that, without further engagement with users and potential users. There is a measurement strategy and an adequately resourced delivery mechanism for the new measures as official statistics. The technical quality of the statistics, and their fitness for use in rather broad terms, has been confirmed, albeit within established procedures rather than by the full range of potential users

Methods and opportunities for effective communication and use of the new statistics and official statistics in general still need further development. A good starting point will be better communication and engagement with actual and potential stakeholders and improving awareness and quantitative skills of policy-makers, the media, and the public. Users of UK official statistics have been pressing for this for decades. In response to recommendations from a Parliamentary Committee looking at official statistics (PACAC, 2019), the recent announcement that the ONS and the UK Government Statistical Service "will develop a stakeholder engagement strategy and implementation plan" (Athow, 2019, para. 9) is to be welcomed.

Conclusion

The ONS program to measure well-being, launched in November 2010, continues to generate masses of data. These data are corralled in two sets: a set of anonymized microdata collected in response to the four subjective well-being questions in the APS; and a set of indicators of national well-being, which includes a number of subjective and objective measures drawn from other statistical sources, as well as measures derived from the subjective well-being data. There are regular outputs of summary statistics based on these data, including a dashboard (e.g., ONS, 2019a) and a series of statistical releases on subjective and economic well-being (e.g., ONS 2019b). The ONS subjective well-being data are also analyzed by external researchers (e.g., Bangham, 2019). Further secondary analysis of the ONS data is being encouraged by the UK economic and social research funding body, in cooperation with the What Works Centre for Wellbeing.

Some progress in policy take-up is being made. This chapter is not primarily a review of well-being in policy, a topic covered more fully elsewhere (e.g., Allin, 2014). A helpful and reassuring snapshot comes from the OECD working paper mentioned earlier (Exton & Shinwell, 2018) reporting relevant work in 19 countries, including the United Kingdom. The paper contains case studies of 15 countries with extensive well-being measurement frameworks and 10 countries with specific mechanisms for embedding

well-being metrics in central government policy. The working paper is a reminder that well-being measurement and policy is being driven forward by
the devolved governments within the United Kingdom, not just at the UK
government level that is the focus of this chapter. There is also a strong exemplar in the form of the implementation of a well-being framework into
policy in New Zealand, where "The Living Standards Framework is 'intended to help Treasury consistently provide Ministers robust, theoretically-
grounded and evidence-based advice that aims to improve the lives of all
New Zealanders'" (Exton & Shinwell, 2018, p. 38). The journey reported
includes the initial development of a framework within the Treasury in co-
operation with the New Zealand national statistics offices and other minis-
tries, followed by a stage of "identifying ways in which the Framework could
be used as a practical tool for day-to-day use by Treasury staff in making
policy evaluations and decisions." In a phrase that echoes the need for practical utility of official statistics, New Zealand officials learned that "The importance of prioritising practical usefulness was also emphasised by staff
from the Australian Treasury, based on their own experience of developing a
broader well-being framework" (Exton & Shinwell, 2018, p. 40). A number of
uses of the framework have been logged, and more are under way.

In this chapter I have also not explored how well-being is being taken up
under other broad policy initiatives, most notably the universal commitment to the UN's goals for sustainable development by 2030. These include
the development of more than 240 indicators (e.g., see the UK's current state
of play at https://sdgdata.gov.uk/). Only four of these indicators are subjective assessments, and they are about, for example, satisfaction with public
services, rather than subjective well-being questions covered in this chapter.
The UN's goals also include a general—but unexplained—commitment "to
developing broader measures of progress to complement gross domestic
product (GDP)" (UN, 2015, para. 48). There are clearly opportunities here
for the further development of well-being measures and, especially, further
ways in which measures could and should be used.

Apart from around the time of the launch of the ONS program, there
has been little media coverage in the United Kingdom of well-being statistics. It is still GDP that features in media headlines, rather than the wider
measures. One indication of the continuing prevalence of GDP is that,
at the time of writing, the ONS lists 463 upcoming releases of statistics, of
which 23 are GDP statistics and only 1 is about well-being (www.ons.gov.uk/
releasecalendar). There is a lack of evidence that more people are thinking

differently about their goals and their well-being based on well-being measures. Anecdotally, it is television programs such as the BBC TV *Blue Planet* series that appear to be most effective in increasing awareness of harm to the environment and the natural world from human economic activity. Research into how information is used in decision-making rarely looks specifically at the role of official statistics. I have yet to find any research about how people and businesses use official statistics on well-being (as opposed to views and aspirations from outside about how they might use well-being statistics), a gap that we suggest urgently needs filling.

It would be tempting to conclude that it is still early days and that wider usage will emerge from what is a huge and growing set of data on personal well-being. For example, the role of evidence translators, such as the What Works Centre for Wellbeing, is to provide more material that is relevant to policy, commercial, and public audiences. Even this is not without challenges as evidence may be of varying quality and a definitive view, say, of the association between income, financial satisfaction, and life satisfaction, may not yet have been reached.

However, I suggest that is too complacent a view to wait for change to occur based on a perfect set of well-being data. The aim should be for well-being evidence that is good enough and accessible enough to help inform decisions and choices and draw attention to the benefits of looking more broadly than just at GDP growth. Part of this is about transitioning to considering tradeoffs, say, between current economic activity and environmental impact, and between current and future well-being, rather than simply judging success as an increase in the value of one statistic.

I suggest that more should be done to encourage decisions and actions to be taken informed by well-being measures. The work undertaken by the UK's national statistics office is essentially supply-side, helping to develop and maintain a robust, national data infrastructure. This is necessary but not sufficient. In building the infrastructure, official statisticians must engage more with politics, policy, businesses, academia, and public opinion, thereby helping to stimulate demand for personal well-being measures.

The decision for national statistics offices to collect and publish subjective measures of personal well-being as well as objective measures has been widely accepted across the European Union and in some other countries. The ONS's four subjective well-being questions are also now found in a range of UK social surveys (ONS, 2018c). The questions are at the heart of the OECD guidelines on measuring subjective well-being (2013): the core question, on life satisfaction, is the same apart from a minor change in wording; the "worthwhile" question is the same; the "yesterday" affect questions are slightly different, though still rated on a 0–10 scale.

Other countries appear to be embracing the OECD guidelines. Durand and Smith (2013, table 7.1) listed, as part of the 2013 World Happiness Report, how official national statistics on subjective well-being were, or would shortly be, available in nine countries, mostly on a regular basis. The OECD life satisfaction question appeared in 10 of the 13 surveys in these countries, with the "affect" and "worthwhile" questions in around half of the surveys. In addition, the EU-SILC ad hoc module on well-being, including all the OECD questions, was being carried out in each of the 28 EU Member States and in four other European countries. More recently, a further five countries in the Asia-Pacific region reported their developments at a 2015 workshop (OECD, 2015), and there will be other examples. However, at least until the 2019 edition of the World Happiness Report (Helliwell et al., 2019), the latest available at the time of writing, global analyses of subjective well-being have remained based on the nonofficial Gallup World Poll because Gallup carries out fieldwork around the world.

Equally important is that subjective well-being is now included in a fuller assessment of how the United Kingdom as a country is doing, beyond GDP, as recommended by Stiglitz et al. (2010). A similar exercise for the United Kingdom and other countries is undertaken by the OECD, along with other data. The OECD phrases the question as "how's life?" and answers this with evidence from 50 indicators (e.g., OECD, 2017).

However, clearly, the story is not finished. At this point, three reflections might be made. The first is about the proliferation of official and nonofficial measures of well-being. Allin and Hand (2014, pp. 252–268) identified more than 130 indicator projects relating to the well-being of various nations or communities around the world, and this was almost certainly not an exhaustive list. Since then, further indicators have appeared (though no doubt others have been discontinued). One recent UK example from the commercial sector is the Sainsbury's Living Well Index (www.about.sainsburys.co.uk/about-us/live-well-for-less/living-well-index). This seeks to address what the company calls "unanswered questions," such as what does it mean to live well, and how are we really living as a nation? These are good questions. However, with this index and with all the other indicator projects, it is difficult to ascertain who is using them and how they are being used. It is probably safe to assume that they are being underutilized and that there is potentially more use to be made, whether to stimulate discussion on the state of well-being across the population or to design research and policy to increase well-being.

Moreover, the example of the Sainsbury's Index prompts the observation that there appears to be already a number of other well-being measures that could be used to answer these questions. It is perhaps understandable that a desire to make a change is invariably manifest through the production of a new measure. This demonstrates commitment and can help raise awareness. There may also be a preference for using a measure that is specific to the area or community in question. However, the producers of new indices and well-being studies may wish at least to consider whether to incorporate existing and tested measures for well-being, as proposed in the recommendations chapter of this volume (Chapter 14, in this volume). It turns out that the on-line Living Well Quiz associated with the Sainsbury's Index was compiled using a survey that included the ONS's four subjective well-being questions.

Generally, it is seen to be helpful to have a market in ideas and information, but perhaps an overconcentration on the supply-side in this market raises the possibility of confusing rather than clarifying the situation. We have come a long way from the simple idea that there are facts about the world in which we live and on which we can all agree. The UN's fundamental principles for official statistics, referred to in earlier sections, recognize that official statistics are one element in a national information system, although they also characterize official statistics as an *indispensable* element. I referred earlier to the two contrary views of official statistics reported by Davies (2017). In this chapter I have attempted to make the case for official statistics as a public good, available to all. But this is not a given, and it may be too simplistic to say that the trustworthiness, quality, and societal value of official statistics will win through. All these aspects have to be justified by the actions and activities of official statisticians. These pillars are all interconnected, and there are, for example, aspects of quality, such as timeliness, where there are nuanced differences between official statistics and those from other sources. Also, there is a premium on maintaining at least some statistics and indicators over time and maintaining their comparability over time. While this may be a desired feature of official statistics, there are also examples of long runs of nonofficial sources.

A second reflection concerns the balance between international comparability and meeting national needs. To take the United Kingdom's relationship with the OECD as an example, the UK measures of personal well-being are closely reflected in the OECD international guidelines. Formulating the UK questions helped with compilation of international guidance for national statistics offices should they wish to begin measuring subjective well-being in this way. This prompts a question: Are developments of subjective and wider national well-being measures something to be left to each nation to consider, or are there benefits in encouraging international cooperation and exchange of good practice, which is generally valued in the fundamental principles for official statistics?

Currently, there are two versions of the wider set of national well-being measures for the United Kingdom: the ONS dashboard and the OECD How's Life? Index. Each meets different needs. National well-being measures should include the things that matter to people in the country. However, international comparisons or aggregate measures for regions of the world need to be produced on a harmonized basis, as is done in the Gallup World Poll. Both needs are recognized in the UN fundamental principles, but they have to be addressed by each producer and in ways that do not lead to confusion or to gaming over the choice of which source to use. It is not clear that this issue has been fully considered.

The third reflection is to seek to move the focus from the supply-side. It seems clear that well-being can be measured, and it is being measured in many of its dimensions. There is depth, breadth, and longevity in many well-being datasets. But that still leaves the challenge of using these better data for better lives. Here there is more to do to stimulate the demand-side of this information market. Behavior change does not naturally follow from a change in the ways in which economic performance is measured. It is turning out to be more difficult than that, or at least to be subject to a considerable lag. There is progress in policy take-up of well-being evidence, not only in raising awareness of well-being measures and evidence, but also of implementing well-being in policy, but this appears slow. Well-being measures could be used in so many more helpful ways, as a number of reports have urged. O'Donnell, Deaton, Durand, Halpern, and Layard (2014, p. 14) set out "how governments and individuals can take account of wellbeing and use it for everyday decisions," for example, but note that they say "can" not "do."

More needs to be done to change the culture among politicians, policymakers, and business and civic leaders. Decisions should be based on wider well-being metrics and not just on the bottom line of economic profitability. All of us, as consumers, investors, voters, and members of civil society, should play our part. We should recognize and act in light of the picture of the world that appears from well-being measures that go way beyond GDP, even though the picture is more complex than just looking at the value of overall economic activity as measured by GDP. Well-being measures are necessary but not sufficient to improve our understanding of well-being. We then have to move on from trying to understand well-being to do more about trying to improve it.

About the Author

Paul V. Allin is Visiting Professor in statistics at the Department of Mathematics, Imperial College London, and coauthor of *The Wellbeing of Nations: Meaning, Motive and Measurement* (Wiley). He also chairs the UK Statistics User Forum and the Advisory Panel of the What Works Centre for Wellbeing, following a career as a professional statistician, researcher, and policy analyst in various UK government departments and agencies, latterly as the first director of the Measuring National Wellbeing Programme. His current research interests are the measurement of national well-being and progress and the use of these measures in politics, policy, business, and everyday life.

Author Note

The author gratefully acknowledges advice and information kindly provided by colleagues in the What Works Centre for Wellbeing and former colleagues in the ONS. Thanks also to Jonathan Michie, for insights into behavior change, to John Helliwell for a reminder about Statistics Canada's General Social Survey, to the Carnegie UK Trust for the opportunity to raise some of these issues in a blog, and to all participants in the Workshop on Happiness, Well-Being, and Measurement at Harvard University in April 2018, for interest in and helpful responses to my presentation. Thanks, too, for the encouragement and helpful suggestions provided by the editors of this book and the reviewers of the draft of this chapter. This work was supported in part by a grant from the John Templeton Foundation and by the Lee Kum Sheung Center for Health and Happiness. The views expressed in this chapter represent the perspective of the author and do not reflect the opinions or endorsement of any organization. I have no known conflict of interest to disclose. Correspondence concerning this chapter should be directed to Paul Allin, Department of Mathematics, Imperial College London, South Kensington Campus, London SW7 2AZ, United Kingdom (p.allin@imperial.ac.uk).

References

Allin, P. (2014). Measuring wellbeing in modern societies. In P. Y. Chen & C. L. Cooper (Eds.), *Work and wellbeing: Wellbeing: A complete reference guide, volume III.* (pp. 409–463). Chichester, UK: John Wiley and Sons.

Allin, P., & Hand, D. J. (2014). *The wellbeing of nations: Meaning, motive and measurement*. Chichester, UK: John Wiley and Sons.

Athow, J. (2019). Governance of official statistics: Appendix 4: Office for National Statistics and Government Statistical Service response. https://publications.parliament.uk/pa/cm201719/cmselect/cmpubadm/2656/265605.htm

Bangham, G. (2019). *Happy now? Lessons for economic policy makers from a focus on subjective well-being*. London: Resolution Foundation. https://www.resolutionfoundation.org/publications/happy-now-lessons-for-economic-policy-makers-from-a-focus-on-subjective-well-being/

Bryson, B. (2015). *The road to Little Dribbling: More notes from a small island*. London: Transworld.

Cameron, D. (2010). PM speech on wellbeing. www.gov.uk/government/ speeches/pm-speech-on-wellbeing

Clark, A. E. (2018). Four decades of the economics of happiness: Where next? *Review of Income and Wealth, 64*, 245–269.

Davies, W. (2017). *How statistics lost their power—and why we should fear what comes next*. www.theguardian.com/politics/2017/jan/19/crisis-of-statistics-big-data-democracy

Dorling, D. (2016). *A better politics: How government can make us happier*. London: London Publishing.

Durand, M., & Smith, C. (2013). The OECD approach to measuring subjective well-being. In J. F. Helliwell, R. Layard, & J. D. Sachs (Eds.). *World happiness report 2013*. (pp. 112–137). New York: Sustainable Development Solutions Network. https://worldhappiness.report/ed/2013/

Eurostat. (2013). EU-SILC description of target variables: Cross-sectional and longitudinal 2013 operation (version May 2013). https://circabc.europa.eu/sd/a/d7e88330-3502-44fa-96ea-eab5579b4d1e/SILC065%20operation%202013%20VERSION%20MAY%202013.pdf

Exton, C., & Shinwell, M. (2018). *Policy use of well-being metrics: Describing countries' experiences*. Paris: OECD Statistics Working Papers 2018/07. https://doi.org/10.1787/d98eb8ed-en

Fioramonti, L. (2013). *Gross domestic problem: The politics behind the world's most powerful number*. London: Zed.

Fioramonti, L. (2017). *The world after GDP*. Cambridge: Polity Press.

Helliwell, J. F., Layard, R., & Sachs, J. D. (Eds.). (2019). *World happiness report 2019*. New York: Sustainable Development Solutions Network. https://worldhappiness.report/ed/2019/

Huppert, F. A., & So, T. T. (2013). Flourishing across Europe: Application of a new conceptual framework for defining well-being. *Social Indicators Research, 110*, 837–861.

Kahneman, D., & Ris, J. (2005). Living and thinking about it: Two perspectives on life. In F. A. Hubbert, N. Baylis, & B. Keverne (Eds.), *The science of well-being* (pp. 285–304). Oxford: Oxford University Press.

O'Donnell G., Deaton A., Durand M., Halpern D., & Layard R. (2014). *Wellbeing and policy*. London: Legatum Institute.

OECD. (2013). Guidelines on measuring subjective well-being. www.oecd.org/statistics/oecd-guidelines-on-measuring-subjective-well-being-9789264191655-en.htm

OECD. (2015). Asia-Pacific workshop on subjective well-being: Measurement and policy use. http://www.oecd.org/statistics/Workshop%20on% 20Subjective%20Well-Being%20November%202015%20agenda.pdf

OECD. (2017). How's life? 2017: Measuring well-being. www.oecd.org/statistics/how-s-life-23089679.htm

ONS. (2018a). Personal well-being user guidance. www.ons.gov.uk/peoplepopulation andcommunity/wellbeing/methodologies/personalwellbeingsurveyuserguide

ONS. (2018b). Personal well-being frequently asked questions. www.ons.gov.uk/peoplepopulationandcommunity/wellbeing/methodologies/personalwellbeingfreque ntlyaskedquestions

ONS. (2018c). Surveys using our four personal well-being questions. www.ons.gov.uk/peoplepopulationandcommunity/wellbeing/methodologies/surveysusingthe4officefo rnationalstatisticspersonalwellbeingquestions

ONS. (2019a). Measures of national well-being dashboard. www.ons.gov.uk/peoplepopulationandcommunity/wellbeing/articles/measuresofnationalwellbeingdas hboard/2018-04-25

ONS. (2019b). Personal and economic well-being in the UK: April 2019. www.ons.gov.uk/peoplepopulationandcommunity/wellbeing/bulletins/personalandeconomicwellb eingintheuk/april2019

Pavot, W., & Diener, E. (1993). Review of the satisfaction with life scale. *Psychological Assessment, 5*, 164–172.

PACAC. (2019). Public Administration and Constitutional Affairs Committee: Governance of statistics inquiry. http://data.parliament.uk/writtenevidence/committee evidence.svc/evidencedocument/public-administration-and-constitutional-affairs-committee/governance-of-statistics/written/96403.html

Statistics User Forum. (2019). Written evidence from the Statistics User Forum (GOS 24). https://ec.europa.eu/eurostat/web/ess/forum

Stiglitz, J. E., Sen, A., & Fitoussi, J-P. (2010). *Mismeasuring our lives: Why GDP doesn't add up.* New York: New Press.

UK Statistics Authority. (2014). Statistics on personal well-being. www.statisticsauthority.gov.uk/publication/statistics-on-personal-well-being/

UK Statistics Authority. (2018). Code of practice for statistics. www.statisticsauthority.gov.uk/code-of-practice/

UN. (2014). Fundamental principles of official statistics (A/RES/68/261 from 29 January). https://unstats.un.org/unsd/dnss/gp/fundprinciples.aspx

UN. (2015). Transforming our world: The 2030 Agenda for Sustainable Development, 2015. https://sustainabledevelopment.un.org/post2015/transformingourworld

VanderWeele, T. J. (2017). On the promotion of human flourishing. *Proceedings of the National Academy of the United States, 114,* 8148–8156.

3

Assessments of Societal Subjective Well-Being

Ten Methodological Issues for Consideration

Louis Tay, Andrew T. Jebb, and Victoria S. Scotney

Abstract

This chapter examines 10 methodological issues when assessing and analyzing societal well-being using self-reports. First, there are unit-of-analysis issues: deciding the appropriate level of analysis, accounting for individual-level score variability in societal-level scores, testing isomorphism across levels, and finding ways of aggregating and accounting for score variability. Second, there are comparability issues: researchers have sought to homogenize well-being scales with different response scales or use translated measures to compare across nations. Furthermore, there is the concern of whether well-being measures can capture the full range of well-being (both positive and negative aspects). The final set of issues are prediction issues: well-being measures may be more sensitive to negative than positive events/experiences, societal well-being may not always be linearly related to variables of interest, and domain-specific measures may be more sensitive than general measures of well-being, especially when tracking specific changes in well-being or comparing subgroups.

The topic of well-being has been one of the perennial concerns in human history, although its definition and manifestations across time and cultures have varied (McMahon, 2006). In this day and age, individuals and governments continue to care deeply about well-being, and we have come to a consensus that, despite the different philosophical, cultural, and historical traditions concerning it, different psychological dimensions of well-being can be

Louis Tay, Andrew T. Jebb, and Victoria S. Scotney, *Assessments of Societal Subjective Well-Being* In: *Measuring Well-Being*. Edited by: Matthew T. Lee, Laura D. Kubzansky, and Tyler J. VanderWeele, Oxford University Press (2021). © Oxford University Press. DOI: 10.1093/oso/9780197512531.003.0004 empirically assessed (Diener, 1994). These scientific advances have prompted the use of well-being assessments as part of national accounting among governments and intergovernmental agencies (Diener, Oishi, & Tay, 2018). For example, in 2010, the former Prime Minister of the United Kingdom, David Cameron, advocated for well-being as the key indicator of progress rather than the gross domestic product (GDP). In 2011, the United Nations General Assembly adopted historic Resolution 65/309 that recognized the limitations of GDP as an index of societal progress and encouraged member nations to develop new indicators for measuring happiness and well-being.

While well-being can be assessed in any given society, there remain multiple issues that can limit its use and usefulness. For example, Paul Allin (Chapter 2, in this volume) notes that even though well-being is being tracked, such information is not readily used in policy-making. In this chapter, we focus on methodological issues that should be highlighted and considered when examining societal levels of subjective well-being. We believe that awareness of these methodological issues will better enable us to address potential limitations in its assessment and analysis. We use the term "subjective well-being" to refer to *self-reported* well-being given that such methods have a long history (Schwarz, 1999) and continue to be the primary way for assessing well-being. Other newer data science methods such as internet searches (e.g., Ford, Jebb, Tay, & Diener, 2018) and deriving assessments of well-being from social media data (e.g., Schwartz et al., 2013) will not be directly discussed here due to space limitations, although many of the issues raised are also applicable to such approaches. Furthermore, we do not cover psychological processes, such as retrospective biases or survey techniques such as scale response labeling (e.g., Kahneman, 1999; Schwarz & Strack, 1999) as these are well-known and have been discussed elsewhere (e.g., Tay, Chan, & Diener, 2014). In this regard, we seek to raise methodological issues that are less studied. For each issue, we provide recommendations for addressing them and make suggestions for future research.

Unit-of-Analysis Issues

Much of the research on the reliability and validity of subjective well-being indicators has emerged from the psychological literature (e.g., Diener, 1984; Ryff & Keyes, 1995). The psychological focus and a methodological reliance on individual respondents to provide self-reported subjective well-being scores has naturally led to an examination of the psychometric properties of well-being measures at the *individual* level of analysis. Calculating the properties of these well-being measures does not take into consideration group-level units (e.g., communities, countries). For example, an internal consistency reliability of 0.82 and a 2-month test-retest reliability of 0.82 for the Satisfaction with Life Scale (SWLS) is calculated using individual-level scores (Diener, Emmons, Larsen, & Griffin, 1985). Yet, in seeking to assess subjective well-being at a societal level, we need to use a different level as the primary unit of analysis to understand reliability and factorial validity and even to aggregate different distributions of individual subjective well-being scores. These are all unit-of-analysis issues.

Issue 1: The Importance of Different Societal Levels (Not Just the Nation)

When considering different levels of societal subjective well-being, the first units that come to mind are usually countries. One's national identity is a salient part of personal psychological identity, making the nation level a very important level to address when considering well-being (e.g., Morrison, Tay, & Diener, 2011). However, at the same time, there are other important societal levels that can be considered. Imagine an individual living in a borough of New York City. This person will exist within and relate to many important societal levels beneath the nation. A particularly important one is the *community level*. Steps above the community level for this person will be the greater *metropolitan level* (e.g., the greater New York City area), the *state and province level* (New York), and the *regional* level (Eastern United States). At any one of these levels, subjective well-being assessments can be made by aggregating individual ratings of well-being, which may reveal observable differences between units existing at that level. These differences may reveal important events or circumstances at that level that are occurring and impacting individuals collectively.

In addition to societal levels below the nation, there are also societal levels above it. Examples occur when countries are aggregated into world regions, as seen in the *CIA Factbook*, and, of course, the broadest societal level: human civilization as a whole. As one advances to higher levels, accurate assessment is usually more time-consuming because of the increased scope, but the benefit is that these measurements provide a greater overall summary of human well-being. Thus, well-being assessments at lower and higher societal levels complement one another: lower levels have a smaller span that may be more directly relevant to the lives of the member individuals, whereas higher level assessments provide broader summaries due to their larger scope. This means that although countries are psychologically important, societal well-being can be conceived at many other levels of analysis, and any of these may be fruitful and meaningful to measure. For example, at the community level, one may be interested in the characteristics of the neighborhood that could impact well-being (Luttmer, 2005); however, at the regional level, one may be interested in the impact of culture on well-being (Diener, Oishi, & Lucas, 2003).

There are two senses of the term "societies": one based on individuals living in proximity to one another; the other based on individuals who share a common purpose. Therefore, apart from societal levels that are distinguished or based on regions, another societal level is the *organizational level*, where the interest is organizational units such as schools, companies, or institutions. In this regard, individuals are sampled across multiple organizations to make comparisons, such as the well-being of schools within the United States. At the organizational level, members in the units of interest can be situated within a specific region. However, these members can also be situated across different regions. For instance, organizations such as multinational companies have organizational members than span across multiple nations. Therefore they may not necessarily be nested, unlike levels based on regions.

Methodologically, delineating these different types of societal levels can also be helpful in deciding the types of analysis to use. When regions are used as the unit of analysis, there is a clear nested structure: communities are nested within states, states are nested within nations, and nations nested within broader regions. Critically, we need to recognize that these effects across multiple levels occur concomitantly to potentially influence subjective well-being. It is important to consider the use of statistical techniques that account for the nested structure of the data, such as multilevel modeling (Snijders & Bosker, 1999) if we are to parse the extent that these different levels exert effects on well-being. At the organizational level, members of these groups may have multiple shared groupings (e.g., multinational companies have members in different nations but share a common company). However, statistical techniques such as (generalized) linear mixed modeling (Berridge & Crouchley, 2011) can similarly be considered to account for these different types of groupings in the data.

Recommendation: When examining societal-level well-being, researchers should be very mindful of the different collective levels that exist and can be assessed. They should avoid thinking that the nation level is the only important societal level. Many important assessments can be seen at lower (e.g., communities, states/provinces) or higher levels (e.g., world regions). Furthermore, given that multiple levels exist, analysis of societal subjective well-being data at a specific level (e.g., community level) may need to account for other possible levels (e.g., nation level) through appropriate statistical modeling.

Issue 2: Variance Attributable to a Societal Level and Reliability

When we are using individual-level self-reports aggregated to a societal level, it is important to ask whether well-being measures discriminate between societal units of interest (e.g., countries, communities). One way to assess this is by examining the variability, or variance, of aggregated (to a societal level) well-being scores. Intuitively, if there is substantial variability across these aggregated scores, then one can tell which societies have higher well-being and which have lower well-being. If there is minimal variability or variance in aggregated scores, then the well-being measure is less useful in differentiating societies.

Recommendation: Where possible, we should consider examining the absolute variability (e.g., standard deviation) of societal-level scores.

For simplicity, let us consider two primary levels—individuals and nations. A more appropriate way of examining this issue is not merely assessing the absolute variability of national scores but also assessing how much of the total variability of a measure is due to the individual versus national level. This represents the extent we can expect national-level factors to influence a specific measure of well-being and is substantively important for researchers seeking to understand relative influences of national-level factors versus individual-level factors. For example, researchers often calculate *intraclass correlations* (ICCs), which are defined as the between-group variability (i.e., national-level variability) divided by total variability (i.e., national-level variability + individual-level variability). In one study, different well-being measures on a sample of 123 nations showed that the ICC (specifically ICC(1)) for life satisfaction was 0.24, meaning that 24% of the variance of life satisfaction was attributable to the national level (Tay & Diener, 2011). By contrast, ICCs for positive and negative emotions were 0.06 and 0.04, respectively. Because the ICC represents the proportion of variance attributable to the national level, we expect that the measure of life satisfaction may be relatively more sensitive to national-level factors (e.g., GDP per capita) than positive and negative emotion measures. Notably, the ICC index is also the basis for computing reliability of individual self-report measures aggregated to the national level. Having greater reliability at the national level means that we are more likely to be sensitive to picking up effects at the national level (Bliese, 1998).

> Recommendation: Where possible, we should consider examining the proportion of variability attributable to the societal level(s) of interest (or higher level of aggregation), usually quantified using the ICC(1). Similarly, where possible, we should calculate the reliability of societal-level subjective well-being scores.

Issue 3: Isomorphism and Factorial Validity

Another significant point to consider is whether the factorial structure of a measure at the individual level holds when scores are aggregated. We do not necessarily know if the same factor structure will hold at a societal level. For instance, a measure of well-being may be composed of several latent variables, but what if there is a different number of factors when the scores are aggregated to a higher societal level? This would mean that distinguishing these different dimensions may be only viable at the individual level but not at a societal level; that is, that the concept being measured is fundamentally different. If this is the case, the score averages using individual-level factorial structures cannot be compared across different societies. Furthermore, we may not be able to appropriately label the different dimensions of subjective well-being (i.e., life evaluations, positive emotions, negative emotions) given that we do not know if they are similarly distinct dimensions at a societal level. We often assume that the factor structure remains preserved when making score aggregations, but we do not often directly examine it. This issue has been recognized in other domains of research such as the isomorphism of values between individual and societal levels. Past research on values iso-morphism has found high similarity between the two levels but that they are not strictly isomorphic (Fischer, Vauclair, Fontaine, & Schwartz, 2010).

Examining whether the factor structure remains constant across levels is called testing for *psychometric isomorphism* (Tay, Woo, & Vermunt, 2014). Psychometric isomorphism is essentially a kind of measurement invariance. Classic measurement invariance seeks to show that a measure has the same factor structure across groups at the same level of analysis (e.g., between men and women or respondents from different countries) to show that the same construct is being measured. Testing for psychometric isomorphism does the same thing but with regard to different levels of analysis. One can conveniently think of classic measurement invariance as testing the measure's factor structure "horizontally," whereas psychometric isomorphism tests it "vertically." The reader should note that this only needs to be done when scores are aggregated using a method like taking the mean (not when aggregating to get a measure of variability like the variance; Jebb, Tay, Ng, & Woo, 2019).

Recommendation: Where possible, tests of psychometric isomorphism should be conducted between the individual level and a societal level that the scores are being aggregated to (Tay, Woo, & Vermunt, 2014). This is done to ensure that the factor structures hold across levels so that the same well-being construct(s) can be said to be measured.

Issue 4: Limitations in Measures of Central Tendency

Researchers and policy-makers often rely on the statistical mean values of individual scores to represent societal-level scores. This may be done out of habit or convenience because there are other statistical parameters that can be used to assess the center of the distribution, such as the mode or median. More critically, all of these are simply measures of the distribution's *central tendency* and do not show how the scores within a particular level of society are distributed.

In addition to central tendency, there are measures of well-being distributions that could be examined. This is substantively informative to consider, as what matters is not only the average happiness levels for a society, but also the degree of *dispersion* (or spread) in well-being scores. Whether there is a large or a small spread can indicate important things about that society, such as an unequal distribution of resources or inequality among societal members. Such distributions are critical for researchers and policymakers to understand because they can shed light on who may have substantially lower and higher levels of well-being and what types of factors may be at play. Indeed, Veenhoven (1990) notes that there are different types of inequalities that may exist in societies (e.g., income, power, prestige, etc.) and that statistics of the well-being distribution, rather than central tendency, may better reveal these. Specifically, in addition to central tendency, other measures that can be used are dispersion measures (e.g., standard deviation, range, variance) or measures of skew (for examples, see Jebb, Tay, Ng, & Woo, 2019). Like the mean, measures of dispersion can serve as a relevant outcome or predictor in statistical modeling. Considering the societal-level of the nation, past research shows that the Gini coefficient calculated on life satisfaction scores (which is a measure of dispersion in the distribution) predicts average levels of enjoyment, anger, sadness, and stress over and above average annual household income (Diener & Tay, 2015). Moreover, Ovaska and Takashima (2014) have found income inequality and health inequality to be related to higher levels of life satisfaction dispersions within countries.

> Recommendation: Researchers examining societal-level well-being should recognize the limitations of central tendency measures for describing the well-being distribution and the importance of other statistics, such as dispersion and skew measures. Visualizations of the full distribution (e.g., histograms, kernel densities) can be an effective way to see or communicate the full picture of well-being at that level of society.

Comparability Issues

The next set of issues are collectively organized under comparability issues, where we discuss how past work has sought to create comparable well-being scores across societies—typically nations. We examine some of these methods and provide recommendations. Furthermore, we also consider whether subjective well-being measures capture the full range of well-being (i.e., equivalence in assessing positive and negative aspect of well-being in a measure).

Issue 5: Scale Homogenization via Linear Stretch

In survey research, it is common to see different measures for the same well-being construct. Sometimes researchers simply develop or use different measures because they are working independently (e.g., there are many slightly different life satisfaction measures). At other times, this occurs with archival data from different countries that have assessed well-being at different time periods in that nation. In any case, because scales are not always standardized over research studies, it is hard to know whether these scores can be compared. Scales of the same construct might have different numbers of response options (e.g., 1–5 vs. 1–10 response options) or types of response options (e.g., Not at all/A little bit/Somewhat/Very much/extremely vs. strongly agree/Agree/Disagree/Strongly disagree). Are two 1–5 scales with different response options perfectly comparable?

The different types and wording of the items notwithstanding, researchers have sought to use transformations to create a common metric to compare different measures across countries and over time. In other words, researchers seek to conduct *scale homogenization* (de Jonge, Veenhoven, & Arends, 2014) to either "stretch out" scores to a common standard (e.g., 1–5 response scale to a 1–10 response scale) or to "compress" them (e.g., 1–11 response scale to a 1–10 response scale). One conventional scale homogenization method has been the *linear stretch* method, which takes the lowest scale response option (e.g., 1 on a 1–5 response scale) and projects it onto the lowest number on a common scale (e.g., 0 on a 0–10 response scale) and the highest response option (e.g., 5 on a 1–5 response scale) and projects it onto the highest number on the common scale (e.g., 10 on a 0–10 response scale). All intermediate scale response options are then transformed to equally distanced scores (e.g., 2 on a 1–5 response scale projected as 2.5 on a 0–10 response scale; de Jonge et al., 2014).

Past research has shown that the linear stretch method for scale homogenization does not lead to equivalence. Using the World Database of Happiness of 67 nations between 1945 and 2013, it was found that when scales were equivalized to a 0–10 scale, those with fewer scale response options on the original scale (e.g., 3 response options vs. 7) had lower rescaled scores (Batz, Parrigon, & Tay, 2016). This trend held for both life satisfaction and other happiness scales. In other words, the linear stretch method may *artifactually* score nations lower if they used self-reported well-being scales that had few response options. In addition to distorting raw scores, this can also affect substantive relationships. In the same study, GDP per capita predicting happiness had linear regression coefficients that were significantly larger when not accounting for the number of scale response options ($\beta = 0.65$, 95% confidence interval [CI] [0.49, 0.81]) as compared to accounting for the scale response options ($\beta = 0.33$, 95% CI [0.22, 0.44]; Batz et al., 2016).

Instead of the conventional linear stretch method of scale homogenization, past work has shown that other more sophisticated methods may be more appropriate, although with limitations (de Jonge et al., 2014). Our suggestion is that researchers interested in societal well-being should strive to use scales that are homogenous in the first place rather than rely on mathematical transformations.

Recommendation: For comparisons of societal-level well-being, researchers must be aware that when different scales are being used, especially if the number of response options differs, there may not be equivalence. Ideally, research should rely on common, equivalently worded scales, scale responses, and scale response wording for accurate comparisons.

Issue 6: Measurement Equivalence

Even with the use of equivalently worded measures—both in item content and scale responses—there can be differences in the language(s) spoken and understood by respondents in a society that may lead to nonequivalence in measurement. In other words, language differences can lead to potential measurement bias in well-being scales; *measurement bias* means that respondents in a society are systematically scored higher or lower than their "true" level (Tay, Meade, & Cao, 2015). Therefore, we may observe score differences on well-being scales between societies not because of "true" construct differences but because the well-being scales are not equivalent. Aside from language, there are other reasons for measurement bias that include differences in culture (even with the same language; e.g., culture of modesty), differences in response context (e.g., phone poll vs. face to face), and other factors (Robert, Lee, & Chan, 2006).

Therefore, it is important to not merely use equivalently worded measures and have appropriate translations into different languages, but to also empirically determine if there is measurement equivalence across societal units of interest (e.g., communities, countries, organizations). There are well-established statistical procedures for assessing measurement equiva-lence (Tay et al., 2015; Vandenberg & Lance, 2000). A key requirement is that the scale have multiple items and not be made up of a single item. Multi-item scales make it statistically possible to disentangle potential measurement bias from true differences, whereas a single item cannot. Moreover, with multi-item measures we are able to ascertain if there are specific items that may be causing any nonequivalence. For example, it has been shown that even within the United States, a negatively scored item for negative affect (i.e., "full of life") was not equivalent between Hispanics/Latinos and non-Hispanic whites (Kim, Wang, & Sellbom, 2020). Identifying these nonequivalent items will allow researchers to later exclude them from the analysis. This can only be done if multi-item measures are used.

For example, our research group examined the measurement equivalence of the Comprehensive Inventory of Thriving (CIT; Su, Tay, & Diener, 2014), which assesses a large number of dimensions of well-being (e.g., relationship, engagement, mastery, autonomy, meaning, optimism, subjective well-being). Measurement equivalence was assessed at the societal level of nations: United States, Argentina, Australia, China, Germany, India, Mexico, Russia, Singapore, Spain, and Turkey (Wiese, Tay, Su, & Diener, 2018). It was found that there was measurement equivalence of the CIT measure across the different countries but not in Argentina, Mexico, and China. Specifically, it was found that the dimen-sion of "engagement" did not fit well across these nations. This finding can serve to prompt further research on whether the translation of "engagement" may be interpreted differently in these countries. It can also guard against reading too much into national differences on the "engagement" dimension.

> Recommendation: Where possible, researchers should use multi-item well-being measures and assess their measurement equivalence when different societies are examined. This is not possible with a single-item measure. Additionally, it can be beneficial to use scales that have already been exam-ined and validated for measurement equivalence across nations as this can help forestall potential problems in nonequivalence prior to data collection.

Issue 7: Equivalence in Well-Being Poles

One issue that has been more recently considered in the literature is whether our measures adequately assess the full range of well-being (i.e., from suffering to flourishing; Tay & Jebb, 2018). While positive aspects of well-being have long been considered and valued, positive psychology (Seligman & Csikszentmihalyi, 2000) has focused measurement efforts to go explicitly beyond the negative aspects (e.g., depression, stress, suicide). A comprehensive assessment of societal subjective well-being should consider whether our administered measures equivalently assess both positive and negative aspects.

In our work on continuum specification, we discuss the importance of defining and operationalizing *construct continua* (Tay & Jebb, 2018). In its application to societal subjective well-being, we need to determine whether we are adequately capturing one end of well-being to the lack of inclusion of the other. We also need to be clear about the nature of the gradations on the continuum (i.e., the quality that separates high from low scores; e.g., intensity of positive feelings; frequency of positive feelings). Continuum specification enables greater measurement validity, where we explicitly define the full span of a concept and are confident that our scale content and scale response options operationally assess this full span. For example, in claims that most people are happy (Diener & Diener, 1996), it is important to consider if the well-being scale administered adequately captures the full span in the purported well-being poles.

Continuum specification also exists at a broader conceptual analysis beyond a single self-report scale. In this regard, the continuum does not refer to the continuum of any given single construct (e.g., meaning, life satisfaction, social support). Rather, the continuum refers to the full range of the well-being concept (i.e., from suffering to flourishing). Different types of measures that index ill-being and well-being are required in the suite of societal subjective well-being measures. This may include pairings such as loneliness and social connection, positive feelings and negative feelings, depression and awe, distress and eustress, optimism and pessimism.

Recommendation: Researchers should be mindful of all the degrees and the overall span that well-being can take. If a full measure of well-being is desired, one must ensure that the full range of well-being is encompassed or is at least included in the suite of measures that are used.

Prediction Issues

The initial set of issues was concerned with the assessment of societal well-being itself. This final set of issues is concerned with how these assessments of societal well-being are typically used in research and analysis which form the basis of scientific conclusions and policy recommendations. If societal well-being is measured, one interest will simply be in the levels that are observed. This information is important because it gives a direct summary about the well-being of a particular level of society. However, researchers will often want to go beyond examining just these differences in levels. They will often want to also examine what predicts well-being (e.g., GDP per capita, employment) and what is predicted by well-being (e.g., physical health, different social attitudes; Diener et al., 2018). We label these as *prediction issues*. In some cases, prediction will be important because one is trying to establish a causal relationship, and correlation is a necessary condition for causation. In others, prediction itself will be the goal; a variable might be able to predict societal well-being even though it is not a direct cause, and the ability to anticipate future well-being levels can be important in its own right (see Shmueli, 2010, for distinctions between causal and predictive modeling).

In this section, we touch on several issues related specifically to building statistical models that include societal well-being. However, because statistical modeling is an extensive topic, the reader should note that there are many more issues that we do not touch on here, such as consideration of interaction effects, appropriate use of control variables, and fulfilling the assumptions of these models (e.g., homogeneity of variance). These more general issues are important and are discussed in many other resources (e.g., Gelman & Hill, 2007).

Issue 8: Bad May Be Stronger Than Good

One important consideration in assessing the predictors of well-being is that negative and positive events have an asymmetrical relationship to well-being. Specifically, negative events are known to generally be more strongly related to well-being than are positive events (Baumeister, Bratslavsky, Finkenauer, & Vohs, 2001). For instance, when local businesses or factories close, people are more emotionally affected than when they are preserved or added to. Empirically, pivotal research in behavioral economics has shown that people are more sensitive to losses than gains (i.e., loss aversion; Kahneman & Tversky, 1979). In psychology, there is evidence that negative events (e.g., divorce, job loss, loss of spouse) tend to exert stronger and longer lasting effects on subjective well-being than are positive events (e.g., marriage, lottery wins;

Tay & Kuykendall, 2013). These effects have also recently been demonstrated at higher societal levels; a recent study by De Neve et al. (2018) showed that negative economic change is more strongly related to national subjective well-being than is positive economic change. This negativity bias has been observed even in early development (Vaish, Grossmann, & Woodward, 2008). When positive events happen, there is less of a reason to feel strong emotions because events are unfolding as they "ought to." However, when negative events occur, strong emotions are needed to draw attention to the problems and correct them. Indeed, many theorists agree that this is a standard purpose of emotion: to direct our attention and motivate us to deal with life events (Izard, 2010).

These considerations are useful when constructing a statistical model where well-being is conceived as an outcome of societal-level indicators. From this psychological theory, we think it is likely that societal well-being is better predicted by negative indicators. Knowing this provides guidance in constructing better models of societal well-being and helps avoid looking for important predictors in the dark. For example, rather than examining very broad societal-level factors like GDP or housing rates, one might have better success looking at variables that directly quantify problems, such as the percentage of the unemployed or the percentage of those who have difficulty affording housing. That is, one interesting strategy is to look at *societal problems* rather than just broad societal factors. This approach is informed by a consistent finding that negative and positive events have an asymmetrical relationship to well-being. We can apply this to different societal levels by examining specific problems at that level (e.g., community- or state-level problems).

> Recommendation: When constructing models of societal-level well-being, researchers should recognize that positive and negative events may not be equally related to well-being. Using this psychological theory, researchers may be able to more efficiently identify the key predictors, which might be problems that exist at that societal level.

To clarify, we are not stating that bad will *always* be stronger than good or that protective or positive factors will have nugatory effects. Rather, when we are seeking to model predictors of well-being from a large number of variables at a specific societal level, it is worth considering negative events or conditions. Certainly, researchers may be interested in comparing different types of positive conditions and their differential effects on well-being or the different types of positive well-being dimensions and their differential effects on outcomes (e.g., Chapters 4 and 5, both in this volume). Even when seeking to assess positive conditions, one can assess it alongside negative conditions or variables, as when comparing between positive and negative economic changes on societal well-being (De Neve et al., 2018). This also extends to modeling outcomes of well-being where positive and negative emotions have been found to have independent effects on future physical health (Wiese, Chen, Tay, Friedman, & Rector, 2018).

Issue 9: Curvilinear Effects

Linear models are prevalent in the social sciences. Part of this is due to the fact that they are both conceptually and mathematically simple. Conceptually, *linearity* means that the slope between the variables remains constant, and mathematically, any linear relationship can be represented by simple arithmetic terms (e.g., multiplication and addition). However, the popularity of linear models is not just due to convenience, but also because they are often accurate. Linearity is often a useful approximation for real-life processes (Cowpertwait & Metcalfe, 2009). For example, it is natural to think of well-being as increasing linearly with things like amount of leisure time or financial security. However, because well-being cannot increase infinitely (Diener, Lucas, & Scollon, 2006), it is likely that it will have many associations that are not fully linear. With the examples of leisure time and financial security, one can easily imagine that, after an individual has enough leisure time or financial security, then more of either of these does not increase well-being. Indeed, recent research has given evidence that the relationship between subjective well-being and income is linear but only up to a point. When income is high enough to satisfy basic needs and higher order desires, then the relationship becomes flat (Jebb, Tay, Diener, & Oishi, 2018). Instead of linearity, this is an example of a *monotonic* relationship, which is simply any relationship between variables where the slope maintains the same sign (but is not necessarily linear because the magnitude of the slope can change). In addition to monotonicity, there are also *curved relationships* where the sign of the slope *does* change (from positive to negative or vice versa). One can easily imagine a scenario where all of a person's time is *leisure*, which can lead to feelings of a lack of meaning and negatively impact well-being. One empirical example can be found in the individual-level association between well-being and age. Substantial research has shown that the association between well-being and age has a slight curve such that, prior to middle age, the slope is negative, but after middle age, the slope is positive (Blanchflower & Oswald, 2017; López Ulloa, Møller, & Sousa-Poza, 2013). At a societal level, GDP per capita does not increase linearly with national subjective well-being (e.g., Inglehart, Foa, Peterson, & Welzel, 2008).

The key point we hope to make is that just because linearity often holds at some levels of the variables, researchers should not be lured into thinking that the *entire* relationship is necessarily linear. In this regard, we may want to consider some alternatives to the standard linear model, such as polynomial models (Cohen, Cohen, West, & Aiken, 2003), regression splines (Harrell, 2015), or nonlinear models (Motulsky & Ransnas, 1987) when modeling societal-level well-being.

Recommendation: Carefully consider whether a relation may be linear when analyzing societal well-being. One may need to utilize other models aside from standard linear regression to accurately estimate and understand the predictors and outcomes of societal well-being.

Issue 10: Level of Specificity

Because well-being can be considered to encompass many aspects of life, assessments of well-being will vary in whether they are *broad* (e.g., satisfaction with life in general, negative emotions) or *specific* (e.g., satisfaction with work, the presence of worry). This is called the *level of specificity* of the measure, and it is an important factor to consider when assessing or modeling societal well-being. First, in terms of assessment, a greater level of specificity helps respondents focus on a specific domain of well-being in question (e.g., Cummins, 2005; Oishi & Diener, 2001). This makes that domain the source of their well-being, making it arguably more sensitive to that source. Second, when including well-being as a variable in statistical models, specificity is important to consider because, in general, specific outcomes tend to be predicted better by specific predictors, whereas broader outcomes are better predicted by broader predictors (Cronbach & Gleser, 1965). When the outcome is broad, many aspects are measured as part of it, and if this content is not matched to the content in a predictor, the correlation will be driven down. Conversely, if the outcome is specific and the predictor is broad, the association will be reduced by the content in the predictor that is simply irrelevant to the outcome. For instance, an overall measure of physical health includes many components (e.g., illnesses, quality of diet), and a broad predictor like an overall happiness score may be a good fit because it is also a function of many things (e.g., satisfaction with one's job, social life, and leisure activities). However, as the outcome becomes narrower in scope, more and more of a broad predictor will become irrelevant. Thus, predicting a specific aspect of physical health, like exercise habits, will have a lower correlation to overall happiness. In this case, a better predictor would be a more specific measure, such as vitality.

The idea that associations are maximized when outcomes and predictors are matched in their level of specificity is referred to as the *bandwidth-fidelity* distinction (Cronbach & Gleser, 1965). This is just an observation to consider when planning a research study, and it should not determine what the researcher does. Predictors included in a statistical model can be broad even if the outcome is narrow (and vice versa); it depends on the context and aims of the research (e.g., maybe the researchers is genuinely interested in how overall well-being relates to a specific narrow variable). However, we note this because, to our knowledge, this is not an issue often considered explicitly in well-being research. Our research group sought to examine this issue by comparing the sensitivity of life satisfaction (very broad) and job satisfaction (more specific) to gender inequality and found preliminary evidence that job satisfaction may be more sensitive to gender inequality than overall life satisfaction (Batz-Barbarich, Tay, Kuykendall, & Cheung, 2018). This suggests, when looking at specific factors that might reduce (or promote) well-being, that one should consider using more specific well-being measures.

> Recommendation: For a given research question or topic, one should consider the level of specificity at play. If the outcome or predictor is narrow, this means its content will also be narrow. Generally, broad outcomes tend to have stronger associations with broad predictors, and the same is true for narrower outcomes and predictors. When investigating what best predicts narrower aspects of well-being, researchers may want to consider narrower predictors.

Conclusion

The assessment of societal well-being is a growing and active area, important not only to researchers, but to government leaders and policy-makers as well. We have summarized some of the key issues for consideration and proposed specific recommendations for addressing—or at least being mindful of—these issues. We presented several suggestions to consider when assessing well-being when societies are the unit of interest. For example, researchers may want to consider the use of measures of dispersion, rather than central tendency, in order to address the range of well-being experienced within a society (e.g., What is the significance of a country where most people have similar levels of well-being [low dispersion] versus a country where there are many people experiencing well-being extremes [high dispersion]?). Furthermore, we discussed issues in comparing well-being across societies where different measurement scales are used or when items in a scale do not have the same interpretation by people of different cultures, language, or other demographics. Addressing these issues is foundational to making comparisons between societies that are not confounded by measurement artifacts. Finally, we discussed issues in prediction of and by societal well-being that include the valence of well-being measures, the linearity of relations with well-being, and the specificity of well-being measures. We hope the issues we presented encourage researchers to expand their thinking about the measurement and analysis of societal subjective well-being. We believe that the consideration of these issues could help develop new research ideas and clarify the phenomena of interest. In this regard, we hope that this chapter can serve to highlight areas that require more active research.

About the Authors

Louis Tay is Associate Professor of Industrial-Organizational Psychology at Purdue University. His research interests are in well-being, methodology, and measurement. He is the co-editor of the books *Handbook of Well-Being* (DEF Publishers) and *Big Data in Psychological Research* (APA Books). He serves as an associate editor at *Organizational Research Methods*.

Andrew T. Jebb is a research scientist at the University of Oklahoma's Institute for the Study of Human Flourishing. He is a graduate of Purdue University's Department of Psychological Sciences (in industrial–organizational psychology). He is interested in happiness and well-being, the employee–organization relationship, and psychological measurement and statistics.

Victoria S. Scotney is a graduate student in industrial–organizational psychology at Purdue University. She has published in outlets such as *Psychological Bulletin* and *Frontiers* *in Psychology*. Her current research interests include prosocial giving and receiving, well-being, research methods, and measurement.

Author Note

This work was supported in part by a grant from the John Templeton Foundation and by the Lee Kum Sheung Center for Health and Happiness. The views expressed in this chapter represent the perspectives of the authors and do not reflect the opinions or endorsement of any organization. We have no known conflict of interest to disclose. Correspondence concerning this chapter should be directed to Louis Tay, Department of Psychological Sciences, Purdue University, 703 Third Street, West Lafayette, Indiana, 47907 (stay@purdue.edu).

References

Batz, C., Parrigon, S., & Tay, L. (2016). The impact of scale transformations on national subjective well-being scores. *Social Indicators Research, 129*, 13–27.

Batz-Barbarich, C., Tay, L., Kuykendall, L., & Cheung, H. K. (2018). A meta-analysis of gender differences in subjective well-being: Estimating effect sizes and associations with gender inequality. *Psychological Science, 29*(9), 1491–1503.

Baumeister, R. F., Bratslavsky, E., Finkenauer, C., & Vohs, K. D. (2001). Bad is stronger than good. *Review of General Psychology, 5*(4), 323–370.

Berridge, D. M., & Crouchley, R. (2011). *Multivariate generalized linear mixed models using R*. Cleveland, OH: CRC Press.

Blanchflower, D. G., & Oswald, A. J. (2017). Do humans suffer a psychological low in mid-life? Two approaches (with and without controls) in seven data sets. Bonn: Institute of Labor Economics (IZA). Https://www.econstor.eu/bitstream/10419/170942/1/dp10958.pdf

Bliese, P. D. (1998). Group size, ICC values, and group-level correlations: A simulation. *Organizational Research Methods, 1*(4), 355–373.

Cohen, J., Cohen, P., West, S. G., & Aiken, L. S. (2003). *Applied multiple regression/correlation analysis for the behavioral sciences* (3rd ed.). Mahwah, NJ: Lawrence Erlbaum Associates.

Cowpertwait, P. S., & Metcalfe, A. (2009). *Introductory time series with R*. New York: Springer-Verlag.

Cronbach, L. J., & Gleser, G. C. (1965). *Psychological tests and personnel decisions*. Champaign: University of Illinois Press.

Cummins, R. A. (2005). The domains of life satisfaction: An attempt to order chaos. In A. C. Michalos (Ed.), *Citation classics from social indicators research: The most cited articles edited and introduced by Alex C. Michalos* (pp. 559–584). Dordrecht: Springer Netherlands.

de Jonge, T., Veenhoven, R., & Arends, L. (2014). Homogenizing responses to different survey questions on the same topic: Proposal of a scale homogenization method using a reference distribution. *Social Indicators Research, 117*, 275–300.

De Neve, J. E., Ward, G., De Keulenaer, F., Van Landeghem, B., Kavetsos, G., & Norton, M. I. (2018). The asymmetric experience of positive and negative economic growth: Global evidence using subjective well-being data. *Review of Economic Statistics, 100*(2), 362–375.

Diener, E. (1984). Subjective well-being. *Psychological Bulletin, 95*, 542–575.

Diener, E. (1994). Assessing subjective well-being: Progress and opportunities. *Social Indicators Research, 31*, 103–157.

Diener, E., & Diener, C. (1996). Most people are happy. *Psychological Science, 7*, 181–185.

Diener, E., Emmons, R. A., Larsen, R. J., & Griffin, S. (1985). The satisfaction with life scale. *Journal of Personality Assessment, 49*, 71–75.

Diener, E., Lucas, R. E., & Scollon, C. N. (2006). Beyond the hedonic treadmill: Revising the adaptation theory of well-being. *American Psychologist, 61*(4), 305–314.

Diener, E., Oishi, S., & Lucas, R. E. (2003). Personality, culture and subjective well-being: Emotional and cognitive evaluations of life. *Annual Review of Psychology, 54*, 403–425.

Diener, E., Oishi, S., & Tay, L. (2018). Advances in subjective well-being research. *Nature Human Behavior, 2*, 253–260.

Diener, E., & Tay, L. (2015). Subjective well-being and human welfare around the world as reflected in the Gallup World Poll. *International Journal of Psychology, 50*, 135–149.

Fischer, R., Vauclair, C.-M., Fontaine, J. R. J., & Schwartz, S. H. (2010). Are individual-level and country-level value structures different? Testing Hofstede's legacy with the Schwartz value survey. *Journal of Cross-Cultural Psychology, 41*, 135–151.

Ford, M. T., Jebb, A. T., Tay, L., & Diener, E. (2018). Internet searches for affect-related terms: An indicator of subjective well-being and predictor of health outcomes across US states and metro areas. *Applied Psychology: Health and Well-Being, 10*(1), 3–29.

Gelman, A., & Hill, J. (2007). *Data analysis using regression and multilevel/hierarchical models.* Cambridge: Cambridge University Press.

Harrell Jr, F. E. (2015). *Regression modeling strategies: With applications to linear models, logistic and ordinal regression, and survival analysis.* New York: Springer.

Inglehart, R., Foa, R., Peterson, C., & Welzel, C. (2008). Development, freedom, and rising happiness: A global perspective (1981-2007). *Perspectives on Psychological Science, 3*, 264–285.

Izard, C. E. (2010). The many meanings/aspects of emotion: Definitions, functions, activation, and regulation. *Emotion Review, 2*(4), 363–370.

Jebb, A. T., Tay, L., Diener, E., & Oishi, S. (2018). Happiness, income satiation, and turning points around the world. *Nature Human Behavior, 2*, 33–38.

Jebb, A. T., Tay, L., Ng, V., & Woo, S. (2019). Construct validation in multilevel studies. In S. E. Humphrey & J. M. LeBreton (Eds.), *The handbook of multilevel theory, measurement, and analysis* (pp. 253–278). American Psychological Association. https://doi.org/10.1037/0000115-012

Kahneman, D. (1999). Objective happiness. In D. Kahneman, E. Diener, & N. Schwarz (Eds.), *Well-being: The foundations of hedonic psychology* (pp. 3–25). New York: Russell Sage Foundation.

Kahneman, D., & Tversky, A. (1979). Prospect theory: An analysis of decision under risk. *Econometrica*, 47, 263–291.

Kim, G., Wang, S. Y., & Sellbom, M. (2020). Measurement Equivalence of the Subjective Well-Being Scale Among Racially/Ethnically Diverse Older Adults. *The Journals of Gerontology: Series B*, 75(5), 1010–1017.

López Ulloa, B. F., Møller, V., & Sousa-Poza, A. (2013). How does subjective well-being evolve with age? A literature review. *Journal of Population Ageing*, 6(3), 227–246.

Luttmer, E. F. P. (2005). Neighbors as negatives: Relative earnings and well-being. *The Quarterly Journal of Economics*, 120, 963–1002.

McMahon, D. M. (2006). *Happiness: A history*. New York: Grove.

Morrison, M., Tay, L., & Diener, E. (2011). Subjective well-being and national satisfaction. *Psychological Science*, 22, 166–171.

Motulsky, H. J., & Ransnas, L. A. (1987). Fitting curves to data using nonlinear regression: A practical and nonmathematical review. *FASEB Journal*, 1, 365–374.

Oishi, S., & Diener, E. (2001). Re-examining the general positivity model of subjective well-being: The discrepancy between specific and global domain satisfaction. *Journal of Personality*, 69, 641–666.

Ovaska, T., & Takashima, R. (2014). Does a rising tide lift all the boats? Explaining the national inequality of happiness. *Journal of Economic Issues*, 44(1), 205–224.

Robert, C., Lee, W. C., & Chan, K.-Y. (2006). An empirical analysis of measurement equivalence with the INDCOL measure of individualism and collectivism: Implications for valid cross-cultural inference. *Personnel Psychology*, 59, 65–99.

Ryff, C. D., & Keyes, C. L. M. (1995). The structure of psychological well-being revisited. *Journal of Personality and Social Psychology*, 69, 719–727.

Schwartz, H. A., Eichstaedt, J. C., Kern, M. L., Dziurzynski, L. A., Lucas, R. E., Agrawal, M., . . . Ungar, L. H. (2013). *Characterizing geographic variation in well-being using tweets*. Paper presented at the Proceedings of the Seventh International AAAI Conference on Weblogs and Social Media (ICWSM), Boston, MA.

Schwarz, N. (1999). Self-reports: How the questions shape the answer. *American Psychologist*, 54, 93–105.

Schwarz, N., & Strack, F. (1999). Reports of subjective well-being: Judgmental processes and their methodological implications. In D. Kahneman, E. Diener, & N. Schwarz (Eds.), *Well-being: The foundations of hedonic psychology* (pp. 61–84). New York: Russell Sage Foundation.

Seligman, M. E. P., & Csikszentmihalyi, M. (2000). Positive psychology: An introduction. *American Psychologist*, 55, 5–14.

Shmueli, G. (2010). To explain or predict? *Statistical Science*, 25, 289–310.

Snijders, T., & Bosker, R. (1999). *Multilevel analysis: An introduction to basic and advanced multilevel modeling*. Thousand Oaks, CA: Sage.

Su, R., Tay, L., & Diener, E. (2014). The development and validation of the Comprehensive Inventory of Thriving (T) and the Brief Inventory of Thriving (BIT). *Applied Psychology: Health and Well-Being*, 6, 251–279.

Tay, L., Chan, D., & Diener, E. (2014). The metrics of societal happiness. *Social Indicators Research*, 117, 577–600.

Tay, L., & Diener, E. (2011). Needs and subjective well-being. *Journal of Personality and Social Psychology*, 101, 354–365.

Tay, L., & Jebb, A. T. (2018). Establishing construct continua in construct validation: The process of continuum specification. *Advances in Methods and Practices in Psychological Science*, 1(3), 375–388.

Tay, L., & Kuykendall, L. (2013). Promoting happiness: The malleability of individual and societal-level happiness. *International Journal of Psychology*, 159–176.

Tay, L., Meade, A. W., & Cao, M. (2015). An overview and practical guide to IRT measurement equivalence analysis. *Organizational Research Methods*, 18, 3–46.

Tay, L., Woo, S. E., & Vermunt, J. K. (2014). A conceptual and methodological framework for psychometric isomorphism: Validation of multilevel construct measures. *Organizational Research Methods*, 17, 77–106.

Vaish, A., Grossmann, T., & Woodward, A. (2008). Not all emotions are created equal: The negativity bias in social-emotional development. *Psychological Bulletin*, 134(3), 383–403.

Vandenberg, R. J., & Lance, C. E. (2000). A review and synthesis of the measurement invariance literature: Suggestions, practices, and recommendations for organizational research. *Organizational Research Methods*, 3, 4–70.

Veenhoven, R. (1990). Inequality in happiness: Inequality in countries compared across countries. https://mpra.ub.unimuenchen.de/11275/1/MPRA_paper_11275.pdf

Wiese, C. W., Chen, Z. J., Tay, L., Friedman, E. M., & Rector, J. L. (2018). The role of affect on physical health over time: A cross-lagged panel analysis over 20 years. *Applied Psychology: Health and Well-Being*, 11, 202–222.

Wiese, C. W., Tay, L., Su, R., & Diener, E. (2018). Measuring thriving across nations: Examining the measurement equivalence of the Comprehensive Inventory of Thriving (CIT) and the Brief Inventory of Thriving (BIT). *Applied Psychology: Health and Well-Being*, 10(1), 127–148.

4

Eudaimonic and Hedonic Well-Being

An Integrative Perspective with Linkages to Sociodemographic Factors and Health

Carol D. Ryff, Jennifer Morozink Boylan, and Julie A. Kirsch

Abstract

This chapter provides an overview of two prominent approaches to well-being, the hedonic and the eudaimonic, both with roots traceable to the ancient Greeks. We first examine the distant history of each approach and then describe scientific endeavors seeking to translate the ideas to empirical assessment tools. We then review how these two varieties of well-being are distributed in the general population by attending to their associations with major demographic factors (age, socioeconomic status, gender, race) as well as the interplay (intersectionality) of such factors. Such information contextualizes what is known about who reports they are or are not experiencing various aspects of well-being. The third section then examines how hedonic and eudaimonic well-being are linked with multiple indicators of health (self-reported, morbidity, mortality, biological systems). Although extensive research exists, there is a paucity of studies that have jointly examined both types of well-being. The fourth section draws attention to changing historical conditions and what that means for the future study of well-being and health.

Two prominent varieties of well-being, namely hedonic and eudaimonic well-being, are the focus of this chapter. Because extensive research over multiple decades has grown up around these two approaches, the objective is to distill what has been learned from prior studies in hopes of building a cumulative science of well-being. We begin by reviewing the conceptual meanings and philosophical origins of hedonia and eudaimonia, followed

Carol D. Ryff, Jennifer Morozink Boylan, and Julie A. Kirsch, *Eudaimonic and Hedonic Well-Being* In: *Measuring Well-Being*. Edited by: Matthew T. Lee, Laura D. Kubzansky, and Tyler J. VanderWeele, Oxford University Press (2021).
DOI: 10.1093/oso/9780197512531.003.0005

by consideration of how the ideas were translated to scientific tools needed to assess the two broad approaches to well-being. Not included in our coverage are more recent perspectives on well-being (e.g., Goodman, Disabato, Kashdan et al., 2017; Su, Tay, & Diener, 2014; VanderWeele, 2017), given that limited research has been assembled on these relative to hedonic and eudaimonic approaches.

Following definitional beginnings, the second section summarizes evidence on how hedonic and eudaimonic well-being are distributed in the general population. Specifically, we examine how they are associated with key sociodemographic variables (age, socioeconomic status [SES], gender, race). Although frequently included in analytic models as covariates, these mostly assigned variables warrant careful consideration in their own right because they afford critical windows into life contexts. That is, they situate human lives within broader social structural realities that are critical for understanding experiences of well-being. We also draw attention to the interplay (intersectionality) of these defining attributes and call for further work of this nature in future studies. Again, we note that our look at correlates of hedonic and eudaimonic well-being is not exhaustive. For example, we do not include personality or relational correlates (e.g., Marks & Lambert, 1998; Pavot, Diener, & Fujita, 1990; Schmutte & Ryff, 1997), nor do we consider how religiosity and spirituality matter for well-being and health (e.g., Greenfield, Vaillant, & Marks, 2009; Koenig, King, & Carson, 2012), even though several chapters in this volume (Chapters 10, 11, and 16, all in this volume) address religion and spirituality.

Maintaining a selective focus on hedonic and eudaimonic well-being, the third section then examines how they are linked with multiple indicators of health. Our coverage includes self-reported health, morbidity, mortality, and biological systems. Although only limited studies have included measures of both types of well-being, those that have underscore the independent effects of each. Tracking these associations longitudinally, as is done in the chapter by Trudel-Fitzgerald, Kubzansky, and VanderWeele (Chapter 5, in this volume) linking well-being to mortality, is a key future direction.

Because economic, social, and political change has been prominent in recent times, a fourth section then calls for greater attention to historical dynamics in future research on well-being. We consider how heightened job, financial, and housing hardships, which unfolded during the Great Recession, matter for people's subjective views about their lives and for their health. Building on evidence of increased experiences of despair, particularly among disadvantaged segments of society, we call for future inquiries that address growing problems of inequality.

What Is Psychological Well-Being?

There are multiple ways to conceptualize and measure what it is to be well. Interestingly, the definitional challenges have distant philosophical roots. The ancient Greeks, for example, were interested in fundamental questions about how to live—effectively, what constitutes a good life. Aristippus (435–356 BCE) taught that the goal of life is to experience the maximum amount of pleasure and that happiness consists of the totality of one's hedonic moments (Laertius, 1925). He took pride in extracting enjoyment from many circumstances and, relatedly, in controlling both adversity and prosperity. Epicurus (341–270 BCE), in turn, founded the school of philosophy known as epicureanism, which sought to attain a happy, tranquil life, one characterized by peace and freedom from fear and pain. Living a self-sufficient life surrounded by friends was also part of his view (Barnes, 1986). In notable contrast, Aristotle's (384–322 BCE) *Nichomachean Ethics,* written in 350 BCE, stated that the highest of all human goods achievable by human action was "eudaimonia," which he defined as activity of the soul in accord with virtue. The highest virtue for Aristotle was thus a kind of personal excellence; that is, achieving the best that is within us.

These contrasting conceptions of well-lived lives continue to have resonance in our own era. Ryan and Deci's (2001) integrative review of the field of well-being, in fact, organized it in terms of two broad traditions: one dealing with happiness (hedonic well-being) and the other dealing with human potential (eudaimonic well-being). Both formulations have been fundamental in current efforts to understand the nature of human well-being (Huta & Waterman, 2014; Vitterso, 2013; Waterman, 1993). Although other psychological characteristics (e.g., optimism, sense of control, conscientiousness) constitute valued aspects of positive functioning, as noted in our introduction, coverage in this chapter is restricted to hedonic and eudaimonic well-being.

The Hedonic Approach

Kahneman, Diener, and Schwarz (1999) defined hedonic psychology as the study of what makes experiences in life pleasant and unpleasant, thus aligning themselves with certain conceptions from the ancient Greeks. Nonetheless, it is important to underscore that multiple additional terms (and related assessment items)—subjective well-being, life satisfaction, happiness, positive and negative affect—are exemplars of the hedonic approach. In addition, it is useful to recognize that many "indicators" in this arena had little, if any, conceptual or philosophical foundation. For example, in the middle of the past century, interest in subjective well-being emerged not in an effort to illuminate meanings of hedonic psychology, but rather in pursuit of ideas about quality of life that could serve as a window on social change (Land, 1975). The argument at the time (Andrews & Withey, 1976; Campbell, Converse, & Rodgers (1976) was that even though people live in objectively defined environments (e.g., income), it is their *subjective experience* that offers uniquely relevant information on quality of life.

Others from that era (Bradburn, 1969; Cantril, 1965; Gurin, Veroff, & Feld, 1960) considered life satisfaction and happiness to be key components of well-being. According to Bradburn (1969), happiness results from a balance between positive and negative affect. This distinction between pleasant and unpleasant aspects of personal experience continued to be fundamental in subsequent conceptions of hedonic well-being (Diener, Smith, & Fujita, 1995), along with life satisfaction, which came to be seen as the more evaluative and judgmental assessment of one's life. While the social indicators movement was unfolding, the early field of social gerontology also gave prominence to life satisfaction (Neugarten, Havighurst, & Tobin, 1961). A 30-year review (Larson, 1978) designated life satisfaction as the most frequently studied variable in gerontological studies.

Decades later, the threefold structure of life satisfaction, positive affect, and negative affect remains core in defining what constitutes subjective well-being (Lucas, Diener, & Suh, 1996). These three components thus comprise the contemporary formulation of hedonia (Ryan & Deci, 2001) (see Box 4.1 for illustrative definitions and items). For present purposes, it is important to emphasize that these operational definitions of hedonic well-being were not grounded in a priori theory about what constitutes positive functioning. Rather, they exemplified relatively straightforward and useful questions intended to probe people's evaluations of their well-being, such as the degree to which they were satisfied with life as a whole or with specific domains of life, such as work, health, or family relationships. Similarly, questions about positive and negative affect used differing temporal frames (now, last week, past year)

Box 4.1 Components of Hedonic Well-Being

Life Satisfaction

Typically assessed by a rating of overall satisfaction with life, sometimes accompanied by domain-specific assessments (e.g., satisfaction with work, health, partner relationship, relationship with children).[a,b] Viewed as a more enduring, long-term aspect of well-being.

Sample item: "From 0 (worst possible) to 10 (best possible), how would you rate your life overall?"

Positive Affect

Typically assessed with frequency ratings (how often in the past week, month, year) one felt cheerful, in good spirits, extremely happy, calm and peaceful, full of life).[c]

Sample item: "During the past 30 days, how much of the time did you feel cheerful?"

Negative Affect

Typically assessed with frequency ratings (how often in the past week, month, year) one felt hopeless, so sad nothing could cheer you up, nervous, restless or fidgety, that everything was an effort, worthless.[c]

Sample item: "During the past year, how much of the time did you feel hopeless?"

[a] Sources of above positive and negative affect items are detailed in Mroczek & Kolarz (1998).

[b] Another source of high-arousal positive affect (enthusiastic, attentive, proud, active) and negative affect (afraid, jittery, irritable, ashamed, upset) items is the PANAS scale (Watson, Clark, & Tellegen, 1988).

[c] Response options: 1 (all of the time), 2 (most of the time), 3 (some of the time), 4 (a little of the time), 5 (none of the time).

to inquire about the frequency with which respondents experienced an array of positive or negative emotions.

Extensive research has grown up around these aspects of hedonic well-being, such as how they change with age (Charles, Reynolds, & Gatz, 2001; Diener & Suh, 1997; Mroczek & Kolarz, 1998; Shmotkin, 1990), how they vary across cultures (Suh, Diener, Oishi, & Triandis, 1998), and are linked with heredity (Lykken & Tellegen, 1996), personality (McCrae & Costa, 1994), living conditions (Veenhoven, 1991), or differential life opportunities (Graham,

2017). More recently, as distilled in a subsequent section, investigators have probed links between components of the hedonic well-being and health.

The Eudaimonic Approach

Whereas the hedonic tradition in contemporary science had little conceptual or theoretical foundation, the eudaimonic tradition emerged from numerous formulations in clinical, developmental, existential, and humanistic psychology, along with Aristotle's distant writings. For example, lifespan theorists such as Erikson (1959) and Neugarten (1973a) elaborated how people negotiate the tasks and challenges of different life periods, including whether they do so successfully or unsuccessfully. Other psychologists sought to articulate the full growth and development of the individual, formulated in terms of self-actualization (Maslow, 1968), the fully functioning person (Rogers, 1961), maturity (Allport, 1961), and individuation (Jung, 1933). Frankl's (1959) classic, *Man's Search for Meaning*, offered further insight into the importance of finding purpose in significant life challenge. Drawing on these views, Jahoda (1958) distilled criteria of positive mental health that were fundamentally positive in nature, in contrast to the absence of illness (e.g., depression, anxiety) definitions found in most mental health research and practice at the time.

Reviewing the preceding literature, Ryff (1989; Ryff & Keyes, 1995) proposed a multidimensional model of eudaimonic well-being built on points of convergence in the varying perspectives (for a philosophical engagement with this model, see Chapter 9, by Baril; for a theological perspective, see Chapter 10, by Messer, both in this volume). Six key dimensions emerged from this integration, which is fundamentally about well-being as challenged thriving. Each dimension of psychological well-being thus articulates different challenges that individuals encounter as they strive to function positively. People attempt to feel good about themselves even while being aware of their own limitations (*self-acceptance*). They also seek to develop and maintain warm and trusting interpersonal relationships (*positive relations with others*) and to shape their surrounding environments to meet personal needs and desires (*environmental mastery*). In sustaining their individuality in diverse social contexts, they also seek a sense self-determination and personal authority (*autonomy*). A vital endeavor is to find meaning in their endeavors and challenges (*purpose in life*). Last, making the most of personal talents and capacities (*personal growth*) is central to this model of well-being and comes closest to Aristotle's conception of personal excellence as realization of one's unique talents and capacities.

Detailed definitions of the six constructs are found in Box 4.2. Importantly, these definitions served as the basis for writing self-descriptive items to operationalize each dimension. Thus, drawing on the descriptions of high and low scorers for each dimension (derived from the underlying theoretical formulations), self-report items were generated. The decision to operationalize both what it means to have or not have (high scorer vs. low scorer) added conceptual and empirical rigor to the measures, such that receiving a high score on any of the six dimensions requires respondents to strongly agree with positively worded items as well as strongly disagree with negatively worded items. Further analyses evaluated and refined the item pools (see Ryff, 1989). For example, to be retained, all items had to correlate more highly with their own scale than with another scale. Confirmatory factor analyses were also conducted to examine the multidimensional structure of the model. Findings supported the intended six-factor model (Ryff & Keyes, 1995). Detailed summaries of this theory-guided approach to eudaimonic well-being and the findings that have grown up around it are available elsewhere (e.g., Ryff, 2014, 2018; Ryff & Singer, 2008).

Given emphasis on both hedonic and eudaimonic well-being herein, a key empirical finding from the baseline assessments in the Midlife in the United States (MIDUS) national sample of US adults was that eudaimonic and hedonic well-being (operationalized as previously described) were found to be *related but distinct* aspects of what it means to be psychologically well (Keyes, Shmotkin, & Ryff, 2002). That is, the indicators were positively intercorrelated with each other, as would be expected given that all assess aspects of positive psychological functioning, but the best fitting model was one that maintained the distinction between eudaimonic and hedonic well-being. This first empirical assessment of both approaches also showed differing varieties of how the hedonia and eudaimonia come together in individual lives. Although many participants had jointly low (or high) profiles on both indicators, others showed notably higher hedonic than eudaimonic well-being, or the reverse, notably higher eudaimonia than hedonia. In addition, this initial study documented differing sociodemographic and personality correlates for the various combinations of well-being.

Box 4.2 Definitions of Theory-Guided Dimensions of Eudaimonic Well-Being

Autonomy

High scorer: Is self-determining and independent; able to resist social pressures to think and act in certain ways; regulates social pressures to think and act in certain ways; regulates behavior from within; evaluates self by personal standards.[a]

Sample item: "I have confidence in my own opinions, even if they are different from the way most other people think."

Low scorer: Is concerned about the expectations and evaluations of others; relies on judgments of others to make important decisions; conforms to social pressures to think and act in certain ways.

Sample item: "I tend to be influenced by people with strong opinions."

Environmental Mastery

High scorer: Has a sense of mastery and competence in managing the environment; controls complex array of external activities; makes effective use of surrounding opportunities; able to choose or create contexts suitable to personal needs and values.

Sample item: "I am quite good at managing the many responsibilities of my daily life."

Low scorer: Has difficulty managing everyday affairs; feels unable to change or improve surrounding context; is unaware of surrounding opportunities; lacks sense of control over external world.

Sample item: "The demands of everyday life often get me down."

Personal Growth

High scorer: Has a feeling of continued development; sees self as growing and expanding; is open to new experiences; has sense of realizing his or her potential; sees improvement in self and behavior over time; is changing in ways that reflect more self-knowledge and effectiveness.

Sample item: "For me, life has been a continuous process of learning, changing, and growth."

Low scorer: Has a sense of personal stagnation; lacks sense of improvement or expansion over time; feels bored and uninterested with life; feels unable to develop new attitudes or behaviors.

Sample item: "When I think about it, I haven't really improved much over the years."

Positive Relations with Others

High scorer: Has warm, satisfying, trusting relationships with others; is concerned about the welfare of other others; capable of strong empathy, affection, and intimacy; understands give and take of human relationships.

Sample item: "I enjoy personal and mutual conversations with family and friends."

Low scorer: Has few close, trusting relationships with others; finds it difficult to be warm, open, and concerned about others; is isolated and frustrated in interpersonal relationships; not willing to make compromises to sustain important ties with others.

Sample item: "I have not experienced many warm and trusting relationships with others."

Purpose in Life

High scorer: Has goals in life and a sense of directedness; feels there is meaning to present and past life; holds beliefs that give life purpose; has aims and objectives for living.

Sample item: "I have a sense of direction and purpose in life."

Low scorer: Lacks a sense of meaning in life; has few goals or aims; lacks sense of direction; does not see purpose of past life; has no outlook or beliefs that give life meaning.

Sample item: "I don't have a good sense of what it is I'm trying to accomplish in life."

Self-Acceptance

High scorer: Possesses a positive attitude toward the self; acknowledges and accepts multiple aspects of self, including good and bad qualities; feels positive about past life.

Sample item: "When I look at the story of my life, I'm pleased with how things have turned out."

Low scorer: Feels dissatisfied with self; is disappointed with what has occurred in past life; is troubled about certain personal qualities; wishes to be different from what he or she is.

Sample item: "My attitude about myself is probably not as positive as most people feel about themselves."

[a] Response options for all above items: 1 (*strongly disagree*) to 7 (*strongly agree*).

Sociodemographic Correlates of Hedonic and Eudaimonic Well-Being

Dimensions of hedonic and eudaimonic well-being are meaningfully contoured by sociodemographic factors; that is, age, SES, gender, and race/ethnicity play important roles in predicting *who* is happy and living a meaningful life. Summarized here are distilled findings for hedonic and eudaimonic well-being, organized separately by age, SES, gender, and race. We attend to the current state of the science of well-being and these four sociodemographic factors by examining cross-sectional and longitudinal findings drawn from nationally representative samples of adults. Notably, a large body of literature on sociodemographic factors and well-being is limited to cross-sectional data. More comprehensive longitudinal studies are emerging in the field (see Bastarache et al., 2019).

Although other social identities are important for well-being (e.g., sexual identity, culture), this summary is restricted to the aforementioned categories, which encompass a sizable literature for both hedonic and eudaimonic well-being. The section concludes with recommendations for future research on the intersectionality of sociodemographic characteristics and how they jointly contour hedonic and eudaimonic well-being profiles.

Hedonic Well-Being

Age. Movement from specific life stages (e.g., adolescence to young adulthood; midlife to old age) presents new challenges that impact well-being (Neugarten, 1973b; Ryff, 1989). For hedonic well-being, studies have shown that as individuals grow older they tend to prioritize positive emotions over negative emotions, a phenomenon referred to as the *positivity effect* (Carstensen & Mikels, 2005; Stone, Schwartz, Broderick, & Deaton, 2010). The relationship between age and positive affect may, however, be nonlinear. In a national sample of adults (aged 25–74), the cross-sectional association between age and positive affect strengthened with each 1-year increase in age (Mroczek & Kolarz, 1998). The positivity effect may also level off in older adulthood. In a cross-sectional study of a select sample of younger to older aged cohorts, middle-aged adults (mean age = 49.9) experienced greater positive affect than younger adults (mean age = 19.5), but older adults (mean age = 75.0) did not significantly differ from middle-aged adults (Ryff, 1989).

Furthermore, longitudinal studies restricted to adults older than 70 found that positive affect *declined* (see Smith, Fleeson, Geiselmann et al., 1999).

Cross-sectional studies have shown that life satisfaction follows a U-shaped pattern by age wherein satisfaction tends to reach its lowest point at midlife between the ages of 30 and 60 and then peaks in older adulthood (Blanchflower & Oswald, 2008). The midlife dip in life satisfaction is posited to result from multiple role demands and life stressors, including raising adolescents while providing care for elderly parents (Aldwin & Levenson, 2001; Almeida & Horn, 2004). Alternatively, researchers have posited that the dip in life satisfaction may reflect cohort or period effects, rather than age effects.

Longitudinal findings from the MIDUS study documented that midlife adults (aged 40–59) were similarly satisfied with life as younger adults (aged 24–39) and showed increments in life satisfaction over a 10-year span. Older adults (aged 60–75) did not show significant increments in life satisfaction (Lachman, Teshale, & Agrigoroaei, 2015). In the English Longitudinal Study of Aging, which measures well-being and health every 2 years, adults aged 50 and older initially reported declines in life satisfaction over time, but in later waves the trend reversed and life satisfaction increased over time (Shankar, Rafnsson, & Steptoe, 2015). In a comprehensive analysis of 11 population-based longitudinal studies, positive affect was best characterized by an inverted U trajectory across the lifespan, peaking at about the mid to late 50s and then declining. Relatedly, negative affect was best characterized by a U-shaped curve over the lifespan, with levels starting higher in younger adulthood, declining until the late 60s, and then increasing afterward (Bastarache et al., 2019). In summary, increments in age are associated with increments in both positive affect and life satisfaction, at least until older adulthood. More longitudinal studies spanning diverse age cohorts are needed to disentangle the effects of age from period and/or cohort effects.

Socioeconomic Status. SES represents position in the social hierarchy and, relatedly, access to material goods and resources. SES is theorized to influence individual factors, including well-being. The relationship between SES and hedonic well-being has been extensively studied in multinational, cross-sectional studies. In many countries, life satisfaction, compared to positive affect, is consistently linked with higher income (see Diener, Oishi, & Tay, 2018). Higher education is also associated with higher levels of life satisfaction (Fernández-Ballesteros, Zamarrón, & Ruíz, 2001). Boehm, Chen,

Williams, Ryff, and Kubzansky (2015) examined cross-sectional associations between education and income gradients in life satisfaction and positive affect in the MIDUS study. Satisfied individuals tended to be more highly educated and had higher incomes. Positive affect, however, was not associated with income or education. Ethnographic research also revealed that those who lack socioeconomic advantage are able to maintain high levels of positive affect (Markus, Ryff, Curhan, & Palmersheim, 2004) and high levels in specific domains of life satisfaction (Biswas-Diener, & Diener, 2001). As noted earlier, most findings on the relationship between SES and hedonic well-being are from cross-sectional data, thus requiring more longitudinal research to determine the directionality and lasting influences of SES on hedonic well-being.

Gender. The large literature on gender differences in hedonic well-being is complex and lacks a coherent conclusion. Focusing on large-scale nationally representative studies and meta-analyses, gender differences are more consistently found for life satisfaction than for positive affect, but the direction of the difference varies (Batz & Tay, 2018). Studies of younger to older age cohorts found that women reported *higher* life satisfaction than men (Blanchflower & Oswald, 2004; Inglehart, 2002; Tay, Ng, Kuykendall, & Diener, 2014). However, in cross-sectional studies restricted to adults aged 55 and older, women reported *lower* levels of life satisfaction than men (Pinquart & Sorensen, 2001). A meta-analysis of 281 multinational studies documented that women reported significantly lower levels of life satisfaction than men (Batz-Barbarich, Tay, Kuykendall, & Cheung, 2018). Zuckerman, Li, and Diener (2017) examined gender differences in a multi-item scale of positive and negative affect from the Gallup World Poll. Although gender differences were not evident for positive affect, women reported significantly higher levels of negative affect than men.

In summary, gender differences for hedonic well-being are varied and likely depend on additional individual and social factors. Other studies show that controlling for other demographic factors besides gender (e.g., age, SES, or marital status) reduces the gender difference in hedonic well-being to nonsignificance (Shmotkin, 1990; White, 1992). Most of the preceding findings are cross-sectional or time-series data (repeated, but different samples). More longitudinal studies of within-person change are needed.

Race. Racial and ethnic inequality is a major social issue in the United States. Black–White divisions in income and wealth remain entrenched and are widening (Shapiro, Meschede, & Osoro, 2013). Furthermore, minority groups experience structural and interpersonal racism. Minority racial status is thus a social identity and sociodemographic characteristic usually conceptualized as a risk factor for mental and physical health problems (Link & Phelan, 2002). Black–White disparities in hedonic well-being have been widely documented. Drawing on 1972–1985 time-series data from the General Social Survey (GSS), Thomas and Hughes (1986) showed that Black adults were less satisfied and less happy than White adults. The findings have been replicated with more recent time-series data from the GSS and other national studies in the United States (Beatty & Tuch, 1997; Coverdill, Lopez, & Petrie, 2011; Hughes & Thomas, 1998; Iceland & Ludwig-Dehm, 2019; Yang, 2008). Even though there is some evidence that the Black–White racial gap in happiness and life satisfaction has narrowed over time (e.g., Blanchflower & Oswald, 2004; Coverdill et al., 2011), the difference still remains large according to recent analyses of GSS data (Iceland & Ludwig-Dehm, 2019).

Socioeconomic inequality is theorized to account for racial disparities in well-being (Link & Phelan, 2002). However, disparities in hedonic well-being persist even when controlling for other sociodemographic factors, such as education, income, and marital status (Barger, Donoho, & Wayment, 2009; Hughes & Thomas, 1998). Beatty and Tuch (1997) examined Black–White differences in domain-specific life satisfaction among those holding similar middle-class occupations. Middle-class Black adults expressed lower levels of life satisfaction across multiple domains (e.g., residence, family, friends, health) compared to middle-class White adults. Furthermore, controlling for education, area of residence, and social participation did not explain racial differences in domain-specific life satisfaction. However, after adjusting for discrimination, Black adults reported higher positive affect and life satisfaction than White adults (Keyes, 2009). In summary, these findings underscore that, despite improvements in civil rights for Black adults, effects of social disadvantage linger and negatively impact hedonic well-being. That said, racial disparities in hedonic well-being do not always translate to other domains of mental health: Black adults are *not* more likely than White adults to have psychiatric disorders, and in some studies Black adults have lower rates than White adults on indicators of depression, affective disorders, and substance use disorders (Keyes, 2009; Williams & Harris-Reid, 1999). These findings offer further support that indicators of ill-being are distinct from indicators of well-being.

Eudaimonic Well-Being

Age. Supporting the idea that eudaimonic well-being is multidimensional in nature, different facets of eudaimonic well-being show varying associations with age. With cross-sectional data, Ryff and Keyes (1995) found that age was positively associated with environmental mastery and autonomy but unassociated with self-acceptance, and inconsistently associated with positive relations. The most reliable evidence of age-related change pertains to purpose in life and personal growth. Cross-sectional and longitudinal studies from MIDUS and the Wisconsin Longitudinal Study (WLS) have found that among adults aged 25–75, increasing age predicts declines in purpose in life and personal growth (Ryff & Keyes, 1995; Springer, Pudrovska, & Hauser, 2011). Declines may reflect the "structural lag" problem, which posits that social institutions are not keeping up with the added years of life that many older adults now experience (Riley, Kahn, Foner, & Mack, 1994). As social roles diminish with age, fewer opportunities may be available for older individuals to contribute to society, thus limiting opportunities for personal growth and purposeful engagement. Nonetheless, there is notable variability in purpose in life and personal growth among older adults, with some showing considerably higher scores than their same-aged peers. Subsequent sections examine the import of such variability for health.

Socioeconomic Status. Eudaimonic well-being is patterned by indicators of SES (education, income, occupation; Marmot et al., 1998; Marmot, Ryff, Bumpass, Shipley, & Marks, 1997), with most analyses focused on education. All six dimensions of eudaimonic well-being were positively associated with education (Ryff, 2016; Ryff et al., 2015). Other work showed education to be positively associated with most aspects of eudaimonic well-being, except positive relations with others and autonomy (Curhan et al., 2014). Similar to age, the two dimensions most strongly correlated with education were personal growth and purpose in life. Findings for educational differences in eudaimonic well-being have been based primarily on cross-sectional data, thus longitudinal work is needed to tease apart the directional nature of the relationship between eudaimonia and education. Additionally, as with age, there is notable heterogeneity within SES strata (see Markus et al., 2004; Ryff, 2016), suggesting that social structural constraints on well-being are not uniform.

Gender. In contrast to hedonic well-being, studies on gender differences in eudaimonic well-being are more limited even though gender is a common covariate in eudaimonic studies. In the 1992–1993 WLS survey wave (age ~50), the largest gender differences were found for positive relations with others and personal growth, with higher values for women compared to men (Marks, 1996). These findings were evident in another small-scale study (Ryff & Heidrich, 1997), but other dimensions of well-being did not show consistent gender differences (Ryff, 1995). In contrast, using a composite measure of eudaimonic well-being, Bookwala and Boyar (2008) found that women reported significantly lower values than men, although the effect size was small. Longitudinal findings focusing on gender and eudaimonic well-being are lacking.

   Race. Studies on racial differences in eudaimonic well-being contrast with findings for hedonic well-being, showing that Black adults are lower on hedonic well-being than White adults. For eudaimonic well-being, however, Black adults reported higher levels of eudaimonic well-being across every dimension (Ryff, Keyes, & Hughes, 2003). Furthermore, experiences of discrimination suppressed the minority group advantage in eudaimonic well-being (Keyes, 2009). Selection bias was viewed as an unlikely explanation for higher eudaimonic well-being among Black compared to White adults. The minority group advantage in eudaimonic well-being may suggest that experiences of social disadvantage contribute to the building of psychological strengths, such as purpose in life and personal growth. Positive group identification (Branscombe, Schmitt, & Harvey, 1999) and religious attendance (Ellison, 1995) have been proposed as plausible pathways to promote resilience and flourishing in the face of adversity. Positive group identification may help some cope with racism and instill self-acceptance and a sense of meaning and commitment to fulfill life goals. Religious practices are prominent in the Black community (Taylor, Chatters, Jayakody, & Levin, 1996) and may be one such way that positive group identification is nurtured.

Intersectionality of Sociodemographic Correlates of Well-Being

It is increasingly evident that multiple social categories intersect with each other to shape human behavior, health, and well-being (Cole, 2009). Kimberlé Crenshaw, a legal scholar and critical race theorist, formulated the term "intersectionality" to draw attention to the meaning and consequences of multiple social group identities. For example, Black women may experience additive or multiplicative discrimination as a result of being both a person of color and a woman, or they could experience a unique form of discrimination specific to their identity as a Black woman (Crenshaw, 1991).

The unique experiences resulting from multiple intersecting social identities may have different consequences for hedonic and eudaimonic well-being. Ryff et al. (2003) studied intersections of race and gender and their relationship with eudaimonic well-being in the baseline MIDUS sample. Minority group status was positively associated with multiple dimensions of eudaimonic well-being, but more so for African American men than for African American women. In a study focused on autonomy in the work place, Black females reported the least autonomy compared to their Black male and White female counterparts, whereas White men reported the most autonomy (Petrie & Roman, 2004). Jackson and Williams (2006) illustrated the intersections among race, gender, and SES in relation to mental and physical health. High suicide rates among higher SES Black men relative to their White counterparts were attributed to increased exposure to discriminatory stressors in the workplace and lack of advancement in occupational status despite high educational achievement. In contrast, recent Gallup data showed that, among the SES disadvantaged, Blacks reported higher life satisfaction than Whites (Graham, 2017). In summary, the intersecting forces of race, gender, and SES draw attention to the different ways in which multiple group identities shape individual well-being outcomes. Future work needs to examine how specific dimensions of hedonic and eudaimonic well-being are differentially impacted by multiple social identities.

Race, gender, and SES differences in well-being may also vary by age. According to cumulative inequality theory, health and well-being inequalities are hypothesized to widen with age (Ferraro & Shippee, 2009). Whites, men, and higher SES individuals, compared to racial minorities, women, and lower SES persons, respectively, have greater access to social capital and financial resources. These resources likely cumulate over time and thereby play a role in maintaining or promoting well-being through old age. More advantaged individuals may be more likely to show the positivity effect, experience age-related increases in hedonic well-being, and be less vulnerable to age-related declines in purpose in life and personal growth. As a result, SES, gender, and racial gaps in well-being may increase with age. In contrast to cumulative inequality theory, the *age-as-leveler hypothesis* predicts that the challenges of aging will produce less heterogeneity in well-being, thus reducing inequalities (Dupre, 2007; Yang, 2008).

Some evidence suggests that well-being differences by gender change with age. Two large national studies of age and gender differences in positive affect found that younger women tended to be happier than younger men, but the gender difference reversed in older age, such that older women were significantly less happy than older men (Easterlin, 2003; Inglehart, 2002). This shift resulted from women's larger declines in happiness in response to worsening health and men's larger increases in happiness post-retirement compared to women. According to happiness ratings in the GSS, White men over the age of 50 were the happiest of all age, gender, and racial groups, whereas Black women of the same age were the least happy (Yang, 2008). This research needs to be extended to other dimensions of hedonic and eudaimonic well-being and to longitudinal surveys.

Summary

The existing literature on sociodemographic correlates of well-being offers empirical support for the distinction between hedonic and eudaimonic concepts. That prior work includes both cross-sectional and longitudinal findings is valuable. The former document differences that may be attributable aging processes or variation across cohorts, both of which are informative. The latter documents cross-time dynamics, often revealing that putative antecedents and consequents are both changing in time. That is, longitudinal inquiry is not always definitive about the causal directionality of influences.

Nonetheless, these prior studies show that increasing age predicts increments in hedonic well-being but decrements in some dimensions of eudaimonic well-being, particularly purpose in life and personal growth. Other dimensions of eudaimonic well-being remain relatively stable with age, such as positive relations with others, autonomy, and self-acceptance. These findings align with prior work showing that age trajectories in well-being depend on the dimension examined and on the period of the life course considered (Lachman, Lewkowicz, Marcus, & Peng, 1994; Staudinger & Bluck, 2001).

For SES, income and education are most strongly positively associated with life satisfaction, but inconsistently associated with positive affect. Education is most strongly positively associated with purpose in life and personal growth but less robustly associated with positive relations with others and autonomy. These findings suggest that certain dimensions of hedonic and eudaimonic well-being are more sensitive to socioeconomic forces than others. Gender differences in hedonic and eudaimonic well-being are varied and are sensitive to sampling and methodological differences. Although minority group status is theorized to be detrimental to health and well-being, the literature shows that racial differences are nuanced and vary by hedonic and eudaimonic well-being. Despite the existence of a Black–White "happiness gap," Black adults evidence *higher* levels of eudaimonic well-being than do White adults. These patterns bring to light subgroup differences in vulnerability and resilience, which may depend on intersecting group identities. Future research needs to attend to the interplay between multiple sociodemographic predictors and their combined influences on well-being. The next section examines the linkages between hedonic and eudaimonic well-being and health.

Linking Well-Being to Health

A growing literature documents how hedonic and eudaimonic well-being predict health outcomes. In this section, evidence that well-being is associated with improved physical health and may offset health risks attendant to socioeconomic disadvantage is reviewed. Separately for hedonic and eudaimonic well-being, evidence first focuses on links between well-being and self-reported health, followed by evidence linking well-being to objective measures of health, including functional capacities, morbidity, mortality, and biological measures. Most studies utilize well-being as an antecedent variable, but some include well-being as a moderator of sociodemographic gradients in health. Moderation analyses capitalize on the heterogeneity in well-being within sociodemographic subgroups, as described in the previous section. The final section discusses studies that include both hedonic and eudaimonic well-being in the same analytic models. Although rarely done, these studies are necessary to discern if their psychological distinctiveness translates to differential health outcomes. We note that Trudel-Fitzgerald et al. (Chapter 5, in this volume) likewise review literature linking specific dimensions of well-being (e.g., purpose in life, life satisfaction, positive affect) to mortality, specifically focusing on longitudinal studies that adjust for sociodemographic factors, medical status, and health behaviors.

Hedonic Evidence

Self-Reported Health. Hedonic well-being has been prospectively linked to better self-rated health (Benyamini, Idler, Leventhal, & Leventhal, 2000; Segerstrom, 2014), fewer chronic conditions (Friedman & Ryff, 2012), fewer cold symptoms among volunteers exposed to the cold virus (Cohen, Doyle, Turner, Alper, & Skoner, 2003), and less pain among patients with rheumatoid arthritis and fibromyalgia (Zautra, Johnson, & Davis, 2005). In the Health and Retirement Study (HRS), a nationally representative sample of older adults, those with high life satisfaction had fewer doctor visits over a 4-year period than did those with low life satisfaction, net of covariates (Kim, Park, Sun, Smith, & Peterson, 2014). A recent systematic review and meta-analysis found that trait positive affect was associated with better sleep outcomes in healthy populations, although most studies provided relatively weak evidence or contained a high risk of bias (Ong, Kim, Young, & Steptoe, 2017).

Other evidence supports the reciprocal relationship between hedonic well-being and health such that individuals with major illnesses report lower levels of positive affect and life satisfaction than healthy controls (e.g., Çeliker & Borman, 2001; Elkins, Pollina, Scheffer, & Krupp, 1999; Knox, Svensson, Waller, & Theorell, 1988). Gana and colleagues (2016) tested competing models of whether positive affect predicted functional health or whether health predicted changes in positive affect in a longitudinal study of older adults (aged 62–101). Good functional health was associated with higher positive affect over time, but positive affect did not predict changes in health, thus highlighting the utility of examining cross-time dynamics between hedonic well-being and health status. In the UK Million Women Study, poor self-rated health prospectively predicted unhappiness, and happiness was not associated with mortality over a 10-year follow-up, net of covariates. However, happiness predicted lower mortality when self-rated health was not included as a covariate (Liu et al., 2016), suggesting that overlap between happiness and self-rated health is relevant in interpreting these findings. There are concerns regarding the potential overlap among indicators of hedonic well-being and subjective health. For example, some adjectives used to assess hedonic well-being may themselves reflect health, such as *energetic* and *vigorous* (Cohen & Pressman, 2006). Such concerns underscore the need to link hedonic well-being with objective health outcomes.

Morbidity. Positive affect, life satisfaction, and happiness prospectively predict numerous disease outcomes, including fewer clinical colds (Cohen et al., 2003), lower hospital readmission rates (Middleton & Byrd, 1996), lower body mass index (BMI) among adolescents (Saloumi & Plourde, 2010), lower risk of stroke (Ostir, Markides, Peek, & Goodwin, 2001), and lower risk of incident coronary heart disease and hypertension (Boehm, Peterson, Kivimaki, & Kubzansky, 2011; Davidson, Mostofsky, & Whang, 2010; Shirai et al., 2009; Trudel-Fitzgerald, Boehm, Kivimaki, & Kubzansky, 2014; Yanek et al., 2013). These salubrious effects remained significant after controlling for baseline disease status. As reviewed in Boehm and Kubzansky (2012) and Steptoe (2019), effect sizes are clinically significant, although not all studies have yielded significant results, and there is variability in the quality of hedonic well-being assessments. For instance, some studies utilize measures of depression to assess hedonic well-being despite widespread recognition that positive and negative affect are distinct constructs. Furthermore, the health-protective role of hedonic well-being is stronger among initially healthy adults than in patient populations (Boehm & Kubzansky, 2012).

Mortality. Positive affect and life satisfaction have widely been shown to protect against mortality risk (Boehm & Kubzansky, 2012; Chida & Steptoe, 2008; Diener & Chan, 2011; Lamers, Bolier, Westerhof, Smit, & Bohlmeijer, 2012; Pressman & Cohen, 2005; Steptoe, Dockray, & Wardle, 2009; Steptoe & Wardle, 2011, 2012; Xu & Roberts, 2010). Hedonic well-being also reduces the risk of multiple causes of death, including all-cause mortality, cardiovascular mortality, and mortality caused by renal failure or HIV (Chida & Steptoe, 2008; Pressman & Cohen, 2005). A recent meta-analysis of population-based studies found that adults reporting more happiness had lower all-cause mortality independent of confounding factors (Martín-María et al., 2017). Positive affect also predicted lower mortality among patients with ischemic heart disease, with the relationship mediated by patients' engagement in exercise (Hoogwegt et al., 2013). In extant reviews of hedonic well-being and mortality, findings were stronger in healthy compared to disease populations and in middle-aged and older adults (over the age of 55). These studies have led to growing interest in relationships between hedonic well-being and biological mechanisms of disease, as described in the next section.

Biological Health. Measures of multiple physiological systems, including the cardiovascular, neuroendocrine, immune, and metabolic systems, have been linked to hedonic well-being in cross-sectional (Bacon et al., 2004; Bhattacharyya, Whitehead, Rakhit, & Steptoe, 2008; Prather, Marsland,

Muldoon, & Manuck, 2007; Stellar et al., 2015; Steptoe, O'Donnell, Badrick, Kumari, & Marmot, 2008; Tsenkova, Love, Singer, & Ryff, 2008; Yoo, Miyamoto, Rigotti, & Ryff, 2017; Yoo, Miyamoto, & Ryff, 2016) and longitudinal studies (Boehm, Chen, Williams, Ryff, & Kubzansky, 2016; Boylan & Ryff, 2015; Matthews, Zhu, Tucker, & Whooley, 2006). Not all support better functioning, with null effects reported as well (Friedman, Hayney, Love, Singer, & Ryff, 2007; Paschalides et al., 2004; Ryff et al., 2006).

Hedonic well-being may buffer the effects of stress on biological risk. Among healthy adults, those with high trait positive affect showed faster wound healing after an acute psychological stressor, with no effects found in the no-stress condition (Robles, Brooks, & Pressman, 2009). Similarly, positive affect was associated with lower C-reactive protein (CRP), but only among individuals reporting high perceived stress (Blevins, Sagui, & Bennett, 2017). Some evidence suggests that the health-protective effects of hedonic well-being is stronger among older women (Korkeila, Kaprio, Rissanen, Koshenvuo, & Sörensen, 1998; Steptoe, Demakakos, de Oliveira, & Wardle, 2012). Finally, positive affect predicted reduced risk of diabetes among individuals with a family history of diabetes but not among those with no family history (Tsenkova, Karlamangla, & Ryff, 2016). Overall patterns indicate that positive affect, life satisfaction, happiness, and other aspects of hedonic well-being are associated with better health across many domains, including self-reported outcomes, disease incidence and severity, mortality, and biological risk factors.

Eudaimonic Evidence

Self-Reported Health. As with hedonic well-being, measures of eudaimonic well-being have been associated with subjective health in both cross-sectional and longitudinal studies (Keyes, 2005; Keyes & Grzywacz, 2005). Evidence also supports bidirectional relationships between subjective health and eudaimonic well-being (Heidrich & Ryff, 1993a, 1993b). Chang, Hong, and Charles (2018) used cross-lagged path models to show bidirectional relationships between purpose in life and self-rated health across the three waves (i.e., nearly 30 years) of MIDUS. Profiles of eudaimonic well-being in MIDUS also reveal notable stability over a 9- to 10-year period—some were persistently high in their levels of eudaimonic well-being across time, while others were persistently low. These differing profiles predicted cross-time changes in health: those with persistently high well-being showed gains in subjective health along with better profiles in chronic conditions, health symptoms, and functional health over time compared to those with persistently low well-being (Ryff et al., 2015). Healthcare utilization may be a relevant pathway through which eudaimonic well-being is related to health outcomes. For example, those with higher levels of purposeful engagement were more likely to engage in preventive health behaviors, such as cholesterol tests and cancer screenings (Kim, Strecher, & Ryff, 2014); have lower healthcare utilization and expenditures (Musich, Wang, Kraemer, Hawkins, & Wicker, 2018); and they also show better objective functional capacities (i.e., grip strength, walking speed; Kim, Kawachi, Chen, & Kubzansky, 2017).

Further evidence supports eudaimonic well-being as a protective influence on health changes associated with aging. Friedman and Ryff (2012) showed that purpose in life and positive relations with others buffered against adverse physiological consequents of later life comorbidity (multiple chronic conditions). A related study found that among older women who reported higher levels of eudaimonic well-being (all dimensions except autonomy), lower levels of disrupted sleep (a common problem of aging) were evident (Phelan, Love, Ryff, Brown, & Heidrich, 2010).

Morbidity Outcomes. Numerous studies have linked diagnosed disease or disability statuses to eudaimonic well-being, with particular attention paid to purpose in life. In the Rush Memory and Aging Project, higher purpose in life at baseline was associated with reduced incidence of Alzheimer's disease and mild cognitive impairment 7 years later (Boyle, Buchman, & Bennett, 2010) as well as lower odds of subsequent hospitalization for ambulatory care-sensitive conditions (e.g., asthma, diabetes, hypertension; Wilson et al., 2018). In the HRS, high purpose in life was linked with reduced risk of stroke (Kim, Sun, Park, & Peterson, 2013) and myocardial infarction among those with coronary heart disease (Kim, Sun, Park, Kubzansky, & Peterson, 2013). Though studies adjust for multiple covariates, disentangling the direction of effects between well-being and disease status is challenging, especially in cross-sectional research. Indicators of poor health or the presence of disease have also been associated with compromises in eudaimonic well-being (Andrew, Fisk, & Rockwood, 2012; Costanzo, Ryff, & Singer, 2009; Guidi, Rafanelli, Roncuzzi, Sirri, & Fava, 2013; Kashubeck-West & Meyer, 2008; Pusswald et al., 2012; Schleicher et al., 2005). As such, longitudinal research is needed to test possible bidirectional relationships and also model mediating pathways.

Mortality Outcomes. Two longitudinal community samples of older adults without dementia (Rush Memory and Aging Project, Minority Aging Research Study) showed that high purpose in life predicted reduced rates of mortality over 7 years (Boyle, Barnes, Buchman, & Bennett, 2009). Findings from MIDUS (Hill & Turiano, 2014) replicated and extended these prior findings by showing greater survival 14 years later among those with higher purpose in life at baseline after adjusting for numerous covariates. This work underscored that longevity benefits were not conditional on respondents' age but applied across the adult years. A meta-analysis of 10 prospective studies involving more than 136,000 participants reported significant associations between purpose in life and reduced all-cause mortality and reduced cardiovascular events (R. Cohen, Bavishi, & Rozanski, 2016). The protective effects remained significant in adjusted models. These results are notable given that older adults are at heightened risk of losing their sense of purpose in life. Studies pursuing associations between eudaimonic well-being and biology offer insights into mechanisms that may underlie theses protective effects on morbidity and mortality.

Biological Health. Initial studies examined whether eudaimonic well-being predicted reduced biological risk factors in small community samples. Those with higher well-being (particularly for personal growth, positive relations with others, and purpose in life) had better neuroendocrine regulation, better inflammatory profiles, lower cardiovascular risk factors, and better sleep profiles (Friedman et al., 2005; Hayney et al., 2003; Lindfors & Lundberg, 2002; Ryff et al., 2006; Ryff, Singer, and Love, 2004; Singer, Friedman, Seeman, Fava, & Ryff, 2005). Over the past two decades, biological assessments have been added to several national surveys that also included measures of well-being. In these studies, purpose in life has been associated with better glycemic regulation (lower HbA1c) (Boylan, Tsenkova, Miyamoto, & Ryff, 2017; Hafez et al., 2018) and lower allostatic load, a composite of biomarkers representing multisystem biological dysregulation (Zilioli, Slatcher, Ong, & Gruenewald, 2015), while personal growth was associated with lower risk of metabolic syndrome (Boylan & Ryff, 2015). Cross-time profiles of well-being were also associated with lipid profiles such that those with persistently high environmental mastery and self-acceptance had higher HDL cholesterol and lower triglycerides as compared to individuals with persistently low well-being (Radler, Rigotti, & Ryff, 2017). Not all studies have found significant associations between eudaimonic well-being and biological risk factors (see Feldman & Steptoe, 2003; Sloan et al., 2017).

Eudaimonic well-being may also moderate health effects patterned by socioeconomic disadvantage. Multiple studies have shown evidence of mitigating between SES and health, including self-rated health (Ryff et al., 2015), chronic conditions (O'Brien, 2012), inflammatory markers (Elliot & Chapman, 2016; Morozink, Friedman, Coe, & Ryff, 2010), diurnal cortisol (Zilioli, Imami, & Slatcher, 2015), HbA1c (Tsenkova, Love, Singer, & Ryff, 2007), and cardiovascular recovery following an acute stressor (Boylan, Jennings, & Matthews, 2016). The general pattern is that lower SES is more weakly associated with poor health outcomes for those with high eudaimonic well-being. Instead, lower SES individuals with high well-being show health outcomes that are more comparable to their higher SES counterparts, suggesting that well-being may counteract some risks attendant to socioeconomic disadvantage. Given that developing and maintaining high hedonic and eudaimonic well-being may be less common or more difficult in lower SES contexts, it is important to interrogate within-group variability to understand the multitude of ways in which lower SES individuals with high well-being come to exhibit better physical health.

In summary, linkages between eudaimonic well-being and health are extensive. Epidemiological studies document the protective influence of well-being (especially purpose in life) on disease outcomes as well as length of life, while other studies show that those diagnosed with disease or disability often have compromised well-being. Numerous studies show that higher well-being predicts better biological regulation measured in terms of stress hormones, inflammatory markers, and cardiovascular risk factors, although more longitudinal research is needed. Importantly, hedonic and eudaimonic well-being are rarely examined in the same study.

Studies Incorporating Both Eudaimonic and Hedonic Well-Being

Incorporating measures of both hedonic and eudaimonic well-being in the same statistical models is necessary to compare relative effect sizes and determine independence of effects as they relate to health. Despite evidence of psychometric independence between eudaimonic and hedonic well-being assessments, it is unknown whether such distinctiveness translates at the level of the brain, peripheral biology, or morbidity and mortality outcomes.

Overall, the studies that have investigated both types of well-being generally show that relationships between well-being dimensions and health are independent and relatively equivalent in effect size. That is, when measures of well-being are included as covariates, the association between the focal well-being dimension and health is not attenuated (Friedman & Ryff, 2012; Morozink et al., 2010; Steptoe et al., 2012; Tsenkova et al., 2007). Two studies using MIDUS data have demonstrated that, relative to eudaimonic well-being, hedonic well-being dimensions more strongly predict insomnia (Hamilton et al., 2007) and metabolic syndrome (Boylan & Ryff, 2015) when measures are included in the same models. However, cross-sectional findings from the Gallup World Poll suggest that eudaimonic well-being, assessed with an ad hoc seven-item measure of positive psychosocial experiences, is a stronger predictor of subjective health than is hedonic well-being, measured with two items reflecting enjoyment and the frequency of smiling and laughing (Joshanloo & Jovanović, 2018). Additional evidence from studies of gene expression (i.e., modifications to genes that change the likelihood that a gene is transcribed) support the distinction between hedonic and eudaimonic well-being, both assessed with high-quality measures. Specifically, eudaimonic well-being predicted down-regulation of the conserved transcriptional response to adversity (CTRA; Cole, 2013), marked by higher expression of pro-inflammatory genes and lower expression of antibody synthesis genes across multiple studies (Cole et al., 2015; Fredrickson et al., 2013, 2015). Furthermore, eudaimonic well-being interventions have likewise shown down-regulation of pro-inflammatory genes and up-regulation of antibody synthesis genes (Nelson-Coffey, Fritz, Lyubomirsky, & Cole, 2017; Seeman, Merkin, Goldwater, & Cole, 2019). Hedonic well-being was associated with up-regulation of the CTRA, marked by pro-inflammatory genes and down-regulation of antibody synthesis genes in one study (Fredrickson et al., 2013) and uncorrelated with the CTRA in another (Fredrickson et al., 2015).

More research that integrates hedonic and eudaimonic well-being with assessments of health is needed. Whether life contentment or life engagement (or both) are health-protective may ultimately depend on the health outcome of interest and possible subgroups defined by age, gender, race, and/or SES. The overall conclusion from this section is that both hedonic and eudaimonic well-being are associated with better health profiles across many health domains, including self-reported outcomes, incidence, disease incidence and severity, mortality, and biological risk factors. Tracking these associations longitudinally to determine which varieties of well-being are most consequential for physical health, as well as the pathways underlying such salubrious relationships, is key for future work. How relationships between varieties of well-being and health are situated in broader social, cultural, and historical contexts is covered in the final section below.

Historical Change, Well-Being, and Health: An Integrative Approach

The previous sections highlighted sociodemographic factors and well-being along with studies of well-being and diverse health outcomes. The relationships among sociodemographic factors, well,-being and health may vary over time and thus requires an integration with other fields as well. Cultural, social, economic, and political trends (i.e., historical change) can alter personal life circumstances and influence well-being (see Diener et al., 2018, for review). This section highlights key historical changes that have occurred in the past few decades and discusses their implications for linkages of well-being with health.

In the United States, positive social changes beginning in the 1960s, including greater gender equality, improvements in the social welfare system, and the civil rights movement, were thought to improve the well-being of historically marginalized sociodemographic groups, including women, lower SES populations, and minorities (Yang, 2008). There is evidence, however, that ratings of life satisfaction and happiness among marginalized groups have not significantly improved nor converged with the advantaged (Hughes & Thomas, 1998; Iceland & Ludwig-Dehm, 2019; Yang, 2008). Other historical changes in the United States may undermine the well-being and health of the disadvantaged relative to the advantaged. There has been a dramatic increase in income and wealth inequality over the past few decades (Piketty & Saez, 2014). The American dream, defined by continued improvement of the younger generation's standard of living relative to their parents' generation, has diminished. Only 50% of children born in the 1980s achieved a higher income than their parents, compared to 90% for children born in the 1940s (Chetty et al., 2017).

The Great Recession of 2007–2009 was also a formative historical event that resulted in a period of extreme socioeconomic adversities (e.g., job loss, financial loss, housing loss). Furthermore, people exposed to greater job, financial, and housing hardship during the Great Recession were at increased risk for symptoms of depression, generalized anxiety, panic attacks, or problems associated with substance use (Forbes & Krueger, 2019) and had higher allostatic load (Patel, 2019). Less advantaged groups (low SES and minorities) experienced more adversities and had more difficulty recovering from the Great Recession than their more advantaged counterparts (Carnevale, Jayasundera, & Gulish, 2016; Hoynes, Miller, & Schaller, 2012). Historical trends in socioeconomic inequality may therefore have downstream influences on well-being and health.

The growing socioeconomic divide, exacerbated by the Great Recession, could lead to declines in well-being, particularly among marginalized groups. Cross-time and longitudinal surveys of MIDUS participants from 1990s to early 2010s documented increasing economic distress for those at the bottom of the SES hierarchy compared to those at the top (Glei, Goldman, & Weinstein, 2018, 2019). Over the same period, average levels of hedonic and eudaimonic well-being declined (Kirsch, Love, Radler, & Ryff, 2019). Furthermore, declines in well-being were more pronounced for the SES disadvantaged relative to the advantaged (Goldman, Glei, & Weinstein, 2018). However, some aspects of eudaimonic well-being, such as purpose in life, did not change, suggesting that certain indicators of well-being may be more sensitive to economic shocks than others. Additional research needs to attend to historical changes in well-being, possibly intersecting with social identities defined by race, age, and gender.

Historical changes in well-being could be implicated in historical trends in health and health disparities. From 2001 to 2014, the life expectancy gap between the richest 1% and poorest 1% has widened (Chetty et al., 2016). Mortality rates for educationally disadvantaged, middle-aged Whites have increased over the past three decades. Increases in mortality were primarily driven by "deaths of despair," that is, deaths caused by suicide, drug overdose, and alcohol poisoning (Case & Deaton, 2015, 2017) and by cardiovascular disease mortality (Case & Deaton, 2017). A separate literature has shown that times with greater socioeconomic inequality correspond to less happiness, particularly among individuals with lower income (Oishi, Kesebir, & Diener, 2011) and those facing financial scarcity (Sommet, Morselli, & Spini, 2018). Such widening disparities in well-being could contribute to widening disparities in physical health. Alternatively, historical trends in well-being and health could be a symptom of other social changes, such as declines in the social safety net, and may not be causally related. Furthermore, many studies on historical changes in socioeconomic inequality and well-being are limited to single-item indicators of happiness, anxiety, or social trust (i.e., Buttrick & Oishi, 2017). More time-series and longitudinal studies of theory-driven, multi-item indicators of hedonic and eudaimonic well-being are thus necessary to test historical changes in the associations between well-being and physical health.

Conclusion and Future Directions

The goal of this chapter is to build a cumulative science of well-being that attends to the past as it examines the present and anticipates the future. In the first section, we examined the conceptual and philosophical histories of hedonic and eudaimonic well-being, the two most prominent approaches in extant science. We showed that both perspectives are traceable to the ancient Greeks, although their presence in current empirical work shows notable differences between them. Hedonic indicators first entered population-based assessments in the 1960s and were largely without theoretical foundations. The focus rather was on relatively straightforward questions about life satisfaction, happiness, and positive affect. Eudaimonia, in contrast, drew extensively on formulations in clinical, developmental, existential, and humanistic psychology, along with Aristotle's distant writings, to identify multiple dimensions of what it means to be well (autonomy, environmental mastery, personal growth, positive relationships with others, purpose in life, self-acceptance). Detailed definitions of these components of hedonic and eudaimonic well-being were provided; they constitute the foundation from which empirical assessments tools were generated, which lead to decades of scientific research.

The second section provided a descriptive look at how the two broad types of well-being are distributed in the general population, focusing on age, SES, gender, and race/ethnicity. These sociodemographic factors situate human lives within broader social structural contexts and thereby afford valuable windows by which to understand variation in reported levels of well-being. Drawing on both cross-sectional and longitudinal evidence, hedonic and eudaimonic well-being were found to vary in their associations with sociodemographic factors. Regarding age, hedonic well-being was shown in some studies to increase with age, although eudaimonic well-being, especially purpose in life and personal growth, was shown to decline.

Both types of well-being were positively linked with higher SES, although stronger patterns were evident for some dimensions (e.g., purpose in life, personal growth) than others. Gender differences in hedonic well-being show varied patterns that likely intersect with other social factors. Some investigations showed women to have higher profiles than men on two aspects of eudaimonia: positive relations with others and personal growth. Racial disparities in hedonic well-being have shown lower reports of life satisfaction and happiness among Blacks compared to Whites, but such patterns were reversed after adjusting for perceived discrimination. Black adults have also reported higher levels of eudaimonic well-being (all dimensions) compared to Whites. Of increasing interest is the intersectionality among these sociodemographic factors. Examples of the combined effects of age, race, gender, and SES in shaping well-being outcomes were noted. Some draw attention to changes in gender differences that may unfold with age as well as to the cumulative impact with age of inequalities tied to gender, race, and SES status.

Our third section examined links between hedonic and eudaimonic well-being with self-rated health, morbidity, mortality, and biological health outcomes. Reciprocal relationships between well-being and subjective health were evident for both hedonic and eudaimonic well-being. Longitudinal evidence supports protective effects of higher life satisfaction as well as purpose in life and positive relations with others on multiple health outcomes (doctor visits, chronic conditions). Multiple prospective studies show that hedonic and eudaimonic well-being, specifically positive affect, life satisfaction, and purpose in life, reduce risk for all-cause and cardiovascular-specific mortality, independent of confounding factors. Multiple prospective studies have also shown that higher purpose in life reduces risk of cognitive impairment, Alzheimer's disease, stroke, and myocardial infarction, net of confounds. Considerable research has linked both hedonic and eudaimonic well-being to better physiological functioning across cardiovascular, neuroendocrine, immune, and metabolic systems. Similarly, evidence shows that eudaimonic well-being buffers against the adverse effects of low SES status on inflammatory markers and diurnal cortisol.

Going forward, there is a clear need for studies that incorporate both hedonic and eudaimonic measures so that their independent and relative effect sizes can be examined. The little work that has been done underscores effects that are, in fact, independent and relatively equivalent in effect size, a pattern that also pertains to growing research linking well-being to brain-based measures and gene expression involved in inflammatory and antibody processes. Bridging our first two sections, future work, especially longitudinal designs, is needed to illuminate how health and well-being linkages may vary depending on sociodemographic factors (age, gender, SES, race/ethnicity).

Our fourth section underscored that the literature on well-being and health has unfolded on a changing historical stage influenced by cultural, social, economic, and political trends. Here we gave attention to dramatic increases in income and wealth inequality over recent decades. How hardships of the Great Recession, which continue to linger for some, are linked with reports of well-being as well depression and anxiety was noted. Of concern is what these macro-level economic changes will mean for the well-being of future cohorts of adults, particularly those in disadvantaged segments of society. These are important questions going forward.

In conclusion, growing interest in human well-being, political and scientific, calls for a deeper understanding of how sociodemographic and contextual factors influence people's inner sense of how their lives are going and the associated health implications. Future research requires theoretically informed studies that draw on the corpus of scientific evidence described herein to explicate hypothesized antecedents and consequents as well as mediating and moderating influences. Such comprehensive science on what it means to be well, for whom opportunities of wellness are available, and what health consequences well-being may have is critical to inform public policy as well as guide future research. We emphasize that unique contexts, such as widening social inequalities, racial disparities in health, and different sociocultural contexts, may uniquely affect distinct dimensions of hedonic and eudaimonic well-being. The literature reviewed in this chapter thus provides a foundation on which next generations of research can build.

About the Authors

Carol D. Ryff is Director of the Institute on Aging and Hilldale Professor of Psychology at the University of Wisconsin-Madison. She studies psychological well-being—how it varies by sociodemographic factors and how it matters for health, including diverse disease outcomes, length of life, physiological regulation, and neural circuitry. She is Principal Investigator of the Midlife in the United States (MIDUS) longitudinal study and its sister study in Japan, Midlife in Japan (MIDJA). An integrative theme across these studies is resilience—the capacity to maintain or regain well-being and health in the face of adversity.

Jennifer Morozink Boylan is Assistant Professor of Health and Behavioral Sciences at the University of Colorado Denver. She received her PhD in biological psychology from the University of Wisconsin-Madison and completed postdoctoral fellowships in the Health Disparities Research Scholars Program at the University of Wisconsin-Madison School of Medicine and Public Health and in the Cardiovascular Behavioral Medicine Program at the University of Pittsburgh. Her program of research centers on conceptualizing positive psychological characteristics and their potential influence on physical health, situating psychological risk and protective factors within broader social contexts (e.g., SES, race, and culture), and examining biological mechanisms underlying how the social environment affects disease pathophysiology.

Julie A. Kirsch is a postdoctoral fellow at the University of Wisconsin-Madison Center for Tobacco Research and Intervention. She studies the intersections among inequality, health, and well-being and psychosocial pathways to mitigating the consequences of socioeconomic adversity. Her research reflects integrative work that spans psychological and health sciences.

Author Note

This work was supported by the John D. and Catherine T. MacArthur Foundation Research Network and National Institute on Aging (P01-AG020166, U19-AG051426), with additional support provided by the John Templeton Foundation and the Lee Kum Sheung Center for Health and Happiness. The views expressed in this chapter represent the perspectives of the authors and do not reflect the opinions or endorsement of any organization. We have no known conflict of interest to disclose. Correspondence concerning this chapter should be directed to Carol D. Ryff, Institute on Aging, 2245 Medical Science Center, University of Madison, WI 53706 (cryff@wisc.edu).

References

Aldwin, C. M., & Levenson, M. R. (2001). Stress, coping, and health at mid-life: A developmental perspective. In M. E. Lachman (Ed.), *The handbook of midlife development* (pp. 188–214). New York: John Wiley & Sons.

Allport, G. W. (1961). *Pattern and growth in personality*. New York: Holt, Rinehart, & Winston.

Almeida, D. M., & Horn, M. C. (2004). Is daily life more stressful during middle adulthood? In O. G. Brim, C. R., Ryff & R. C. Kessler (Eds.), *How healthy are we? A national study of well-being at midlife* (pp. 425–451). Chicago, IL: University of Chicago Press.

Andrew, M. K., Fisk, J. D., & Rockwood, K. (2012). Psychological well-being in relation to frailty: A frailty identity crisis? *International Psychogeriatrics, 24*(8), 1347–1353.

Andrews, F. M., & Withey, S. B. (1976). *Social indicators of well-being: America's perception of life quality.* New York: Plenum Press.

Aristotle. (1925). *The Nicomachean ethics* (D. Ross, Trans). New York: Oxford University Press.

Bacon, S. L., Watkins, L. L., Babyak, M., Sherwood, A., Hayano, J., Hinderliter, A. L., . . . Blumenthal, J. A. (2004). Effects of daily stress on autonomic cardiac control in patients with coronary artery disease. *American Journal of Cardiology, 93*(10), 1292–1294.

Barger, S. D., Donoho, C. J., & Wayment, H. A. (2009). The relative contributions of race/ ethnicity, socioeconomic status, health, and social relationships to life satisfaction in the United States. *Quality of Life Research, 18*(2), 179–189.

Barnes, J. (1986). Hellenistic philosophy and science. In J. Boardman, J. Griffin, & O. Oswyn (Eds.), *The Oxford history of the classical world* (pp. 365–385). Oxford: Oxford University Press.

Bastarache, E. D., Graham, E. K., Estabrook, R., Ong, A., Piccinin, A., Hofer, S., Spiro, A. III., & Mroczek, D. K. (2019). Trajectories of positive and negative affect: A coordinated analysis of 11 longitudinal samples. *Innovation in Aging, 3*, S696–S696.

Batz, C., & Tay, L. (2018). Gender differences in subjective well-being. *Handbook of Well-Being*, 1–15. https://www.nobascholar.com/chapters/30/download.pdf

Batz-Barbarich, C., Tay, L., Kuykendall, L., & Cheung, H. K. (2018). A meta-analysis of gender differences in subjective well-being: Estimating effect sizes and associations with gender inequality. *Psychological Science, 29*(9), 1491–1503.

Beatty, P., & Tuch, S. A. (1997). Race and life satisfaction in the middle class. *Sociological Spectrum, 17*(1), 71–90.

Benyamini, Y., Idler, E. L., Leventhal, H., & Leventhal, E. A. (2000). Positive affect and function as influences on self-assessments of health: Expanding our view beyond illness and disability. *Journals of Gerontology, Series B: Psychological Sciences and Social Sciences, 55*(2), P107–16.

Bhattacharyya, M. R., Whitehead, D. L., Rakhit, R., & Steptoe, A. (2008). Depressed mood, positive affect, and heart rate variability in patients with suspected coronary artery disease. *Psychosomatic Medicine, 70*(9), 1020–1027.

Biswas-Diener, R., & Diener, E. (2001). Making the best of a bad situation: Satisfaction in the slums of Calcutta. *Social Indicators Research, 55*, 329–352.

Blanchflower, D. G., & Oswald, A. J. (2004). Well-being over time in Britain and the USA. *Journal of Public Economics, 88*(7–8), 1359–1386.

Blanchflower, D. G., & Oswald, A. J. (2008). Is well-being U-shaped over the life cycle? *Social Science and Medicine, 66*(8), 1733–1749.

Blevins, C. L., Sagui, S. J., & Bennett, J. M. (2017). Inflammation and positive affect: Examining the stress-buffering hypothesis with data from the National Longitudinal Study of Adolescent to Adult Health. *Brain, Behavior, and Immunity, 61*, 21–26.

Boehm, J. K., Chen, Y., Williams, D. R., Ryff, C., & Kubzansky, L. D. (2015). Unequally distributed psychological assets: Are there social disparities in optimism, life satisfaction, and positive affect? *PLoS ONE, 10*(2), 1–17.

Boehm, J. K., Chen, Y., Williams, D. R., Ryff, C. D., & Kubzansky, L. D. (2016). Subjective well-being and cardiometabolic health: An 8–11 year study of midlife adults. *Journal of Psychosomatic Research, 85*, 1–8.

Boehm, J. K., & Kubzansky, L. D. (2012). The heart's content: The association between positive psychological well-being and cardiovascular health. *Psychological Bulletin, 138*(4), 655–691.

Boehm, J. K., Peterson, C., Kivimaki, M., & Kubzansky, L. (2011). A prospective study of positive psychological well-being and coronary heart disease. *Health Psychology, 30*(3), 259–267.

Bookwala, J., & Boyar, J. (2008). Gender, excessive body weight, and psychological well-being in adulthood. *Psychology of Women Quarterly, 32*(2), 188–195.

Boylan, J. M., Jennings, J. R., & Matthews, K. A. (2016). Childhood socioeconomic status and cardiovascular reactivity and recovery among black and white men: Mitigating effects of psychological resources. *Health Psychology, 35*(9), 957–966.

Boylan, J. M., & Ryff, C. D. (2015). Psychological well-being and metabolic syndrome: Findings from the Midlife in the United States national sample. *Psychosomatic Medicine, 77*(5), 548–558.

Boylan, J. M., Tsenkova, V. K., Miyamoto, Y., & Ryff, C. D. (2017). Psychological resources and glucoregulation in Japanese adults: Findings from MIDJA. *Health Psychology, 36*(5), 449–457.

Boyle, P. A., Barnes, L. L., Buchman, A. S., & Bennett, D. A. (2009). Purpose in life Is associated with mortality among community-dwelling older persons. *Psychosomatic Medicine, 71*(5), 574–579.

Boyle, P. A., Buchman, A. S., & Bennett, D. A. (2010). Purpose in life is associated with a reduced risk of incident disability among community-dwelling older persons. *The American Journal of Geriatric Psychiatry, 18*(12), 1093–1102.

Bradburn, N. M. (1969). *The structure of psychological well-being.* Chicago: Aldine.

Branscombe, N. R., Schmitt, M. T., & Harvey, R. D. (1999). Perceiving pervasive discrimination among African-Americans: Implications for group identification and well being. *Journal of Personality and Social Psychology, 77*(1), 135–149.

Buttrick, N. R., & Oishi, S. (2017). The psychological consequences of income inequality. *Social and Personality Psychology Compass, 11*(3), 1–12.

Campbell, A., Converse, P. E., & Rodgers, W. L. (1976). *The quality of American life: Perceptions, evaluations, and satisfactions.* New York: Russell Sage Foundation.

Cantril, H. (1965). *The pattern of human concerns.* New Brunswick, NJ: Rutgers University Press.

Carnevale, A. P., Jayasundera, T., & Gulish, A. (2016). America's divided recovery: College haves and have-nots. cew.georgetown.edu/dividedrecovery

Carstensen, L. L., & Mikels, J. A. (2005). At the intersection of emotion and cognition. *Current Directions in Psychological Science, 14*(3), 117–121.

Case, A., & Deaton, A. (2015). Rising morbidity and mortality in midlife among white non-Hispanic Americans in the 21st century. *Proceedings of the National Academy of Sciences, 112*(49), 15078–15083.

Case, A., & Deaton, A. (2017). Mortality and morbidity in the 21st century HHS Public Access. *Brookings Papers on Economic Activity, Spring 201*, 397–476.

Çeliker, R., & Borman, P. (2001). Fibromyalgia versus rheumatoid arthritis: A comparison of psychological disturbance and life satisfaction. *Journal of Musculoskeletal Pain, 9*(1), 35–45.

Chang, S., Hong, J., & Charles, S. (2018). Purpose in life and self-rated health across adulthood: The importance of the bidirectional relationship. *Innovation in Aging, 2,* 309.

Charles, S. T., Reynolds, C., & Gatz, M. (2001). Age-related differences and changes in positive and negative affect over 23 years. *Journal of Personality and Social Psychology, 80,* 136–151.

Chetty, R., Grusky, D., Hell, M., Hendren, N., Manduca, R., & Narang, J. (2017). The fading American dream: Trends in absolute income mobility since 1940. *Science, 356*(April), 398–406.

Chetty, R., Stepner, M., Abraham, S., Lin, S., Scuderi, B., Turner, N., . . . Cutler, D. (2016). The association between income and life expectancy in the United States, 2001–2014. *Journal of the American Medical Association, 315*(16), 1750–1766.

Chida, Y., & Steptoe, A. (2008). Positive psychological well-being and mortality: A quantitative review of prospective observational studies. *Psychosomatic Medicine, 70*(7), 741–756.

Cohen, R., Bavishi, C., & Rozanski, A. (2016). Purpose in life and its relationship to all-cause mortality and cardiovascular events: A meta-analysis. *Psychosomatic Medicine, 78,* 122.

Cohen, S., Doyle, W. J., Turner, R. B., Alper, C. M., & Skoner, D. P. (2003). Emotional style and susceptibility to the common cold. *Psychosomatic Medicine, 65*(4), 652–657.

Cohen, S., & Pressman, S. D. (2006). Positive affect and health. *Current Directions in Psychological Science, 15*(3), 122.

Cole, E. R. (2009). Intersectionality and research in psychology. *American Psychologist, 64*(3), 170–180.

Cole, S. W. (2013). Social regulation of human gene expression: Mechanisms and implications for public health. *American Journal of Public Health, 103.* Suppl 1:S84–S92.

Cole, S. W., Levine, M. E., Arevalo, J. M. G., Ma, J., Weir, D. R., & Crimmins, E. M. (2015). Loneliness, eudaimonia, and the human conserved transcriptional response to adversity. *Psychoneuroendocrinology, 62,* 11–17.

Costanzo, E. S., Ryff, C. D., & Singer, B. H. (2009). Psychosocial adjustment among cancer survivors: Findings from a national survey of health and well-being. *Health Psychology, 28*(2), 147–156.

Coverdill, J. E., Lopez, C. A., & Petrie, M. A. (2011). Race, ethnicity and the quality of life in America, 1972–2008. *Social Forces, 89*(3), 783–805.

Crenshaw, K. (1991). Mapping the margins: Intersectionality, identity politics, and violence against women of color. *Stanford Law Review, 43*(6), 1241.

Curhan, K. B., Levine, C. S., Markus, H. R., Kitayama, S., Park, J., Karasawa, M., . . . Ryff, C. D. (2014). Subjective and objective hierarchies and their relations to psychological well-being: A US/Japan comparison. *Social Psychological and Personality Science, 5*(8), 855–864.

Davidson, K. W., Mostofsky, E., & Whang, W. (2010). Don't worry, be happy: Positive affect and reduced 10-year incident coronary heart disease: The Canadian Nova Scotia Health Survey. *European Heart Journal, 31*(9), 1065–1070.

Diener, E., & Chan, M. Y. (2011). Happy people live longer: Subjective well-being contributes to health and longevity. *Applied Psychology: Health and Well-Being, 3*(1), 1–43.

Diener, E., Oishi, S., & Tay, L. (2018). Advances in subjective well-being research. *Nature Human Behaviour, 2*(4), 253–260.

Diener, E., Smith, E., &Fujita, F. (1995). The personality structure of affect. *Journal of Personality and Social Psychology, 69*, 130–141.

Diener, E., & Suh, E. (1997). Measuring quality of life: Economic, social, and subjective indicators. *Social Indicators Research, 40*, 189–216.

Dupre, M. E. (2007). Educational differences in age-related patterns of disease: Reconsidering the cumulative disadvantage and age-as-leveler hypotheses. *Journal of Health and Social Behavior, 48*, 1–15.

Easterlin, R. A. (2003). Explaining happiness. *Proceedings of the National Academy of Sciences, 100*(19), 11176–11183.

Elkins, L. E., Pollina, D. A., Scheffer, S. R., & Krupp, L. B. (1999). Psychological states and neuropsychological performances in chronic Lyme disease. *Applied Neuropsychology, 6*(1), 19–26.

Elliot, A. J., & Chapman, B. P. (2016). Socioeconomic status, psychological resources, and inflammatory markers: Results from the MIDUS study. *Health Psychology, 35*(11), 1205–1213.

Ellison, C. G. (1995). Race, religious involvement and depressive symptomatology in a southeastern US Community. *Social Science and Medicine, 40*(11), 1561–1572.

Erikson, E. (1959). Identity and the life cycle. *Psychological Issues, 1*, 1–171.

Feldman, P. J., & Steptoe, A. (2003). Psychosocial and socioeconomic factors associated with glycated hemoglobin in nondiabetic middle-aged men and women. *Health Psychology, 22*(4), 398–405.

Fernández-Ballesteros, R., Zamarrón, M. D., & Ruíz, M. A. (2001). The contribution of socio-demographic and psychosocial factors to life satisfaction. *Ageing and Society, 21*(1), 25–43.

Ferraro, K. F., & Shippee, T. P. (2009). Aging and cumulative inequality: How does inequality get under the skin? *Gerontologist, 49*(3), 333–343.

Forbes, M. K., & Krueger, R. F. (2019). The great recession and mental health in the United States. *Clinical Psychological Science, 7*(5), 900–913.

Frankl, V. (1959). *Man's search for meaning.* Boston, MA: Beacon Press.

Fredrickson, B. L., Grewen, K. M., Algoe, S. B., Firestine, A. M., Arevalo, J. M. G., Ma, J., & Cole, S. W. (2015). *Psychological well-being and the human conserved transcriptional response to adversity. PLos ONE, 10*(3), e0121839.

Fredrickson, B. L., Grewen, K. M., Coffey, K. A., Algoe, S. B., Firestine, A. M., Arevalo, J. M. G., . . . Cole, S. W. (2013). A functional genomic perspective on human well-being. *Proceedings of the National Academy of Sciences of the United States of America, 110*(33), 13684–13689.

Friedman, E. M., Hayney, M., Love, G. D., Singer, B. H., & Ryff, C. D. (2007). Plasma interleukin-6 and soluble IL-6 receptors are associated with psychological well-being in aging women. *Health Psychology, 26*(3), 305–313.

Friedman, E. M., Hayney, M. S., Love, G. D., Urry, H. L., Rosenkranz, M. A., Davidson, R. J., . . . Ryff, C. D. (2005). Social relationships, sleep quality, and interleukin-6 in aging women. *Proceedings of the National Academy of Sciences, 102*(51), 18757–18762.

Friedman, E. M., & Ryff, C. D. (2012). Living well with medical comorbidities: A biopsychosocial perspective. *Journals of Gerontology, Series B: Psychological Sciences and Social Sciences*, 1–10.

Gana, K., Saada, Y., Broc, G., Quintard, B., Amieva, H., & Dartigues, J.-F. (2016). As long as you've got your health: Longitudinal relationships between positive affect and functional health in old age. *Social Science & Medicine, 150*, 231–238.

Glei, D. A., Goldman, N., & Weinstein, M. (2018). Perception has its own reality: Subjective versus objective measures of economic distress. *Population and Development Review, 44*(4), 695–722.

Glei, D. A., Goldman, N., & Weinstein, M. (2019). A growing socioeconomic divide: Effects of the Great Recession on perceived economic distress in the United States. *PLoS ONE, 14*(4), 1–25.

Goldman, N., Glei, D. A., & Weinstein, M. (2018). Declining mental health among disadvantaged Americans. *Proceedings of the National Academy of Sciences, 115*(28), 7290–7295.

Goodman, F., Disabato, D., Kashdan, T., & Kauffman, S. (2017). Measuring well-being: A comparison of subjective well-being and PERMA. *Journal of Positive Psychology, 13*, 321–332.

Graham, C. (2017). *Happiness for all? Unequal lives and hopes in pursuit of the American Dream*. Princeton, NJ: Princeton University Press.

Greenfield, E. A., Vaillant, G. E., & Marks, N. F. (2009). Do formal religious participation and spiritual perceptions have independent linkages with diverse dimensions of psychological well-being? *Journal of Health and Social Behavior, 50*, 196–212.

Gurin, G., Veroff, J., & Feld, S. (1960). *Americans view their mental health*. New York: Basic Books.

Guidi, J., Rafanelli, C., Roncuzzi, R., Sirri, L., & Fava, G. A. (2013). Assessing psychological factors affecting medical conditions: Comparison between different proposals. *General Hospital Psychiatry, 35*(2), 141–146.

Hafez, D., Heisler, M., Choi, H., Ankuda, C. K., Winkelman, T., & Kullgren, J. T. (2018). Association between purpose in life and glucose control among older adults. *Annals of Behavioral Medicine, 52*(4), 309–318.

Hamilton, N. A., Gallagher, M. W., Preacher, K. J., Stevens, N., Nelson, C. A., Karlson, C., & McCurdy, D. (2007). Insomnia and well-being. *Journal of Consulting and Clinical Psychology, 75*(6), 939–946.

Hayney, M. S., Love, G. D., Buck, J. M., Ryff, C. D., Singer, B., & Muller, D. (2003). The association between psychosocial factors and vaccine-induced cytokine production. *Vaccine, 21*(19–20), 2428–2432.

Heidrich, S. M., & Ryff, C. D. (1993a). Physical and mental health in later life: The self-system as mediator. *Psychology and Aging, 8*, 327–338.

Heidrich, S. M., & Ryff, C. D. (1993b). The role of social comparisons processes in the psychological adaptation of elderly adults. *Journal of Gerontology, 48*(3), P127–P136.

Hill, P. L., & Turiano, N. A. (2014). Purpose in life as a predictor of mortality across adulthood. *Psychological Science, 25*, 1482–1486.

Hoogwegt, M. T., Versteeg, H., Hansen, T. B., Thygesen, L. C., Pedersen, S. S., & Zwisler, A.-D. (2013). Exercise mediates the association between positive affect and 5-year mortality in patients with ischemic heart disease. *Circulation. Cardiovascular Quality and Outcomes, 6*(5), 559–566.

Hoynes, H., Miller, D. L., & Schaller, J. (2012). Who suffers during recessions? *Journal of Economic Perspectives, 26*(3), 27–48.

Hughes, M., & Thomas, M. S. (1998). The continuing significance of race revisited : A study of race, class, and quality of life in America, 1972 to 1996. *American Sociological Review, 63*(6), 785–795.

Huta, V., & Waterman, A. S. (2014). Eudaimonia and its distinction from hedonia: Developing a classification and terminology for understanding conceptual and operational definitions. *Journal of Happiness Studies: An Interdisciplinary Forum on Subjective Well-Being, 15*, 1425–1456.

Iceland, J., & Ludwig-Dehm, S. (2019). Black-white differences in happiness, 1972–2014. *Social Science Research, 77*(October 2018), 16–29.

Inglehart, R. (2002). Gender, aging, and subjective well-being. *International Journal of Comparative Sociology, 43*(3–5), 391–408.

Jahoda, M. (1958). *Current concepts of positive mental health.* New York: Basic Books.

Jackson, P. B., & Williams, D. R. (2006). The Intersection of Race, Gender, and SES: Halth Pradoxes. In A. J. Schulz & L. Mullings (Eds.), *Gender, race, class, & health: Intersectional approaches* (pp. 131–162). Jossey-Bass/Wiley.

Joshanloo, M., & Jovanović, V. (2018). Subjective health in relation to hedonic and eudaimonic wellbeing: Evidence from the Gallup World Poll. *Journal of Health Psychology,* 135910531882010.

Jung, C. G. (1933). *Modern man in search of a soul.* (W. S. Dell & C. F. Baynes, Trans.). New York: Harcourt, Brace, & World.

Kahneman, D., Diener, E., & Schwarz, N. (Eds.). (1999). *Well-being? The foundations of hedonic psychology.* New York: Russell Sage Foundation.

Kashubeck-West, S., & Meyer, J. (2008). The well-being of women who are late deafened. *Journal of Counseling Psychology, 55*(4), 463–472.

Keyes, C. L. M. (2005). Mental illness and/or mental health? Investigating axioms of the complete state model of health. *Journal of Consulting and Clinical Psychology, 73*(3), 539–548.

Keyes, C. L. M. (2009). The black-white paradox in health: Flourishing in the face of social inequality and discrimination. *Journal of Personality, 77*(6), 1677–1706.

Keyes, C. L. M., & Grzywacz, J. G. (2005). Health as a complete state: The added value in work performance and healthcare costs. *Journal of Occupational and Environmental Medicine, 47*(5), 523–532.

Keyes, C. L. M., Shmotkin, D., & Ryff, C. D. (2002). Optimizing well-being: The empirical encounter of two traditions. *Journal of Personality and Social Psychology, 81*, 1007–1022.

Kim, E. S., Kawachi, I., Chen, Y., & Kubzansky, L. D. (2017). Association between purpose in life and objective measures of physical function in older adults. *JAMA Psychiatry, 74*(10), 1039.

Kim, E. S., Park, N., Sun, J. K., Smith, J., & Peterson, C. (2014). Life satisfaction and frequency of doctor visits. *Psychosomatic Medicine, 76*(1), 86–93.

Kim, E. S., Strecher, V. J., & Ryff, C. D. (2014). Purpose in life and use of preventive health care services. *Proceedings of the National Academy of Sciences of the United States of America, 111*(46), 16331–16336.

Kim, E. S., Sun, J. K., Park, N., Kubzansky, L. D., & Peterson, C. (2013). Purpose in life and reduced risk of myocardial infarction among older US adults with coronary heart disease: A two-year follow-up. *Journal of Behavioral Medicine, 36*(2), 124–133.

Kim, E. S., Sun, J. K., Park, N., & Peterson, C. (2013). Purpose in life and reduced incidence of stroke in older adults: "The Health and Retirement Study." *Journal of Psychosomatic Research, 74*(5), 427–432.

Kirsch, J. A., Love, G. D., Radler, B. T., & Ryff, C. D. (2019). Scientific imperatives vis-à-vis growing inequality in America. *American Psychologist, 74*(7), 764.

Knox, S., Svensson, J., Waller, D., & Theorell, T. (1988). Emotional coping and the psychophysiological substrates of elevated blood pressure. *Behavioral Medicine, 14*(2), 52–58.

Koenig, H. G., King, D. E., & Carson, V. B. (2012). *Handbook of religion and health* (2nd ed.). Oxford: Oxford University Press.

Korkeila, M., Kaprio, J., Rissanen, A., Koshenvuo, M., & Sörensen, T. I. (1998). Predictors of major weight gain in adult Finns: Stress, life satisfaction and personality traits. *International Journal of Obesity & Related Metabolic Disorders, 22*(10), 949–957.

Lachman, M. E., Lewkowicz, C., Marcus, A., & Peng, Y. (1994). Images of midlife development among young, middle-aged, and older adults. *Journal of Adult Development, 1*(4), 201–211.

Lachman, M. E., Teshale, S., & Agrigoroaei, S. (2015). Midlife as a pivotal period in the life course: Balancing growth and decline at the crossroads of youth and old age. *International Journal of Behavioral Development, 39*(1), 20–31.

Laertius, D. (1925). Socrates, with predecessors and followers: Aristippus. In *Lives of the Eminent Philosophers* (Translated by R. D. Hicks). Cambridge, MA: Loeb Classical Library.

Lamers, S. M. A., Bolier, L., Westerhof, G. J., Smit, F., & Bohlmeijer, E. T. (2012). The impact of emotional well-being on long-term recovery and survival in physical illness: A meta-analysis. *Journal of Behavioral Medicine, 35*(5), 538–547.

Land, K. C. (1975). Social indicator models: An overview. In K. C. Land & S. Spilerman (Eds.), *Social indicator models* (pp. 5–35). New York: Russell Sage Foundation.

Larson, R. (1978). Thirty years of research on subjective well-being of older Americans. *Journal of Gerontology, 33*, 109–125.

Lindfors, P., & Lundberg, U. (2002). Is low cortisol release an indicator of positive health? *Stress and Health, 18*(4), 153–160.

Link, B. G., & Phelan, J. C. (2002). McKeown and the idea that social conditions are fundamental causes of disease. *American Journal of Public Health, 92*(5), 730–732.

Liu, B., Floud, S., Pirie, K., Green, J., Peto, R., Beral, V., & Million Women Study Collaborators. (2016). Does happiness itself directly affect mortality? The prospective UK Million Women Study. *Lancet, 387*(10021), 874–881.

Lucas, R. E., Diener, E, & Suh, E. (1996). Discriminant validity of well-being measures. *Journal of Personality and Social Psychology, 71*, 616–628.

Lykken, D., & Tellegen, A. (1996). Happiness is a stochastic phenomenon. *Psychological Science, 7*, 186–189.

Marks, N. F. (1996). Flying solo at midlife: Gender, marital status, and psychological well-being. *Journal of Marriage and Family, 58*(4), 917–932.

Marks, N. F., & Lambert, J. D. (1998). Marital status continuity and change among young and midlife adults. *Journal of Family Issues, 19*, 652–686.

Markus, H. R., Ryff, C. D., Curhan, K. B., & Palmersheim, K. A. (2004). In their own words: Well-being a midlife among high school-educated and college-educated adults. In R. Brim, O. G. Ryff, & C. D. Kessler (Ed.), *How healthy are we? A national study of well-being at midlife* (Vol. 2004, pp. 273–319). Chicago, IL: University of Chicago Press.

Marmot, M. G., Fuhrer, R., Ettner, S. L., Marks, N. F., Bumpass, L. L., & Ryff, C. D. (1998). Contribution of psychosocial factors to socioeconomic differences in health. *Milbank Quarterly, 76*(3), 403–448, 305.

Marmot, M., Ryff, C. D., Bumpass, L. L., Shipley, M., & Marks, N. F. (1997). Social inequalities in health: Next questions and converging evidence. *Social Science & Medicine, 44*(6), 901–910.

Martín-María, N., Miret, M., Caballero, F. F., Rico-Uribe, L. A., Steptoe, A., Chatterji, S., & Ayuso-Mateos, J. L. (2017). The impact of subjective well-being on mortality. *Psychosomatic Medicine, 79*(5), 565–575.

Maslow, A. H. (1968). *Toward a psychology of being* (2nd ed.). New York: Van Nostrand.

Matthews, K. A., Zhu, S., Tucker, D. C., & Whooley, M. A. (2006). Blood pressure reactivity to psychological stress and coronary calcification in the Coronary Artery Risk Development in Young Adults Study. *Hypertension, 47*(3), 391–395.

McCrae, R. R., & Costa, P. (1994). The stability of personality: Observations and evaluations. *Current Directions in Psychological Science, 3*, 173–175.

Middleton, R. A., & Byrd, E. K. (1996). Psychosocial factors and hospital readmission status of older persons with cardiovascular disease. *Journal of Applied Rehabilitation Counseling, 27*(4), 3–10.

Morozink, J. A., Friedman, E. M., Coe, C. L., & Ryff, C. D. (2010). Socioeconomic and psychosocial predictors of interleukin-6 in the MIDUS national sample. *Health Psychology, 29*(6), 626–635.

Mroczek, D. K., & Kolarz, C. M. (1998). The effect of age on positive and negative affect. *Journal of Personality and Social Psychology, 75*(5), 1333–1349.

Musich, S., Wang, S. S., Kraemer, S., Hawkins, K., & Wicker, E. (2018). Purpose in life and positive health outcomes among older adults. *Population Health Management, 21*(2), 139–147.

Nelson-Coffey, S. K, Fritz, M. M., Lyubomirsky, S., & Cole, S. W. (2017). Kindness in the blood: A randomized controlled trial of the gene regulatory impact of prosocial behavior. *Psychoneuroendocrinology, 81*, 8–13.

Neugarten, B. L. (1973a). Patterns of aging: Past, present, and future. *Social Service Review, 47*(4), 571–580.

Neugarten, B. L. (1973b). Personality change in late life: A developmental perspective. In C. Eisdorfer & M. P. Lawton (Eds.), *The psychology of adult development and aging* (pp. 311–335). Washington, DC: American Psychological Association.

Neugarten, B. L., Havighurst, R., & Tobin, S. (1961). The measurement of life satisfaction. *Journal of Gerontology, 16*, 134–143.

O'Brien, K. M. (2012). Healthy, wealthy, wise? Psychosocial factors influencing the socioeconomic status-health gradient. *Journal of Health Psychology, 17*(8), 1142–1151.

Oishi, S., Kesebir, S., & Diener, E. (2011). Income inequality and happiness. *Psychological Science, 22*(9), 1095–1100.

Ong, A. D., Kim, S., Young, S., & Steptoe, A. (2017). Positive affect and sleep: A systematic review. *Sleep Medicine Reviews, 35*, 21–32.

Ostir, G. V, Markides, K. S., Peek, M. K., & Goodwin, J. S. (2001). The association be-tween emotional well-being and the incidence of stroke in older adults. *Psychosomatic Medicine, 63*(2), 210–215.

Paschalides, C., Wearden, A. J., Dunkerley, R., Bundy, C., Davies, R., & Dickens, C. M. (2004). The associations of anxiety, depression and personal illness representations with glycaemic control and health-related quality of life in patients with type 2 diabetes mellitus. *Journal of Psychosomatic Research, 57*(6), 557–564.

Patel, P. C. (2019). The Great Recession and allostatic load in the United States. *International Journal of Stress Management, 26*, 411–417.

Pavot, W., Diener, E., & Fujita, F. (1990). Extraversion and happiness. *Personality and Individual Differences, 11*, 1299–1306.

Petrie, M., & Roman, P. M. (2004). Race and gender differences in workplace autonomy: A research note. *Sociological Inquiry, 74*(4), 590–603.

Phelan, C. H., Love, G. D., Ryff, C. D., Brown, R. L., & Heidrich, S. M. (2010). Psychosocial predictors of changing sleep patterns in aging women: A multiple pathway approach. *Psychology and Aging, 25*(4), 858–866.

Piketty, T., & Saez, E. (2014). Income inequality in Europe and the United States. *Science, 344*(6186), 838–843.

Pinquart, M., & Sorensen, S. (2001). Gender differences in self-concept and psychological well-being in old age. *Journal of Gerontology: Psychological Sciences, 56B*(4), 195–213.

Prather, A. A., Marsland, A. L., Muldoon, M. F., & Manuck, S. B. (2007). Positive affective style covaries with stimulated IL-6 and IL-10 production in a middle-aged community sample. *Brain, Behavior, and Immunity, 21*(8), 1033–1037.

Pressman, S. D., & Cohen, S. (2005). Does positive affect influence health? *Psychological Bulletin, 131*(6), 925–971.

Pusswald, G., Fleck, M., Lehrner, J., Haubenberger, D., Weber, G., & Auff, E. (2012). The "Sense of Coherence" and the coping capacity of patients with Parkinson disease. *International Psychogeriatrics, 24*(12), 1972–1979.

Radler, B. T., Rigotti, A., & Ryff, C. D. (2017). Persistently high psychological well-being predicts better HDL cholesterol and triglyceride levels: Findings from the midlife in the US (MIDUS) longitudinal study. *Lipids in Health and Disease, 17*(1), 1.

Riley, M. W., Kahn, R. L., Foner, A., & Mack, K. A. (Eds.). (1994). *Age and structural lag: Societies failure to provide meaningful opportunities in work, family, and leisure.* John Wiley & Sons.

Robles, T. F., Brooks, K. P., & Pressman, S. D. (2009). Trait positive affect buffers the effects of acute stress on skin barrier recovery. *Health Psychology, 28*(3), 373–378.

Rogers, C. R. (1961). *On becoming a person.* Boston: Houghton Mifflin.

Ryan, R. M., & Deci, E. L. (2001). On happiness and human potentials: A review of re-search on hedonic and eudaimonic well-being. *Annual Review of Psychology, 52*, 141–166.

Ryff, C. D. (1989). Happiness is everything, or is it?: Explorations on the meaning of psy-chological well-being. *Journal of Personality and Social Psychology, 57*, 1068–1081.

Ryff, C. D. (1995). Psychological well-being in adult life. *Current Directions in Psychological Science, 4*(4), 99–104.

Ryff, C. D. (2014). Psychological well-being revisited: Advances in the science and prac-tice of eudaimonia. *Psychotherapy and Psychosomatics, 83*, 10–28.

Ryff, C. D. (2016). Eudaimonic well-being education: Probing the connections. In D. W. Harward (Ed.), *Well-being and higher education: A strategy for change and the realization of education's greater purposes* (pp. 37–48). Washington, DC: Association of American Colleges and Universities.

Ryff, C. D. (2018). Well-being with soul: Science in pursuit of human potential. *Perspectives in Psychological Science, 13,* 242–248.

Ryff, C. D., & Heidrich, S. M. (1997). Experience and well-being: Explorations on domains of life and how they matter. *International Journal of Behavioral Development, 20*(2), 193–206.

Ryff, C. D., & Keyes, C. L. M. (1995). The structure of psychological well-being revisited. *Journal of Personality and Social Psychology, 69*(4), 719–727.

Ryff, C. D., Keyes, C. L. M., & Hughes, D. L. (2003). Status inequalities, perceived discrimination, and eudaimonic well-being: Do the challenges of minority life hone purpose and growth? *Journal of Health and Social Behavior, 44*(3), 275.

Ryff, C. D., Love, G. D., Urry, H. L., Muller, D., Rosenkranz, M. A., Friedman, E. M., . . . Singer, B. (2006). Psychological well-being and ill-being: Do they have distinct or mirrored biological correlates? *Psychotherapy and Psychosomatics, 75*(2), 85–95.

Ryff, C. D., Miyamoto, Y., Boylan, J. M., Coe, C. L., Karasawa, M., Kawakami, N., . . . Kitayama, S. (2015). Culture, inequality, and health: Evidence from the MIDUS and MIDJA comparison. *Culture and Brain, 3*(1), 1–20.

Ryff, C. D., & Singer, B. H. (2008). Know thyself and become what you are: A eudaimonic approach to psychological well-being. *Journal of Happiness Studies, 9,* 13–39.

Ryff, C. D., Singer, B. H., & Love, G. D. (2004). Positive health: Connecting well-being with biology. *Philosophical Transactions: Biological Sciences, 359*(1449), 1383–1394.

Saloumi, C., & Plourde, H. (2010). Differences in psychological correlates of excess weight between adolescents and young adults in Canada. *Psychology, Health and Medicine, 15*(3), 314–325.

Schleicher, H., Alonso, C., Shirtcliff, E. A., Muller, D., Loevinger, B. L., & Coe, C. L. (2005). In the face of pain: The relationship between psychological well-being and disability in women with fibromyalgia. *Psychotherapy and Psychosomatics, 74*(4), 231–239.

Schmutte, P., & Ryff, C. D. (1997). Personality and well-being? Reexamining methods and meaning. *Journal of Personality and Social Psychology, 73,* 549–559.

Seeman, T., Merkin, S. S., Goldwater, D., & Cole, S. W. (2019). Intergenerational mentoring, eudaimonic well-being and gene regulation in older adults: A pilot study. *Psychoneuroendocrinology, 111,* 104468.

Segerstrom, S. C. (2014). Affect and self-rated health: A dynamic approach with older adults. *Health Psychology, 33*(7), 720.

Shankar, A., Rafnsson, S. B., & Steptoe, A. (2015). Longitudinal associations between social connections and subjective wellbeing in the English Longitudinal Study of Ageing. *Psychology and Health, 30*(6), 686–698.

Shapiro, T., Meschede, T., & Osoro, S. (2013). The roots of the widening racial wealth gap: Explaining the black white economic divide. *Institute on Assets and Social Policy, 48*(202), 238. https://heller.brandeis.edu/iasp/pdfs/racial-wealth-equity/racial-wealth-gap/roots-widening-racial-wealth-gap.pdf

Shirai, K., Iso, H., Ohira, T., Ikeda, A., Noda, H., Honjo, K., . . . Japan Public Health Center-Based Study Group. (2009). Perceived level of life enjoyment and risks of cardiovascular disease incidence and mortality. *Circulation, 120*(11), 956–963.

Shmotkin, D. O. V. (1990). Subjective well-being as a function of age and gender: A multi-variate look for differentiated trends. *Social Indicators Research, 23*, 201–230.

Singer, B., Friedman, E., Seeman, T., Fava, G. A., & Ryff, C. D. (2005). Protective environments and health status: Cross-talk between human and animal studies. *Neurobiology of Aging, 26*(Suppl 1), 113–118.

Sloan, R. P., Schwarz, E., McKinley, P. S., Weinstein, M., Love, G., Ryff, C., . . . Seeman, T. (2017). Vagally-mediated heart rate variability and indices of well-being: Results of a nationally representative study. *Health Psychology, 36*(1), 73–81.

Smith, F., Fleeson, W., Geiselmann, B., Settersten, R. A. Jr., & Kunzmann, U. (1999). Sources of well-being in very old age. In P. B. Baltes & K. U. Mayer (Eds.), *The Berlin Aging Study: Aging from 70 to 100* (pp. 450–471). New York: Cambridge University Press.

Sommet, N., Morselli, D., & Spini, D. (2018). Income inequality affects the psychological health of only the people facing scarcity. *Psychological Science, 29*(12), 1911–1921.

Springer, K. W., Pudrovska, T., & Hauser, R. M. (2011). Does psychological well-being change with age? Longitudinal tests of age variations and further exploration of the multidimensionality of Ryff's model of psychological well-being. *Social Science Research, 40*(1), 392–398.

Staudinger, U. M., & Bluck, S. (2001). A view on midlife development from life-span theory. In M. E. Lachman (Ed.), *Handbook of midlife development* (pp. 3–39). New York: Wiley.

Stellar, J. E., John-Henderson, N., Anderson, C. L., Gordon, A. M., McNeil, G. D., & Keltner, D. (2015). Positive affect and markers of inflammation: Discrete positive emotions predict lower levels of inflammatory cytokines. *Emotion, 15*(2), 129–133.

Steptoe, A. (2019). Happiness and health. *Annual Review of Public Health, 40*(1), 339–359.

Steptoe, A., Demakakos, P., de Oliveira, C., & Wardle, J. (2012). Distinctive biological correlates of positive psychological well-being in older men and women. *Psychosomatic Medicine, 74*(5), 501–508.

Steptoe, A., Dockray, S., & Wardle, J. (2009). Positive affect and psychobiological processes relevant to health. *Journal of Personality, 77*(6), 1747–1776.

Steptoe, A., O'Donnell, K., Badrick, E., Kumari, M., & Marmot, M. (2008). Neuroendocrine and inflammatory factors associated with positive affect in healthy men and women: The Whitehall II study. *American Journal of Epidemiology, 167*(1), 96–102.

Steptoe, A., & Wardle, J. (2011). Positive affect measured using ecological momentary assessment and survival in older men and women. *Proceedings of the National Academy of Sciences of the United States of America, 108*(45), 18244–18248.

Steptoe, A., & Wardle, J. (2012). Enjoying life and living longer. *Archives of Internal Medicine, 172*(3), 273–275.

Stone, A. A., Schwartz, J. E., Broderick, J. E., & Deaton, A. (2010). A snapshot of the age distribution of psychological well-being in the United States. *Proceedings of the National Academy of Sciences, 107*(22), 9985–9990.

Suh, E., Diener, E., Oishi, S., & Triandis, H. D. (1998). The shifting basis of life satisfaction judgments across cultures: Emotions versus norms. *Journal of Personality and Social Psychology, 74*, 482–493.

Su, R., Tay, L., & Diener, E. (2014). The development and validation of the Comprehensive Inventory of Thriving (CIT) and the Brief Inventory of Thriving (BIT). *Applied Psychology: Health and Well-Being, 6*(3), 251–279.

Tay, L., Ng, V., Kuykendall, L., & Diener, E. (2014). Demographic factors and worker well-being: An empirical review using representative data from the United States and across the world. *Research in Occupational Stress and Well Being, 12*(September), 235–283.

Taylor, R. J., Chatters, L. M., Jayakody, R., & Levin, J. S. (1996). Black and white differences in religious participation: A multisample comparison. *Journal for the Scientific Study of Religion, 35*(4), 403–410.

Thomas, M. E., & Hughes, M. (1986). The continuing significance of race: A study of race, class, and quality of life in America, 1972–1985. *American Sociological Association, 51*(6), 830–841.

Trudel-Fitzgerald, C., Boehm, J. K., Kivimaki, M., & Kubzansky, L. D. (2014). Taking the tension out of hypertension: A prospective study of psychological well being and hypertension. *Journal of Hypertension, 32*(6), 1222–1228.

Tsenkova, V. K., Karlamangla, A. S., & Ryff, C. D. (2016). Parental history of diabetes, positive affect, and diabetes risk in adults: Findings from MIDUS. *Annals of Behavioral Medicine, 50*(6), 836–843.

Tsenkova, V. K., Love, G. D., Singer, B. H., & Ryff, C. D. (2007). Socioeconomic status and psychological well-being predict cross-time change in glycosylated hemoglobin in older women without diabetes. *Psychosomatic Medicine, 69*(8), 777–784.

Tsenkova, V. K., Love, G. D., Singer, B. H., & Ryff, C. D. (2008). Coping and positive affect predict longitudinal change in glycosylated hemoglobin. *Health Psychology, 27,* S163–S171.

VanderWeele, T. J. (2017). On the promotion of human flourishing. *Proceedings of the National Academy of Sciences, 114*(31), 8148–8156.

Veenhoven, R. (1991). Is happiness relative? *Social Indicators Research, 24,* 1–34.

Vittersø, J. (2013). Happiness, inspiration, and the fully functioning person: Separating hedonic and eudaimonic well-being in the workplace. *Journal of Positive Psychology, 7,* 387–398.

Waterman, A. S. (1993). Two conceptions of happiness: Contrasts of personal expressiveness (eudaimonia) and hedonic enjoyment. *Journal of Personality and Social Psychology, 64,* 678–691.

Watson, D., Clark, L. A., & Tellegen, A. (1988). Development and validation of brief measures of positive and negative affect: The PANAS scales. *Journal of Personality and Social Psychology, 54,* 1063–1070.

White, J. M. (1992). Marital Status and Well-Being in Canada. *Journal of Family Issues, 13*(3), 390–409.

Williams, D. R., & Harris-Reid, M. (1999). Race and mental health: Emerging patterns and promising approaches. In A. V. Horwitz & T. L. Scheid (Eds.), *A handbook for the study of mental health: Social contexts, theories, and systems* (pp. 295–314). Cambridge University Press.

Wilson, R. S., Capuano, A. W., James, B. D., Amofa, P., Arvanitakis, Z., Shah, R., . . . Boyle, P. A. (2018). Purpose in life and hospitalization for ambulatory care-sensitive conditions in old age. *American Journal of Geriatric Psychiatry, 26*(3), 364–374.

Xu, J., & Roberts, R. E. (2010). The power of positive emotions: It's a matter of life or death—Subjective well-being and longevity over 28 years in a general population. *Health Psychology, 29*(1), 9–19.

Yanek, L. R., Kral, B. G., Moy, T. F., Vaidya, D., Lazo, M., Becker, L. C., & Becker, D. M. (2013). Effect of positive well-being on incidence of symptomatic coronary artery disease. *American Journal of Cardiology, 112*(8), 1120–1125.

Yang, Y. (2008). Social inequalities in happiness in the United States, 1972 to 2004: An age-period cohort analysis. *American Sociological Review, 73*, 204–226.

Yoo, J., Miyamoto, Y., Rigotti, A., & Ryff, C. D. (2017). Linking positive affect to blood lipids: A cultural perspective. *Psychological Science, 28*(10), 1468–1477.

Yoo, J., Miyamoto, Y., & Ryff, C. D. (2016). Positive affect, social connectedness, and healthy biomarkers in Japan and the US. *Emotion, 16*(8), 1137–1146.

Zautra, A. J., Johnson, L. M., & Davis, M. C. (2005). Positive affect as a source of resilience for women in chronic pain. *Journal of Consulting and Clinical Psychology, 73*(2), 212–220.

Zilioli, S., Imami, L., & Slatcher, R. B. (2015). Life satisfaction moderates the impact of socioeconomic status on diurnal cortisol slope. *Psychoneuroendocrinology, 60*, 91–95.

Zilioli, S., Slatcher, R. B., Ong, A. D., & Gruenewald, T. L. (2015). Purpose in life predicts allostatic load ten years later. *Journal of Psychosomatic Research, 79*(5), 451–457.

Zuckerman, M., Li, C., & Diener, E. F. (2017). Societal conditions and the gender difference in well-being: Testing a three-stage model. *Personality and Social Psychology Bulletin, 43*(3), 329–336.

5

A Review of Psychological Well-Being and Mortality Risk

Are All Dimensions of Psychological Well-Being Equal?

Claudia Trudel-Fitzgerald, Laura D. Kubzansky,
and Tyler J. VanderWeele

Abstract

Increasing evidence suggests that psychological well-being (PWB) is associated with lower chronic disease and mortality risk and may be enhanced with relatively low-cost interventions. While many interventions are targeted at specific dimensions of PWB (e.g., optimism, purpose in life), limited research has evaluated rigorously whether distinct PWB dimensions may differentially impact physical health outcomes. Without clear understanding of which dimensions of PWB are most relevant for physical health, effectiveness of PWB interventions to improve physical health will be limited and difficult to assess. A growing body of research has considered multiple PWB dimensions in relation to mortality risk, but a comparison of findings across studies has not been done. This chapter summarizes the empirical evidence regarding specific relationships between all-cause mortality and multiple dimensions of PWB (e.g., life purpose, mastery, positive affect, life satisfaction, optimism). It also reviews possible biological (e.g., inflammation, antioxidants) and behavioral (e.g., smoking, physical activity) mechanistic pathways that could explain these associations. Methodological considerations for epidemiological studies targeting the potential protective role of psychological well-being in risk of mortality (and other health-related outcomes) are discussed, and recommendations for future directions in this field are provided.

Claudia Trudel-Fitzgerald, Laura D. Kubzansky, and Tyler J. VanderWeele, *A Review of Psychological Well-Being and Mortality Risk* In: *Measuring Well-Being*. Edited by: Matthew T. Lee, Laura D. Kubzansky, and Tyler J. VanderWeele, Oxford University Press (2021). © Oxford University Press. DOI: 10.1093/oso/9780197512531.003.0006

Over the past decades, evidence for the physical health benefits of enhanced psychological well-being (PWB) has expanded dramatically (Boehm & Kubzansky, 2012; Pressman, Jenkins, & Moskowitz, 2019). Notably, research in the fields of behavioral and psychosomatic medicine as well as health psychology have substantially contributed to this body of work (Boehm & Kubzansky, 2012; Folkman & Moskowitz, 2000; Kobau et al., 2011; Pressman et al., 2019; Seligman & Csikszentmihalyi, 2000; Steptoe, 2019; Van Cappellen, Rice, Catalino, & Fredrickson, 2018). Yet such work is still neglected by the public health community. For instance, the discipline of epidemiology maintains a primary focus on risk, deficits, and problems rather than on identifying and promoting factors that might serve as assets to enhance health and longevity (VanderWeele et al., 2020). Similarly, although it is well accepted that PWB represents more than the absence of psychological distress (e.g., depressive and anxiety symptoms; Boehm & Kubzansky, 2012; Ryff et al., 2006), in medicine, PWB assessment is not part of usual care (VanderWeele, McNeely, & Koh, 2019). Nonetheless, associations of PWB with subsequent physical health outcomes have been well-documented, with findings generally suggesting that higher PWB is associated with reduced risk of chronic diseases like cardiovascular disease and diabetes, as well as increased likelihood of healthy aging and longevity (Boehm & Kubzansky, 2012; Pressman et al., 2019; Steptoe, 2019). However, there are some conflicting results in this literature that may explain, at least in part, ongoing skepticism among the broader scientific community as to the importance of PWB as a health asset (Miller, Sherman, & Christensen, 2010).

Until recently, most investigators have not carefully distinguished between dimensions of PWB regarding their impact on physical health or considered whether all dimensions have similar effects (Diener, Lucas, & Oishi, 2018), even though PWB is clearly comprised of distinct dimensions (e.g., positive affect, optimism, life satisfaction). While distinct dimensions of PWB may share common variance, they could differentially impact physical health, thereby explaining certain conflicting findings (Pressman et al., 2019). If PWB is to be embraced by the public health community as a health asset and incorporated into decision-making and policies along with efforts targeting other established social determinants of physical health like poverty, education, discrimination, and social capital (Berkman, Kawachi, & Glymour, 2014; Marmot & Wilkinson, 2005), these distinctions need to be made clear.

In this chapter, we review the empirical evidence from the most rigorous methods available on associations of multiple PWB dimensions with all-cause mortality, an objective endpoint and the aftermath of various chronic diseases. We consider those dimensions that have received some attention in the literature and have been captured by leading theoretical perspectives in PWB research (described later); these dimensions include life purpose, personal growth, mastery, autonomy, *ikigai*, life satisfaction, positive affect, sense of coherence, optimism, and emotional vitality. We further consider potential behavioral and biological mechanisms that could underlie these associations and whether such mechanisms are likely to be similar across different dimensions of PWB. Finally, we discuss future avenues for research in this field.

Defining Well-Being

Well-being is a complex and multifactorial construct. Measures of well-being are sometimes divided into objective measures that mostly seek to capture "standard of living," as reflected by levels of education or income, physical health; and subjective measures that seek to capture psychological, social, and spiritual experiences based on an individual's perceptions (Lee Kum Sheung Center for Health and Happiness, 2017; National Research Council, 2013). When these measures concern psychological aspects (e.g., happiness) and are derived from cognitive and affective judgments a person makes about his or her life, they are often referred to as *measures of psychological well-being* (PWB). PWB has been a central area of research in psychology for decades (Kobau et al., 2011; Seligman & Csikszentmihalyi, 2000), most commonly used in studies as an outcome in its own right. It is also increasingly taken up in epidemiologic research to understand its contribution to health outcomes and, more broadly, to public health, notably to implement country-level monitoring and policies promoting overall health (Diener & Seligman, 2018; Kobau et al., 2011).

Distinct theoretical perspectives have been proposed to characterize PWB research thus far (for more details, see Boehm & Kubzansky, 2012; Hernandez et al., 2018; National Research Council, 2013; Ryff, 2017; Steptoe, 2019): hedonic well-being (e.g., feeling happy), evaluative well-being (e.g., being satisfied with life, although life satisfaction is also sometimes categorized as an hedonic dimension), eudaimonic well-being (e.g., finding purpose in life, having a sense of mastery and autonomy in one's own decisions), and other constructs that contribute to feeling whole or well (e.g., optimism).

While some of these dimensions may be conceptualized as more stable over time, like psychological attributes (e.g., optimism, life satisfaction), others may be more variable or transient states (e.g., positive affect, happiness).

Research has documented statistically significant associations between PWB constructs themselves. For instance, pioneering work showed magnitude of estimates varying from small (e.g., $r = 0.13$ between purpose in life and autonomy) to moderate (e.g., $r = 0.46$ between self-acceptance and mastery) when evaluated among a nationally representative sample of 1,108 US adults, aged 46 years on average (Ryff & Keyes, 1995). Since then, various studies have aimed to replicate these results using the same scales. Stronger correlations have been observed in both larger US samples and non-US representative samples: for example, $r = 0.60$ between self-acceptance and mastery in a nationally representative sample of 3,487 midlife adults in the US (Hsu, Hsu, Lee, & Wolff, 2017), whereas $r = 0.57$ between purpose in life and autonomy among 1,179 midlife women in the United Kingdom (Abbott et al., 2006). However, in some cases estimates were somewhat weaker: for example, $r = 0.39$ between self-acceptance and mastery among 4,960 older adults in Canada (Clarke, Marshall, Ryff, & Wheaton, 2001). Research conducted in younger adults, such as colleges students, also revealed significant but moderate correlations between various measures of life satisfaction and positive affect (i.e., r values from 0.43 to 0.52; Lucas, Diener, & Suh, 1996). Overall, these findings suggest that although some variation may exist across samples, PWB dimensions may both share a latent factor and also represent distinct constructs.

Psychological Well-Being and All-Cause Mortality

Psychological Well-Being as a Determinant of Physical Health

Given that various PWB dimensions, as measured with self-reported scales in most cases, have been linked with myriad health-related outcomes, it is plausible that PWB would be reliably associated with all-cause mortality. In prior research conducted in the general population (i.e., nonmedical samples), greater PWB levels have been related to lower risk of various chronic conditions (e.g., cardiometabolic diseases, infectious illness, arthritis) and of physical and cognitive decline, although results with cancer are less clear (Boehm & Kubzansky, 2012; Kim et al., 2017; Okely, Cooper, &

Gale, 2016; Okely & Gale, 2016; Pressman et al., 2019; Ryff, Heller, Schaefer, van Reekum, & Davidson, 2016). Emerging evidence also suggests that various PWB dimensions, particularly higher levels of optimism, positive affect, and life satisfaction, are associated with lifespan (i.e., life duration) and exceptional longevity (Lee et al., 2019; Liu et al., 2014), which is typically defined as survival to 85 years or beyond (Newman & Murabito, 2013; Revelas et al., 2018). Life extension in individuals who experience greater levels of PWB could be explained, at least in part, by compressed morbidity and aging in health. This hypothesis is in fact supported by recent prospective study results showing that midlife adults with higher levels of optimism and mastery, respectively, are more likely to be healthy agers compared to their counterparts with lower PWB levels (James et al., 2019; Kim et al., 2019; Latham-Mintus, Vowels, & Huskins, 2018).

Existing Methodological Concerns

Although the PWB–health relationship is likely to be bidirectional, whereby PWB influences physical health outcomes and vice versa, the primary interest of this body of research is to determine whether PWB is causally related to health outcomes. Such examination is crucial from a primary or primordial prevention perspective; in fact, if such effects exist, subsequent efforts should develop and implement specific policy and interventions that target PWB to improve physical health and longevity. However, even when studies use longitudinal data to examine relationships, whereby PWB precedes subsequent health outcomes, due to methodological limitations it is not always clear whether observed associations (1) would remain after more rigorous confounder control (i.e., a third factor influencing both PWB and health) and (2) do not capture reverse causation (i.e., health status driving PWB levels). Considering mortality risk, an objective endpoint, offers some methodological strengths, such as virtually no misclassification and research that requires a longitudinal design by nature of the outcome.

Overview of Meta-Analyses Targeting Mortality

Recent meta-analyses have suggested that distinct PWB dimensions are protective against mortality (Cohen, Bavishi, & Rozanski, 2016; Martin-Maria et al., 2017; Rozanski, Bavishi, Kubzansky, & Cohen, 2019; Zhang & Han, 2016). For instance, after pooling 10 studies (total N = 136,265), higher versus lower levels of purpose in life were associated with a multivariate-adjusted 17% reduced mortality risk (relative risk [RR] = 0.83, 95% confidence intervals [CI] [0.75, 0.91]) over a mean follow-up of 7 years (Cohen et al., 2016). Results from nine pooled studies comprising 188,599 participants further suggested a 14% decreased risk in all-cause mortality (RR = 0.86, CI [0.80, 0.92] over 8–40 years for individuals with highest versus lowest levels of optimism (Rozanski et al., 2019). Another meta-analysis combined 22 studies with sample sizes ranging from 101 to 97,253 participants (Zhang & Han, 2016); each included study assessed the risk of mortality for higher versus lower levels of either a PWB dimension (i.e., optimism, life satisfaction, happiness, and positive affect) or a related well-being construct (i.e., attitude toward aging) as the exposure. The authors evaluated first the association of mortality risk with overall well-being (all exposures pooled) and then examined mortality risk with each exposure separately. Results from unadjusted models indicated a 25% decreased risk of mortality for elevated levels of overall well-being, as well as 46%, 28%, 29%, and 16% decreased risk of mortality for elevated levels of life satisfaction, happiness, optimism, and positive affect, respectively, over 17 years on average. Interestingly, effect estimates from individual exposures evaluated independently were statistically significantly different from one another (p <0.05), but, after adjustment for covariates, the differences in the magnitude of associations was attenuated and nonsignificant. However, it was unclear whether each individual exposure remained associated with mortality after such statistical control since the multivariate estimates were reported for overall well-being only (showing a 15% reduced risk of mortality; Zhang & Han, 2016). Findings from another meta-analysis of 90 studies (N = 1,309,527; 50% of studies with at least 10 years of follow-up) examining life satisfaction, positive affect, and purpose in life also suggested that estimates of mortality associations across these three PWB dimensions did not significantly differ (Martin-Maria et al., 2017). Moreover, in this meta-analysis, the associations with mortality remained statistically significant after covariate control: compared to participants with lower levels, those with higher levels of life satisfaction, positive affect, and purpose in life had a 12%, 8%, and 7% decreased risk of mortality, respectively, over the follow-up periods across studies.

However, in all of these meta-analyses the quality of statistical adjustment for potential confounders in the included studies was variable and the cause of death was heterogeneous (e.g., all-cause and some cause-specific deaths pooled), which prevent more precise conclusions. Moreover, certain PWB dimensions have received more attention than others, probably due to data availability across selected samples. Notably, numerous individual studies have considered life satisfaction (Martin-Maria et al., 2017; Zhang & Han, 2016). There have also been sufficient studies on purpose in life and optimism to conduct meta-analyses on these PWB dimensions (Cohen et al., 2016; Rozanski et al., 2019); of note, in the purpose in life meta-analysis, the inclusion criteria was fairly large and comprised studies on closely related construct such as *ikigai*, which conceptually captures more than life purpose (as detailed later). Conversely, fewer focused on positive affect (Martin-Maria et al., 2017), or, when they did, some of the included studies used lower levels of negative affect (e.g., sadness, depressive symptoms) as an indicator of higher levels of positive affect (Zhang & Han, 2016). This is problematic because the absence of psychological distress does not necessarily denote the presence of PWB (Boehm & Kubzansky, 2012; Ryff et al., 2006), and depression scales were not developed to measure positive affect per se (Ryff et al., 2006; Ryff & Singer, 2007).

Criteria for Selecting Studies Included in This Chapter

Here, we provide an overview of the evidence of whether and how various PWB dimensions are associated with reduced risk of all-cause mortality in follow-up. Literature searches within PubMed and PsycInfo databases targeted individual prospective and longitudinal studies evaluating the role of at least one PWB dimension with all-cause mortality risk, written in English or French. Dimensions needed to be evaluated with a PWB scale rather than one aimed at measuring psychological distress. Additional studies were obtained through bibliographies of eligible articles. Individual studies included in this narrative review were selected for their methodological rigor, with some of them being included in the meta-analyses cited previously, whereas others were published subsequently. In considering rigorous studies, we retained studies that adjusted for all the following categories of potential covariates at baseline (i.e., when PWB was measured): sociodemographic factors (e.g., age, sex, education), medical status (e.g., blood pressure, body mass index, chronic conditions), and health behaviors (e.g., smoking, physical activity). Therefore, all reported estimates (e.g., hazard ratios, relative risk) in this chapter are multivariate estimates from studies that statistically adjusted for at least one indicator of each of these three categories of covariates in their analytic models.[1] Some studies further adjusted for psychological distress to account for its potentially confounding role between PWB and mortality as well as to determine PWB's role on mortality beyond any effects of ill-being (e.g., anxiety and depression symptoms; as depicted in Figure 5.1). Some studies also additionally controlled for self-rated health, which is one of the strongest predictors of future morbidity and mortality risk and is usually assessed via one item asking whether individuals perceive their health as excellent, very good, good, fair, or poor (Jylha, 2009; Picard, Juster, & Sabiston, 2013). We explicitly mention in the following sections when studies performed further statistical adjustment for psychological distress and/or self-rated health beyond the sociodemographics, medical, and behavioral covariates just mentioned.

Results of the Narrative Review

Dimensions Related to Eudaimonic Well-Being
Purpose in Life. Experiencing a sense of purpose and direction in one's life has been studied substantially, with results indicating a consistent association with reduced mortality over each study's follow-up period. The three studies described here have all used the purpose in life subscale from the Scales of Psychological Well-Being (Ryff, 1989). In one of the most rigorous studies included in the meta-analysis cited earlier (Cohen et al., 2016), every standard deviation (*SD*) increase in life purpose was associated with 40% decreased hazard of 5-year mortality (hazard ratio [HR] = 0.60; CI [0.42, 0.87] among 1,236 older US adults from the Rush Memory and Aging Project, and Minority Aging Research Study (mean age = 78 years; Boyle, Barnes, Buchman, & Bennett, 2009). In the Women's Health Initiative cohort, after additional statistical control for psychological distress in multivariable models, greater life purpose was also associated with lower likelihood of death over a 2-year period in 7,675 US women aged 65 years and older (Zaslavsky et al., 2014). Interestingly, in a recent study of 6,985 older adults from the nationally representative Health and Retirement Study conducted after publication of the meta-analysis, the association was maintained not only after adjustment for traditional covariates and psychological distress, but also after further controlling for other PWB dimensions including

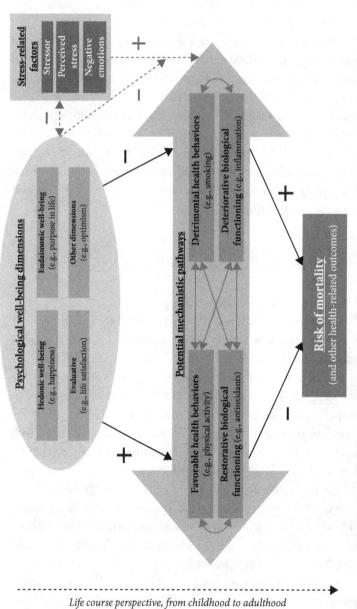

Figure 5.1 Potential biobehavioral pathways relating psychological well-being (PWB) to risk of mortality.

For the purpose of this chapter, other psychosocial assets (e.g., social integration, emotional support) are omitted from this figure. Likewise, while bidirectional effects between psychological well-being and biobehavioral processes are likely, in keeping with the focus of the chapter, only single-direction arrows are shown. For a more in-depth explanation of the role of stress-related factors in the PWB–health associations, see Pressman et al. (2019).

Model adapted from Boehm & Kubzansky (2012), Kubzansky et al. (2018), Trudel-Fitzgerald, Qureshi, Appleton, & Kubzansky (2017).

optimism, positive affect, and social participation (lowest vs. highest quintiles of life purpose: HR = 2.43, CI [1.57, 3.75]; Alimujiang et al., 2019).

Some research has examined the role of *meaning* in life, but the results are less convincing than those assessing purpose. "Purpose in life" and "meaning in life" are two terms that some studies have treated interchangeably as referring to the same underlying construct. However, emerging theoretical and empirical work has led to greater distinction between the terms and the recent development of a tripartite model of meaning in life, which consists of three subconstructs: (1) *purpose* in life, (2) coherence/comprehension (the degree to which people perceive that their lives make sense), and (3) significance/mattering (the degree to which people feel their existence is of significance, importance, and value in the world; George & Park, 2017; Chapter 12, in this volume; Martela & Steger, 2016). These constructs may be differentially associated with mortality. A study of 1,361 older US adults (mean age = 79 years) over 5 years evaluated meaning in life with a shortened version of Krause's scale (Krause, 2004), which captures four domains (i.e., values, purpose, goals, and reconciliation with the past) that can be related to the three subconstructs reported earlier. No relationship of meaning in life with all-cause mortality (odds ratio [OR] = 0.97; CI [0.93, 1.01]) was found in multivariable models adjusting for self-rated health, although it is worth noting that in the sociodemographics-adjusted model, the association was small but statistically significant (OR = 0.92; CI [0.89, 0.96]; Krause, 2009). These results could also raise the question of whether "meaning" and "purpose," often used interchangeably, might indeed capture constructs that relate differently to mortality.

Personal Growth. To our knowledge, personal growth—that is, whether individuals seek to realize their full potential and recognize that the self is constantly developing (Boehm & Kubzansky, 2012; Ryff & Keyes, 1995)—has been explored in relation to mortality risk in only one study. In the Women's Health Initiative investigation described earlier, using items from the Scales of Psychological Well-Being (Ryff, 1989), personal growth levels were associated with lower 2-year mortality rates when personal growth was considered as a continuous (per 1-unit increase: HR = 0.95; CI [0.93, 0.98]) or categorical variable (lower vs. higher [reference group] quartile: OR = 2.10, CI [1.42, 3.08]; Zaslavsky et al., 2014). As mentioned earlier, this study also evaluated life purpose, and a comparison of multivariable-adjusted estimates for life purpose versus personal growth (ORs = 3.55 vs. 2.10) suggested stronger associations of purpose with mortality in these women aged 65 years and older.

Mastery. Mastery—whether individuals effectively manage their environments or perceive life as being under their control (Boehm & Kubzansky, 2012; Ryff & Keyes, 1995)—has been well-studied in relation to mortality, although not all investigations have rigorously taken into account key potential confounders (e.g., sociodemographics, medical status). Among those who did, an early investigation followed 2,829 Dutch adults (aged 55–85) from the Longitudinal Aging Study Amsterdam for up to 3 years (Penninx et al., 1997). In this study, each 1-unit rise in mastery as captured by an abbreviated 5-item version of the Pearlin Mastery Scale (Pearlin & Schooler, 1978) was associated with 6% lower mortality odds (OR = 0.94, CI [0.89, 0.99]), even after extensive adjustment of covariates including PWB correlates such as self-rated health, social support, self-efficacy, and self-esteem. Likewise, among English adults from the EPIC-Norfolk Study (*N* = 20,495; aged 41–80), every 1-*SD* increase in mastery based on a modified 7-item version of the Pearlin Mastery Scale was associated with an 18% lower rate of death (RR = 0.82, CI [0.76, 0.89]) over 5 years, after further controlling for psychological distress (Surtees, Wainwright, Luben, Khaw, & Day, 2006). Similar results have also been obtained in US samples and with alternative measures of mastery. For example, in the Midlife in the United States study (MIDUS), authors developed several additional items and combined them with some items from the Pearlin Mastery Scale (Turiano, Chapman, Agrigoroaei, Infurna, & Lachman, 2014).

Autonomy. Although research is sparse, available evidence to date has not found consistent associations of mortality risk with autonomy, characterized as the extent to which individuals act independently without concern for external pressures (Boehm & Kubzansky, 2012; Ryff & Keyes, 1995). For example, in a relatively large study of 9,420 midlife British adults (mean age = 58 years), the autonomy subscale from the Control, Autonomy, Self-Realization, and Pleasure (CASP) scale (Hyde, Wiggins, Higgs, & Blane, 2003) was considered in relation to mortality risk over a 5-year period (Netuveli, Pikhart, Bobak, & Blane, 2012). Autonomy scores were modestly but significantly related to the hazard of death in the unadjusted model (per 1-*SD* increase: HR = 1.07, CI [1.00, 1.13]) but were attenuated and no longer statistically significant in multivariate models that further controlled for self-rated health and psychological distress (per 1-unit increase: HR = 1.02; CI [0.96, 1.09]; although health behaviors were not assessed in this study; Netuveli et al., 2012). While these results may reflect a true null association, different findings may be obtained with the use of a different autonomy scale. In fact, the 19-item CASP scale (Hyde et al., 2003) includes general statements such as "I can do the things that I want to do," which could be conflated with a sense of physical autonomy. By contrast, the autonomy subscale from the Scales of Psychological Well-Being (Ryff, 1989) refers more to the psychological facet of autonomy (e.g., "My decisions are not usually influenced by what everyone else is doing"), which may relate differently to mortality. To our knowledge, no studies have examined a measure that solely captures psychological autonomy in relation to mortality risk among non-medical samples.

Ikigai. This term is uniquely Japanese and does not directly translate to a single English term that has been examined in non-Japanese samples. *Ikigai* has been defined as having a sense of happiness, worth, and benefit of being alive (Sone et al., 2008; Tanno et al., 2009). While it largely captures eudaimonic well-being (e.g., life purpose), it also encompasses aspects of hedonic well-being (e.g., pleasure), although usually assessed with only one item (Sone et al., 2008; Tanno et al., 2009). Findings obtained from a handful of published studies are generally positive. For example, using data from the nationwide Japan Collaborative Cohort Study for Evaluation of Cancer Risk (N = 73,272; aged 40–79), adults with versus without *ikigai* had a reduced hazard of mortality over 5 years (HR_{men} = 0.80; CI [0.72, 0.89]; HR_{women} = 0.80; CI [0.69, 0.92]; Tanno et al., 2009). In another Japanese cohort, the Ohsaki National Health Insurance Cohort Study (N = 43,391; aged 40–79), lower and moderate *ikigai* levels (vs. higher) were related to an increased 7-year hazard of death ($HR_{moderate}$ = 1.1; CI [1.0, 1.2]; HR_{lower} = 1.5; CI [1.3, 1.7]), with further adjustment for self-rated health not altering these results (Sone et al., 2008).

Dimensions Related to Hedonic Well-Being
Positive Affect. Feeling happy, joyful, cheerful, excited, and proud are often included in the construct of positive affect. As mentioned earlier, there has been a substantial number of studies conducted on positive affect's role in mortality risk, although the number is somewhat reduced after excluding studies that measured (the absence of) negative affect because it does not truly capture positive affect. In one study using data from the German Aging Survey (N = 3,124; aged 40–85), every unit increase in positive affect, as assessed with 10 items from the Positive and Negative Affect Schedule (PANAS) measure (Watson, Clark, & Tellegen, 1988), was associated with a 19% lower 14-year mortality risk after adjusting for sociodemographics,

medical status, psychological distress, and also life satisfaction (HR = 0.81, CI [0.70, 0.93]); further controlling for self-rated health and physical activity attenuated the association (HR = 0.88, CI [0.76, 1.02]; Wiest, Schuz, Webster, & Wurm, 2011). However, in a recent study of adults from Norway (N = 5,554; aged 47–74) that also used the 10 PANAS items, even after adjusting for sociodemographics, medical status, health behaviors (smoking, alcohol use, and physical activity), and psychological distress, positive affect remained significantly associated with mortality risk (Petrie et al., 2018). Specifically, individuals categorized in the lower versus higher tertile of positive affect scores had a 38% increased risk of death (HR = 1.38; CI [1.12, 1.71]) over an average of 16.5 years of follow-up. No significant association was obtained for participants in the moderate tertile, and results were robust to further adjustment for psychological distress (Petrie et al., 2018).

Happiness. Although happiness is a pleasurable feeling that is sometimes included in positive affect, it has also been studied as a separate construct in prior PWB–mortality research. In a subset of the Million Women Study (N = 719,617; aged 53–72), English women who said they were "unhappy" or "usually happy" on a 1-item measure did not differ in mortality risk in 10-year follow-up compared to those who said they were "happy most of the time" (RR = 0.98, CI [0.94, 1.01]; RR = 0.99, CI [0.96, 1.01], respectively; Liu et al., 2016). While this study has drawn media attention because of its methodological strengths (e.g., large sample size, statistical control for multiple covariates), its conclusions obtained from the use of a single happiness item have also has generated some controversy within the scientific community based on this and other methodological limitations and concerns (e.g., Diener, Pressman, & Lyubomirsky, 2015; Kubzansky, Kim, Salinas, Huffman, & Kawachi, 2016). Moreover, the thin distinction between some levels of exposure (i.e., "happy most of the time" [reference group] vs. "usually happy") could also have contributed to the null results. Likewise, another rigorous study of 861 older adults from the Arnhem Elderly Study found no association between happiness assessed with two items (i.e., "I have many moments of happiness" and "I often laugh happily") and mortality over a 15-year follow-up period (Koopmans, Geleijnse, Zitman, & Giltay, 2010). Taken together, findings from studies on positive affect and happiness as a unitary construct may suggest that the comprehensive experience of various types of positive affect, rather than the sole experience of feeling happy as captured by single items, matters more in terms of longevity.

Dimensions Related to Evaluative Well-Being

Life Satisfaction. Life satisfaction can be measured either globally, capturing the extent to which individuals judge their life as a whole to be satisfactory, or specifically, by individual life domains (e.g., work, family). Although a handful of studies have investigated the role of specific life domains in mortality risk, they were not included in the current narrative review either because they considered mortality from coronary heart disease solely (Boehm, Peterson, Kivimaki, & Kubzansky, 2011) or did not adjust for health behaviors (St John, Mackenzie, & Menec, 2015). Yet these preliminary results suggest that some, but not all, dimensions of life satisfaction could relate to mortality risk, thus supporting the need for further research in this area. Global life satisfaction is frequently measured with a single item. As a result, it has been included in various epidemiological cohorts and other long-standing population-based studies, which have provided follow-up periods long enough to ascertain death cases in multiple studies on this topic. Unlike happiness, the use of single life satisfaction items has been validated in three large studies and has shown a substantial degree of criterion validity with multi-item, validated scales of life satisfaction (Cheung & Lucas, 2014).

A Canadian population-based study ($N = 73,904$; aged 18 to >80) revealed that "very dissatisfied" versus "very satisfied or satisfied" individuals had an increased mortality risk over 6 years (HR = 1.70, CI [1.16, 2.51]) after controlling for numerous relevant covariates (Rosella, Fu, Buajitti, & Goel, 2018). These results were consistent with other studies conducted among different samples using single life satisfaction items, including among 4,458 Australian adults over 9 years (Boehm, Winning, Segerstrom, & Kubzansky, 2015) and 10,957 German adults over 20 years (Hulur et al., 2017). In the German Aging Survey described earlier, mortality risk was reduced by 11% for each unit increase in life satisfaction, as measured with the 5-item Satisfaction with Life Scale (Pavot, Diener, Colvin, & Sandvik, 1991), after further adjusting for sociodemographics, medical status, psychological distress and also positive affect (HR = 0.89, CI [0.79, 1.00]), but the association was substantially attenuated and became not statistically significant after additional control for self-rated health and physical activity (Wiest et al., 2011). Although the estimate appears stronger with positive affect than life satisfaction in this study (even when both were included simultaneously in the statistical models), these dimensions were assessed with distinct scales and scores were not standardized, which precludes formal comparison. Other authors have reported an elevated 12-year risk of mortality with lower life satisfaction (assessed using the 20-item Life Satisfaction Index A [LSI-A]) among 1,939 Korean men and women from the Kangwha Cohort (Kimm, Sull, Gombojav, Yi, & Ohrr, 2012). However, a closer look at the 20 items composing the LSI-A revealed that, while most captured life satisfaction, some queried other PWB dimensions (e.g., "I expect some interesting and pleasant things to happen to me in the future"), as well as physical states (e.g., "I feel old and somewhat tired"; Neugarten, Havighurst, & Tobin, 1961), which raises the question of whether the association obtained in this study was truly driven by life satisfaction per se.

Other Psychological Well-Being Dimensions

Sense of Coherence. Sense of coherence is a fairly stable personality disposition that encompasses three constructs: the belief that what happens in individuals' lives is rational, predictable, structured, and understandable (comprehensibility); that adequate and sufficient resources are perceived to be available to help resolve difficulties as they arise (manageability); and that the demands created by exposure to adversity are seen as challenges and are worthy of engagement (meaningfulness; Antonovsky, 1987). It may be worth mentioning that, when looking more closely at the items usually used to measure these constructs, the meaningfulness items (e.g., "Do you usually feel that your daily life is a source of personal satisfaction?"; "How often do you have a feeling that there's little meaning in the things you do in your daily life?") seem to overlap with other PWB dimensions, such as life satisfaction and meaning in life. For this reason, future studies about sense of coherence should consider associations by constructs separately, to disentangle whether any protective effects on mortality risk might instead be attributed to other PWB constructs captured by this construct. Models that include other PWB dimensions in addition to sense of coherence as the exposure would also speak to whether sense of coherence may uniquely contribute to morality risk.

That said, sense of coherence, when taken as a whole, appears to be related to reduced mortality risk over time in several studies that have been conducted on the topic. One of the most rigorous early studies evaluating its role in mortality risk was conducted in the EPIC-Norfolk Study among 16,668 men and women aged 41–80 at baseline (Surtees, Wainwright, Luben, Khaw, & Day, 2003). Sense of coherence was captured by the sum of three items each measuring one of the three primary constructs in the theory (i.e., manageability, comprehensibility, and meaningfulness;

Lundberg & Peck, 1995). Adults with higher (vs. lower) sense of coherence had a 24% reduced risk of 6-year mortality (RR = 0.76, CI [0.64, 0.90]) after control for multiple covariates including psychological distress. These results were replicated among 10,863 Dutch adults aged 20–65 from the Monitoring Project on Chronic Risk Factors (MORGEN) who completed the same three items in a subsequent study with an average follow-up of 14 years (Super, Verschuren, Zantinge, Wagemakers, & Picavet, 2014). Findings with this longer follow-up period showed that, compared to participants with moderate levels of sense of coherence, those with lower levels had a 27% increased risk of mortality (HR = 1.27; CI [1.01, 1.59]) even after further adjustment for self-rated health (Super et al., 2014). Somewhat surprisingly, no significant differences were observed between moderate and higher levels, perhaps hinting at a threshold effect at which lower sense of coherence levels can be harmful for longevity. Alternatively, some authors have reported poorer psychometric properties, including lack of discrimination across higher scores, for this 3-item version of the Antonovsky's scale compared to the longer 13- and 29-item versions (Olsson, Gassne, & Hansson, 2009).

When researchers did use these more comprehensive assessments of the three sense of coherence constructs, results were generally consistent, albeit more nuanced. For instance, one study of 585 men from the Israel Study of Glucose Intolerance, Obesity, and Hypertension Study followed for 22 years used the original Antonovsky 29-item scale (Antonovsky, 1993): results showed that men with the highest versus lowest tertile of scores had a 34% reduced risk of mortality (HR = 0.66, CI [0.46, 0.94]; Geulayov, Drory, Novikov, & Dankner, 2015). Although the association was not statistically significant among men with an intermediate versus lower level of sense of coherence, every 1-unit increase in sense of coherence was modestly but significantly associated with reduced mortality risk (HR = 0.99, CI [0.99, 1.00]; Geulayov et al., 2015). In another investigation using an abbreviated 13-item version of Antonosky's scale among 7,933 adults from the National FINRISK Study, every 1-SD increase was related to 10% lower risk of death (HR = 0.90; CI [0.84, 0.97]) over 14 years follow-up on average (Haukkala, Konttinen, Laatikainen, Kawachi, & Uutela, 2010). These findings might suggest that a smaller, monotonic increase in sense of coherence also matters for reducing mortality risk. However, because further adjustment in this study for depressive symptoms attenuated associations whereby they were no longer statistically significant, it remains unclear whether sense of coherence has an independent effect or is distinct from the lack of psychological distress (Haukkala et al., 2010).

Optimism. Optimism has been conceptualized either as a dispositional trait—a person's general expectation that the future will turn out well or that good things will happen in the future—or an explanatory style, in this case a person's tendency to make internal, stable, and global attributions for good events (Scheier & Carver, 2018; Tennen & Affleck, 1987). Prior work suggests these forms of optimism are moderately to highly correlated (Kubzansky et al., 2002; Scheier, Carver, & Bridges, 2001). While dispositional optimism has been considered in multiple investigations of both chronic disease and mortality risk, explanatory style optimism has not been assessed in relation to mortality risk specifically thus far. Evidence indicates that higher dispositional optimism is associated with lower mortality risk. A study of 97,253 women aged 50–79 participating in the Women's Health Initiative showed that scoring in the highest versus lowest quartile of optimism, as defined by the 6-item Life Orientation Test-Revised (LOT-R) scale (Scheier, Carver, & Bridges, 1994), was related to a 14% reduced hazard of mortality over 8 years (HR = 0.86, CI [0.79, 0.93]) even after adding psychological distress to multivariable models (Tindle et al., 2009). Analyses conducted in another cohort of midlife US women, the Nurses' Health Study, replicated these results using the same research design (Kim et al., 2017). Additionally, a Netherlands-based study among men and women aged 65–85 ($N = 941$; from the Arnhem Elderly Study) found a similar pattern over a 9-year period ($HR_{\text{highest vs. lowest quartiles}} = 0.71$; CI [0.52, 0.97]) despite using a different optimism measure (seven items derived from the Dutch Scale of Subjective Well-Being for Older Persons scale). However, these results were not adjusted for psychological distress (Giltay, Geleijnse, Zitman, Hoekstra, & Schouten, 2004).

Because of the lack of studies considering explanatory style optimism in relation to mortality, we cannot directly compare mortality findings across the two forms of optimism. However, in a very recent investigation, researchers used the Revised Optimism-Pessimism (PSM-R) index derived from the Minnesota Multiphasic Personality Inventory (Malinchoc, Offord, & Colligan, 1995) to measure explanatory-style optimism among 1,429 US men from the VA Normative Aging Study and assess its association with longevity (Lee et al., 2019). Results suggested that those in the highest versus lowest quartile of optimism scores were significantly more likely to reach the age of 85 over a 30-year period (OR = 1.5, CI [1.0, 2.3]) after adjustment for sociodemographics, medical status, health behaviors, and further control for psychological distress (Lee et al., 2019). Such findings provide promising preliminary evidence that the explanatory style of optimism is also related to mortality risk.

Emotional Vitality. Emotional vitality is a positive state characterized by feelings of enthusiasm, energy, and interest combined with an ability to effectively regulate emotions, thoughts, and behavior (Kubzansky & Thurston, 2007; Ryan & Frederick, 1997). Although no studies to date have evaluated its association with all-cause mortality risk while adjusting for sociodemographics, medical status, and health behaviors, secondary results reported in a study of emotional vitality and risk of coronary heart disease provide some preliminary evidence (Kubzansky & Thurston, 2007). Using data from the National Health and Nutrition Examination Survey (NHANES) cohort with 6,265 adults, researchers created an emotional vitality index using six items from the General Well-Being Schedule (Fazio, 1977). Findings suggested that moderate and higher versus lower levels of emotional vitality were associated with a 19% and 24% reduced risk of mortality, respectively, over a mean of 15 years of follow-up (HR = 0.81, CI [0.72, 0.91]; HR = 0.76; CI [0.68, 0.85]) when controlling for sociodemographics (Kubzansky & Thurston, 2007).

Overall Psychological Well-Being. A few other studies have investigated effects of global measures of psychological well-being in relation to mortality risk. For instance, in a subset of the MIDUS cohort (N = 3,032; aged 25–74), scores on items assessing positive affect, life satisfaction, eudaimonic well-being, and social well-being were combined to capture positive mental health—also labeled *flourishing* by the authors (Keyes & Simoes, 2012). Multivariable results indicated that those who were not versus were flourishing according to this composite had significantly greater odds of 10-year mortality (OR = 1.62; CI [1.00, 2.62]). Similar results were obtained from a recent 10-year study conducted as part of a larger cohort grouping 12 European countries (the Survey of Health Ageing and Retirement in Europe [SHARE]), in which the 19-item CASP scale capturing a sense of control, autonomy, pleasure, and self-realization (Hyde et al., 2003) was administered to 13,596 adults aged 50 years and older (Okely, Weiss, & Gale, 2018). Specifically, for every 1-SD increase on the index score, mortality risk was reduced by 8% (HR = 0.92; CI [0.86, 0.97]) after additional control for psychological distress and country-level health care (Okely et al., 2018).

Summary

Consistency of Associations. Overall, this narrative review of the existing literature indicates that several PWB dimensions are associated with a reduced risk of all-cause mortality among the general population, with small to medium effects. These relationships were observed in studies with large sample sizes and over a range of follow-up period durations. Associations were robust to adjustment for numerous covariates, including potential mechanisms that could explain associations (e.g., health behaviors); for some dimensions, associations were consistently evident regardless of which scale was used to assess the same PWB construct (e.g., optimism). Among the dimensions reviewed for which at least a few studies were available, purpose in life, optimism, and life satisfaction most consistently showed a significant association with reduced mortality risk, independent of covariates, followed by *ikigai*, positive affect, mastery, and sense of coherence. Available results with happiness, personal growth, and autonomy suggested no effect or were too limited to draw firm conclusions.

Other potentially important PWB dimensions, including self-acceptance, joy, and awe, have not been investigated with all-cause mortality risk using prospective research designs and rigorous control for traditional medical and behavioral risk factors. Whether studies of PWB and mortality will benefit from using a combined (e.g., flourishing) versus specific (e.g., life purpose) measure of PWB has not been sufficiently evaluated in prior work. Based on findings reported throughout this chapter, we suggest that retaining an understanding of how individual components of PWB relate to mortality (and other physical health outcomes) remains a valuable endeavor. Nonetheless, some research questions will clearly benefit from combining various components of PWB. For example, if investigators are considering PWB as an outcome and trying to assess ways to optimize individuals' overall sense of well-being, a combined measure may be highly valuable (VanderWeele, 2017). However, when trying to understand whether some dimensions may play a stronger/independent role in longevity, these composite scores also limit our understanding of the specific dimensions that matter and further constrain our ability to make appropriate recommendations for future interventions (Scheier & Carver, 2018; VanderWeele, 2017).

Quality of Statistical Adjustment for Covariates. Nearly all studies described in our review carefully controlled for baseline sociodemographics, medical status, and health behaviors, and, even after further adjustment for psychological distress, associations were generally evident. When adjusting for self-rated health, some of these studies of certain domains (i.e., purpose in life, autonomy, positive affect, life satisfaction), though not all (i.e., mastery, *ikigai*), indicated null estimates. However, controlling for self-rated health may sometimes be an overadjustment (Diener et al., 2018; Kubzansky et al., 2016) because this rating is both defined and influenced by functional health, physical conditions, and, most importantly, psychological distress and well-being (Jylha, 2009; Picard et al., 2013). Nevertheless, those PWB dimensions that are associated with lower mortality even after adjustment for self-rated health arguably manifest even stronger evidence for an independent relationship.

Comparison of Effect Estimates Across Dimensions. Only a handful of the cited studies have considered more than one PWB dimensions permitting direct comparisons within study. For instance, the British study of 9,420 adults followed over 5 years (Netuveli et al., 2012) evaluated four domains of PWB (sense of control, self-realization, autonomy, pleasure), and results suggested that only a sense of control and self-realization were significantly associated with mortality risk in separate models. However, in most studies, even when more than one PWB dimension was investigated, few authors evaluated their independent roles by including dimensions simultaneously in the analytic models. One exception is the German Aging Survey study in which independent effects of life satisfaction and positive affect with all-cause mortality were reported (Wiest et al., 2011). Yet PWB scores came from different scales and were not standardized, which precludes comparing their respective estimates vis-à-vis magnitude since they are not on the same scale. In Alimujiang and colleagues' study, the fully adjusted estimate of the relationship between purpose in life and all-cause mortality remained statistically significant beyond adjustment for optimism and positive affect; however, estimates for these two other PWB dimensions were not reported (Alimujiang et al., 2019). Thus, while these PWB factors appear conceptually distinct, it remains uncertain whether they independently reduce all-cause mortality, and, if so, what is the relative magnitude of their effects.

Potential Mechanistic Pathways

There are various theoretical models explaining how PWB can potentially influence health outcomes, including mortality. We will focus on biological and behavioral processes here, as depicted in Figure 5.1. Also shown in this figure are the potential effects of PWB on stress-related processes. Briefly, it is postulated that another way that PWB influences physical health is by reducing the frequency/severity of stress-related factors, such as perceived stress and negative emotions, and their harmful impact on health outcomes. For more details on this stress-buffering effect, we refer the readers to a recent article on the topic (Pressman et al., 2019).

Both observational and interventions studies targeting PWB's role on biobehavioral processes are reported here. Examples of observational studies were selected for their rigorous research design, analogous to those used in the mortality studies described earlier. Interventions studies cited in the current section are primarily at the individual level, derived from research in positive psychology, which generally shows modest but positive changes in PWB levels following interventions aiming to enhance one or multiple PWB dimensions (Bolier et al., 2013; Chakhssi, Kraiss, Sommers-Spijkerman, & Bohlmeijer, 2018; Sin & Lyubomirsky, 2009; Trudel-Fitzgerald et al., 2019b). While the contribution of biological and societal factors in one's PWB has been widely documented (Bartels, 2015; Kobau et al., 2011; Kubzansky et al., 2018; Patel et al., 2018; Steptoe, 2019), individual choices and behaviors, such as self-regulation and lifestyle habits, are also important determinants of PWB (Kubzansky et al., 2018; Van Cappellen et al., 2018). Readers interested in examples of institution-level interventions and policies to increase dimensions of well-being are referred to a recent narrative review by Trudel-Fitzgerald and colleagues (2019b).

Behavioral Factors

Observational Studies. Results obtained in the general population have shown that individuals experiencing greater levels of PWB are more likely to engage in favorable health behaviors and less likely to adopt detrimental ones (Boehm, Chen, et al., 2018; Boehm & Kubzansky, 2012; Hernandez et al., 2018; Kubzansky et al., 2018; Pressman et al., 2019; Scheier & Carver, 2018) that are important for extending lifespan (Loef & Walach, 2012; Song & Giovannucci, 2016). Yet almost all prospective studies have investigated only one behavior or have focused on only one PWB dimension, with optimism being the most frequent (Baruth et al., 2011; Boehm, Chen, et al., 2018; Boehm, Soo, et al., 2018; Giltay, Geleijnse, Zitman, Buijsse, & Kromhout,

2007; Haller, 2016; Hernandez et al., 2020; Hingle et al., 2014; Kim, Kubzansky, Soo, & Boehm, 2016; Progovac, Chang, et al., 2017; Progovac, Donohue, et al., 2017). Nonetheless, a recent prospective study considered both happiness and optimism in relation to the adoption of multiple health behaviors in more than 35,000 midlife women from the Nurses' Health Study cohort who were free of chronic disease at baseline (Trudel-Fitzgerald et al., 2019a). Results indicated that women with moderate and higher levels of dispositional optimism compared to those with lower levels were 22% and 40% more likely to report sustaining a healthy lifestyle, respectively, over a 10-year period and after adjusting for demographics and psychological distress. This dose-response relationship was also obtained when evaluating associations with each single health-related behavior included in the lifestyle index separately (i.e., physical activity, diet, smoking, alcohol consumption, and body mass index). Highly comparable findings were observed with happiness levels, captured with a 1-item measure, over a 22-year period (Trudel-Fitzgerald et al., 2019a). Importantly, although bidirectional associations were found between PWB and lifestyle levels, estimates were larger when happiness and optimism were considered as the exposures/predictors rather than the outcomes (Trudel-Fitzgerald et al., 2019a). Aside from conventional lifestyle factors, medical adherence could also mediate the association of PWB with mortality and chronic disease risk. For instance, a prospective study among 7,168 midlife adults from the Health and Retirement Study suggested that higher levels of purpose in life were related to a greater likelihood of using preventive health care services, such as obtaining a cholesterol test or colonoscopy over 6 years (Kim, Strecher, & Ryff, 2014). Associations were maintained even after adjusting for psychological distress and positive affect (Kim et al., 2014).

Intervention Studies. Several studies have evaluated whether interventions to modify PWB will affect subsequent lifestyle habits to test more directly whether PWB causally contributes to health behaviors, with most of them conducted in medical patient samples. Even fewer investigations have targeted multiple PWB dimensions, but available results suggest specificity, whereby either (1) some but not all PWB dimensions (targets of intervention) impacted the outcome, or (2) some but not all health behaviors (outcomes) were effectively altered by the intervention. For example, a recent clinical trial evaluated changes in positive affect and in dispositional optimism across the 4-month window following a positive psychology intervention generally targeting gratitude, personal strengths, and meaning in life among 128 patients with an acute coronary syndrome (Duque, Brown, Celano, Healy, & Huffman, 2019). Results indicated that increases in positive affect but not optimism led to greater adherence to multiple health behaviors (e.g., diet, physical activity). Although these findings hint at a distinct influence by separate PWB dimensions, replication of this study is needed as these findings could be a methodological artifact influenced by the small sample size and related limited statistical power. Moreover, a recent randomized controlled trial ($N = 159$) showed that HIV patients who received a positive psychology intervention aimed at increasing positive affect specifically were more likely to adhere to their antiretroviral therapy in the following 15-month period compared to the control group, whereas no differences between groups over time were observed on the adoption of risky sexual behaviors (Moskowitz et al., 2017). However, the intervention was composed of eight strategies targeting multiple PWB dimensions, leaving it unclear whether some dimensions might be more potent with regard to improving medical adherence. Overall, evidence that health behaviors substantially change after an intervention to enhance specific components of PWB (or PWB more generally) is still limited and mixed. Whether such changes are maintained over time is also uncertain, even though a few studies to date have sought to examine this directly. The field will benefit from additional randomized controlled trials with longer follow-up periods (Hernandez et al., 2018; Pressman et al., 2019).

Biological Factors

Although biological factors are often considered as potential mechanistic pathways, relative to studies of behavioral pathways fewer biological factors have been investigated in prospective longitudinal studies despite their direct association with age-related processes (Castagne et al., 2018; Sebastiani et al., 2017). Because collection of biospecimens and biomarker data is resource-intensive, most studies to date are based on cross-sectional data. While such findings can provide preliminary information, they also generally preclude interpretation about directionality/causality. Most studies that do include elements of time ordering are conducted within short-term experimental settings, and, as a result, they cannot inform understanding of natural, secular trends over time.

Observational Studies. Several prospective studies of PWB and health-relevant biological processes that controlled for sociodemographics, medical status, and health behaviors have been conducted, and findings are suggestive. Notably, higher levels of PWB were associated with reduced future risk of dysregulated levels of blood pressure (Richman et al., 2005; Trudel-Fitzgerald, Boehm, Kivimaki, & Kubzansky, 2014) and glucose control (Hafez et al., 2018; Okely & Gale, 2016; Tsenkova, Karlamangla, & Ryff, 2016) and slower progression of carotid intima medial thickness (Matthews, Raikkonen, Sutton-Tyrrell, & Kuller, 2004), as well as with healthier levels of lipids (Radler, Rigotti, & Ryff, 2018; Soo, Kubzansky, Chen, Zevon, & Boehm, 2018) over time. Interestingly, several of these studies have considered more than one PWB dimension. In some cases, methodological artifacts, such as the use of a limited 1-item measure of the exposure (Trudel-Fitzgerald et al., 2014) or a very small number of outcomes (Richman et al., 2005), constrains more definite conclusions as to whether distinct PWB dimensions impact subsequent biological processes differently. A recent MIDUS study is worth mentioning in which *trajectories* of six distinct PWB dimensions, all measured with the Scales of Psychological Well-Being (Ryff, 1989), were investigated in relation to lipids over up to 10 years among 1,054 midlife adults (Radler et al., 2018). Results indicated that adults with persistently high (vs. low) levels of mastery and self-acceptance had significantly healthier levels of HDL cholesterol and triglycerides, whereas no association was found when evaluating trajectories of the other PWB dimensions as exposures (e.g., autonomy, personal growth, purpose in life) nor when considering LDL-cholesterol as the outcome.

PWB has been examined in relation to several markers of other health-related biological processes in prospective studies. For instance, higher PWB levels based on the CASP scores were associated with lower levels of C-reactive protein (CRP) but not fibrinogen, two inflammation markers that were assessed 2 years after PWB among 5,622 British adults 50 years and older from the English Longitudinal Study of Ageing (ELSA; Okely, Weiss, & Gale, 2017). Evidence also indicates that both hedonic and eudaimonic dimensions of PWB are significantly associated with greater likelihood of maintaining healthy functioning in these biological processes (Boylan & Ryff, 2015; Zilioli, Slatcher, Ong, & Gruenewald, 2015). More specifically, in a sample of 1,205 midlife US adults followed for 10 years in MIDUS, for every 1-*SD* increase in life satisfaction there was an 18% lower odds (OR = 0.82; CI [0.69, 0.97]) of developing metabolic syndrome (e.g., unhealthy levels of triglycerides, cholesterol, blood pressure, glucose, and central obesity). The effect estimate was even larger (per 1-SD increase, OR = 0.77; CI [0.65, 0.93]) for a eudaimonic well-being measure (a composite of autonomy, environmental mastery, personal growth, positive relationships, purpose in life, and self-acceptance; Boylan & Ryff, 2015). However, the authors did not report whether these two PWB indicators were associated with the outcome independently of one another. In this study, authors also observed comparable estimates between overall life satisfaction and eudaimonic well-being, respectively, in relation to the number of dysregulated metabolic components exhibited by the participants 10 years later but did not assess the likelihood of developing each component separately (Boylan & Ryff, 2015). Another longitudinal investigation within MIDUS and using the same PWB measure examined a different index of biological function, *allostatic load*, which captures biological wear-and-tear (Zilioli et al., 2015). In this study allostatic load was measured by dysregulated functioning in cardiometabolic parameters, inflammatory processes, and activity of the sympathetic nervous system [SNS], parasympathetic nervous system [PNS], and hypothalamic pituitary adrenal [HPA] axis. Results obtained in 985 midlife adults suggested that higher levels of purpose in life were significantly related to lower levels of allostatic load 10 years later, even after adjusting for sociodemographics, psychological distress, and positive affect (Zilioli et al., 2015).

Preliminary research on several other potential biological pathways are worth mentioning as well, although few studies compared multiple PWB dimensions, and, most importantly, nearly all were cross-sectional. First, investigators are increasingly conducting research using genetic markers. For instance, authors evaluated the association of optimism with telomere length in several samples of European men with n's varying from 101 to 178 and reported null findings (Rius-Ottenheim et al., 2012). However, these studies used a 4-item optimism measure that was not previously validated. Another line of work has reported more positive findings considering dispositional optimism in relation to gene expression among 114 Japanese men (Uchida, Kitayama, Akutsu, Park, & Cole, 2018). Using a genomic approach, other investigators reported separate gene regulation profiles associated with hedonic versus eudaimonic PWB dimensions among 84 US adults (Fredrickson et al., 2013). While these findings seem to hint at critical biological variations underlying PWB dimensions, they have been somewhat controversial, notably because of the substantial overlap between the scores obtained from psychological scales used and the numerous covariates included in the statistical models (Coyne, 2013), suggesting the need for future replication. Second, one study has considered PWB in relation to antioxidants, posited to server as a marker of a restorative health-promoting process. Results obtained in 982 midlife men and women from MIDUS suggested that dispositional optimism was associated with some (e.g., α-carotene and lycopene [carotenoids]) but not all (e.g., α-tocopherol [vitamin E], lutein [carotenoid]) antioxidant indicators on average 2 years later (Boehm, Williams, Rimm, Ryff, & Kubzansky, 2013). Longitudinal studies targeting these biological processes are clearly needed.

Intervention Studies. From a clinical trial perspective, only a handful of studies have investigated whether changes in various PWB dimensions induced by an intervention translate into changes in biomarkers levels. Most of this work has been done in patient populations. In the randomized controlled trial among 159 HIV patients described earlier (Moskowitz et al., 2017), substantial improvement on viral load levels were obtained from pre- to post-assessment in the intervention group (vs. the control group), but no effects were observed on changes in CD4 cell levels. While these results may hint at the possibility of outcome-specificity, exposure-specificity cannot be disentangled due to the multicomponent nature of the intervention, during which multiple dimensions of PWB were manipulated.

Interestingly, another randomized controlled trial among 69 cardiac patients compared levels of biomarkers obtained from blood sample before and after three positive psychology interventions to the levels obtained in a wait-list condition (Nikrahan et al., 2016). The interventions were each informed by one of three different frameworks and consisted of six weekly 90-minute in-person group manualized sessions. Specifically, as reported by the study authors (Nikrahan et al., 2016), the first strategy aimed to increased optimism, positive affect, identifying and using personal strengths, and finding meaning in life; a second strategy targeted the improvement of optimism and gratitude, as well as religion/forgiveness, social relationships, physical activity, and adaptive coping skills; the third strategy focused on optimism in addition to becoming more present-oriented, reducing negative cognitions/affect, increasing organizational/productivity skills, setting realistic goals, and focusing on positive personality traits like being genuine. While there was moderate overlap among the three interventions, notably with the inclusion of optimism strategies, each had some unique elements. Inflammatory markers were collected at pre- (baseline) and post-intervention (week 7) and at the follow-up assessment (week 15), while markers of the HPA-axis activity were assessed pre- and post-intervention only.

Results for inflammatory markers indicated greater decline in CRP levels, but not interleukin (IL)-1 or IL-6, from pre- to post-intervention among participants in the first or third program versus those in the control group after adjustment for clinical variables and psychological distress ($ps = 0.04$). No significant changes were noted from baseline to 15-week follow-up in these two intervention groups. Conversely, compared to the control group, the second program led to no changes from pre- to post-intervention in inflammation markers but to a marginally significant decline in IL-1 from baseline to follow-up ($p = 0.07$). Results with an HPA axis activity marker similarly distinguished the three programs as only the second one was related to an alteration of the cortisol awakening response ($p = 0.03$) beyond control for clinical variables, psychological distress, and awakening time. The authors postulated that changes in eudaimonic PWB dimensions (e.g., meaning in life), rather than in hedonic ones (e.g., positive affect), might have driven these results (Nikrahan et al., 2016). Of course, caution is warranted when interpreting these exploratory results as they are based on small sample sizes; with groups varying from 13 to 15 participants, significant results may indeed be due to chance rather than true effects. However, we describe this study in detail because of its rigorous design and implementation and its novelty in considering multiples biomarkers and distinct positive psychology interventions in relation to various PWB dimensions, in hopes that work like this will encourage future investigations with larger sample sizes to replicate these results.

Summary

Altogether, prospective observational and intervention research on biological and behavioral processes offers sufficient positive results to suggest that further research is warranted. However, important to note is that most results are small to modest, and it is sometimes unclear whether positive findings from intervention studies are due to strategies that aim to increase overall versus specific dimensions of PWB (e.g., multicomponent interventions to increase overall well-being vs. the "best possible self" exercise to increase optimism). Nonetheless, because even changes of small magnitude at the individual level may translate into large changes at the population level, the potential benefits of such interventions on mental and physical health, including mortality risk and related biobehavioral pathways, may be substantial.

In the future, researchers should prioritize methodologically rigorous studies (either observational or experimental) that are (1) based on larger sample sizes, to obtain more stable (and perhaps larger) estimates, and (2) longitudinal, to lower potential for reverse causation. Explicitly comparing PWB dimensions is also warranted. Specifically, in observational studies, considering multiple PWB dimensions will help clarify whether some relate more strongly than others to these potential biobehavioral mechanistic pathways over time; in intervention studies, clarifying whether strategies *a priori target* and, ultimately, *impact* one or more PWB dimensions will bring a more nuanced understanding of the mechanisms of change. Intervention studies among nonmedical populations are also needed.

Other biological processes that are restorative by nature, such as antioxidant action, should also be investigated in future longitudinal studies. Moreover, given the dynamic nature of these processes, subsequent research should take a deeper look into bidirectional associations (Ryff, 2017; Trudel-Fitzgerald et al., 2019a) to determine whether and when PWB truly acts as either a determinant or outcome of these processes. Additionally, consideration of the interrelations between biological and behavioral factors, as depicted in Figure 5.1, will likely lead to a more complex, but also more realistic, understanding of the extent to which these potential mechanistic pathways influence each other when relating PWB to mortality risk. Preliminary exploration of this issue has been done, notably in the MIDUS study on antioxidants described earlier (Boehm et al., 2013). Findings revealed that health behaviors accounted for nearly half (46%) of the association between optimism and total carotenoid concentrations in particular. Because health behaviors and antioxidant levels were assessed at the same time point in this study, the direction of effects remain unclear. Further examination of the intertwined longitudinal relationships between behavioral and biological processes with optimal temporality is warranted.

Methodological Considerations

Findings from existing epidemiological studies may inform future research. In addition to conducting studies using the most rigorous designs possible (e.g., longitudinal, rigorous control for potential confounders), future work will benefit from considering a number of key issues highlighted here. We consider these issues according to their relation with PWB, mortality, or other physical health-related outcomes or covariates including potential confounders, pathways (mediators), or effect modifiers (moderators). We end by considering potential biases and related issues.

Challenges Related to Studying Psychological Well-Being as an Exposure

Comparison of PWB Dimensions. First, as argued throughout this chapter, a critical task for future studies is to shed light on how various PWB dimensions relate to health, both separately and synergistically (Diener et al., 2018; Pressman et al., 2019; Steptoe, 2019). As of today, it remains difficult to compare the magnitude of the effects because, among the few studies that compared several PWB dimensions in relation to mortality, most did not use standardized and comparable scores of the PWB exposures. Although numerous large-scale studies have administered at least one PWB measure to their participants (e.g., Women's Health Initiative cohort, Nurses' Health Study, MIDUS, Health and Retirement Study, Longitudinal Aging Study Amsterdam, EPIC-Norfolk Study, Japan Collaborative Cohort Study), the various indicators are often queried years apart, which limits direct comparison. Including a richer set of PWB measures simultaneously in these studies to permit comparison across constructs and expanding PWB assessments to other large national cohorts may be a challenge given that questionnaire space is limited, but such inclusion remains highly warranted.

To disentangle the unique versus shared contribution of PWB dimensions more optimally, some authors have suggested setting up studies allowing the contrast of PWB dimensions that rely on the same time frame (e.g., past few days vs. over a lifetime; Pressman et al., 2019). In fact, prior work has demonstrated that using the same time frame for distinct PWB measures, notably positive affect and life satisfaction, increased the strength of the correlation between scores but did not fully account for their conceptual differences (Luhmann, Hawkley, Eid, & Cacioppo, 2012); however, these authors have not explored whether such nuances are associated with health-related outcomes. Comparing how items within the same scale are associated with health outcomes may also help to capture active ingredients (e.g., across facets of positive affect; Petrie et al., 2018). A related research question of importance is whether prediction of mortality risk is enhanced by assessing two or more PWB dimensions and combining their scores to identify participants who report, for instance, higher levels on all, some, or none of the PWB dimensions.

Temporality. Other methodological concerns pertain to temporal aspects of the exposure, notably how often PWB is measured, the time frame used to capture PWB, and to what extent PWB dimensions are stable constructs over time.

Frequency of Assessment. First, the vast majority of longitudinal studies presented in this chapter have relied on a single assessment of PWB mean levels in relation to mortality risk. However, multiple assessments of PWB over time may provide complementary information via the characterization of PWB dynamics. For instance, *variability* in the experience of PWB may matter for physical health as well. As an example, in a study of 4,458 Australian adults (Boehm et al., 2015), life satisfaction was assessed annually over 9 years, and results suggested that the risk of mortality was elevated in those with lower mean life satisfaction level, averaging all available PWB assessments, and increased even more strongly if participants exhibited high variability in their PWB scores over time (p-value for mean × standard deviation interaction ≤ 0.001). Similarly, studies examining *(in)stability* of PWB levels over time could shed additional light on this question. For instance, German adults who reported less versus more decline in their trajectory of life satisfaction scores had a reduced risk of mortality over a 20-year follow-up period (Hulur et al., 2017). Other markers of PWB dynamics, such as *inertia,* the resistance to affective change (Ong & Ram, 2017), have not been studied yet in relation to mortality to our knowledge.

Time Frame and Cognitive Orientation to PWB Constructs. A related, albeit distinct, issue is that some PWB dimensions rely on individuals' assessment of their past experiences (e.g., life satisfaction), while others capture their present (e.g., positive affect), or future/predicted experiences (e.g., optimism).[2] Whether different dimensions of PWB differentially predict mortality or other health-related outcomes may relate in part to what individuals are assessing when they self-report PWB. In a 3-year study conducted in nationally representative Spanish sample of adults aged 18 and older (Martin-Maria et al., 2016), positive and negative affect was assessed with the Day Reconstruction Method (DRM; Kahneman, Krueger, Schkade, Schwarz, & Stone, 2004), which restricts evaluation of affect to the prior day during various activities. In the same study, the Cantril Self-Anchoring Striving Scale (Cantril, 1965) was also used to determine the extent to which individuals thought they were living the worst versus best possible life (on a 11-point Likert scale); this measure is highly correlated with life satisfaction (Helliwell, Barrington-Leigh, Harris, & Huang, 2010). Results indicated that a 1-unit increase in positive affect based on an individual's experience of 1 day was related to an 18% decreased risk (HR = 0.82, CI [0.68, 0.99]) of mortality over the follow-up, but life evaluation based on an individual's assessment of their current and past experiences more generally was not associated with mortality risk (Martin-Maria et al., 2016). These findings were evident after including both PWB indicators in the analytic model as well as adjusting for conventional covariates and negative affect. Such results may suggest that assessment of current PWB levels predicts mortality risk more strongly than retrospective levels, but replication is warranted. In fact, effects of positive affect and life evaluation might also differ between, for instance, Spanish versus American participants, as well as individuals in early versus late adulthood.

Stability of PWB Constructs. Furthermore, some PWB dimensions may be conceptualized as more stable (trait-like; e.g., optimism, life satisfaction) than others (state-like; e.g., positive affect, happiness) over days or weeks. The magnitude of changes as a response to external events, called *affective reactivity* (Ong & Ram, 2017), could vary across PWB dimensions depending on whether they are more trait-like or state-like. For instance, 181 men from the VA Normative Aging Study included in an 8-day daily diary study reported every evening various information like daily stressors along with positive and negative affect (Mroczek et al., 2015). While daily average positive affect was not related to mortality risk over the 10-year follow-up, every 1-unit *decrease* in positive affect *following the experience of a daily stressor* was related to 132% increased risk of mortality (HR = 2.32, CI [1.32, 4.00]) after adjusting for sociodemographics, medical status, and psychological distress. Whether changes in PWB dimensions that are believed to be more stable (e.g., optimism) following a minor or major stressor (e.g., argument with a loved one, accident/illness) is related to mortality has not been well studied.

Altogether, considering temporal aspects of PWB suggests the potential importance of studies that include not only repeated measures of PWB levels over many years, but also intensive measurement of PWB levels over consecutive days or weeks. Such measures can be obtained via methods such as Experience Sampling Methods (ESM) and Emotional Momentary Assessment (EMA; Diener et al., 2018; Steptoe, 2019); novel metrics, including recurrence quantification analysis (Jenkins, Hunter, Richardson, Conner, & Pressman, 2019), could also help characterize PWB dynamics in future health-related research (Pressman et al., 2019). However, according to some authors, it remains unclear whether these strategies provide significantly greater advantages over more traditional approaches, such as using the average and standard deviation calculated from scores obtained on self-reported scales and EMA metrics (Dejonckheere et al., 2019; Diener et al., 2018). Regardless, considering these temporal aspects of how PWB is experienced might provide additional information about aspects that distinguish PWB dimensions. Further research needs to determine whether and to what extent the use of dynamic measures can add to our understanding of PWB's role in health outcomes and mortality.

Potential Detrimental Effects. Another methodological issue of note is whether extreme PWB levels might have a detrimental influence on subsequent health-related outcomes (Diener et al., 2018). For example, it is possible that unrealistic optimism (e.g., "I am convinced I won't get lung cancer") or extreme positive affect (e.g., being overly excited) may be followed by adverse health consequences such as smoking habits or increased blood pressure, respectively. Few authors have examined this question empirically, especially within longitudinal research designs, mostly investigating the question with optimism as a predictor of future health behaviors. For instance, a study on unrealistic optimism reported that overly optimistic expectations led to greater alcohol consumption 1 year later in college freshmen (Dillard, Midboe, & Klein, 2009). Conversely, in the study of more than 35,000 midlife women described previously (Trudel-Fitzgerald et al., 2019a), those who had the highest score on the optimism scale (19% of the sample) were still significantly *more likely* to sustain an healthy lifestyle over the 10-year follow-up period compared to their least optimistic counterparts. This discrepancy could be due, at least partly, to the age group under examination, with younger individuals more prone to extreme levels of PWB that can lead to being unrealistic.

Some detrimental effects of PWB on biological factors have been documented. Much of this work was conducted among college students in a series of naturalistic studies of short duration (less than a year; Segerstrom, 2005). While greater optimism levels generally had a protective association with markers of cellular immunity (e.g., number of CD4+ T cells in peripheral blood), a detrimental effect was observed when optimistic individuals persisted in rather than disengaged from a challenge, such as trying to balance extramural commitments with school requirements (Segerstrom, 2005). These findings suggest that not only *extreme levels* of some PWB dimensions could potentially have a detrimental impact on health-related outcomes for certain populations, but also potentially the *context* in which PWB dimensions are experienced and their *duration* could have an effect, even when levels are not extreme. To our knowledge, no mortality studies have specifically tackled this issue of potential detrimental effects by distinct dimensions of PWB. Additionally, much less is known about extreme levels of other PWB exposures and other health-related outcomes in various populations.

Challenges Related to Studying Mortality or Other Physical Health Endpoints as Outcomes

Objective Data. While the methodological issues identified earlier are largely related to methods for assessing, conceptualizing, and evaluating the exposure (PWB), another key element for the PWB-health research pertains to the importance of using objective outcomes. This may seem obvious for mortality, which cannot be self-reported and is usually obtained from medical registers; yet favoring objectively defined chronic disease diagnoses (e.g., as validated by a physician blinded to the study hypotheses or hospital records) whenever possible will lower risk of bias whereby individuals with higher PWB levels may report their physical health more favorably.

Reverse Causation. Along the same lines, reverse causation—whereby participants' declining physical health preceding mortality might impact the assessment or report of PWB levels—is a critical concern that should be addressed in all studies. Increasingly, researchers conduct sensitivity analyses among individuals who survived for at least 1–2 years post-baseline to address this issue. In the few studies cited earlier that included such lagged models, associations were robust and yielded similar results (e.g., Boyle et al.,

2009; Rosella et al., 2018; Sone et al., 2008), which strengthens the evidence that PWB may causally contribute to health outcomes.

Causes of Death. Differences in associations of PWB with varying causes of death have been noted in the handful of studies that had sufficient statistical power to explore this research question. In distinct studies that all controlled for sociodemographics, medical status, and health behaviors and considered either life purpose (Alimujiang et al., 2019), mastery (Surtees et al., 2006), sense of coherence (Surtees et al., 2003), *ikigai* (Tanno et al., 2009), optimism (Tindle et al., 2009), or overall PWB (Okely et al., 2018) in relation to cause-specific mortality, all obtained estimates suggesting stronger associations of PWB with cardiometabolic-related mortality compared to cancer-related mortality over follow-up periods of less than 10 years (except Tanno et al., 2009). As for cancer incidence, the smaller, often null estimates may truly reflect the absence of an association. However, methodological artifacts might also contribute to these findings. First, if the magnitude of the linkages is smaller for PWB with cancer than with cardiovascular outcomes, a larger sample size will be required to detect an effect with cancer. Second, because many cancers are relatively rare, resulting in small case counts, studies often combine cases across cancer sites to increase power. Yet it is well documented that different cancer sites represent different disease processes, with some being potentially more sensitive to psychosocial and behavioral factors than other (e.g., lung vs. pancreas; Poirier et al., 2019; Trudel-Fitzgerald, Chen, Singh, Okereke, & Kubzansky, 2016). Third, unlike cardiometabolic outcomes, carcinogenesis development and progression are long-term processes, sometimes occurring over more than a decade (Conner et al., 2014; Labidi-Galy et al., 2017), which may not be captured adequately over shorter follow-up periods.

Challenges Related to Covariates

Confounding and Mediation. Another concern is the adequate adjustment for potential confounders, especially with regard to third variables that influence both the exposure and the outcome. Although most recent studies have carefully controlled for conventional potential confounders (e.g., sociodemographics, medical status), it is not always the case. Failure to do so not only overlooks possible confounding effects, but also limits comparisons of effect estimates across studies even when they are obtained from the same PWB scales.

The issue of confounding is particularly important when considering the role of behavioral factors in the relationship of PWB with mortality or other physical health outcomes. Health behaviors can act either as confounders in the association or as mechanisms linking PWB to mortality risk (Hernandez et al., 2018). Most studies to date have treated health behaviors as potential confounders, adjusting for baseline health behaviors. However, such studies cannot evaluate the possibility that health behaviors are one mechanism by which PWB may influence subsequent physical health outcomes because baseline behavioral factors do not provide optimal temporality for evaluating mediation. Since few studies have explicitly examined such mediation patterns (see Okely et al., 2017, as one of the exceptions), it remains unclear the extent to which such behavioral factors may lie on the pathway between PWB and mortality risk. Such distinction remains important when trying the understand processes of change to inform intervention strategies (Czajkowski et al., 2015; Nielsen et al., 2018). With multiple waves of data, such issues can, however, be addressed by controlling for health behaviors that are measured *prior* to PWB assessment and by treating as mediator those health behaviors that are measured *subsequent* to the PWB assessment (VanderWeele, 2015). Due to developments within the causal inference framework, there is also growing awareness among scholars that exposure–mediator interactions may exist (Valeri & Vanderweele, 2013) and should be considered in future research investigating PWB's role in mortality risk.

Moderation by Sociodemographic Factors. Moreover, associations have been rarely investigated across sociodemographic groups, and most studies were conducted in Western countries, which may not be generalizable to other subgroups.

> *Race and Culture.* Differences in the experience, value, and understanding of PWB dimensions across various countries, races, and cultures have been documented (Choi & Chentsova-Dutton, 2017; Diener et al., 2018; Ma, Tamir, & Miyamoto, 2018; Ryff, 2017; Weziak-Bialowolska, McNeely, & VanderWeele, 2019; Wirtz, Chiu, Diener, & Oishi, 2009). In fact, preliminary observational findings obtained in the studies described previously hint that various sociodemographic factors may modify the PWB–mortality relationship. For instance, in the Women's Health Initiative study of optimism and mortality (Tindle et al., 2009), race/ethnicity modified the association, whereby the estimates were larger in blacks versus white participants (HR_{Blacks} = 0.67; CI [0.50,

0.90] vs. HR_{Whites} = 0.87; CI [0.80, 0.96]; interaction test, p-value = 0.02).
However, the vast majority of studies cited earlier were conducted
in high-income countries and circumscribed to certain races and
cultures, which may not be generalizable to other populations. Hence,
it remains unclear whether findings obtained from existing rigorous
studies assessing the PWB–mortality association would translate into
similar results across race and cultures worldwide given documented
differences in the experience, value, and understanding of PWB.
Although a relationship between PWB and reduced mortality risk is
likely evident across many different populations (Pressman, Gallagher,
& Lopez, 2013), some PWB dimensions may not translate or be relevant in certain cultures or population settings. Thus, careful assessment of which PWB dimensions are appropriate for study in different
populations will be critical.

In an attempt to tackle potential cultural differences, the recent
multicountry study described earlier (Okely et al., 2018) evaluated the
interaction of overall PWB with levels of individualism within each
European country, hypothesizing that the association of PWB with
mortality would be stronger in more individualistic countries because of
the emphasis they place on well-being. The authors relied on Hofstede's
definition of individualism, which applies to a society "in which the
ties between individuals are loose: everyone is expected to look after
him- or herself and his or her immediate family," and on his related
Individualism Index[3] (Hofstede et al., 2010). The 11 European countries, with 13,596 adults 50 years and older from the SHARE cohort,
were categorized in tertiles based on their score on the Individual Index
(e.g., the Netherlands was in the highest and Greece was in the lowest
tertile). Multivariable models further controlled for psychological distress and, importantly, country-level healthcare to rule out influences
other than individualism that might be due to country differences.

Although the PWB–individualism interaction term was not statistically
significantly related to all-cause mortality within the whole sample (p-
value = 0.15), when considering cardiovascular mortality specifically,
PWB remained significantly associated with mortality only among
adults with the highest level of individualism (HR = 0.64, CI [0.50,
0.84]). As reported by the authors (Okely et al., 2018), it is unclear
whether these findings reflect greater value placed on PWB in individualistic versus collectivistic cultures or, instead, a failure to measure

PWB accurately in collectivistic cultures. Nonetheless, such results remain intriguing, especially when contrasted with the large body of evidence showing that stronger and larger social networks, which are more closely related to collectivism than individualism, are consistently related to lower risk of death (Holt-Lunstad, Robles, & Sbarra, 2017; Holt-Lunstad, Smith, & Layton, 2010).

Sex, Education, and Age. Other sociodemographic factors beyond race and culture may also impact PWB's association with mortality. Sex may be an important consideration because some studies have noted sex differences in these associations while others have not. For example, in one of studies considering *ikigai* (Tanno et al., 2009), although men and women with higher (vs. lower) levels of *ikigai* had reduced mortality risk within 5 years of follow-up (HR_{men} = 0.80; CI [0.72, 0.89] vs. HR_{women} = 0.80; CI [0.69, 0.72]) of similar magnitude, beyond 5 years the estimates became stronger for men compared to women (HR_{men} = 0.85; CI [0.80, 0.90] vs. HR_{women} = 0.93; CI [0.86, 1.00]; interaction test, p-value < 0.05). Socioeconomic status may also modify associations of PWB with mortality. For instance, in a study evaluating mastery levels in relation to mortality risk, positive associations were evident in those with low, but not high, educational attainment; while stratified HRs were not reported, the interaction test was statistically significant with p-value < 0.01 (Turiano et al., 2014). Age may also be relevant. When considered in stratified analyses, estimates are generally similar among younger and older individuals regardless of the PWB dimension studied in relation to mortality (e.g., Petrie et al., 2018; Sone et al., 2008; Tanno et al., 2009; Wiest et al., 2011). That said, few studies systematically considered this factor as a potential effect modifier, often because studies from epidemiological cohorts are based in midlife and older adults and given that health-related outcomes investigated are more often evident in older populations. In fact, participants in the "young" group of these stratified analyses are generally 40 years and older. Yet evidence suggests that levels of certain PWB dimensions, as well as cognitive processes involved in these psychological factors (e.g., emotion regulation), vary by life stages (Lockenhoff & Carstensen, 2004; Scheibe & Carstensen, 2010). As proposed in Figure 5.1, considering PWB early in the life course, as well as its interaction with biobehavioral processes during that period, may be an important time window for investigating these associations to facilitate developing and evaluating primary prevention strategies likely to impact lifelong physical health and mortality risk. Thus, we strongly recommend future research considers age as a modifier, as well as other sociodemographic factors, more comprehensively.

Potential Biases and Related Issues

Survivor Bias. In epidemiological cohorts where PWB measures were queried later in the life course, it is possible that individuals who were included in PWB–mortality studies because they completed the exposure measure are in fact different from those who did not survive to this assessment, also known as *survivor bias* or *left truncation* (Banack, Kaufman, Wactawski-Wende, Troen, & Stovitz, 2019). Participants from a larger cohort who are excluded from a specific analytic sample because they chose to not complete a specific scale (here, the one used to measure the PWB exposure) may be different from participants who did complete the scale and, in turn, were included in the analytic sample. Reporting descriptive statistics of eligible and ineligible participants can hint to the presence of such bias, yet other more precise methods, including inverse probability weights (IPW) whereby individuals included in the analytic sample are up-weighted to account for themselves as well as for those with similar characteristics who are unable to make it to the exposure assessment, could be included in future studies to help reduce concerns about this potential selection bias (Banack et al., 2019). In addition, it is worth briefly mentioning the potential influence of attrition over the follow-up period. For instance, while survival is the outcome of interest in mortality studies, it is not the case in investigations that focus on chronic disease incidence or potential biobehavioral pathways. When death occurs during follow-up, this can lead to "selection bias due to loss to follow-up" or *right truncation* (Banack et al., 2019), which may impact a study's results and conclusions. In addition to mortality, someone may no longer participate in a study because of major psychological distress, cognitive decline, or health-related problems, for example. Such reasons for dropout remain conceptually challenging because they likely relate to either the exposure or outcome of interest. Here again, various strategies can be implemented to assess the presence of such bias, ranging from descriptive statistics to identify potential differences, IPW to be included in the models, or sensitivity analyses that are conducted among non-dropouts only (Banack et al., 2019).

Internal Versus External Validity. Another concern relates to who participates in studies of PWB and mortality or other physical health outcomes. As noted previously, most studies have been conducted in Western population and midlife to older individuals. Although the homogeneity of a population can enhance a study's internal validity, results cannot necessarily be generalized to other populations, including Eastern and younger individuals. This field of research will benefit highly from future work on the association of PWB with risk of mortality and other health-related outcomes among more diverse or understudied populations.

Summary

In brief, prioritizing methodological rigor in future studies will help to provide more compelling evidence regarding whether PWB is a causal contributor of health-related outcomes and will facilitate more accurate comparison across PWB dimensions as well as replication of studies in this field. Systematically incorporating well-being scales in large national cohort studies that provide follow-up periods long enough to tackle outcomes such as chronic diseases and mortality risk will be required. Such inclusion in recurring surveys would also permit investigation of more complex research questions, such as exploring the association between temporal dynamics of PWB with mortality risk. Including psychosocial measures in these multiuse samples has never been a simple task, given that most of these scales comprehensively capture constructs with numerous items and such studies are often highly sensitive to participant burden. Yet taking into consideration constraints commonly encountered in such specific contexts (e.g., space limitations), certain items have recently been recommended to guide selection of measures and stimulate work in this area (Chapter 17, in this volume).

Conclusion

In this chapter, we summarized studies that have rigorously investigated the association between various dimensions of PWB and mortality risk. The most consistent evidence was obtained for purpose in life, optimism, and life satisfaction, further supporting their systematic inclusion in large national cohorts, followed by *ikigai*, positive affect, mastery, and sense of coherence.

In these prospective studies, small to moderate associations were observed even beyond rigorous control for traditional sociodemographic, medical, and behavioral risk factors. Available multivariable results with other PWB dimensions suggested no effect (e.g., happiness) or were too limited (e.g., personal growth, autonomy, emotional vitality) to draw firm conclusions. We also reviewed biological and behavioral mechanistic pathways that could explain the PWB–mortality linkage. Current findings from both epidemiological studies and clinical trials suggest that PWB dimensions are associated with health behaviors (e.g., smoking, diet, physical activity), with the strength of the associations varying depending on the behavior; analogous results were noted for biomarkers (e.g., inflammation, HPA axis activity). We concluded with various methodological considerations that we suggest may guide subsequent research that can most effectively inform the field.

Recommendations for Future Studies

Based on these considerations, we conclude with 12 recommendations for future work in this area. From a study design perspective, when feasible, researchers should consider (1) including an understudied population, (2) including more than one PWB dimension per study, (3) administering repeated measures of distinct PWB dimensions, and (4) combining traditional self-reported scales with intensive longitudinal assessment (e.g., EMA). From an analytic perspective, whenever possible we suggest (1) standardizing scores if obtained from different PWB scales; (2) exploring the potential detrimental effect of extreme PWB levels in health-related outcomes; (3) considering the role of relevant covariates as potential confounders (i.e., sociodemographics, medical status, health behaviors, psychological distress); (4) implementing strategies to overcome potential selection bias; (5) evaluating PWB–mortality associations by cause of death; (6) examining the potential mediating role of biobehavioral pathways with accurate analytic techniques and optimal temporality in the sequence of construct assessments; (7) using stratified analyses to verify the PWB–mortality association by sociodemographic characteristics; and (8) determining the robustness of the association by excluding early deaths (or disease cases). Building evidence in this way would generate stronger evidence for a causal association and could guide the selection of PWB dimensions for randomized controlled trials conducted in specific populations and for specific outcomes. It would also contribute to the development of more targeted interventions that could be broadly disseminated at the population level. Such interventions could improve not only PWB, but may have the potential to promote and maintain physical health as well (Kobau et al., 2011; Chapter 17, in this volume).

Notes

1. In two cases—autonomy and emotional vitality—cited studies included some but not all of the mentioned covariates at baseline. The selection of studies was less strict for these two PWB dimensions because of the scarcity of mortality studies available in the literature. We make note of which covariates were considered when describing the studies.
2. Other authors have referred to these various timeframes by distinguishing "experiential" from "evaluative" measures, where the former captures in situ reports of emotional experiences while the latter captures global retrospective evaluations (Diener et al., 2018).
3. This index provides a score for each country that captures its relative position against other countries. As examples, the United States is ranked in first position with a score of 91, the Netherlands is found to be slightly lower with a score of 80, whereas Greece is ranked 45th with a score of 35 and Guatemala is in last position (76th) with a score of 6 (Hofstede, Hofstede, & Minkov, 2010).

About the Authors

Claudia Trudel-Fitzgerald is Research Scientist at the Lee Kum Sheung Center for Health and Happiness and the Department of Social and Behavioral Sciences at the Harvard T. H. Chan School of Public Health. She is also a licensed clinical psychologist specializing in cognitive-behavioral therapy. Her research projects target the role of positive and negative emotions, and their regulation, in the maintenance and decline of physical health as well as longevity.

Laura D. Kubzansky is Lee Kum Kee Professor of Social and Behavioral Sciences and co-Director of the Lee Kum Sheung Center for Health and Happiness at the Harvard T. H. Chan School of Public Health. Dr. Kubzansky has published extensively on the role of psychological and social factors in health. Ongoing research includes studying biobehavioral mechanisms linking emotions, social relationships, and health; defining, measuring, and modifying aspects of well-being; and workplace conditions in relation to well-being. She has served on the leadership team for multiple training programs for junior scholars and is PI or co-investigator on numerous grants.

Tyler J. VanderWeele is the John L. Loeb and Frances Lehman Loeb Professor of Epidemiology in the Departments of Epidemiology and Biostatistics at the Harvard T. H. Chan School of Public Health, Director of the Human Flourishing Program, and Co-Director of the Initiative on Health, Religion and Spirituality at Harvard University. His research concerns methodology for distinguishing between association and causation in observational studies, and his empirical research spans psychiatric, perinatal, and social epidemiology; the science of happiness and flourishing; and the study of religion and health, including both religion and population health and the role of religion and spirituality in end-of-life care. He has published more than 300 papers in peer-reviewed journals and is author of the book *Explanation in Causal Inference* (Oxford University Press, 2015).

Author Note

This work was supported in part by a grant from the John Templeton Foundation and by the Lee Kum Sheung Center for Health and Happiness, as well as the Fonds de Recherche du Québec–Santé (postdoctoral fellowships) to the first author. We thank Dr. Matthew T. Lee and Dr. Ying Chen for prior comments on this chapter. The views expressed in this chapter represent the perspectives of the authors and do not reflect the opinions or endorsement of any organization. We have no known conflict of interest to disclose. Correspondence concerning this chapter should be directed to Claudia Trudel-Fitzgerald, Department of Social and Behavioral Sciences, Harvard T. H. Chan School of Public Health, 677 Huntington Avenue, 6th floor, Room 612 Kresge Building, Boston, MA 02115 (ctrudel@hsph.harvard.edu).

References

Abbott, R. A., Ploubidis, G. B., Huppert, F. A., Kuh, D., Wadsworth, M. E., & Croudace, T. J. (2006). Psychometric evaluation and predictive validity of Ryff's psychological well-being items in a UK birth cohort sample of women. *Health and Quality of Life Outcomes, 4*, 76.

Alimujiang, A., Wiensch, A., Boss, J., Fleischer, N. L., Mondul, A. M., McLean, K., . . . Pearce, C. L. (2019). Association between life purpose and mortality among US adults older than 50 years. *JAMA Network Open, 2*(5), e194270.

Antonovsky, A. (1987). *Unraveling the mystery of health.* San Francisco, CA: Jossey-Bass.

Antonovsky, A. (1993). The structure and properties of the sense of coherence scale. *Social Science & Medicine, 36*(6), 725–733.

Banack, H. R., Kaufman, J. S., Wactawski-Wende, J., Troen, B. R., & Stovitz, S. D. (2019). Investigating and remediating selection bias in geriatrics research: The selection bias toolkit. *Journal of the American Geriatric Society, 67*(9), 1970–1976.

Bartels, M. (2015). Genetics of wellbeing and its components satisfaction with life, happiness, and quality of life: A review and meta-analysis of heritability studies. *Behavioral Genetics, 45*(2), 137–156.

Baruth, M., Lee, D. C., Sui, X., Church, T. S., Marcus, B. H., Wilcox, S., & Blair, S. N. (2011). Emotional outlook on life predicts increases in physical activity among initially inactive men. *Health Education & Behavior, 38*(2), 150–158.

Berkman, L. F., Kawachi, I., & Glymour, M. M. (2014). *Social epidemiology* (2nd ed.). New York: Oxford University Press.

Boehm, J. K., Chen, Y., Koga, H., Mathur, M. B., Vie, L. L., & Kubzansky, L. D. (2018). Is optimism associated with healthier cardiovascular-related behavior? Meta-analyses of 3 health behaviors. *Circulation Research, 122*(8), 1119–1134.

Boehm, J. K., & Kubzansky, L. D. (2012). The heart's content: The association between positive psychological well-being and cardiovascular health. *Psychological Bulletin, 138*(4), 655–691.

Boehm, J. K., Peterson, C., Kivimaki, M., & Kubzansky, L. D. (2011). Heart health when life is satisfying: Evidence from the Whitehall II cohort study. *European Heart Journal, 32*(21), 2672–2677.

Boehm, J. K., Soo, J., Zevon, E. S., Chen, Y., Kim, E. S., & Kubzansky, L. D. (2018). Longitudinal associations between psychological well-being and the consumption of fruits and vegetables. *Health Psychology, 37*(10), 959–967.

Boehm, J. K., Williams, D. R., Rimm, E. B., Ryff, C., & Kubzansky, L. D. (2013). Association between optimism and serum antioxidants in the midlife in the United States study. *Psychosomatic Medicine, 75*(1), 2–10.

Boehm, J. K., Winning, A., Segerstrom, S., & Kubzansky, L. D. (2015). Variability modifies life satisfaction's association with mortality risk in older adults. *Psychological Science, 26*(7), 1063–1070.

Bolier, L., Haverman, M., Westerhof, G. J., Riper, H., Smit, F., & Bohlmeijer, E. (2013). Positive psychology interventions: A meta-analysis of randomized controlled studies. *BMC Public Health, 13*, 119.

Boylan, J. M., & Ryff, C. D. (2015). Psychological well-being and metabolic syndrome: Findings from the midlife in the United States national sample. *Psychosomatic Medicine, 77*(5), 548–558.

Boyle, P. A., Barnes, L. L., Buchman, A. S., & Bennett, D. A. (2009). Purpose in life is associated with mortality among community-dwelling older persons. *Psychosomatic Medicine, 71*(5), 574–579.

Cantril, H. (1965). *The pattern of human concerns.* New Brunswick, NJ: Rutgers University Press.

Castagne, R., Gares, V., Karimi, M., Chadeau-Hyam, M., Vineis, P., Delpierre, C., . . . Lifepath, C. (2018). Allostatic load and subsequent all-cause mortality: Which biological markers drive the relationship? Findings from a UK birth cohort. *European Journal of Epidemiology, 33*(5), 441–458.

Chakhssi, F., Kraiss, J. T., Sommers-Spijkerman, M., & Bohlmeijer, E. T. (2018). The effect of positive psychology interventions on well-being and distress in clinical samples with psychiatric or somatic disorders: A systematic review and meta-analysis. *BMC Psychiatry, 18*(1), 211.

Cheung, F., & Lucas, R. E. (2014). Assessing the validity of single-item life satisfaction measures: Results from three large samples. *Quality of Life Research, 23*(10), 2809–2818.

Choi, E., & Chentsova-Dutton, Y. E. (2017). The relationship between momentary emotions and well-being across European Americans, Hispanic Americans, and Asian Americans. *Cognition & Emotion, 31*(6), 1277–1285.

Clarke, P. J., Marshall, V. W., Ryff, C. D., & Wheaton, B. (2001). Measuring psychological well-being in the Canadian Study of Health and Aging. *International Psychogeriatrics, 13 Supp 1*, 79–90.

Cohen, R., Bavishi, C., & Rozanski, A. (2016). Purpose in life and its relationship to all-cause mortality and cardiovascular events: A meta-analysis. *Psychosomatic Medicine, 78*(2), 122–133.

Conner, J. R., Meserve, E., Pizer, E., Garber, J., Roh, M., Urban, N., . . . Feltmate, C. (2014). Outcome of unexpected adnexal neoplasia discovered during risk reduction salpingo-oophorectomy in women with germ-line BRCA1 or BRCA2 mutations. *Gynecologic Oncology, 132*(2), 280–286.

Coyne, J. C. (2013). Highly correlated hedonic and eudaimonic well-being thwart genomic analysis. *Proceedings of the National Academy of Sciences of the United States of America, 110*(45), E4183.

Czajkowski, S. M., Powell, L. H., Adler, N., Naar-King, S., Reynolds, K. D., Hunter, C. M., . . . Charlson, M. E. (2015). From ideas to efficacy: The ORBIT model for developing behavioral treatments for chronic diseases. *Health Psychology, 34*(10), 971–982.

Dejonckheere, E., Mestdagh, M., Houben, M., Rutten, I., Sels, L., Kuppens, P., & Tuerlinckx, F. (2019). Complex affect dynamics add limited information to the prediction of psychological well-being. *Nature Human Behavior, 3*(5), 478–491.

Diener, E., Lucas, R. E., & Oishi, S. (2018). Advances and open questions in the science of subjective well-being. *Collabra: Psychology, 4*(1).

Diener, E., Pressman, S. D., & Lyubomirsky, S. (2015). Can 1 million women be wrong about happiness and health? https://www.latimes.com/opinion/op-ed/la-oe-lyubomirsky-et-al-happiness-affects-health-20151217-story.html

Diener, E., & Seligman, M. E. P. (2018). Beyond money: Progress on an economy of well-being. *Perspectives on Psychological Science, 13*(2), 171–175.

Dillard, A. J., Midboe, A. M., & Klein, W. M. (2009). The dark side of optimism: Unrealistic optimism about problems with alcohol predicts subsequent negative event experiences. *Personality and Social Psychology Bulletin, 35*(11), 1540–1550.

Duque, L., Brown, L., Celano, C. M., Healy, B., & Huffman, J. C. (2019). Is it better to cultivate positive affect or optimism? Predicting improvements in medical adherence following a positive psychology intervention in patients with acute coronary syndrome. *General Hospital Psychiatry, 61*, 125–129.

Fazio, A. F. (1977). A concurrent validational study of the NCHS General Well-Being Schedule. *Vital Health Statistics 2*(73), 1–53.

Folkman, S., & Moskowitz, J. T. (2000). Positive affect and the other side of coping. *American Psychologist, 55*(6), 647–654.

Fredrickson, B. L., Grewen, K. M., Coffey, K. A., Algoe, S. B., Firestine, A. M., Arevalo, J. M., . . . Cole, S. W. (2013). A functional genomic perspective on human well-being. *Proceedings of the National Academy of Sciences of the United States of America, 110*(33), 13684–13689.

George, L. S., & Park, C. L. (2017). The Multidimensional Existential Meaning Scale: A tripartite approach to measuring meaning in life. *The Journal of Positive Psychology, 126*, 613–627.

Geulayov, G., Drory, Y., Novikov, I., & Dankner, R. (2015). Sense of coherence and 22-year all-cause mortality in adult men. *Journal of Psychosomatic Research, 78*(4), 377–383.

Giltay, E. J., Geleijnse, J. M., Zitman, F. G., Buijsse, B., & Kromhout, D. (2007). Lifestyle and dietary correlates of dispositional optimism in men: The Zutphen Elderly Study. *Journal of Psychosomatic Research, 63*(5), 483–490.

Giltay, E. J., Geleijnse, J. M., Zitman, F. G., Hoekstra, T., & Schouten, E. G. (2004). Dispositional optimism and all-cause and cardiovascular mortality in a prospective cohort of elderly Dutch men and women. *Archives of General Psychiatry, 61*(11), 1126–1135.

Hafez, D., Heisler, M., Choi, H., Ankuda, C. K., Winkelman, T., & Kullgren, J. T. (2018). Association between purpose in life and glucose control among older adults. *Annals of Behavioral Medicine, 52*(4), 309–318.

Haller, C. S. (2016). Trajectories of smoking behavior as a function of mood and satisfaction with life: What matters most? *Journal of Affective Disorders, 190,* 407–413.

Haukkala, A., Konttinen, H., Laatikainen, T., Kawachi, I., & Uutela, A. (2010). Hostility, anger control, and anger expression as predictors of cardiovascular disease. *Psychosomatic Medicine, 72*(6), 556–562.

Helliwell, J. F., Barrington-Leigh, C. P., Harris, A., & Huang, H. (2010). International evidence on the social context of well-being. In E. Diener, J. F. Helliwell, & D. Kahneman (Eds.), *International differences in wellbeing* (pp. 291–327). New York: Oxford University Press.

Hernandez, R., Bassett, R. M., Boughton, S. W., Schuette, S. A., Shiu, E. W., & Moskowitz, J. T. (2018). Psychological well-being and physical health: Associations, mechanisms, and future directions. *Emotion Review, 10*(1), 1–12.

Hernandez, R., Vu, T. T., Kershaw, K. N., Boehm, J. K., Kubzansky, L. D., Carnethon, M., . . . Liu, K. (2020). The association of optimism with sleep duration and quality: Findings from the Coronary Artery Risk and Development in Young Adults (CARDIA) study. *Behavioral Medicine, 46*(2), 100–111.

Hingle, M. D., Wertheim, B. C., Tindle, H. A., Tinker, L., Seguin, R. A., Rosal, M. C., & Thomson, C. A. (2014). Optimism and diet quality in the Women's Health Initiative. *Journal of the Academy of Nutrition and Dietetics, 114*(7), 1036–1045.

Hofstede, G., Hofstede, G. J., & Minkov, M. (2010). *Cultures and organizations: Software of the mind* (3rd ed.). New York: McGraw Hill.

Holt-Lunstad, J., Robles, T. F., & Sbarra, D. A. (2017). Advancing social connection as a public health priority in the United States. *American Psychologist, 72*(6), 517–530.

Holt-Lunstad, J., Smith, T. B., & Layton, J. B. (2010). Social relationships and mortality risk: A meta-analytic review. *PLoS Medicine, 7*(7), e1000316.

Hsu, H., Hsu, T., Lee, K., & Wolff, L. (2017). Evaluating the construct validity of Ryff's scales of psychological well-being using exploratory structural equation modeling. *Journal of Psychoeducational Assessment, 35*(6), 633–638.

Hulur, G., Heckhausen, J., Hoppmann, C. A., Infurna, F. J., Wagner, G. G., Ram, N., & Gerstorf, D. (2017). Levels of and changes in life satisfaction predict mortality hazards: Disentangling the role of physical health, perceived control, and social orientation. *Psychology and Aging, 32*(6), 507–520.

Hyde, M., Wiggins, R. D., Higgs, P., & Blane, D. B. (2003). A measure of quality of life in early old age: The theory, development and properties of a needs satisfaction model (CASP-19). *Aging and Mental Health, 7*(3), 186–194.

James, P., Kim, E. S., Kubzansky, L. D., Zevon, E. S., Trudel-Fitzgerald, C., & Grodstein, F. (2019). Optimism and healthy aging in women. *American Journal of Preventive Medicine, 56*(1), 116–124.

Jenkins, B. N., Hunter, J. F., Richardson, M. J., Conner, T. S., & Pressman, S. D. (2019). Affect variability and predictability: Using recurrence quantification analysis to better understand how the dynamics of affect relate to health. *Emotion.* doi:10.1037/emo0000556

Jylha, M. (2009). What is self-rated health and why does it predict mortality? Towards a unified conceptual model. *Social Science & Medicine, 69*(3), 307–316.

Kahneman, D., Krueger, A. B., Schkade, D. A., Schwarz, N., & Stone, A. A. (2004). A survey method for characterizing daily life experience: The day reconstruction method. *Science, 306*(5702), 1776–1780.

Keyes, C. L., & Simoes, E. J. (2012). To flourish or not: Positive mental health and all-cause mortality. *American Journal of Public Health, 102*(11), 2164–2172.

Kim, E. S., Hagan, K. A., Grodstein, F., DeMeo, D. L., De Vivo, I., & Kubzansky, L. D. (2017). Optimism and cause-specific mortality: A prospective cohort study. *American Journal of Epidemiology, 185*(1), 21–29.

Kim, E. S., James, P., Zevon, E. S., Trudel-Fitzgerald, C., Kubzansky, L. D., & Grodstein, F. (2019). Optimism and healthy aging in women and men. *American Journal of Epidemiology, 188*(6), 1084–1091.

Kim, E. S., Kubzansky, L. D., Soo, J., & Boehm, J. K. (2016). Maintaining healthy behavior: A prospective study of psychological well-being and physical activity. *Annals of Behavioral Medicine, 51*(3), 337–347.

Kim, E. S., Strecher, V. J., & Ryff, C. D. (2014). Purpose in life and use of preventive health care services. *Proceedings of the National Academy of Sciences of the United States of America, 111*(46), 16331–16336.

Kimm, H., Sull, J. W., Gombojav, B., Yi, S. W., & Ohrr, H. (2012). Life satisfaction and mortality in elderly people: The Kangwha Cohort Study. *BMC Public Health, 12,* 54.

Kobau, R., Seligman, M. E., Peterson, C., Diener, E., Zack, M. M., Chapman, D., & Thompson, W. (2011). Mental health promotion in public health: Perspectives and strategies from positive psychology. *American Journal of Public Health, 101*(8), e1–e9.

Koopmans, T. A., Geleijnse, J. M., Zitman, F. G., & Giltay, E. J. (2010). Effects of happiness on all-cause mortality during 15 years of follow-up: The Arnhem Elderly Study. *Journal of Happiness Studies, 11,* 113–124.

Krause, N. (2004). Stressors arising in highly valued roles, meaning in life, and the physical health status of older adults. *Journal of Gerontology B Series: Psychological Sciences and Social Sciences, 59*(5), S287–S297.

Krause, N. (2009). Meaning in life and mortality. *Journal of Gerontology B Series: Psychological Sciences and Social Sciences, 64*(4), 517–527.

Kubzansky, L. D., Huffman, J. C., Boehm, J. K., Hernandez, R., Kim, E. S., Koga, H. K., . . . Labarthe, D. R. (2018). Positive psychological well-being and cardiovascular disease: JACC Health Promotion Series. *Journal of the American College of Cardiology, 72*(12), 1382–1396.

Kubzansky, L. D., Kim, E. S., Salinas, J., Huffman, J. C., & Kawachi, I. (2016). Happiness, health, and mortality. *Lancet, 388*(10039), 27.

Kubzansky, L. D., & Thurston, R. C. (2007). Emotional vitality and incident coronary heart disease: Benefits of healthy psychological functioning. *Archives of General Psychiatry, 64*(12), 1393–1401.

Kubzansky, L. D., Wright, R. J., Cohen, S., Weiss, S., Rosner, B., & Sparrow, D. (2002). Breathing easy: A prospective study of optimism and pulmonary function in the Normative Aging Study. *Annals of Behavioral Medicine, 24*(4), 345–353.

Labidi-Galy, S. I., Papp, E., Hallberg, D., Niknafs, N., Adleff, V., Noe, M., . . . Velculescu, V. E. (2017). High grade serous ovarian carcinomas originate in the fallopian tube. *Nature Communications, 8*(1), 1093.

Latham-Mintus, K., Vowels, A., & Huskins, K. (2018). Healthy aging among older Black and White men: What is the role of mastery? *Journal of Gerontology B Series: Psychological Sciences and Social Sciences, 73*(2), 248–257.

Lee Kum Sheung Center for Health and Happiness. (2017). Measurement of well-being. https://www.hsph.harvard.edu/health-happiness/research-new/positive-health/measurement-of-well-being/

Lee, L. O., James, P., Zevon, E. S., Kim, E. S., Trudel-Fitzgerald, C., Spiro, A., 3rd, . . . Kubzansky, L. D. (2019). Optimism is associated with exceptional longevity in 2 epidemiologic cohorts of men and women. *Proceedings of the National Academy of Sciences of the United States of America, 116*(37), 18357–18362.

Liu, B., Floud, S., Pirie, K., Green, J., Peto, R., & Beral, V. (2016). Does happiness itself directly affect mortality? The prospective UK Million Women Study. *Lancet, 387*(10021), 874–881.

Liu, Z., Li, L., Huang, J., Qian, D., Chen, F., Xu, J., . . . Wang, X. (2014). Association between subjective well-being and exceptional longevity in a longevity town in China: A population-based study. *Age (Dordr), 36*(3), 9632.

Lockenhoff, C. E., & Carstensen, L. L. (2004). Socioemotional selectivity theory, aging, and health: The increasingly delicate balance between regulating emotions and making tough choices. *Journal of Personality, 72*(6), 1395–1424.

Loef, M., & Walach, H. (2012). The combined effects of healthy lifestyle behaviors on all cause mortality: A systematic review and meta-analysis. *Preventive Medicine, 55*(3), 163–170.

Lucas, R. E., Diener, E., & Suh, E. (1996). Discriminant validity of well-being measures. *Journal of Personality and Social Psychology, 71*(3), 616–628.

Luhmann, M., Hawkley, L. C., Eid, M., & Cacioppo, J. T. (2012). Time frames and the distinction between affective and cognitive well-being. *Journal of Research on Personality, 46*(4), 431–441.

Lundberg, O., & Peck, M. N. (1995). A simplified way of measuring sense of coherence: Experiences from a population survey in Sweden. *European Journal of Public Health, 5*, 56–59.

Ma, X., Tamir, M., & Miyamoto, Y. (2018). A socio-cultural instrumental approach to emotion regulation: Culture and the regulation of positive emotions. *Emotion, 18*(1), 138–152.

Malinchoc, M., Offord, K. P., & Colligan, R. C. (1995). PSM-R: Revised Optimism-Pessimism Scale for the MMPI-2 and MMPI. *Journal of Clinical Psychology, 51*(2), 205–214.

Marmot, M., & Wilkinson, R. G. (2005). *Social determinants of health*. New York: Oxford University Press.

Martela, F., & Steger, M. F. (2016). The three meanings of meaning in life: Distinguishing coherence, purpose, and significance. *Journal of Positive Psychology, 11*(5), 531–545.

Martin-Maria, N., Caballero, F. F., Olaya, B., Rodriguez-Artalejo, F., Haro, J. M., Miret, M., & Ayuso-Mateos, J. L. (2016). Positive affect is inversely associated with mortality in individuals without depression. *Frontiers in Psychology, 7*, 1040.

Martin-Maria, N., Miret, M., Caballero, F. F., Rico-Uribe, L. A., Steptoe, A., Chatterji, S., & Ayuso-Mateos, J. L. (2017). The impact of subjective well-being on mortality: A meta-analysis of longitudinal studies in the general population. *Psychosomatic Medicine, 79*(5), 565–575.

Matthews, K. A., Raikkonen, K., Sutton-Tyrrell, K., & Kuller, L. H. (2004). Optimistic attitudes protect against progression of carotid atherosclerosis in healthy middle-aged women. *Psychosomatic Medicine, 66*(5), 640–644.

Miller, S. M., Sherman, A. C., & Christensen, A. J. (2010). Introduction to special series: The great debate--evaluating the health implications of positive psychology. *Annals of Behavioral Medicine, 39*(1), 1–3.

Moskowitz, J. T., Carrico, A. W., Duncan, L. G., Cohn, M. A., Cheung, E. O., Batchelder, A., . . . Folkman, S. (2017). Randomized controlled trial of a positive affect intervention for people newly diagnosed with HIV. *Journal of Consulting and Clinical Psychology, 85*(5), 409–423.

Mroczek, D. K., Stawski, R. S., Turiano, N. A., Chan, W., Almeida, D. M., Neupert, S. D., & Spiro, A., 3rd. (2015). Emotional reactivity and mortality: Longitudinal findings from the VA Normative Aging Study. *Journal of Gerontology B Series: Psychological Sciences and Social Sciences, 70*(3), 398–406.

National Research Council. (2013). *Subjective well-being: Measuring happiness, suffering, and other dimensions of experience* (Panel on Measuring Subjective Well-Being in a Policy-Relevant Framework, A. A. Stone, & C. Mackie Eds.). Committee on National Statistics, Division on Behavioral and Social Sciences & Education National Research Council. Washington, DC: National Academies Press.

Netuveli, G., Pikhart, H., Bobak, M., & Blane, D. (2012). Generic quality of life predicts all-cause mortality in the short term: Evidence from British Household Panel Survey. *J Journal of Epidemiology and Community Health, 66*(10), 962–966.

Neugarten, B. L., Havighurst, R. J., & Tobin, S. S. (1961). The measurement of life satisfaction. *Journal of Gerontology, 16*, 134–143.

Newman, A. B., & Murabito, J. M. (2013). The epidemiology of longevity and exceptional survival. *Epidemiological Review, 35*, 181–197.

Nielsen, L., Riddle, M., King, J. W., Team, N. I. H. S. o. B. C. I., Aklin, W. M., Chen, W., . . . Weber, W. (2018). The NIH Science of Behavior Change Program: Transforming the science through a focus on mechanisms of change. *Behaviour Research and Therapy, 101*, 3–11.

Nikrahan, G. R., Laferton, J. A., Asgari, K., Kalantari, M., Abedi, M. R., Etesampour, A., . . . Huffman, J. C. (2016). Effects of positive psychology interventions on risk biomarkers in coronary patients: A randomized, wait-list controlled pilot trial. *Psychosomatics, 57*(4), 359–368.

Okely, J. A., Cooper, C., & Gale, C. R. (2016). Wellbeing and arthritis incidence: The Survey of Health, Ageing and Retirement in Europe. *Annals of Behavioral Medicine, 50*(3), 419–426.

Okely, J. A., & Gale, C. R. (2016). Well-being and chronic disease incidence: The English Longitudinal Study of Ageing. *Psychosomatic Medicine, 78*(3), 335–344.

Okely, J. A., Weiss, A., & Gale, C. R. (2017). Well-being and arthritis incidence: The role of inflammatory mechanisms. findings from the English Longitudinal Study of Ageing. *Psychosomatic Medicine, 79*(7), 742–748.

Okely, J. A., Weiss, A., & Gale, C. R. (2018). The interaction between individualism and wellbeing in predicting mortality: Survey of Health Ageing and Retirement in Europe. *Journal of Behavioral Medicine, 41*(1), 1–11.

Olsson, M., Gassne, J., & Hansson, K. (2009). Do different scales measure the same construct? Three Sense of Coherence scales. *Journal of Epidemiology and Community Health, 63*(2), 166–167.

Ong, A. D., & Ram, N. (2017). Fragile and enduring positive affect: Implications for adaptive aging. *Gerontology, 63*(3), 263–269.

Patel, V., Saxena, S., Lund, C., Thornicroft, G., Baingana, F., Bolton, P., . . . UnUtzer, J. (2018). The Lancet Commission on global mental health and sustainable development. *Lancet, 392*(10157), 1553–1598.

Pavot, W., Diener, E., Colvin, C. R., & Sandvik, E. (1991). Further validation of the Satisfaction with Life Scale: Evidence for the cross-method convergence of well-being measures. *Journal of Personality Assessment, 57*(1), 149–161.

Pearlin, L. I., & Schooler, C. (1978). The structure of coping. *Journal of Health & Social Behavior, 19*(1), 2–21.

Penninx, B. W., van Tilburg, T., Kriegsman, D. M., Deeg, D. J., Boeke, A. J., & van Eijk, J. T. (1997). Effects of social support and personal coping resources on mortality in older age: The Longitudinal Aging Study Amsterdam. *American Journal of Epidemiology, 146*(6), 510–519.

Petrie, K. J., Pressman, S. D., Pennebaker, J. W., Overland, S., Tell, G. S., & Sivertsen, B. (2018). Which aspects of positive affect are related to mortality? Results from a general population longitudinal study. *Annals of Behavioral Medicine, 52*(7), 571–581.

Picard, M., Juster, R. P., & Sabiston, C. (2013). Is the whole greater than the sum of the parts? Self-rated health and transdisciplinarity. *Health, 5*(12), 24–30.

Poirier, A. E., Ruan, Y., Volesky, K. D., King, W. D., O'Sullivan, D. E., Gogna, P., . . . Com, P. S. T. (2019). The current and future burden of cancer attributable to modifiable risk factors in Canada: Summary of results. *Preventive Medicine, 122*, 140–147.

Pressman, S. D., Gallagher, M. W., & Lopez, S. J. (2013). Is the emotion-health connection a "first-world problem"? *Psychological Science, 24*(4), 544–549.

Pressman, S. D., Jenkins, B. N., & Moskowitz, J. T. (2019). Positive affect and health: What do we know and where next should we go? *Annual Review of Psychology*. doi:10.1146/annurev-psych-010418-102955

Progovac, A. M., Chang, Y. F., Chang, C. H., Matthews, K. A., Donohue, J. M., Scheier, M. F., . . . Tindle, H. A. (2017). Are optimism and cynical hostility associated with smoking cessation in older women? *Annals of Behavioral Medicine, 51*(4), 500–510.

Progovac, A. M., Donohue, J. M., Matthews, K. A., Chang, C. H., Habermann, E. B., Kuller, L. H., . . . Tindle, H. A. (2017). Optimism predicts sustained vigorous physical activity in postmenopausal women. *Preventive Medicine Reports, 8*, 286–293.

Radler, B. T., Rigotti, A., & Ryff, C. D. (2018). Persistently high psychological well-being predicts better HDL cholesterol and triglyceride levels: Findings from the midlife in the US (MIDUS) longitudinal study. *Lipids in Health and Disease, 17*(1), 1.

Revelas, M., Thalamuthu, A., Oldmeadow, C., Evans, T. J., Armstrong, N. J., Kwok, J. B., . . . Mather, K. A. (2018). Review and meta-analysis of genetic polymorphisms associated with exceptional human longevity. *Mechanisms of Ageing and Development, 175*, 24–34.

Richman, L. S., Kubzansky, L., Maselko, J., Kawachi, I., Choo, P., & Bauer, M. (2005). Positive emotion and health: Going beyond the negative. *Health Psychology, 24*(4), 422–429.

Rius-Ottenheim, N., Houben, J. M., Kromhout, D., Kafatos, A., van der Mast, R. C., Zitman, F. G., . . . Giltay, E. J. (2012). Telomere length and mental well-being in elderly men from the Netherlands and Greece. *Behavioral Genetics, 42*(2), 278–286.

Rosella, L. C., Fu, L., Buajitti, E., & Goel, V. (2018). Mortality and chronic disease risk associated with poor life satisfaction: A population-based cohort study. *American Journal of Epidemiology.* doi:10.1093/aje/kwy245

Rozanski, A., Bavishi, C., Kubzansky, L. D., & Cohen, R. (2019). Association of optimism with cardiovascular events and all-cause mortality: A systematic review and meta-analysis. *JAMA Network Open, 2*(9), e1912200.

Ryan, R. M., & Frederick, C. (1997). On energy, personality, and health: Subjective vitality as a dynamic reflection of well-being. *Journal of Personality, 65*(3), 529–565.

Ryff, C. D. (1989). Happiness is everything, or is it? Explorations on the meaning of psychological well-being. *Journal of Personality and Social Psychology, 57*(6), 1069–1081.

Ryff, C. D. (2017). Eudaimonic well-being, inequality, and health: Recent findings and future directions. *International Revive of Economics, 64*(2), 159–178.

Ryff, C. D., Dienberg Love, G., Urry, H. L., Muller, D., Rosenkranz, M. A., Friedman, E. M., . . . Singer, B. (2006). Psychological well-being and ill-being: Do they have distinct or mirrored biological correlates? *Psychotherapy and Psychosomatics, 75*(2), 85–95.

Ryff, C. D., Heller, A. S., Schaefer, S. M., van Reekum, C., & Davidson, R. J. (2016). Purposeful engagement, healthy aging, and the brain. *Current Behavioral Neuroscience Reports, 3*(4), 318–327.

Ryff, C. D., & Keyes, C. L. (1995). The structure of psychological well-being revisited. *Journal of Personality and Social Psychology, 69*(4), 719–727.

Ryff, C. D., & Singer, B. (2007). What to do about positive and negative items in studies of psychological well-being and ill-being? *Psychotherapy and Psychosomatics, 76*, 61–62.

Scheibe, S., & Carstensen, L. L. (2010). Emotional aging: Recent findings and future trends. *Journal of Gerontology B Series: Psychological Sciences and Social Sciences, 65B*(2), 135–144.

Scheier, M. F., & Carver, C. S. (2018). Dispositional optimism and physical health: A long look back, a quick look forward. *American Psychologist, 73*(9), 1082–1094.

Scheier, M. F., Carver, C. S., & Bridges, M. W. (1994). Distinguishing optimism from neuroticism (and trait anxiety, self-mastery, and self-esteem): A reevaluation of the Life Orientation Test. *Journal of Personality and Social Psychology, 67*(6), 1063–1078.

Scheier, M. F., Carver, C. S., & Bridges, M. W. (2001). Optimism, pessimism, and psychological well-being. In E. C. Chang (Ed.), *Optimism and pessimism: Implications for theory, research, and practice* (pp. 189–216). Washington, DC: American Psychological Association.

Sebastiani, P., Thyagarajan, B., Sun, F., Schupf, N., Newman, A. B., Montano, M., & Perls, T. T. (2017). Biomarker signatures of aging. *Aging Cell, 16*(2), 329–338.

Segerstrom, S. C. (2005). Optimism and immunity: Do positive thoughts always lead to positive effects? *Brain, Behavior, and Immunity, 19*(3), 195–200.

Seligman, M. E., & Csikszentmihalyi, M. (2000). Positive psychology: An introduction. *American Psychologist, 55*(1), 5–14.

Sin, N. L., & Lyubomirsky, S. (2009). Enhancing well-being and alleviating depressive symptoms with positive psychology interventions: A practice-friendly meta-analysis. *Journal of Clinical Psychology, 65*(5), 467–487.

Sone, T., Nakaya, N., Ohmori, K., Shimazu, T., Higashiguchi, M., Kakizaki, M., . . . Tsuji, I. (2008). Sense of life worth living (ikigai) and mortality in Japan: Ohsaki Study. *Psychosomatic Medicine, 70*(6), 709–715.

Song, M., & Giovannucci, E. (2016). Preventable incidence and mortality of carcinoma associated with lifestyle factors among White adults in the United States. *JAMA Oncology, 2*(9), 1154–1161.

Soo, J., Kubzansky, L. D., Chen, Y., Zevon, E. S., & Boehm, J. K. (2018). Psychological well-being and restorative biological processes: HDL-C in older English adults. *Social Science & Medicine, 209*, 59–66.

St John, P. D., Mackenzie, C., & Menec, V. (2015). Does life satisfaction predict five-year mortality in community-living older adults? *Aging & Mental Health, 19*(4), 363–370.

Steptoe, A. (2019). Happiness and health. *Annual Review of Public Health, 1*(40), 339–359.

Super, S., Verschuren, W. M., Zantinge, E. M., Wagemakers, M. A., & Picavet, H. S. (2014). A weak sense of coherence is associated with a higher mortality risk. *Journal of Epidemiology and Community Health, 68*(5), 411–417.

Surtees, P., Wainwright, N., Luben, R., Khaw, K. T., & Day, N. (2003). Sense of coherence and mortality in men and women in the EPIC-Norfolk United Kingdom prospective cohort study. *American Journal of Epidemiology, 158*(12), 1202–1209.

Surtees, P. G., Wainwright, N. W., Luben, R., Khaw, K. T., & Day, N. E. (2006). Mastery, sense of coherence, and mortality: Evidence of independent associations from the EPIC-Norfolk Prospective Cohort Study. *Health Psychology, 25*(1), 102–110.

Tanno, K., Sakata, K., Ohsawa, M., Onoda, T., Itai, K., Yaegashi, Y., & Tamakoshi, A. (2009). Associations of ikigai as a positive psychological factor with all-cause mortality and cause-specific mortality among middle-aged and elderly Japanese people: Findings from the Japan Collaborative Cohort Study. *Journal of Psychosomatic Research, 67*(1), 67–75.

Tennen, H., & Affleck, G. (1987). The costs and benefits of optimistic explanations and dispositional optimism. *Journal of Personality, 55*(2), 376–393.

Tindle, H. A., Chang, Y. F., Kuller, L. H., Manson, J. E., Robinson, J. G., Rosal, M. C., . . . Matthews, K. A. (2009). Optimism, cynical hostility, and incident coronary heart disease and mortality in the Women's Health Initiative. *Circulation, 120*(8), 656–662.

Trudel-Fitzgerald, C., Boehm, J. K., Kivimaki, M., & Kubzansky, L. D. (2014). Taking the tension out of hypertension: A prospective study of psychological well being and hypertension. *Journal of Hypertension, 32*(6), 1222–1228.

Trudel-Fitzgerald, C., Chen, Y., Singh, A., Okereke, O. I., & Kubzansky, L. D. (2016). Psychiatric, psychological, and social determinants of health in the Nurses' Health Study cohorts. *American Journal of Public Health, 106*(9), 1644–1649.

Trudel-Fitzgerald, C., James, P., Kim, E. S., Zevon, E. S., Grodstein, F., & Kubzansky, L. D. (2019a). Prospective associations of happiness and optimism with lifestyle over up to two decades. *Preventive Medicine, 126*, 105754.

Trudel-Fitzgerald, C., Millstein, R. A., von Hippel, C., Howe, C. J., Tomasso, L. P., Wagner, G. R., & VanderWeele, T. J. (2019b). Psychological well-being as part of the public health debate? Insight into dimensions, interventions, and policy. *BMC Public Health, 19*(1), 1–11.

Trudel-Fitzgerald, C., Qureshi, F., Appleton, A. A., & Kubzansky, L. D. (2017). A healthy mix of emotions: Underlying biological pathways linking emotions to physical health. *Current Opinion in Behavioral Sciences, 15*, 16–21.

Tsenkova, V. K., Karlamangla, A. S., & Ryff, C. D. (2016). Parental history of diabetes, positive affect, and diabetes risk in adults: Findings from MIDUS. *Annals of Behavioral Medicine, 50*(6), 836–843.

Turiano, N. A., Chapman, B. P., Agrigoroaei, S., Infurna, F. J., & Lachman, M. (2014). Perceived control reduces mortality risk at low, not high, education levels. *Health Psychology, 33*(8), 883–890.

Uchida, Y., Kitayama, S., Akutsu, S., Park, J., & Cole, S. W. (2018). Optimism and the conserved transcriptional response to adversity. *Health Psychology, 37*(11), 1077–1080.

Valeri, L., & Vanderweele, T. J. (2013). Mediation analysis allowing for exposure-mediator interactions and causal interpretation: Theoretical assumptions and implementation with SAS and SPSS macros. *Psychological Methods, 18*(2), 137–150.

Van Cappellen, P., Rice, E. L., Catalino, L. I., & Fredrickson, B. L. (2018). Positive affective processes underlie positive health behaviour change. *Psychological Health, 33*(1), 77–97.

VanderWeele, T. J. (2015). *Explanation in causal inference: Methods for mediation and interaction.* New York: Oxford University Press.

VanderWeele, T. J. (2017). On the promotion of human flourishing. *Proceedings of the National Academy of Sciences of the United States of America, 114*(31), 8148–8156.

VanderWeele, T. J., Chen, Y., Long, K., Kim, E. S., Trudel-Fitzgerald, C., & Kubzanksy, L. D. (2020). Positive epidemiology? *Epidemiology, 31*(2), 189–193.

VanderWeele, T. J., McNeely, E., & Koh, H. K. (2019). Reimagining health: Flourishing. *JAMA.* doi:10.1001/jama.2019.3035

Watson, D., Clark, L. A., & Tellegen, A. (1988). Development and validation of brief measures of positive and negative affect: The PANAS scales. *Journal of Personality and Social Psychology, 54*(6), 1063–1070.

Weziak-Bialowolska, D., McNeely, E., & VanderWeele, T. J. (2019). Human flourishing in cross cultural settings: Evidence from the United States, China, Sri Lanka, Cambodia, and Mexico. *Frontiers in Psychology, 10*, 1269. doi:10.3389/fpsyg.2019.01269

Wiest, M., Schuz, B., Webster, N., & Wurm, S. (2011). Subjective well-being and mortality revisited: Differential effects of cognitive and emotional facets of well-being on mortality. *Health Psychology, 30*(6), 728–735.

Wirtz, D., Chiu, C. Y., Diener, E., & Oishi, S. (2009). What constitutes a good life? Cultural differences in the role of positive and negative affect in subjective well-being. *Journal of Personality, 77*(4), 1167–1196.

Zaslavsky, O., Rillamas-Sun, E., Woods, N. F., Cochrane, B. B., Stefanick, M. L., Tindle, H., . . . LaCroix, A. Z. (2014). Association of the selected dimensions of eudaimonic well-being with healthy survival to 85 years of age in older women. *International Psychogeriatrics, 26*(12), 2081–2091.

Zhang, Y., & Han, B. (2016). Positive affect and mortality risk in older adults: A meta-analysis. *PsyCh Journal, 5*(2), 125–138.

Zilioli, S., Slatcher, R. B., Ong, A. D., & Gruenewald, T. L. (2015). Purpose in life predicts allostatic load ten years later. *Journal of Psychosomatic Research, 79*(5), 451–457.

PART 2

CONCEPTUAL REFLECTIONS
ON WELL-BEING MEASUREMENT

6

"Positive Biology" and
Well-Ordered Science

Colin Farrelly

Abstract

Going back to the Ancient Greeks (e.g., Plato and Aristotle), philosophers have long asked profound questions such as "What is knowledge?" and "What is the good life?" Such questions compel us to engage in a deeper level of introspection and examination than most of us are typically accustomed to in our daily lives. The philosophical question contemplated in this chapter is "What constitutes 'well-ordered science'?" Invoking a virtue epistemological construal of knowledge as "success from ability," I argue that the study of pathology must be supplemented by the study of the determinates of exemplary positive phenotypes (e.g., healthy aging and happiness). This requires transcending the limitations of what I call "negative biology," and treating "positive biology" as an integral element of well-ordered science in the twenty-first century. Positive biology can help bring to the fore the importance of understanding the evolutionary and life history of our species, thus helping to provide the intellectual frameworks needed to inspire the development of novel and feasible interventions to improve human health and happiness.

Going back to the Ancient Greeks (e.g., Plato and Aristotle), philosophers have long asked profound questions such as "What is knowledge?" and "What is the good life?" Such questions compel us to engage in a deeper level of introspection and examination than most of us are typically accustomed to in our daily lives. Intellectual curiosity and the challenging of our established beliefs are important because we are prone to cognitive biases and superstitious beliefs which exemplify epistemic *vice* (e.g., simplicity of casual

Colin Farrelly, *"Positive Biology" and Well-Ordered Science* In: *Measuring Well-Being*. Edited by: Matthew T. Lee, Laura D. Kubzansky, and Tyler J. VanderWeele, Oxford University Press (2021). © Oxford University Press.
DOI: 10.1093/oso/9780197512531.003.0007

explanation, confirmation bias, etc.) rather than epistemic *virtue* (Zagzebski, 1996), which includes attention to the relevant facts, intellectual humility, adaptability of intellect, etc.

The introspection that philosophy encourages us to engage in can often be a catalyst to new insights because philosophy requires one to make *explicit* the hidden assumptions behind our beliefs and cultural practices. And then, once these assumptions are explicit, the philosopher will critically assess the soundness of these hidden assumptions.

The philosophical question I would like to contemplate in this chapter is "What constitutes 'well-ordered science'?" In the next section I lay some preliminary foundations for addressing this question by elaborating briefly on the virtue epistemological construal of knowledge as "success from ability" (Greco, 2010). This is achieved by drawing a contrast between superstitious beliefs and scientific knowledge. I then invoke James Flory and Philip Kitcher's (2004) definition of well-ordered science (an account that prioritizes asking the most significant questions) and link this to the medical sciences and the fixation on the question "what causes disease?" Drawing a contrast (detailed in a later section) between what I have described elsewhere (Farrelly, 2012a) as "negative biology" and "positive biology," I urge that the study of pathology be supplemented by the study of the determinates of exemplary positive phenotypes (e.g., healthy aging and happiness). Two subsequent sections then detail how this has already been be applied, respectively, to the fields of geroscience and positive psychology. I conclude that positive biology can help bring to the fore the importance of understanding the evolutionary and life history of our species, thus helping to provide the intellectual frameworks needed to inspire the development of novel and feasible interventions to improve human health and happiness that go beyond what is likely to be achieved by functioning solely within the intellectual assumptions of "negative biology."

"Scientia Potentia Est"

"Knock on wood!"
"Find a penny, pick it up; and all day long you'll have good luck!"

These two popular sayings express superstitious beliefs. Beliefs which, if taken seriously as actually possessing *prescriptive* action-guiding advice, would be folly to adhere to. The person who, after knocking on wood or finding a penny, undertakes a risky course of action thinking they will be protected from any potential hazards puts themselves in peril. What is it that separates credulous beliefs from *knowledge*?

Virtue epistemologists define knowledge as "success from ability" (Greco, 2010) or "a state of cognitive contact with reality arising out of acts of intellectual virtue" (Zagzebski, 1996, p. 270). Unlike superstitious beliefs, the insights of epidemiology, agricultural science, physics, and chemistry all have *predictive* power that can be tested and verified in the empirical world. These disciplines constitute "knowledge," even if only provisional and far from complete, because they permit us to enjoy different types of success in navigating through our precarious world. The success science has achieved ranges from protecting populations against infectious disease and providing sufficient water for agriculture, to applying the laws of motion to inform vehicle safety regulations (e.g., speed limits, seat belt requirements) and chemistry to develop safe pharmaceuticals to treat or manage disease.

The word "science" is derived from the Latin *scientia*, which means "knowledge." "*Scientia potentia est*" (or "knowledge is power") is a slogan often attributed to Francis Bacon (1561–1626), and it appears in Thomas Hobbes's *Leviathan*. This motto coheres with the virtue epistemological understanding that knowledge is "success from ability." Acting from a position of knowledge—versus ignorance—permits us to more successfully navigate the perils of the external world so that we may flourish as individual persons and collectively as societies.

The world is a complex and constantly changing environment, and thus knowledge itself will not be fixed or static. The normative value of different types of knowledge will be *context-specific*. In one context certain empirical insights about the world might prove to be vital in helping us protect a population from disease and premature death. But those same empirical insights might be, in a different context, of much more limited use and significance because the most pressing external threats to human populations are different.

This point can be illustrated with the following example. Consider the historical context of fifteenth-century England, where life expectancy at birth would have been less than 40 years of age. If we could travel back in time to the fifteenth century and offer the people living then one—and only one—of the following public health insights to improve population health, which one would we choose to share with them?

1. Edward Jenner's research into cowpox and immunology that helped, eventually, to eradicate smallpox from the world by 1980.

or

2. The knowledge that tobacco is a carcinogen, and that smoking cessation can help prevent lung cancer.

In a world dominated by high rates of early and mid-life mortality and a projected increased risk of infectious diseases like smallpox (as the size of urban populations in cities like London would grow through the seventeenth and eighteenth centuries), Jenner's discovery of the vaccine against small pox would be *significantly* more valuable than a public campaign of smoking cessation in fifteenth-century England. The latter would not offer a significant benefit to population health because other threats, such as infectious disease and poverty, killed most humans before reaching the advanced age when lung cancer would likely develop (which is typically older than 65).

However, today, in the twenty-first century, with smallpox eradicated and life expectancy at birth at age 72 (World Health Organization, n.d.), smoking cessation is a very significant public health priority to help reduce global cancer mortality. The health vulnerabilities facing today's aging populations are different from those that human populations faced in centuries past. And this means that the scientific insights most conducive to health promotion will be constantly evolving as the empirical realities (e.g., risk of disease) facing the world's populations change.

I posit this hypothetical thought experiment of fifteenth-century England to illustrate the point that an empirical insight (or general theoretical framework) can be valuable life-saving knowledge in one context but something that simply satisfies our intellectual curiosity (without being translatable into practical action that could substantively improve population health, happiness, or prosperity) in a different type of context.

Since the rise of epidemiology in the nineteenth century, the central question which has been the primary focus of both clinical medicine and public health is: *What causes disease?* In this chapter I argue that this fixation on *disease-research* (evident in oncology, cardiology, psychiatry, etc.) must now (i.e., in the twenty-first century) be supplemented by a zeal to also invest in and support basic scientific research into the causation of exemplar *positive* phenotypes. These phenotypes range from exceptional healthy aging and HIV resistance to emotional resilience and human happiness. In this chapter I defend and expand upon the intellectual paradigm which unifies these disparate areas of enquiry, what I call "positive biology." I make the case for considering positive biology as an integral part of "well-ordered" science in the twenty-first century.

In the following section, I define what constitutes well-ordered science. I then expand on the contrast between negative and positive biology and the importance the latter places on understanding both the proximate and evolutionary causation of positive phenotypes. The subsequent two sections illustrate the prescriptive potential of positive biology by drawing attention to, respectively, insights from "geroscience" and "positive psychology."

What Constitutes Well-Ordered Science?

I believe a virtue epistemological understanding of knowledge as "success from ability" is helpful because the account of knowledge it champions is one which prescribes that we aspire to achieve a state of cognitive contact with reality that arises from the exercise of *epistemic virtue*. It is only through this cognitive contact with reality that we can hope to flourish in a precarious and uncertain world. For example, with the knowledge of medicine, foreign affairs, and economics we can better secure the desired aims of health, peace, and economic prosperity. Such aims are unlikely to be realized if our actions are guided by mere guesses, flipping a coin, or interpretations of a divine entity's plan for us derived from the celestial movements of the planets (e.g., astrology). Impulsivity or placing faith in chance or dogmatism does not exemplify intellectual virtue. On the contrary, they exemplify epistemic *vice* by ignoring evidence, failing to display an appropriate amount of humility, etc. Belief, for virtue epistemologists, is a kind of performance with a goal (Kelp, 2017, p. 224). *And the ultimate goal or standard for assessing our collective beliefs is their ability to enable us to flourish.*

Conceptualizing knowledge as "success from ability" reminds us that knowledge is not static. Knowledge involves having cognitive contact with an external reality that is constantly changing, sometimes changing in predictable and often unpredictable ways over time. Knowledge that once permitted us to have success against certain extrinsic risks might prove less helpful when new extrinsic risks (e.g., climate change) emerge to pose significant threats to our health and prosperity. And this then compels us to adapt and develop new conceptual tools and innovations if we hope to continue to flourish against new threats.

James Flory and Phillip Kitcher define the idea of well-ordered science as follows: "The pursuit of science in a society is *well-ordered* when the research effort is efficiently directed toward the questions that are most significant" (Flory & Kitcher, 2004, p. 59). Science would fail to be well-ordered, for example, if most of our time, energy and resources were invested in trying to answer trivial or trite questions while ignoring the really significant and pressing questions. In such a scenario our collective intellectual efforts would not yield much in terms of a tangible societal benefit that could improve human health and happiness.

If well-ordered science is defined as the research effort being efficiently directed toward those questions that are most significant, then the obvious place for us to begin our inquiry into the specifics of well-ordered science today is by grappling with the issue of "what makes a question *significant*?" There is a nearly infinite list of questions we could spend our limited time, energy, and resources trying to answer, so what makes some questions more significant than others?

Definitively answering this question goes beyond what I aspire (or could hope) to establish in this chapter. The issue of what constitutes the *most significant* questions in science is of course likely to be contentious, and robust disagreement is no doubt healthy because it helps guard against a society developing persistent epistemic blind spots. At least since the rise of epidemiology in the nineteenth century, one question has clearly dominated most research within the medical sciences—namely, "what causes pathology?" Elsewhere (Farrelly, 2012a, 2012b), I have called the research paradigm that presumes this question is the most significant question to answer the project of "negative biology." This research paradigm explains why the lion's share of money allocated by the National Institutes of Health (NIH; the medical research agency of the United States) goes to disease instead of health research.

With a current annual budget of approximately $39.2 billion (National Institutes of Health, n.d.) the vast majority of this funding is spent on research on disease and disorders. For example, in 2018, $6.6 billion was invested in cancer research, $5.8 billion on brain disorders, $4.9 billion on rare diseases, $3 billion on HIV/AIDS, and $1.7 billion on substance abuse (National Institutes of Health, 2019). Such significant investments are clear evidence of the dominance of the paradigm of negative biology.

The rise of the intellectual framework of negative biology has been one of the most significant achievements of our species. "In 1800, with nearly one billion people alive, life expectancy at birth did not surpass thirty years. By

2000, with more than six billion people alive, life expectancy reached nearly sixty-seven years amidst a continuing rise" (Riley, 2001, p. 1). Many factors account for this dramatic increase in life expectancy over only two centuries, including improved material prosperity, democratization, and birth control. The accomplishments of negative biology (the prevention of disease via public health measures like the sanitation revolution, immunizations, smoking cessation, etc.) coupled with advances in clinical medicine (e.g., treatments for specific disease like HIV, cancer, etc.), are an integral element of the story of this transformation from the "young" world where life was, as Thomas Hobbes described it, "nasty, brutish and short" to the world of today, where a baby born anywhere on the planet can expect to live long enough to become a senior citizen.

In *The Growth of Biological Thought*, Ernst Mayr claims that no biological problem is fully solved until both the proximate and evolutionary causation has been elucidated (Mayr, 1982, p. 73). Scott-Phillips, Dickins, and West (2011) provide the helpful example of a crying baby to explain these two levels of casual explanation. Proximate level explanations of phenotypes "are concerned with the mechanisms that underpin the trait or behavior— that is, how it works" (Scott-Phillips et al., 2011, p. 38). When explaining why an infant cries, for example, a proximate level explanation will invoke the immediate causal triggers that cause infants to cry, such as separation from a caregiver or being hungry or cold. The evolutionary explanation for why infants cry "appeals to the fitness benefits of the trait" (Scott-Phillips et al., 2011, p. 38). Crying behavior is adaptive, it helps improve the probability that vulnerable infants can survive the precarious stages of infancy. Infants who did not cry when in need of assistance were less likely to survive and pass on their genes. Hence the abundance of infants who display this behavior. Darwinian selection favors babies who are able to get their needs met over those that are less capable of doing so.

By emphasizing the importance of the two levels (proximate and evolutionary) of the causal explanation of biological problems, Mayr wanted to ensure that biologists transcended the myopic lens of fixating only on the proximate causation of problems. This myopic lens is something that can limit our study of health and disease. Consider, for instance, cancer. In 2018, approximately 9.6 million people (including my own father) died of cancer worldwide (World Health Organization, 2018). When we ask the question, "What causes cancer?" there are, as there is with infant crying behavior, two levels of explanation on which we might focus our answer. The proximate level of explanation will focus on the factors that immediately contribute to cancer mortality, such as particular genetic mutations and exposure risks to carcinogens like tobacco or UV radiation, etc. And the evolutionary explanation will explain why aging occurs and why senescence makes our mind and body more susceptible to chronic diseases (like cancer) in late life.

Unlike infant crying behavior, cancer is not an adaptive trait. In *Good Reasons for Bad Feelings*, Randolph Nesse describes how when he and George Williams began working on evolutionary medicine they tried to find an evolutionary explanation for disease. Nesse refers to this serious error (which is common in evolutionary medicine) as *viewing diseases as adaptations* (VDAA). But diseases are not adaptations. Late-life diseases like most cancers are not selected for by evolution but are rather "aspects of the body that makes us *vulnerable* to diseases that do have evolutionary explanations" (Nesse, 2019, p. 14). Aging has an evolutionary explanation, known as the *disposable soma theory* (Kirkwood, 1977; Kirkwood & Holliday, 1979), which maintains that biological aging occurs because natural selection favors a strategy in which reproduction is made a higher biological priority (in terms of the utilization of resources) than the somatic maintenance needed for indefinite survival.

Michael Rose explains how the diseases of late life are the product of the "evolutionary neglect" that occurs when reproductive fitness is prioritized by evolution by natural selection.

> Natural selection discards bad genes, genes like those that cause fatal childhood progeria. Bad genes cause these effects by producing inborn errors of metabolism: letting toxins accumulate, impairing brain function, and so on. Many of the diseases that kill infants are the products of such bad genes. . . . Natural selection keeps genes with such devastating early effects rare, because the afflicted individuals die before reproducing. Bad genes destroy themselves when they kill the young. . . . But at later ages, the force of natural selection becomes weak. It leaves genes with late bad effects alone, because natural selection has stopped working. Its force has fallen toward zero. Bad genes that only have late effects will not be removed by natural selection. They can accumulate. There is no more automatic Darwinian screening. (Rose, 2005, p. 42)

This two-level casual explanatory lens could also be applied to human emotions like hedonic well-being (pleasure), anxiety, and romantic love.

One could elucidate the proximate causation of such emotions—the neuro-chemical reactions we experience when eating sugary foods or are exposed to external stressors like job loss or sharing emotional and physical inti-macy with another. When we seek the evolutionary explanation for these same emotions we see that reproductive fitness looms large in explaining the potential adaptive benefits of our emotions, positive and negative. Pleasurable feelings can help motivate us to engage in behavior conducive to our individual and collective survival (e.g., gathering and consuming food, procreation, etc.). Anxiety can help prepare us to deal with threats to our survival and offspring. And love aids in the production and care of offspring.

Proximate-level explanations that focus on the role environment and he-redity play in our susceptibility to disease and behavior are thus only one level of explanation. At best they provide a partial explanation of important phenotypes. A more complete understanding of our susceptibility to cancer, depression, and stroke must also delve into the ultimate, or evolutionary, ex-planation of these phenomenon.

Negative and Positive Biology

Our ability to prevent and treat disease is largely determined by how sound are our intellectual suppositions of well-ordered science. Just as the fixa-tion on the proximate causation of disease can make us susceptible to my-opia (by ignoring the evolutionary causation of disease), focusing exclusively on the question "what causes disease?" can also have myopic consequences. Prioritizing only disease-oriented research threatens to marginalize the study of exemplary positive phenotypes (exceptional healthy aging, resil-ience, and happiness, etc.). Knowledge from these areas of scientific inquiry might prove to be significantly valuable to human health and happiness, of-fering benefits that could not be achieved if we limited ourselves only to the study of pathology.

Elsewhere I draw the contrast between the intellectual suppositions of "negative" and "positive biology" as follows.

Starting Intellectual Assumptions
Negative biology: Health, longevity, and happiness are assumed to be a "given" or part of "normal species functioning" for humans.

Positive biology: There is diverse variation in the genotypes which influence desired phenotypes, such as health. The evolutionary and life histories of different species help explain this variation and the different biological tradeoffs that determine age of reproduction, body size, senescence, complexity of the brain, etc.

What Needs to be Explained?

Negative biology: The proximate causes of disease, frailty, and disability

Positive biology: The proximate and ultimate causes of exceptional health, positive emotions and happiness, high cognitive ability, etc.

Which Kinds of Interventions Ought to be Pursued?

Negative biology: Interventions that help prevent, treat, and cure specific diseases

Positive biology: Interventions that increase the opportunities for health, happiness, and well-being (Farrelly, 2012a, p. 414)

One challenge facing the paradigm of positive biology is that research funding and support within the medical sciences typically flows to the basic research expected to have significant clinical relevance in terms of treating or preventing disease. A cure for one type of cancer or an intervention that reduces the risk of heart disease, for example, has a clear impact that we can measure in terms of mortality reduction. The paradigm of negative biology has helped individuals and populations live longer lives by reducing our susceptibility to early and mid-life mortality (e.g., infectious disease) and manage multimorbidity in late life. What potential benefits can positive biology potentially yield? Are there benefits to be had by studying the *absence* of pathology, something that might escape our attention if we only focus on the development of negative outcomes? And are these potential benefits significant enough to justify buttressing the amount of support invested in positive biology? In other words, is positive biology an integral component of well-ordered science in the twenty-first century?

I believe the answer to this question is a clear "affirmative!" And to make more concrete the specifics of the potential benefits positive biology can yield, I focus on two areas of research that can yield significant benefits in terms of preventative medicine: (1) geroscience and (2) positive psychology. The former studies the determinants of exceptional healthy aging, the latter the determinates of happiness and well-being. Taken together, I believe these two distinct areas of scientific research are essential components of well-ordered science today that could improve the health and happiness of today's aging populations.

Geroscience and the Future of Preventative Medicine

Positive biology prescribes that we seek to understand exceptional positive phenotypes, and healthy aging is perhaps one of the most significant and fascinating examples of positive biology to study. Aging is a major risk factor for chronic disease. And chronic diseases like cancer, heart disease, and stroke are the leading causes of death in the world today. But how persons age can vary significantly. Most people experience at least one (if not several) major chronic disease by their seventh decade of life (Vogeli et al., 2007, 392), and the average life span is estimated to be approximately 85 years (Fries, 2005). Jeffrey Fries explains how estimates of the human life span are arrived at.

> There are several methods of estimating the human life span. One may use the anthropological formulas, reconstruct an ideal survival curve from the tail of the present curve using the assumption that these individuals have been essentially free of disease, make extrapolations from the rectangularizing survival curve, or use estimates based on observed decline in organ reserve. All suggest an average life span of approximately 85 years, with a distribution which includes 99 percent of individuals between the ages of 70 and 100. (Fries, 2005, p. 808)

The maximum human life span is estimated to be around 125 years (Weon & Je, 2009). And there are (rare) individuals who can live a century of disease-free life. Positive biology prescribes that we prioritize the study of the biology of such exemplary healthy aging. Rather than fixating on just the causation of one specific disease of aging, like cancer, heart disease, or stroke, understanding the disease resistance displayed by the longest lived humans (and other species) could offer vital insights into a novel strategy of promoting preventative medicine via an aging intervention.

Not all species biologically age at the same rate. Indeed, even within a species there can be quite a wide variation in the rate of biological aging (e.g., dogs). In *The Long Tomorrow*, Michael Rose notes that many factors can influence the longevity of a species because they impact the force of evolution by natural selection. Size, for example, really does matter in nature.

If a species lives longer in nature, the force of natural selection will be increased at later years. Larger organisms can reproduce at later ages because they are more likely to be alive then, so the force will remain high at later ages. This fosters selection of genes that will tend to keep the larger alive still longer. (Rose, 2005, pp. 64–65)

The bowhead whale can grow to 20 meters in length and has a maximum life span exceeding 200 years. The bowhead whale is an important species to study for positive biology, and its genome has been sequenced. These whales do not become sexually mature until after age 20, and gestation takes more than a year. This can be contrasted with the biology of the tiny field mouse. In the wild, this mouse is vulnerable to many predators, and the winning strategy for the mouse is to reproduce early in life, with a short gestation period and a large litter.

The rate at which a species ages reflects the extrinsic risks it has faced in its evolutionary history. The disposable soma theory predicts that a greater investment in longevity should come at a cost to reproductive fitness. And a variety of studies support that conjecture. In a study (Tabatabaie et al., 2011) comparing the fertility rates of men and women who were young adults in the 1920s, before reliable methods of birth control were widely available, the exceptionally long-lived (both males and females) had an average of 2.01 children versus 2.53 children for the control group. These differences in fertility were not related to gender or education level. But there were developmental differences among the women with exceptional longevity. They tended to reach menarche a year later than average, have their first child 3 years later, and their last child 2.5 years later than average.

Studies examining the impact that castration has on the longevity of men are also evidence of this longevity/reproduction tradeoff. Castrated men residing in a mental hospital lived 14 years longer than intact men in the same hospital (Hamilton & Mestler, 1969). And historical Korean eunuchs had an incidence rate of centenarians at least 130 times higher than that of present-day developed countries (Min, Lee, & Park, 2012). Such findings support what the disposable theory predicts: that longevity comes at a cost to reproductive fitness.

In addition to castration, caloric restriction (CR) has been studied for decades in a variety of species (like mice) and extends life span by altering the rate of biological aging. CR induces stress response pathways in organisms, which results in more than simply longer lives. A longer life is not necessarily desirable, especially if it is achieved by simply keeping an organism alive in a frail and incapacitated state. But CR does the opposite of this. It extends life by keeping an organism *healthy* for a longer period of time (extending the *health span*). Since research in the 1930s, scientists have known "that rats and mice that are given about 40 percent less food than they would eat on their own live about 40 percent longer than do fully fed controls" (Miller, 2002, p. 160).

Castration and CR (which is very burdensome and can be dangerous if a person does not receive enough essential nutrients) are not viable measures for humans to pursue to retard aging, but the genomic era has revealed particular genes that slow down biological aging as well as particular molecules that active those genes (Harrison et al., 2009).

Because positive biology prioritizes the study of exemplar positive phenotypes, well-ordered science ought to entail extensive study of the longest lived humans. This means extensive study of centenarians ought to loom large in the twenty-first century. The longest lived humans are an important biological puzzle to examine not simply because they live so long, but because they typically experience a delay and compression of morbidity. Centenarians are comprised of three different categories: "delayers," "survivors," and "escapers" (Evert, Lawler, Bogan, & Perls, 2007). The "delayers" are people who make it to 100 years with a delay of the onset of common age-associated illness. For "survivors," these are people who were diagnosed with an illness prior to age 80 but survived for at least two more decades. And the third category of centenarians are "escapers," people who escaped the most lethal diseases, such as heart disease, non-skin cancer, and stroke.

The suggestion that we pursue a novel strategy of preventative medicine via an applied gerontological intervention is not science fiction. It may quickly become a reality this century. The launch of targeting aging with meformin (TAME; Barzilai, Crandall, Kritchevsky, & Espeland, 2016), a clinical trial to test the drug metformin as a safe and effective intervention against several age-related diseases, is clear evidence of this. Metformin has been safely utilized as a pharmacological intervention to help control type 2 diabetes for decades. "Metformin exerts its therapeutic effects, through a number of mechanisms and physiological pathways that resemble those generated by caloric restriction (CR), an experimental model known to extend life span and health span in various organisms" (Novelle, Ali, Dieguez, Bernier, & de Cabo, 2016, p. 2).

In experiments on animals, metformin has been shown to slow aging. And now researchers are hoping a similar effect can be shown in humans. "If TAME demonstrates that metformin modulates aging and its diseases, beyond an isolated impact on diabetes, it would pave the way for development of next-generation drugs that directly target the biology of aging" (Barzilai et al., 2016, p. 1060). The researchers undertaking TAME describe the significance of the study as follows:

> In the TAME study, we plan to enroll 3,000 subjects, ages 65–79, in ~14 centers across the US. Rather than study the effects of metformin on each separate condition, we will measure time to a new occurrence of a composite outcome that includes cardiovascular events, cancer, dementia, and mortality. TAME will also assess important functional and geriatric end points.
>
> If successful, TAME will mark a paradigm shift, moving from treating each medical condition to targeting aging per se. We expect this to facilitate the development of even better pharmacologic approaches that will ultimately reduce healthcare costs related to aging. (Barzilai et al., 2016, p. 1063)

By studying exemplar examples of healthy aging in other species and in humans, geroscience could lead to one of the most significant advances in public health this century. Robert Butler (1927–2010), the first Director of the National Institute of Aging in the United States, has urged policy-makers to aspire to slow human aging and to consider this a major priority for public health (Butler et al., 2008). Aspiring to slow the aging process is distinct from the aspiration to treat or cure a specific disease of aging, like cancer, heart disease, or stroke. Supplementing our conception of well-ordered science to include a commitment to positive as well as negative biology might help usher into existence an aging intervention that could promote the health of the 2 billion persons who will be older than 60 by the middle of this century.

Happiness and Psychological Well-Being

Like geroscience's examination of exceptional healthy aging, positive psychology's examination of happiness is another paradigmatic example of positive biology. Rather than making depression and pathology the exclusive focus of psychology, positive psychologists urge that the study of human happiness ought to also be a central focus of research and that the field should aspire to develop empirically valid prescriptions that could improve the well-being of the average person.

In "Positive Psychology: An Introduction," Martin Seligman and Mihaly Csikszentmihalyi make an appeal that the study of the worthwhile life ought to be an integral (instead of neglected) part of well-ordered science when they claim

> Psychology has, since World War II, become a science largely about healing. It concentrates on repairing damage within a disease model of human functioning.
>
> This almost exclusive attention to pathology neglects the fulfilled individual and the thriving community. The aim of positive psychology is to begin to catalyze a change in the focus of psychology from preoccupation only with repairing the worst things in life to also building positive qualities. (Seligman & Csikszentmihalyi, 2000, p. 5)

Positive psychology is perhaps the most prominent research area of positive biology. What Seligman and Csikszentmihalyi are calling for is a shift away from the exclusive focus on negative biology (i.e., pathology) to one that is also committed to positive biology (exemplar phenotypes).

What is happiness? And what are the determinates of happiness? These are deep philosophical and empirical questions, ones not easily answered. I will not attempt to answer them here (for more from philosophy, see Chapter 8 by William A. Lauinger and Chapter 9, by Anne Baril; for social science, see Chapter 13 by Margolis et al. and Chapter 15 by Xi and Lee; for theology, see Chapter 10 by Messer, Chapter 11 by Wynn, and Chapter 16 by VanderWeele, Long, & Balboni, all in this volume). Instead, I seek to make the case that positive psychology is an exemplar example of what positive biology can offer. Quality, and not simply quantity, of life is an integral concern of positive biology.

Happiness has been defined by philosophers, psychologists, and economists, often in different ways. Hedonistic accounts of human happiness, like that of the utilitarian Jeremy Bentham (1784–1832), equate happiness with subjective well-being (or the experience of pleasure). On this account of happiness, a person's "experiencing self" is the authority of a person's well-being. For example, researchers can ask people how happy they feel while performing different types of activities: working, spending time with family, cleaning, exercising, while incarcerated, unemployed, married, divorced, living with a disability, etc. Once researchers accumulate enough responses from different people, particular patterns emerge about the activities associated with high and low levels of well-being.

One surprising and significant finding concerning people's ability to predict their future hedonic responses to events is that we are not very competent at doing this. We are not good at predicting how certain events (e.g., becoming paraplegic, winning the lottery, or moving to California) will impact our well-being. For example, if people are asked to predict how their happiness would be impacted if they became paraplegic, they are likely to answer that it would have a serious, adverse impact on their well-being. Conversely, if asked to predict how happy they would be if they won the lottery, most people would assume this event would have a dramatic impact and substantially increase their happiness. And yet, "in a famous study, the happiness of people 1 year after developing paraplegia was almost indistinguishable from the happiness of people 1 year after winning the lottery" (Ubel et al., 2001, p. 190). When it comes to predicting how happy you would be living in California (Schkade & Kahneman, 1998) or if you were richer (Kahneman, Krueger, Schkade, Schwarz, & Stone, 2006), the actual reports of life satisfaction from people in those circumstances are very different from what people predict the life satisfaction of people in those circumstances must be. When fixating on how the weather or money will impact our well-being we tend to overexaggerate the importance of these factors and ignore other important factors (e.g., the commute to work, relationships, fulfillment with work, etc.).

And this fact reinforces the urgency to derive and promulgate sage prescriptions from positive psychology versus just trusting our individual judgments about what will make us happy in the future as authoritative (especially when the average person is bombarded by consumerist messages daily). We are not reliable predictors of our hedonic states because we suffer from a variety of what Gilbert and Wilson (2007) call "prospection errors." *Prospection* refers to our ability to "pre-experience" the future by simulating it in our minds (Gilbert & Wilson, 2007, p. 1352). Prospection is a unique feature of the cognitive lives of humans. For example, such simulations can be *unrepresentative*. Simulations of the future are constructed from our memories. We retain a memory of extraordinary events (e.g., that time our plane was delayed on the tarmac for 2 hours!) rather than the representative memory (e.g., successfully taking off [approximately] on time). Simulations of the future can also be *abbreviated*. This means that our simulations of the future typically focus on a few, select moments of a future event. For example, when we simulate a potential future where we have won millions in the lottery, we think of all the joy we can get purchasing new homes and automobiles for our family members. But what we do not simulate in our minds is the reality that we can still have interpersonal challenges in our relationships (indeed, winning the lottery might exacerbate those challenges). We fail to internalize how we will, in time, adapt to being much wealthier. Abbreviated simulations are unreliable predictors of our emotional well-being.

Knowledge about our susceptibility to prospection errors and how to minimize making such errors could improve our subjective well-being. But the potential for positive psychology goes much further than simply improving our subjective well-being. Like geroscience, positive psychology extends its scope to the ultimate causation of positive phenotypes like joy, interest, and love. This requires us to consider the type of species *Homo sapiens* actually is, a concern that goes back to at least Aristotle. The function (*ergon*) of a human being, according to Aristotle, consists in activity of the rational part of the soul in accordance with virtue (Aristotle, 1985; NE 1097b22–1098a20). *Eudaimonia* (or happiness) is the highest end, and all other goals—wealth, friendship, health, etc.—are secondary goals that are pursued because they promote eudaimonia.

Positive biology is not simply interested in the proximate causation of happiness; it also adopts an evolutionary lens. The process of evolution by natural selection yielded mental faculties that are much more complex than the picture presumed by Bentham, giving us reason to be skeptical that sage normative prescriptions can be gleamed from the conjecture that it is our nature to be "hedonic maximizers." In *An Introduction to the Principles of Morals and Legislation*, Bentham famously remarked

> Nature has placed mankind under the governance of two sovereign masters, pain and pleasure. It is for them alone to point out what we ought to do, as well as to determine what we shall do. (Bentham, 2008, p. 585)

Evolutionary biologists provide a much more expansive and complex account of our mental life.

> Our evolved natures should be treated with respect, but not with deference. We did not evolve to be happy: rather we evolved to be happy, sad,

miserable, angry, anxious, and depressed, as the mood takes us. We evolved to love and to hate, and to care and be callous. Our emotions are the carrots and sticks that our genes use to persuade us to achieve their ends. But their ends need not be our ends. Goodness and happiness may be goals attainable only by hoodwinking our genes. (Stearns, Nesse, & Haig, 2008, p. 13)

Natural selection did not design us to be "hedonic maximizers." If our species only experienced positive emotions like those of the sensory pleasures (e.g., satiation), we would not have survived for long in the kind of environment that humans have historically faced. Martin Seligman (2002) distinguishes different kinds and levels of happiness. Hedonists who pursue the immediate positive feelings—like the pleasure of a food they enjoy or a compliment—seek the *momentary* happiness of what Seligman calls "the pleasant life." But these pleasures fade quickly and thus do not have a lasting impact on the subjective well-being of actors. Enduring happiness, the kind one enjoys when one lives the truly "excellent life," is realized when one leads a *meaningful life*. Such a life requires we become psychologically connected and continuous with others rather than just our self. After spending years of studying what makes people happy, Seligman remarks

What does Positive Psychology tell us about finding purpose in life, about leading a meaningful life beyond the good life? I am not sophomoric enough to put forward a complete theory of meaning, but I do know that it consists in attachment to something larger, and the larger the entity to which you attach yourself, the more meaning in your life. (Seligman, 2002, p. 14)

A growing body of empirical studies appear to substantiate Seligman's contention. For example, in a study of the daily social behavior of happy people (Mehl, Vazire, Holleran, & Clark, 2010), researchers used an electronically activated recorder (EAR) to record and then later classify participants' daily conversations with others as either "small talk" (e.g., banal conversation) or "substantive talk" (e.g., conversations where meaningful information was exchanged). The study found that higher well-being was associated with having less small talk and having more substantive conversations. While such a study does not establish the factual truth of Socrates's famous claim that the "unexamined life is not worth living," it does suggest that our need to feel attached to something bigger than ourselves plays an important role in our happiness and well-being. And this hypothesis also coheres with the findings of recent studies on spending money and happiness. Elizabeth Dunn et al. (2008) found that when individuals spend more money on *prosocial* goals, like charity, they actually experience greater happiness than when they spend money on themselves.

Taking evolution seriously means we must recognize that positive emotions—like joy, love, and interest—are, like the negative emotions, the result of our evolutionary history. "Negative emotions such as fear, sadness, and anger are our first line of defence against external threats, calling us to battle stations" (Seligman, 2002, p. 31). And the same is true of our positive emotions in that "they help illicit urges to act, though they are usually less specific than the actions urged by negative emotions" (Fredrickson, 1998, p. 303). Furthermore, as Barbara Fredrickson has argued, the positive emotions urge not simply physical action, but rather they also broaden what she describes as our "momentary thought-action repertoire" (Fredrickson, 1998, p. 303). And different positive emotions serve different purposes in broadening this repertoire. Love can foster many different positive emotions—like joy and interest—and permit a person to experience the new stimuli that comes from internalizing the beliefs, information, values, and aspirations of others. Love promotes social connectedness and expands our circle of concern and attention beyond just ourselves. And this connectedness can help provide meaning and purpose in our lives, thus enhancing our well-being.

Like love, play also promotes social connectedness as well as skill acquisition. Play can enrich human capacities in different and diverse ways (Brown, 2009). Physical play (like sports) can raise our awareness of the importance of endurance and strength as well as our physical limitations and vulnerability to injury. Playing sports can help develop balance, speed, and agility. These types of play, which we find intrinsically valuable, also promote other capacities, like bodily health, thought, and the senses.

Most physical play is also a form of *social* play. Playing helps socialize us by helping us internalize the negotiated rules of games, compelling us to control our emotions and providing concrete examples to us of the benefits of social cooperation. Social play helps build trust, communication, empathy, etc. Once a person participates as a member of a team they become psychologically connected and continuous with the team. The player's own cognitive states track the trials and tribulations of the team. A team win can bring the individual player elation, while a loss brings disappointment and a determination to try even harder next time. Indeed, this phenomenon is not limited to just the direct participants in a sport. Even spectators who care passionately about a sport and team often experience similar levels and degrees of "connectedness" to a team.

Play shapes our brain and stimulates many positive emotions. Indeed, some believe that the human capacity to play separates humans from all other animal species. Stuart Brown, for example, argues

> Of all animal species, humans are the biggest players of all. We are built to play and built through play. When we play, we are engaged in the purest expression of our humanity, the truest expression of our individuality. Is it any wonder that often the times we feel most alive, those that make up our best memories, are moments of play? (Brown, 2009, p. 5)

Love and play thus serve to broaden one's "momentary thought-action repertoire," which in turn builds the enduring personal resources necessary for eudaimonia. Understanding the proximate and evolutionary causes of subjective well-being and eudaimonia are an integral element of positive biology.

Like an applied gerontological intervention, the prescriptions generated from positive psychology offer significant potential to function as a form of preventative medicine. Emphasizing the importance of play in our lives is captured eloquently by Brian Sutton in his masterful study of play.

> What is adaptive about play . . . may be not only the skills that are part of it but also the skillful belief in acting out one's own capacity for the future. The opposite of play, in these terms, is not a present reality or work, it is vacillation, or worse, it is depression. (Sutton-Smith, 1997, p. 198)

The eudaimonic understanding of happiness emphasizes the importance of meaning and purpose in our lives. The meaningful life does not consist in simply satisfying our basic primal instincts for food, shelter, and sex. In her examination of what constitutes positive psychological functioning, Carol Ryff (1989; see also Chapter 4, in this volume) identified the following six theory-guided dimensions of well-being:

Self-acceptance: Holding positive attitudes toward oneself emerges as a central characteristic of positive psychological functioning.

Positive relations with others: Self-actualizers are described as having strong feelings of empathy and affection for all human beings and as being capable of greater love, deeper friendship, and more complete identification with others.

Autonomy: Self-determination, independence, and the regulation of behavior from within.

Environmental mastery: One's ability to advance in the world and change it creatively through physical or mental activities.

Purpose in life: The definition of maturity also emphasizes a clear comprehension of life's purpose, a sense of directedness, and intentionality.

Personal growth: Such an individual is continually developing and becoming rather than achieving a fixed state wherein all problems are solved (Ryff, 1989, p. 1071).

These points are reinforced by Seligman and Csikszentmihalyi in their summary of the field of positive psychology.

The field of positive psychology at the subjective level is about valued subjective experiences: well-being, contentment, and satisfaction (in the past); hope and optimism (for the future); and flow and happiness (in the present). At the individual level, it is about positive individual traits: the capacity for love and vocation, courage, interpersonal skill, aesthetic sensibility, perseverance, forgiveness, originality, future mindedness, spirituality, high talent, and wisdom. At the group level, it is about the civic virtues and the institutions that move individuals toward better citizenship: responsibility, nurturance, altruism, civility, moderation, tolerance, and work ethic. (Seligman & Csikszentmihalyi, 2000, p. 5)

The average person's life could be substantively improved when their pursuit of happiness is informed by positive psychology and when the general culture is shaped by the prescriptions of the eudaimonic conception of well-being. Living a life of self-acceptance, healthy relationships, autonomy, environmental mastery, purpose, and personal growth versus a life spent pursuing the insatiable consumption ideals perpetuated by capitalism has the potential to substantively improve our well-being. A culture that celebrates something as basic as play—physical, social, and imaginative—across the human life span, and prosocial activities like philanthropy and volunteerism, could significantly improve the happiness and well-being of its population. For these reasons positive psychology and related approaches, such as humanistic psychology, ought to be considered an integral element of well-ordered science for the twenty-first century.

Conclusion

Science is concerned with creating, and disseminating knowledge. And this knowledge is then the foundation upon which new innovations can be developed to improve human health and happiness. The virtue epistemological construal of knowledge as "success from ability" (Greco, 2010) is useful because it emphasizes the fact that knowledge is always *context-dependent*. Our success in improving human health and happiness will depend on the circumstances of the threats to our health and happiness. The challenges facing human populations in a world dominated by infectious disease and severe poverty are very different from the challenges facing populations living to late life and (at least in developed countries) having access to an excess of material goods.

Historically it made sense for human populations to conceive well-ordered science through the lens of negative biology. Prioritizing the question "What causes disease?" in a world dominated by extreme poverty and infectious diseases (like smallpox) was both a rational and sensible prescription. But now positive biology deserves to take its rightful place within an account of well-ordered science for the twenty-first century. Positive biology encourages us to explore both the proximate and evolutionary causes of exemplary positive phenotypes. Rather than fixating solely on the causation of pathology, positive biology encourages the study of the biology of centenarians, the emotional resilience of those who experience growth and development from adversity (vs. those who become depressed or develop addiction), and the genetic and environmental factors that contribute to self-esteem, healthy relationships, and secure attachment, etc.

What steps need to be taken to ensure that positive biology plays a prominent role in science today? I believe many different courses of action are needed. Conceptually we must overcome the observational bias implicit in negative biology; that is, the assumption that the most important things to explain are the negative outcomes of morbidity and mortality. Science should celebrate a "curiosity-driven" mindset rather than one that predominantly focuses on the prevention and treatment of specific diseases. The success stories of positive biology (e.g., healthy aging, high IQ, emotional resilience, etc.) also deserve serious scientific attention. Elsewhere (Farrelly, 2012b), I argued that the NIH should create a new Institute of Positive Biology, which would help researchers facilitate the novel interdisciplinary research that positive biology can offer. The creation of such an innovative institute would also ensure that research on positive phenotypes can compete on a more level playing field against research on disease. The latter currently enjoys the lion's share of research support. By transcending negative biology's fixation on negative phenotypes, positive biology may be able to yield significant insights and technological advances that help the human populations of the twenty-first century flourish in spite of the fact that we face a potentially precarious and uncertain future.

About the Author

Colin Farrelly is Professor and Queen's National Scholar in the Department of Political Studies at Queen's University, in Kingston, Ontario. He is the author of *Genetic Ethics: An Introduction* (Polity Books, 2018) and *Biologically Modified Justice* (Cambridge University Press, 2016). The themes of reason, science, progress, and optimism inform his curiosity-driven research interests and interdisciplinary focus.

Author Note

I am grateful to the editors of this volume for their helpful comments and suggestions on an earlier version of this chapter. This work was supported in part by a grant from the John Templeton Foundation and by the Lee Kum Sheung Center for Health and Happiness. The views expressed in this chapter represent the perspective of the author and do not reflect the opinions or endorsement of any organization. I have no known conflict of interest to disclose. Correspondence concerning this chapter should be directed to Colin Farrelly, Department of Political Studies, Queen's University, Kingston, ON K7L 3N6, Canada (farrelly@queensu.ca).

References

Aristotle. (1985). *Nicomachean ethics.* (M. Irwin, Trans.). Indianapolis, IN: Hackett.

Barzilai, N., Crandall, J. P., Kritchevsky, S. B., & Espeland, M. A. (2016). Metformin as a tool to target aging. *Cell Metabolism, 23*(6), 1060–1065.

Bentham, J. (2008). *An introduction to the principles of morals and legislation.* In D. Wooton (Ed.), *Modern political thought: Readings from Machiavelli to Nietzsche* (pp. 585–604). Indianapolis, IN: Hackett.

Brown, S. (2009). *Play: How it shapes the brain, opens the imagination, and invigorates the soul.* New York: Penguin Group.

Butler, R., Miller, R. A., Perry, D., Carnes, B. A., Williams, T. F., Cassel, C., & Brody, J. (2008). New model of health promotion and disease prevention for the 21st century. *British Medical Journal, 337,* 149–150.

Dunn, E., Aknin, L., & Norton, M. (2008). Spending money on others promotes happiness. *Science, 319,* 1687–88.

Evert J., Lawler, E., Bogan, H., & Perls, T. (2007). Morbidity profiles of centenarians: Survivors, delayers, and escapers. *Journals of Gerontology: Series A, Biological Sciences and Medical Sciences, 58,* M232–M237.

Farrelly, C. (2012a). Why the NIH should create an Institute of Positive Biology. *Journal of the Royal Society of Medicine, 105,* 412–415.

Farrelly, C. (2012b). "Positive biology" as a new paradigm for the medical sciences. *Nature's EMBO Reports, 13,* 186–188.

Flory, J., & Kitcher, P. (2004). Global health and the scientific research agenda. *Philosophy & Public Affairs, 32*(1), 36–65.

Fredrickson, B. (1998). What good are positive emotions? *Review of General Psychology, 2*(3), 300–319.

Fries, J. (2005). The compression of morbidity. *Milbank Quarterly, 83*(4), 801–823.

Gilbert, D., & Williams, T. (2007). Prospection: Experiencing the future. *Science, 317*(5843), 1351–1354.

Greco, J. (2010). *Achieving knowledge: A virtue-theoretic account of epistemic normativity.* Cambridge: Cambridge University Press.

Hamilton, J., & Mestler, G. (1969). Mortality and survival: Comparison of eunuchs with intact men and women in a mentally retarded population. *Journal of Gerontology, 24,* 395–411.

Harrison, D. E., Strong, R., Sharp, Z. D., Nelson, J. F., Astle, C. M., Flurkey, K., . . . Miller, R. A. (2009). Rapamycin fed late in life extends lifespan in genetically heterogeneous mice. *Nature, 460,* 392–395.

Kahneman, D., Krueger, A. B., Schkade, D., Schwarz, N., & Stone, A. A. (2006). Would you be happier if you were richer? A focusing illusion. *Science, 312*(5782), 1908–1910.

Kelp, C. (2017). Knowledge-first virtue epistemology. In J. Carter, E. Gordon, & B. Jarvis (Eds.), *Knowledge first: Approaches in epistemology and mind* (pp. 223–245). Oxford: Oxford University Press.

Kirkwood, T. (1977). Evolution of aging. *Nature, 270,* 301–304.

Kirkwood, T., & Holliday, R. (1979). The evolution of ageing and longevity. *Proceedings of the Royal Society of London: Biology, 205,* 531–546.

Mayr, E. (1982). *The growth of biological thought: Diversity, evolution, and inheritance.* Cambridge, MA: Harvard University Press.

Mehl, M. R., Vazire, S., Holleran, S. E., & Clark, C. S. (2010). Eavesdropping on happiness: Well-being is related to having less small talk and more substantive conversations. *Psychological Science, 21*(2010): 539–541.

Miller, R. (2002). Extending life: Scientific prospects and political obstacles. *Milbank Quarterly, 80*(1), 155–174.

Min, K. J., Lee, C. K., & Park, H. N. (2012). The lifespan of Korean eunuchs. *Current Biology, 22*(18), R792–R793.

National Institutes of Health. (n. d.). Budget. www.nih.gov/about-nih/what-we-do/budget

National Institutes of Health. (2019). Estimates of funding for various research, condition, and disease categories (RCDC). https://report.nih.gov/categorical_spending.aspx

Nesse, R. (2019). *Good reasons for bad feelings: Insights from the frontier of evolutionary psychiatry.* New York: Penguin Random House.

Novelle, M. G., Ali, A., Diéguez, C., Bernier, M., & de Cabo, R. (2016). Metformin: A hopeful promise in aging research. *Cold Spring Harbor Perspectives in Medicine, 6,* a025932.

Riley, J. (2001). *Rising life expectancy: A global history.* New York: Cambridge University.

Rose, M. (2005). *The long tomorrow: How advances in evolutionary biology can help us postpone aging.* New York: Oxford University.

Ryff, C. (1989). Happiness is everything, or is it? Explorations on the meaning of psychological well-being. *Journal of Personality and Social Psychology, 57*(6), 1069–1081.

Schkade, D., & Kahneman, D. (1998). Does living in California make people happy? A focusing illusion in judgments of life satisfaction. *Psychological Science 9*(5), 340–346.

Scott-Phillips, T., Dickins, T., & West, S. (2011). Evolutionary theory and the ultimate-proximate distinction in the human behavioral sciences. *Perspectives on Psychological Science, 6*(1), 38–47.

Seligman, M. E. (2002). *Authentic happiness: Using the new positive psychology to realize your potential for lasting fulfillment.* New York: Simon and Schuster.

Seligman, M., & Csikszentmihalyi, M. (2000). Positive psychology: An introduction. *American Psychologist, 55*(1), 5–14.

Stearns, S., Nesse, R., & Haig, D. (2008). Introducing evolutionary thinking for medicine. In S. Stearns & J. Koella (Eds.), *Evolution in health and disease* (pp. 3–16). Oxford: Oxford University Press.

Sutton-Smith, B. (1997). *The ambiguity of play.* Cambridge, MA: Harvard University Press.

Tabatabaie, V., Tabatabaie, V., Atzmon, G., Rajpathak, S. N., Freeman, R., Barzilai, N., & Crandall, J. (2011). Exceptional longevity is associated with decreased reproduction. *Aging, 3*(12), 1202–1205.

Ubel, P. A., Loewenstein, G., Hershey, J., Baron, J., Mohr, T., Asch, D. A., & Jepson, C. (2001). Do nonpatients underestimate the quality of life associated with chronic health conditions because of a focusing illusion? *Medical Decision Making, 21*(3), 190–199.

Vogeli, C., Shields, A. E., Lee, T. A., Gibson, T. B., Marder, W. D., Weiss, K. B., & Blumenthal, D. (2007). Multiple chronic conditions: Prevalence, health consequences, and implications for quality, care management, and costs. *Journal of General Internal Medicine, 22*(3), 391–395.

Weon, B., & Je, J. (2009). Theoretical estimation of maximum human lifespan. *Biogerontology, 10,* 65–71.

World Health Organization. (2018). Cancer fact sheet. www.who.int/news-room/fact-sheets/detail/cancer

World Health Organization. (n. d.). Global Health Observatory (GHO). www.who.int/gho/mortality_burden_disease/life_tables/situation_trends/en/

Zagzebski, L. (1996). *Virtues of the mind: An inquiry into the nature of virtue and the ethical foundations of knowledge.* Cambridge: Cambridge University Press.

7

Philosophy of Well-Being for the Social Sciences

A Primer

Guy Fletcher

Abstract

In this chapter I try to provide an introduction to *philosophical* work on well-being. I explain the specific kinds of questions that philosophers are interested in when it comes to well-being. I then seek to explain the role of thought experiments in philosophical work on well-being. I explain why such cases are useful, and non-gratuitous, and the methodological assumptions that underlie their use. Finally, I explain how philosophers seek to preserve a common subject matter for debate—well-being—even in the presence of radical disagreement about which theory is correct.

Socrates famously asked for the real definitions of things, for example and perhaps most famously, "What is Justice?" In asking this question the aim was to discover the fundamental nature of justice—in what does it consist? What needs to be the case in a city or an individual for that city or individual to be just? Answering these questions generated Plato's *Republic* (and a great deal of subsequent philosophical debate).

Philosophers ask the same kind of question about well-being—what is it, exactly? In asking this question philosophers aim to find out the fundamental nature of well-being. In what does it consist? What needs to be in place in an individual's life for that individual to have a high level of well-being?

To those working in other disciplines, work which begins with such abstract and fundamental questions probably seems abstruse and peculiar. In this chapter, I seek to remedy this situation by trying to give a sense of

Guy Fletcher, *Philosophy of Well-Being for the Social Sciences* In: *Measuring Well-Being*. Edited by: Matthew T. Lee, Laura D. Kubzansky, and Tyler J. VanderWeele, Oxford University Press (2021). © Oxford University Press.
DOI: 10.1093/oso/9780197512531.003.0008

what philosophers are doing when they investigate well-being in a distinctively philosophical way. I will proceed by laying out the main distinctions, concepts, debates, and methodologies in philosophical work on well-being. My aim is to make this material more accessible to those working in other academic disciplines rather than trying to break new ground within the philosophy of well-being.

I first explain the specific kinds of questions that philosophers are interested in when they work on well-being and the ways in which these complement, converge with, and diverge from the work done in the social sciences (to the best of my understanding of these other fields). I then seek to explain why philosophical work on well-being so often involves using somewhat recherché thought experiments to test theories. I explain why such cases are useful and nongratuitous and the methodological assumptions that underlie their use. Subsequently, I explain how philosophers preserve a common subject matter for debate even in the presence of radical disagreement.

Philosophy of Well-Being: Questions

When thinking about the fundamental nature of well-being, philosophers typically proceed by first asking a series of sub-questions, questions that we need to address if we are to answer the main overarching question about the fundamental nature of well-being.

A common place to start with these sub-questions is the issue of which things contribute to well-being. This is a natural enough starting point: well-being is, pretty obviously, that quality or state had by a life that is going well. The next question that arises, then, is what makes a life go well? What contributes to well-being?

However, as happens a great deal in philosophy, it turns out that this last question is not a very interesting one because it is not sufficiently precise. To see this, consider that philosophers working on well-being are not much interested in the following question: Which things contribute to well-being *at all*? Indeed, philosophers will typically agree that there is a very wide range of things that contribute to well-being, at least as a general rule. This will include pleasurable experiences, material wealth, education, friendships and relationships, and so on. Philosophers will only start to be interested in the question of which things contribute to well-being once we mark, at the very least, a division between (1) things that contribute to well-being merely instrumentally and (2) things that contribute to well-being noninstrumentally or intrinsically.[1] This marks the divide between things that are *themselves* well-being enhancing in their own right versus things that simply bring about other things that are well-being enhancing. For example, money is *instrumentally* well-being enhancing. That is because with money one can obtain various things that enhance well-being in their own right. But it is nowhere near as plausible that having money makes someone's life go better in its own right. Thus many philosophers will hold that money is *instrumentally* good for us but it is not *intrinsically* good for us.[2] By contrast, one of the questions that philosophers of well-being are interested in, then, is:

Which Things Are Noninstrumentally Well-Being Enhancing?

And here is where we start to get some answers. We find various proposals put forward by different philosophers: well-being is enhanced by pleasure (famously held by both Bentham and Mill), by happiness, by desire satisfaction, by some plurality of goods, or by some complex relation between such goods and desire fulfillment or pleasure, and so on.

Another question that philosophers of well-being are not much interested in is *which* lives are going well and which are going badly with respect to well-being. That is to say, there is much (albeit mostly implicit) agreement about which lives are going well and which are going badly. To give one example, every remotely plausible contender to be the correct philosophical theory of well-being is going to deliver the verdict that Barack Obama's life is going well. However, once we turn to the question of *why* a life is going well, that is when we find a focus of intense philosophical disagreement. One philosopher will think that some life—Barack Obama's for example—is going well precisely in virtue of the presence of one feature of the life (its hedonic quality, for example). Another philosopher will think that the very same life is going well in virtue of the presence of some *other* feature of the life (its perfectionist quality, for example).

How do we adjudicate between these different views? One difficulty that immediately arises here is that there is such a high degree of overlap between the various proposed features that are postulated to explain why a life is going well or going badly. To illustrate this point, consider the following sample of philosophical theories of well-being:

Hedonism: All and only pleasure intrinsically contributes to well-being. All and only pain intrinsically detracts from well-being.[3]

Desire-fulfillment theory: All and only desire fulfillment intrinsically contributes to well-being. All and only desire frustration intrinsically detracts from well-being.[4]

(One particular) objective list theory: All and only pleasure, friendship, and achievement intrinsically contribute to well-being.[5]

Perfectionism: All and only the exercise and development of human capacities intrinsically contributes to well-being.[6,7]

Now imagine a cognitively typical human being, living in a well-functioning society, who spends their time engaged in a job as an architect, who has a loving and supportive family, who enjoys ample leisure time during which they pursue woodwork and team sports. If we add in plausible empirical assumptions about human psychology, we will find that the hedonist theory of well-being says that this person is high in well-being because their life scores well hedonically (it is high in net pleasure over pain). We will also find that the desire fulfillment theory likewise scores the life highly but because it is full of desire satisfaction (again, given plausible auxiliary assumptions). The same will be true of the particular objective list theory and of perfectionism. There is a high degree of overlap. Each theory will say that this life is going well. So they do not disagree in their verdicts about this life. Where they will disagree is (only) on the question of *why* exactly this life is going well.[8]

How, then, do we go about answering our questions? How do we determine which theory ultimately gives us the correct account of the nature of well-being? The lesson of the preceding discussion is that you cannot make progress in adjudicating between the main theories of well-being by thinking about the verdicts that they reach in typical cases (by which I mean those cases of lives that are typical). This leads us on to an important point about the methodology of philosophy of well-being.

Philosophy of Well-Being: Methods

Once we realize the high degree of overlap between the properties deemed relevant by each of the main theories of well-being, we realize that we cannot make progress by looking at what seems plausible in normal cases. The major theories will agree about the question of the *level* of well-being in most regular cases. This motivates philosophers of well-being to try to conjure up scenarios where we can prise apart the well-being determining properties postulated by the theories (hedonic level, desire-satisfaction, objective goods, etc.) to see which one is *really* explaining levels of well-being. Here are two such cases. The first is Nozick's (1974) "experience machine."

> Suppose there was an experience machine that would give you any experience you desired. Super-duper neuropsychologists could stimulate your brain so that you would think and feel you were writing a great novel, or making a friend, or reading an interesting book. All the time you would be floating in a tank, with electrodes attached to your brain. Should you plug into this machine for life, preprogramming your life experiences? . . . Of course, while in the tank you won't know that you're there; you'll think that it's all actually happening. . . . Would you plug in?[9]

Regrettably, Nozick's introduction of the example introduces a lot of distracting complicating factors (for one thing, one might be distracted by practicalities such as the maintenance of the machine). But the basic thought which his case is used to bring out is that we can imagine a life plugged into a sophisticated virtual reality device wherein the life would score very highly with respect to its hedonic profile but which would score badly when evaluated by other theories of well-being. For example, the person might have lots of desires that go unfulfilled due to living life in the machine because, for example, they desire to *actually* write the great American novel, not merely to have the realistic simulation of doing so. Similarly, their life would lack friendship and achievement and would also involve little if any development and exercise of their capacities. This means that while hedonism would ascribe a high level of well-being to someone in an experience machine, each of the main theories aside from hedonism would have a plausible explanation of why someone in the experience machine would *not* have a high level of well-being even if their life in the machine was very pleasurable. Philosophers of well-being thus use cases like the experience machine to tease out our reactions to lives that do well hedonically but not in other respects.

The most common reaction that people have when presented with this case is the judgment that the person plugged into the machine does not have a high level of well-being. This helps to undermine the plausibility of hedonism and drives some to give more credence to other theories of well-being, ones that say life in the experience machine would not have a high level of well-being. Of course, this is not to deny that some continue to find hedonism appealing even when presented with the experience machine example. Rather, it is only to note that many find hedonism less appealing when we move away from the verdict it reaches in normal cases and start to think about the verdicts it is committed to in some other cases.

Another useful case for theorizing about well-being is Derek Parfit's (1984) stranger case. While the experience machine was useful in providing an example of a life that did well hedonically but was lacking in other goods, Parfit builds a case of desire fulfillment in the absence of other goods.

> Suppose that I meet a stranger who has what is believed to be a fatal disease, my sympathy is aroused, and I strongly want this stranger to be cured. Much later, when I have forgotten our meeting, the stranger is cured. On the Unrestricted Desire-Fluffiest Theory, this event is good for me, and makes my life go better. This is not plausible, we should reject this theory.[10]

Many find it plausible, with Parfit, that the mere fact that the stranger was cured does not, by itself, positively impact upon his (Parfit's) well-being in this case. This case thus motivates the idea that having your desires be fulfilled is not what *fundamentally* matters to well-being because, as in this case, desire fulfillment without any associated pleasure or other goods seems not to be beneficial (or, at least, *much* less plausible than for any normal case of desire fulfillment, one accompanied by pleasure). Thus this kind of case puts pressure on the simple desire fulfillment theory of well-being by showing how the theory loses plausibility once we prise desire fulfillment apart from the other properties it typically comes along with (which also happen to be properties deemed to be relevant by other theories of well-being, such as pleasure or achievement). It is a way of arguing that desire fulfillment enhances well-being only instrumentally and not in every case.

These are just two of the cases deployed by philosophers of well-being but, as I hope to have shown, the main dialectical point is common across them: to show how we can prise apart the properties postulated by theories as the fundamental explanation of well-being in order to see how plausible they are in isolation from each other. The weirdness of these cases is thus precisely by design. By thinking of weird possibilities we can prise apart theories which would agree on everyday cases to see which of them is doing the real explanatory work. This is why philosophers tend to downplay what we can learn from everyday cases—because the theories agree so much about ordinary cases—and instead make recourse to recherché thought experiments when testing their views. It also explains why philosophers can seem uninterested in empirical work on well-being, such as that done in positive psychology, given that such empirical work will not isolate each potential explanation in the manner needed to make progress on philosophical questions.[11]

Having explained the distinctive questions within philosophy of well-being and explained how they lead to the use of thought experiments based around unusual cases, let me now move to explaining a more abstract issue in the philosophy of well-being: conceptual questions and substantive questions and how the ideas here might be of use to those doing empirical work on well-being.

Philosophy of Well-Being: Concepts and Conceptions

Something that may have occurred to the reader by this point is to ask why it is that philosophers of well-being take themselves to all be answering the same question, to all be giving an account of the fundamental nature of well-being? Another way to put this is to say that one background question to all theorizing about well-being is, how is it that we can actually disagree about the subject matter? After all, if I subscribe to hedonism about well-being and you subscribe to perfectionism about well-being, what makes it true that we are having a disagreement about some common thing—well-being— as opposed to simply thinking about and talking about different things? Furthermore, if we are thinking about the same thing, how we can we know this to be true?

The standard way that philosophers would think of the situation is that we have a common *concept* of well-being but different *conceptions*, or theories, of it. A concept will be identified with a set of very general high-level claims, whereas the conceptions are much more specific. Thus there will be some very general conceptual claims in common between us that fix the subject matter. Here is an example to illustrate the distinction. Libertarians and socialists disagree vehemently in their theories of distributive justice. Yet we still think that they are disagreeing about something. They are not simply talking past each other. How does that happen? Well, to have a disagreement at all they must agree on some *very* high-level claims—for instance, that justice is concerned with *entitlements* to property and the grounds of such entitlements, or something like that. That is to say, there must be enough agreement between them, on very high-level claims, to provide a subject matter for disagreement.

Before turning to well-being let me note three complications in passing. First, the difference between the high-level conceptual claims and the substantive claims will not always be uncontentious or obvious. Second, the method does not guarantee that we are always disagreeing when we think we are. Perhaps sometimes people really *are* talking about two different things but unfortunately using the same term. Third, it is not necessary for disagreeing parties to accept *all* of the high-level claims. Rather, they must simply accept enough of them; where what counts as enough is going to be difficult to determine.

When it comes to well-being the relevant high-level concept-fixing claims will be things like well-being is a matter of how that subject's life goes *for them* (as opposed to how good their life is for their community or the world); humans have levels of well-being; tables and chairs do not have levels of well-being; and various kinds of non-human animals might have levels of well-being, depending upon their capacities. We will also hold in common claims including that well-being is connected to care and concern, such that caring for someone (a relative, a friend etc.) *is* partly a matter of promoting and preserving that person's well-being, and so on. These platitudinous claims about well-being fix the subject matter, and philosophers then offer competing theories of it. This ensures enough commonality for there to be a subject matter but enough diversity to allow for radical disagreement, as there is between (say) hedonists and objective list theorists about well-being.

Philosophy of Well-Being and Psychology: Differences and Disagreement

Philosophical work on well-being is very relaxed about fundamental disagreement. This is—from what I can tell—quite different from the way in which work on well-being proceeds in psychology. There, it seems, there is a tendency to *generate* subject matters from theories or, put another way, to fix a subject matter using a theory or set of theories. Let me give an example. Psychologists refer to "subjective well-being," "hedonic well-being," and "eudaimonic well-being." This is in stark contrast with philosophy, bracketing some recent work for a moment (but which I discuss later). Philosophers refer to hedonistic *theories of well-being*, eudaimonic *theories of well-being*, and the like. Thus in philosophy it is clear that competing theories of *one and the same thing* are being offered, such that hedonism is the true philosophical theory of well-being or it is false and some other theory is true instead.[12] By contrast, in psychology it seems that those working on *hedonic well-being* are just looking into something different from those investigating *eudaimonist well-being*.[13]

Once we notice this difference, we can ask how these two projects (or sets of projects)—the philosophical and the psychological—relate. One way to reconcile them would be if we were supposed to take the theories from psychology—theories of hedonic well-being and eudaimonist well-being and the like—and then ask whether hedonic well-being or eudaimonist (as understood by the best psychological model of them) fits our ordinary, pretheoretical concept of well-being. That would be to treat work in psychology as providing the best descriptive account of the elements postulated within the philosophical theories of well-being. For example, psychological work on hedonic well-being would thus be contributing to the theory of the nature of the elements postulated by the (philosophical) hedonic theory of well-being (specifically, pleasure and pain). If it is the right way to think of the relation between work on well-being in philosophy and psychology—and I am by no means certain that it is—then it gives a sense of how researchers working in each of these two areas should regard the other.

One complication that arises for the rapprochement just sketched is that recent work in philosophy has postulated genuine conceptual pluralism within thought and talk about "well-being." Anna Alexandrova (2017) and Steve Campbell (2016) have each explored and defended views which hold (roughly) that talk about well-being (and similar expressions such as "good for," "doing well," etc.) exhibit a radical kind of pluralism by not always referring to the same thing. This means, for example, that each of two speakers could both say something true if they say, of the same person: "Jack is doing well" and "Jack is not doing well."[14] If this view is true then it might be that across different conversational contexts different things are meant by "well-being" and that the different referents of the expression are (e.g.) hedonic well-being, eudaimonic well-being, and the like.[15] If this is so, then it would be the job of philosophy to devise a theory of which "kind of well-being" is relevant in different contexts and why, and then work in psychology would be able to provide a theory of what each of these "kinds of well-being" is like.

Conclusion

In this chapter I have attempted to clarify philosophical work on well-being by bringing out its distinctive questions, commitments, and methodologies. Two major points about philosophical theories of well-being were, first, that such theories are typically offered as competing theories of one and the same subject-matter—"well-being"—as opposed to theories of different "types of well-being" or the like. A second major point is that philosophical theories of well-being aim to find explanations of what fundamentally, noninstrumentally contributes to and detracts from well-being.

The aims of philosophical work on well-being lead philosophers to focus away from typical cases and to reflect on cases where the explanatory factors that feature within the major theories of well-being can be prised apart. This is why philosophers use thought experiments about quite unusual cases so that they can see which factors are most plausible candidates for explaining facts about well-being.

Notes

1. For further discussion see Chapters 8 and 9, both in this volume).
2. There is a dense but interesting debate in philosophy about whether all value that is noninstrumental is *intrinsic*. I don't want to introduce those issues here so just read "intrinsic" as "noninstrumental." I choose "intrinsic" just for readability. To learn more about these controversies see, for example, Korsgaard (1983) and Bradley (1998).
3. For discussion of hedonism about well-being see, for example, Gregory (2015).
4. For discussion of desire-fulfillment theories of well-being see, for example, Heathwood (2015).
5. For discussion of objective list theories see, for example, Fletcher (2015a).
6. For discussion of perfectionist theories see, for example, Bradford (2015).
7. The negative side of perfectionist theories is less clear than their positive claim. The same holds for objective list theories. I thus omit formulations of these parts of these theories. For more on the main philosophical theories of well-being, see Fletcher (2015b, 2016).
8. How far this overlap extends into theological conceptions of well-being, I do not know. But see Chapter 10 and 16 (both in this volume) for more on this.
9. Nozick (1974, pp. 44–45). For discussion of the example see, for example, Lin (2016).
10. Parfit (1984, p. 494).
11. This is *not* to say that all philosophers neglect empirical work. For important exceptions see Baril (Chapter 9, in this volume); Besser (2014), Bishop (2015), and Haybron (2008).

12. See Lauinger (Chapter 8, in this volume) for one such attempt.
13. One exception here is Disabato et al. (2016).
14. They would need to be in different conversational contexts, though.
15. For discussion of Alexandrova and Campbell's pluralist theories, see Fletcher (2019), Lin (2018), and Mitchell (2018).

About the Author

Guy Fletcher is Senior Lecturer in Philosophy at the University of Edinburgh. His work examines the nature of moral discourse, philosophical theories of well-being, and theories of prudential discourse. He edited the *Routledge Handbook of Philosophy of Well-Being* (Routledge, 2015) and co-edited *Having It Both Ways: Hybrid Theories in Meta-Normative Theory* (Oxford University Press, 2014). He is author of *An Introduction to the Philosophy of Well-Being* (Routledge, 2016) and *Dear Prudence: The Nature and Normativity of Prudential Discourse* (Oxford University Press, 2021).

Author Note

Many thanks to Debbie Roberts and Steve Loughnan for helpful comments on earlier versions of this chapter. This work was supported in part by a grant from the John Templeton Foundation and by the Lee Kum Sheung Center for Health and Happiness. The views expressed in this chapter represent the perspective of the author and do not reflect the opinions or endorsement of any organization. I have no known conflict of interest to disclose. Correspondence concerning this chapter should be directed to Guy Fletcher, Philosophy, PPLS, Dugald Stewart Building, 3 Charles Street, University of Edinburgh, Edinburgh, EH8 9AD (Guy.Fletcher@ed.ac.uk).

References

Alexandrova, A. (2017). *A philosophy for the science of well-being*. Oxford: Oxford University Press.
Besser, L. (2014). *Eudaimonic ethics: The philosophy and psychology of living well*. New York: Routledge.
Bishop, M. (2015). *The good life: Unifying the philosophy and psychology of well-being*. Oxford: Oxford University Press.
Bradford, G. (2015). Perfectionism. In G. Fletcher (Ed.), *The Routledge handbook of philosophy of well-being* (pp. 124–134). Oxford: Routledge.
Bradley, B. (1998). Extrinsic value. *Philosophical Studies, 91*, 109–126.
Campbell, S. (2016). The concept of well-being. In G. Fletcher (Ed.), *The Routledge handbook of philosophy of well-being* (pp. 402–414). Oxford: Routledge.

Disabato, D., Goodman, F., Kashdan, T., Short, J., & Aaron, J. (2016). Different types of well-being? A cross-cultural examination of hedonic and eudaimonic well-being. *Psychological Assessment, 28*(5), 471–482.

Fletcher, G. (2015a). Objective list theories. In G. Fletcher (Ed.), *The Routledge handbook of philosophy of well-being* (pp. 148–160). Oxford: Routledge.

Fletcher, G. (2015b). *The Routledge handbook of philosophy of well-being*. Oxford: Routledge.

Fletcher, G. (2016). *The philosophy of well-being: An introduction*. Oxford: Routledge.

Fletcher, G. (2019). Against contextualism about prudential discourse. *Philosophical Quarterly, 69*, 699–720.

Gregory, A. (2015). Hedonism. In G. Fletcher (Ed.), *The Routledge handbook of philosophy of well-being* (pp. 113–122). Oxford: Routledge.

Haybron, D. (2008). *The pursuit of unhappiness*. Oxford: Oxford University Press.

Heathwood, C. (2015). Desire-fulfillment theory. In G. Fletcher (ed.), *The Routledge handbook of philosophy of well-being* (pp. 135–147). Oxford: Routledge.

Korsgaard, C. (1983). Two distinctions in goodness. *Philosophical Review, 92*(2). 169–195.

Lin, E. (2016). How to use the experience machine. *Utilitas, 28* (3), 314–332.

Lin, E. (2018). Review of "A philosophy for the science of well-being." *Ethics, 129*, 116–122.

Mitchell, M. (2018). *The construction of well-being*. Doctoral thesis, University College London.

Nozick, R. (1974). *Anarchy, state and utopia*. Oxford: Blackwell.

Parfit, D. (1984). *Reasons and persons*. Oxford: Oxford University Press.

8

Defending a Hybrid of Objective List and Desire Theories of Well-Being

William A. Lauinger

Abstract

This chapter extends previous work of mine on a view of human well-being that is a hybrid of objective list theories and desire theories. Though some of what I say traverses old ground, much of what I say is new—not in terms of ultimate conclusions, but rather in terms of routes toward these ultimate conclusions and certain implications of these ultimate conclusions (e.g., implications concerning the measurement of well-being). There are two different visions of what human beings are that I privilege and attempt to synthesize herein. One of these visions pushes us toward an objective list theory. This vision is a broadly Aristotelian one according to which humans have various capacities that are central to their functioning well as the kinds of things they are, that is, as human beings. Though this broadly Aristotelian vision captures something necessary for well-being, it is, as it were, only half of the story. The other half of the story derives from a vision of human beings as unique individuals with different sets of intrinsic desires, and this desire-focused vision of humans is itself informed by Jacques Lacan and his view that each human self is constituted by a particular and dynamic chains-of-signifiers-plus-desire-flow structure. I start by briefly discussing mental state theories. Then I discuss objective list theories at some length, and, while doing this, I occasionally comment on pro-attitude theories (e.g., desire theories). After that, I present the hybrid theory of well-being that I favor and defend it against some objections. Last, I conclude the chapter.

William A. Lauinger, *Defending a Hybrid of Objective List and Desire Theories of Well-Being* In: *Measuring Well-Being.* Edited by: Matthew T. Lee, Laura D. Kubzansky, and Tyler J. VanderWeele, Oxford University Press (2021). © Oxford University Press. DOI: 10.1093/oso/9780197512531.003.0009

In past work, I argued for a view of human well-being that is a hybrid of objective list theories and desire theories (Lauinger, 2012, pp. 3–120; Lauinger, 2013a).[1] I still accept this view, and, in what follows I will try to provide some support for it. Though some of what I am going to say will traverse old ground, much of what I am going to say will be new—not in terms of ultimate conclusions, but rather in terms of routes toward these ultimate conclusions and certain implications of these ultimate conclusions (e.g., implications concerning the measurement of well-being). There are two different visions of what humans are that I will privilege and attempt to synthesize herein. One is broadly Aristotelian and focuses on the similarities that obtain across humans in terms of their functioning well as the kinds of things they are: that is, as human beings. The other vision focuses on humans as unique selves, with different sets of intrinsic desires. In presenting this latter vision of humans, I will draw on Jacques Lacan's view of human subjectivity. There are, of course, other visions of what humans are that might be privileged when one is constructing a theory of human well-being. For instance, there are theologically informed visions that might be considered (e.g., Chapters 10, 11, and 16, all in this volume). Though I intend for the account of human well-being that I provide in this chapter to be acceptable to theists and non-theists alike, I should perhaps explicitly note that, in my view, a thorough exploration of the metaphysics that best supports this account reveals that it is not only compatible with theism, but actually points us toward theism (for the details concerning why I believe this, see Lauinger, 2012, pp. 123–178).

Here is an outline of what follows. I start by briefly discussing mental state theories. Then I discuss objective list theories at some length, and, while doing this, I will occasionally comment on pro-attitude theories (e.g., desire theories).[2] After that, I present the hybrid theory of well-being that I favor and defend it against some objections. Last, I conclude the paper.

Mental State Theories

Mental state theories come in different types, but all of them centrally claim that nothing can enter the content of any given human's well-being except certain of his or her psychological states.[3] Naturally, the contrast here is with theories that allow for more than just one's mental states to enter the content of one's well-being. Such theories are sometimes called *state-of-the-world theories* because they allow states of the world beyond one's mind (e.g., states of bodily health such as that of having a well-functioning cardiovascular system) to be included within the content of one's well-being (Griffin, 1986, p. 7). Though I will not provide a detailed argument against mental state theories here, I do want to provide a brief sense of why I reject them.

In constructing a mental state theory, it is most common, and also most plausible, to privilege pleasure, understood as positive affect, or instead to privilege favorable beliefs about one's life or the conditions of one's life. Accordingly, a mental state theorist might say (a) that one's well-being consists in, and only in, one's experience of positive affect or, instead, (b) that one's well-being consists in, and only in, one's having favorable beliefs about one's life or the conditions of one's life.

With regard to mental state theories that privilege positive affect, I think that such theories are implausible because we often have experiences that enhance our well-being even though they involve no positive affect or even mildly negative affect. For instance, often when I am teaching or writing, it seems to me that I am intrinsically (i.e., noninstrumentally) gaining in well-being by accomplishing something while my affect is neutral or even mildly negative, if only because of the cognitive exertion involved. And I am not peculiar in this regard. Indeed, people often take themselves to be intrinsically gaining in well-being by accomplishing things through work, but where these accomplishments are not accompanied by positive affect. Similar remarks can be made about time spent with one's children. I sometimes help my 9-year-old daughter with math homework, and this activity is often mildly negative, affect-wise, for me, simply because (a) it requires some cognitive effort on my part and (b) it is mildly unpleasant to see my daughter experience frustration with the math problems (indeed, she sometimes cries!). Still, whether positive affect is present for me or not, I believe that I intrinsically gain in well-being almost every time I help my daughter with her math homework because the relationship between us is strengthened almost every time we do this activity together. And, again here, I am not peculiar. Parents often believe that they are intrinsically gaining in well-being while spending time with their children without there being any positive affect present for themselves.

Turning now to mental state theories that privilege favorable beliefs about one's life or the conditions of one's life, we might ask whether the favorable beliefs in question need to be true in order to be aspects of one's well-being. It seems unpromising to answer "no," for it seems unpromising to make beliefs that need not be true the centerpiece of a theory of well-being. Naturally, we could add the amendment that the favorable beliefs in question must be true in order to be aspects of one's well-being. However, if we do that, I think that we are thereby abandoning the parameters of a mental state theory of well-being. After all, a belief that is true seems to be more than just a state in one's own mind. It seems, that is, to be a state in one's own mind that somehow corresponds to or represents how things are in reality, where "somehow corresponds to or represents how things are in reality" cannot convincingly be spelled out without appealing to something external to one's own mind.

Speaking generally, our minds are not closed in on themselves, as, indeed, our beliefs, desires, and intentions are all typically directed outward (i.e., toward some kind of interaction with the world beyond our minds). In view of this, it might well be a mistake to begin our welfare theorizing with the assumption that well-being is entirely internal to the mind.

Initial Comments on Objective List Theories

Objective list theories are centered on the basic goods—that is, general goods such as friendship (i.e., close personal relationships), accomplishment, and knowledge. Objective list theories claim that something (anything) is an aspect of one's well-being if and only if, and because (a) it is a basic good or (b) it is a state of affairs that instantiates a basic good for oneself.[4] An example will make the instancing relation that is in play here clearer: If I am reading an academic article and learning from it, objective list theorists will say that I am gaining in well-being inasmuch as I am gaining instances of the basic good of knowledge for myself. Importantly, objective list theories are pro-attitude independent theories in that they entail (a) that each basic good is a fixed component of one's well-being regardless of whether one has any kind of pro-attitude toward it and (b) that each state of affairs that instantiates a basic good for oneself is an aspect of one's well-being regardless of whether one has any kind of pro-attitude toward it and, more generally, regardless of whether it connects at all to one's pro-attitudes. Also, as standardly understood, objective list theories are pro-attitude independent theories in that they entail (c) that, for any given thing that is included within the content of one's well-being (be it a basic good or an instance of a basic good), one's pro-attitude(s) toward this thing cannot directly affect the degree to which this thing is intrinsically prudentially good for one. There might be logical space available for objective list theorists to deny (c) from the previous sentence, but, that said, it would be highly unusual for an objective list theorist to make this denial.[5] Thus, in what follows I will use "objective list theories" and "objective list theorists" in ways that assume that objective list theories do indeed entail the immediately preceding (c).

In virtue of being pro-attitude independent theories, objective list theories differ from pro-attitude theories of well-being. The core idea behind pro-attitude theories is to seize on some kind of pro-attitude (e.g., intrinsic desire, enjoyment, or favorable belief) and then to claim that something (anything) is an aspect of one's well-being if and only if and because one has the designated kind of pro-attitude toward it. Pro-attitude theories are often complicated in certain ways. For instance, a desire theorist might claim that one's well-being is composed not of those objects that one actually (intrinsically) desires to obtain, but rather of those objects that one would (intrinsically) desire to obtain if one were better informed with respect to nonevaluative information than one actually is. Complications aside, though, the core idea behind pro-attitude theories is straightforward: it is that something (anything) that is an aspect of one's well-being is so because one has the designated kind of pro-attitude toward it.

Many, though not all, objective list theorists fill their theories out in Aristotelian-perfectionist terms, claiming that the basic goods are not only components of each human's own well-being but are also completing or fulfilling of each human's own human nature.[6] Usually this position is elaborated on by claiming (a) that each of us is a certain kind of thing, namely, a human being; (b) that, in virtue of this being so, each of us has a human nature that he or she can complete or fulfill; (c) that each of us completes or fulfills his or her own human nature by exercising, developing, or actualizing those capacities that he or she has that are constitutive of the well-functioning of the human being as such (e.g., the capacity to deepen or to maintain friendships, the capacity to accomplish worthwhile tasks, and the capacity to gain knowledge of oneself and the world in general); and (d) that, for each of us, the completing or fulfilling of his or her own human nature is the same thing, metaphysically, as his or her gaining in individual well-being. To be clear, the philosophers who accept this metaphysical identity claim are aware that there is a conceptual distinction between well-being (i.e., prudential value) and perfectionist value.[7] They are aware, that is, that (as a conceptual matter) prudential value consists in one's living well or doing well as the *individual* one is, whereas perfectionist value consists in one's living well or doing well as the *kind* of thing one is: namely, a human being. Still, they are

convinced that due reflection reveals that there is a metaphysical identity relationship in play here.

Though objective list theorists agree with each other that there is one true
list of basic goods, they disagree with each other to some extent about which
items are on this one true list. There seems to be a solid consensus among
objective list theorists that knowledge, accomplishment, health, friendship,
and aesthetic experience are basic goods.[8] However, there does not seem
to be much agreement regarding other items, ones such as pleasure, happiness (where this is taken to differ from pleasure even if it involves pleasure),
freedom or autonomy, meaningfulness, life, play, moral virtue, religion, and
self-acceptance. It will help, for this chapter, if we have on hand a working
list of basic goods. We need not hold that this list is set in stone. The point is
simply to have a fairly convincing list on hand so that we can rely on it as a
way of helping us (a) to understand objective list theories well and then later
(b) to understand well the particular hybrid theory that I favor. Here, then, is
a working list of basic goods: knowledge, accomplishment, health (i.e., both
bodily and mental health), friendship, aesthetic experience, and pleasure.[9]

Aside from pleasure, this working list of basic goods does not contain any
items that are purely psychological. Knowledge involves true belief, and, as
I indicated earlier, a belief that is true seems to go beyond the limits of one's
own mind. Accomplishment involves the actual doing of something worthwhile, where this standardly involves moving one's physical body in certain
ways (e.g., as when a basketball player makes a difficult shot). Health involves
the well-functioning of the physical body, and so it is not a purely psychological item. Much of friendship takes one beyond one's own mind, for much of
friendship involves doing things with one's friend, where this itself involves
moving one's physical body (e.g., as when one goes on a walk with one's
friend). Aesthetic experience is the experience of something beautiful, where
what is beautiful is typically something that is (entirely or at least partly) external to one's own mind, as is the case when one witnesses the beauty of a
mountain or hears the beauty of a song on the radio, and thus aesthetic experience typically takes one beyond one's own mind.

Let me now discuss measurement on objective list theories. Start here with
the basic good of friendship and a particular human. We can have this human
provide self-rating scores by answering questions such as "How strong, on a
scale of 1–7 (where 7 stands for "very strong" and 1 stands for "very weak") is
your relationship with (a) your parents, (b) your siblings, (c) your children,
(d) your significant other or spouse, (e) your work colleagues, and (f) other

friends of yours?" I do not know exactly how best to word the questions in play here, but presumably the more narrowly focused they are, the more accurate will be the self-ratings. One obvious problem with these kinds of questions is that recent events can significantly skew self-rating scores. For instance, if the human at issue has just had a bad fight with his or her significant other, this could lead him or her to give a significantly lower rating score than is accurate for the strength of his or her relationship with his or her significant other. I am not sure how best to mitigate this problem, but perhaps it is best (a) to have the human at issue do the self-ratings many times over the course of a year and then (b) to seize on his or her median self-rating scores.

To provide a fuller picture and also to some extent to correct for inaccuracies in self-ratings, we could interview friends and family members to get their evaluations of how well the human in question is doing in his or her personal relationships. We might also have an expert (e.g., a psychologist) interview the human in question, and this expert could provide an assessment of how well this human is doing in his or her personal relationships.[10] Also, if we are worried that the self-ratings might be infected with a high degree of inaccuracy because the questions being asked are too general, then perhaps we could use experience sampling, the day reconstruction method, or brain scanning in order to supplement and, to some extent, correct the measurements arrived at through the self-ratings.[11] With regard to experience sampling, we could text the human at issue at random moments and have him or her provide a self-rating in relation to friendship at these moments (e.g., if this human is at work when we text him or her, he or she could say how things are going with his or her work colleagues, friendship-wise, at that moment). With regard to the day reconstruction method, we could have the human at issue recall the previous day in an episode-by-episode way and then have him or her provide self-ratings for each episode in relation to friendship. With regard to brain scanning, if there are specific areas of the brain that are typically activated when people are engaging in friendship, then perhaps there is a way to use brain scanning to help us in measuring how well the human in question is doing in relation to friendship. As a final comment here, if the culture that the human in question belongs to is known to have a bias of some sort in relation to friendship, then perhaps we could adjust (i.e., discount or inflate) this human's self-rating scores to whatever extent would be needed to correct for the cultural bias in question.

In practice, we would probably never be able to use all of these just mentioned measurement methods and considerations to help us in measuring the well-being of the human in question in relation to the basic good of friendship. In principle, though, we could do this. However, even if we were to do this, there would still be more measurement work to do for we would still need to answer a question about the weightings that are in play here. Indeed, there are various relationships in play here (e.g., relationships with parents, siblings, and children), and, to come up with a fairly accurate measurement of this human's level of well-being in relation to friendship, we would need to know how much each one of these relationships matters for this human's level of well-being in relation to friendship. But suppose, if only for the sake of argument, that we can resolve this worry and in turn come up with a fairly accurate measurement of this human's level of well-being in relation to friendship. Furthermore, suppose (if only for the sake of argument) that, by using the same kinds of measurement methods and considerations discussed in the previous two paragraphs, we can attain a fairly accurate measurement of any given human's well-being in relation to any given basic good. Even then there would still be the question of how well off any given human is *overall* (and so not just in relation to this or that basic good). To answer this question of how well off any given human is *overall*, we would need to know how the basic goods are objectively ordered—that is, we would need to know if the basic goods are arranged in an objective hierarchy and, if so, which basic good is primary, which basic good is secondary, and so on. Most (though not all) present-day objective list theorists maintain that there is no objective ordering or hierarchy among the basic goods.[12] But, if this is correct, how should we proceed? Perhaps the best option is to count each basic good as being of equal weight (i.e., when we are trying to come up with an *overall* measurement of any given human's well-being). A second option is to claim that there is no truth about any given human's *overall* level of well-being (i.e., there are only truths about each human's level of well-being in relation to each basic good). And there might be other options besides these two.

Where Objective List Theories Err

As a start here, it is worth emphasizing that the domain of prudence or well-being seems to be much more personal or individual-focused than other normative or evaluative domains (e.g., the domain of morality and the domain of perfectionist value).[13] How, then, might we capture the especially personal or individual-focused nature of well-being? The most common way to do this is to claim that, in order for something (anything) to count as an aspect of one's well-being, it must be nonvacuously connected to (i.e., dependent on) one's own pro-attitudes.[14] I think that this is the correct thing to do. Indeed, though I disagree with pro-attitude theorists inasmuch as they refuse to place an objective value constraint on well-being, I agree with pro-attitude theorists on the point that well-being is a pro-attitude dependent kind of value. To be clear, in holding that well-being is pro-attitude dependent, I do not have concerns about autonomy or sovereignty over one's own life in mind; rather, I am concerned with capturing the personal psychological fulfillment that seems to be essential to well-being.

To provide some support for (a) the claim that well-being is a pro-attitude dependent kind of value and, in line with this, (b) the claim that objective list theories are inadequate, I will make three distinct but related sets of points. Each focuses on the pro-attitude of intrinsic desire, which is the pro-attitude that I take well-being necessarily to depend on. With regard to these three sets of points: the first concerns prudential deliberation, the second concerns certain cases of tie-breaking, and the third concerns the way in which certain desires are bound up with people's life histories. After I make these three sets of points, I will very briefly consider what objective list theorists might say in response.

Prudential Deliberation

Suppose that someone named Dottie is deciding between buying House A and House B. And suppose that Dottie says the following to her friend: "The price for House A is much lower than the price for House B, and I want the lower priced home, all else equal, since I want to be as free as possible of financial worries. Also, House A is prettier and in a prettier neighborhood, and I do want the aesthetics of my home and neighborhood to be as good as possible. However, there are some reasons to favor House B. House B is closer to work, and I want the shortest possible commute, since that would reduce stress and increase enjoyment in my life. In addition, House B is closer to my friends and family members, and I do want to live as close as possible to them. So, right now, I am torn." I think that, when we engage in prudential deliberation, we do what Dottie is doing here. On the one hand, we consider desire-independent goods such as pleasure, aesthetic experience, and friendship, and we focus on the ways in which and the extents to which these desire-independent goods might be instantiated in our lives; and, on the other hand, we consider our own desires and how strongly we want the different objects that are open to us.

Now imagine that Dottie's friend is a convinced objective list theorist, and imagine that, after hearing Dottie discuss House A and House B, Dottie's friend replies: "Dottie, in deciding between buying House A and buying House B, it is smart to consider factors such as cost, aesthetics, proximity to work, and proximity to friends and family members. But you also keep mentioning your own desires. That is a serious mistake. Since your own desires play no direct role in constituting your well-being, it is important simply to ignore them when you are making decisions about your well-being. This holds true regardless of whether the context is trivial (e.g., as when you are deciding between ice cream flavors or kinds of candy) or weighty (e.g., as when you are deciding between career paths or romantic partners)." This advice seems to me both strange and bad: strange because people do not ignore their own desires when engaging in prudential deliberation, and bad because it seems unwise for people to ignore their own desires when engaging in prudential deliberation.[15]

Tie-Breaking, Desire Strengths, and Well-Being

It is reasonable to think that people sometimes choose between two options, each of which promises them the same amount of well-being as measured from the objective list theory point of view. For example, a high school student might be choosing between playing football or soccer in the fall, and these two options might be equal in terms of how much they would add to his well-being; that is, if we are considering the matter from the objective list theory point of view—which entails our taking into account the degree to which each of these two options would instantiate basic goods such as pleasure, accomplishment, health, and friendship in this high school student's life. But now suppose that this high school student has a significantly stronger intrinsic desire to play soccer than he does to play football, and, in line with this, suppose that he has significantly stronger intrinsic desires for the instances of basic goods that would come to him through playing soccer than he does for the instances of basic goods that would come to him through playing football. In this case, it seems that we should say that the soccer option provides this high school student with more well-being, overall, than the football option does. Yet we cannot say this if we are objective list theorists about well-being. Rather, we can say this only if we admit that desire strengths can directly affect the degree to which states of affairs intrinsically prudentially benefit people.

Desires, Life Histories, and Well-Being

The point that desire strengths can directly affect the degree to which states of affairs intrinsically prudentially benefit people seems to be relevant not only in tie-breaking cases such as the one just discussed, but also in cases involving certain desires that are bound up with people's life histories. In supporting my position on this matter, it will help if I begin by making some background comments about Lacan's view of human subjectivity.

Lacan accepts various claims about human subjectivity. Here are some of them.[16] (1) The real subject (i.e., the real agent) is unconscious and is constituted by a dynamic structure that involves chains of signifiers (i.e., words) and intrinsic desire (i.e., noninstrumental motivational force). (2) Some of these chains of signifiers form the core of the subject in that (a) they somehow govern all of the less central chains of signifiers and (b) they are strongly charged with, or animated by, desire. (3) For each human, his or her childhood—and, more generally, his or her life history—plays a crucial role in determining which chains of signifiers are at the core of his or her subjectivity. (4) From the standpoint of conscious, rational thought, it is extremely difficult to understand why any given human's subjectivity has the particular chains-of-signifiers-plus-desire-flow structure that it has; this is so because the rules that unconscious thought follows (e.g., metonymy) are very different from the rules that are characteristic of conscious, rational thought.[17] (5) Though the conscious ego takes itself to be the real subject, it is in fact a phony gloss that covers the real, unconscious subject. (6) The real, unconscious subject is by no means entirely cut off from consciousness, as, indeed, it often juts into consciousness, making itself known through slips of the tongue, through denegation, through the conversation topics that people are receptive to or that they select as being worthy of discussion, and so on.[18] (7) By talking with an analyst or a lay person who is a good listener, and by not censoring one's thoughts as one talks, one can uncover one's subjectivity—that is, one can bring to consciousness some of the particular chains-of-signifiers-plus-desire-flow structure that constitutes one's subjectivity. (8) Insofar as one's subjectivity is brought to consciousness, one gains in self-knowledge, at which point true healing or growth can begin to occur (e.g., if one has been suffering from a psychological problem, the problem might be eliminated or have its force mitigated).

Though I believe that Lacan's view of human subjectivity places far too much emphasis on the unconscious and not nearly enough emphasis on consciousness, I am nonetheless convinced that there is something right and important about Lacan's view of human subjectivity. Here consider two sets of comments. (1) The way that people conceive of themselves and talk about themselves suggests that there is something right and important about Lacan's view of human subjectivity. A brief anecdote will help to illustrate this point. My wife's parents recently sold their house, and my wife was sad about this. This was the house that she grew up in, and the thought of no more Christmases there, no more summer visits there, no more waking up in her old bedroom, and so on was hard for her to accept. All of this sounds ordinary, but I was struck when my wife said that she felt as though an important part of herself had suddenly been ripped out. Given Lacan's view of the subject, this way of putting the matter is apt. It stands to reason that, for my wife, there are certain chains of signifiers that essentially involve *the being there* of the house that she grew up in and that have long been part of the core of her subjectivity. For the house to be sold is for her suddenly to lose these chains of signifiers and thus suddenly to lose an important part of the chains-of-signifiers-plus-desire-flow structure that constitutes her subjectivity (i.e., for the house to be sold is, in that sense, for her to have an important part of herself suddenly ripped out). (2) Consider the word "Manhattan." For one person, this word might be unconsciously bound up with "so much to do," "electrifying," "the only place I want to live," "full of interesting people," and so on. But, for another person, this word might be unconsciously bound up with "crowded," "smells like urine," "overwhelming," "exorbitantly expensive," "full of mean people who say whatever the hell they want to say," and so on. Now consider the word "golf." For one person, this word might be unconsciously bound up with "happy summer days with my dad," "I wish my dad were still alive, so that I could tell him how much I love him," "miss my dad," and so on. But, for another person, "golf" might be unconsciously bound up with "rich snobs," "men wearing pink polo shirts and talking about their investments," "rich people do not know what hard work is," and so on. The general point here is (a) that words and chains of words can connect to other words and chains of words in one's unconscious in ways that are extremely difficult to understand from the standpoint of conscious, rational thought and (b) that one's beliefs and desire flow can become bound up with these unconscious words and chains of words in such a way as to have a significant influence on how one behaves and, more generally, lives. For example, because of unconscious connections involving words and chains of words, one person can be strongly inclined to stay away from Manhattan, while another person can be strongly inclined to make sure that he or she lives in Manhattan.

Now let us return to the claim that desire strengths can directly affect the degree to which states of affairs intrinsically prudentially benefit people. Objective list theories reject this claim. But if we consider certain desires that are bound up with people's life histories, I think that we can see that the objective list theory position is in error. Consider the person who has positive unconscious associations with the word "Manhattan." If this person lives in Manhattan and gains in well-being from doing so, then objective list theorists can point to the pleasure, aesthetic experience, and so on that this person derives from living in Manhattan. But I doubt that this suffices as a full explanation of the amount of well-being gained here. To provide a full explanation here, it seems to me that we need to reference this person's life history and the various intrinsic desires related to Manhattan that have over time become embedded in this person's subjectivity; that is, in this person's dynamic chains-of-signifiers-plus-desire-flow structure. Similar remarks can be made about the example involving the person who unconsciously associates golf with his dad in positive ways. In accounting for the amount of well-being that this person derives from playing golf, objective list theorists can point to the pleasure, health, and so on that this person derives from playing golf. But, as an explanation, this seems to fall short, for it leaves out this person's life history and the various intrinsic desires related to playing golf that have over time become embedded in this person's subjectivity; that is, in this person's dynamic chains-of-signifiers-plus-desire-flow structure.

Two clarifications are in order here. First, with regard to both the Manhattan case and the golf case, I am not saying that objective list theorists are wrong about *which* states of affairs enter the content of well-being. Indeed, I think that, in both of these cases, objective list theorists are correct about which states of affairs enter the content of well-being. What I am saying is that objective list theorists are wrong about *how much* well-being is contained in the states of affairs that enter the content of well-being in these cases. In the Manhattan case, the states that enter the content of the person's well-being are states that instantiate pleasure, aesthetic experience, and so on for this person; however, the degree to which these states intrinsically prudentially benefit this person seems to depend partly on this person's intrinsic desires for these states, where these intrinsic desires are themselves bound up with this person's life history and with the fact that the word "Manhattan" is strongly charged with intrinsic desire for this person. *Mutatis mutandis*, the same holds for the golf case. Second, objective list theorists can appeal to people's life histories when they are explaining people's well-being. However, in the process of doing this, objective list theorists must bracket (i.e., abstract from) people's desires in such a way as to retain their claim that well-being is a pro-attitude independent kind of value. In bracketing people's desires in this way, objective list theorists are, I think, bracketing something that is essential to people's well-being.

Very Briefly Considering What Objective List Theorists Might Say in Response

In responding to the preceding three sets of points that I have made, objective list theorists might claim that desire fulfillment is on the list of basic goods. Making this claim would go some way toward answering the concerns that I have raised, as, indeed, making this claim would constitute an acknowledgment on the part of objective list theorists that desires should not be ignored in a theory of human well-being. I am not aware of any objective list theorists who *do* claim that desire fulfillment is on the list of basic goods. However, Mark Murphy is an objective list theorist who comes close to doing this.[19] And, in any case, there is no bar, in principle, to an objective list theorist's doing this. If an objective list theorist were to do this, he or she would thereby be claiming that desire fulfillment is an aspect of one's well-being regardless of whether one wants it and, more generally, regardless of whether it connects at all to one's pro-attitudes.[20] This claim might be paradoxical, but, even so, it is not inconsistent. There are, however, two problems with this claim that are worth noting. One: it is difficult to see objective list theorists accepting that desire fulfillment is prudentially beneficial for a person in cases where the desires being fulfilled are defective (e.g., because they are seriously immoral or exceptionally unhealthy). Much of the appeal of objective list theories lies in the fact that they can easily avoid the problem of defective desires that plagues desire theories of well-being. However, if objective list theorists were to claim that desire fulfillment is on the list of basic goods, then the problem of defective desires would become a problem for objective list theories, too.[21] Two: even if objective list theorists were to claim that desire-fulfillment is on the list of basic goods, a lack of psychological fulfillment would still be built into their theory inasmuch as their theory would still entail that all of the basic goods (e.g., health, accomplishment, knowledge, and friendship) are aspects of one's well-being regardless of whether one wants them and, more generally, regardless of whether they connect at all to one's pro-attitudes.

Admittedly, there are other responses that objective list theorists might have to the preceding three sets of points that I have made.[22] For instance, some objective list theorists would note (a) that pleasure is one of the basic goods and (b) that there are other basic goods that necessarily carry with them some degree of psychological fulfillment inasmuch as they necessarily involve pro-attitudes (e.g., the basic good of friendship necessarily involves the desire to spend time with one's friend and care for one's friend). This response would help, for it would go some way toward acknowledging that psychological fulfillment matters for well-being. Still, this response would (in my view) fall short in that it would not ensure that every aspect of one's well-being brings with it some degree of psychological fulfillment. However, Guy Fletcher has advanced an objective list theory that is unique in that it entails that *all* of the basic goods have pro-attitudes as necessary components (2013, pp. 214–216). Thus, on Fletcher's objective list theory, every aspect of one's well-being *would* bring with it some degree of psychological fulfillment. There are, however, two criticisms that I have of Fletcher's objective list theory.[23] One: Fletcher's list of basic goods is as follows: achievement, friendship, happiness, pleasure, self-respect, and virtue (2013, p. 214). This list excludes knowledge and health. But it seems that both knowledge and health should be on any objective list theorist's list of basic goods. Yet neither of these items contains a pro-attitude as a necessary component. Two: Fletcher's objective list theory does not seem to capture the connection between what one intrinsically wants and what is intrinsically prudentially beneficial for one in quite a strong enough way. Here consider the individual-deliberative perspective in relation to well-being. When engaging in prudential deliberation, one *might* consider the question of whether an option that is open to one contains within itself a pro-attitude that one has. But still, the questions "Do I *want* this option that is open to me?" and "*How much* do I want this option that is open to me?" seem to be far more central to prudential deliberation than the question "Does this option that is open to me have a pro-attitude of mine inside it?"

A Hybrid of Objective List and Desire Theories of Well-Being: The Desire-Perfectionism Theory

Most extant hybrid theories of well-being are subjective-objective hybrids in that they incorporate both a pro-attitude constraint and an objective value constraint—that is, they entail that each human's well-being is directly constituted by some kind of pro-attitude and some kind of objective value.[24] The primary aim of incorporating a pro-attitude constraint is to capture (a) the especially personal or individual-focused nature of well-being and, in line with this, (b) the psychological fulfillment that seems to be essential to well-being. And the primary aim of incorporating an objective value constraint is to avoid the problem of defective pro-attitudes that seems to plague all pro-attitude theories. The problem of defective pro-attitudes can be put as follows: it seems that humans sometimes have the relevant kind of pro-attitude (e.g., intrinsic desire, enjoyment, or favorable belief) toward states of affairs that do not seem to be good in any way, including the prudential way. Though pro-attitude theorists have tried hard over the years to come up with ways of avoiding the problem of defective pro-attitudes (e.g., by moving to second-order pro-attitude theories or to idealized pro-attitude theories), I do not think that they have been successful (for a defense of this point that focuses on desire theories in particular, see Lauinger, 2012, pp. 23–57).

I favor a particular subjective-objective hybrid theory of well-being that I refer to as *the desire-perfectionism theory*.[25] This label is appropriate because this theory relies on intrinsic desire for its pro-attitude constraint and on perfectionist value for its objective value constraint.

To begin to understand the desire-perfectionism theory, we can consider Aristotelian-perfectionist objective list theories of well-being. Such theories take the basic goods (e.g., knowledge, friendship, health, and accomplishment), at the start, to be components not only of each human's perfection as a human being, but also of each human's well-being. By contrast, the desire-perfectionism theory does *not* take the basic goods, at the start, to be components of each human's well-being. Indeed, the desire-perfectionism theory takes the basic goods, at the start, *only* to be components of each human's perfection as a human being. The qualification "at the start" matters because the desire-perfectionism theory entails that, once some (any) human being intrinsically desires some (any) basic good, then, at that moment, this basic good becomes a component of this human's well-being.

In line with the foregoing remarks, we can understand the desire-perfectionism theory as centrally claiming the following:

> Something (anything) is intrinsically prudentially beneficial for some (any) human if and only if, and because, (a) this thing is either a basic good or a state of affairs that instantiates a basic good for this human, where the basic goods are items such as knowledge, friendship, health, and accomplishment and where the basic goods are being conceived of as perfectionist goods and not as components of well-being, and (b) this human intrinsically desires this thing (or, if this human does not intrinsically desire this thing, then it is at least true that this thing is, for this person, an instance of a basic good that this human intrinsically desires).

With regard to the parenthetical comment contained in condition (b), the desire condition, my point is this: for any given state of affairs that instantiates a basic good for someone, it need not be true that he or she intrinsically desires this state of affairs in order for this state of affairs to count as an aspect of his or her welfare because it is enough if he or she simply intrinsically desires the basic good that this state of affairs instantiates for him or her. Here consider an undergraduate student named Bob. Suppose that Bob is sitting in his ethics class and that he has no desire to know anything about Sidgwick's ethical views—say, because he has never even heard of Sidgwick.[26] But suppose also that Bob does have an intrinsic desire for knowledge. If the teacher begins lecturing on Sidgwick's ethics, and if Bob in turn gains knowledge of Sidgwick's ethical views, then Bob's intrinsic desire for knowledge is thereby (*pro tanto*) satisfied. Even though Bob here has no antecedent desire for the state *his gaining knowledge of Sidgwick's ethical views*, the obtaining of this state does (*pro tanto*) satisfy an intrinsic desire that Bob antecedently has: namely, the intrinsic desire for knowledge.[27] And that is enough to fulfill the desire condition of the desire-perfectionism theory. In sum, the idea here is that, in order for any given state of affairs to count as an aspect of one's well-being, its obtaining must (at least *pro tanto*) fulfill an intrinsic desire that one has. This is, I believe, enough to secure the psychological fulfillment that is essential to well-being.

There are various objections that might be leveled against the desire-perfectionism theory. Though I will not address all of these objections, I will address some of them.

Objection 1

For its pro-attitude constraint, the desire-perfectionism theory appeals to the pro-attitude of intrinsic desire. But one might object to this. One might think, in particular, that it is better to appeal to enjoyment. Indeed, if we consider currently circulating subjective-objective hybrid theories of well-being, we will see that most of these theories do appeal to enjoyment for their pro-attitude constraint (e.g., Adams, 1999, pp. 93–101; Kagan, 2009). My primary reason for thinking that enjoyment is the wrong pro-attitude to invoke should be clear from the first section of this chapter: people often have experiences that enhance their well-being even though they involve no positive affect and thus no enjoyment (e.g., various working and parenting experiences fit this description). Admittedly, one might use the word "enjoyment" in an extended sense, whereby enjoyment need not involve positive affect. But why would one bother with this move? This is not how we use "enjoyment" in ordinary language. Granted, if we were unable to invoke desires, perhaps invoking enjoyment and then using "enjoyment" in an extended sense would be called for. But, of course, we can invoke desires.

Objection 2

For its objective value constraint, the desire-perfectionism theory appeals to perfectionist value. But anyone who is skeptical of perfectionist value will object to this appeal. The objection in question here could be specified in different ways. For instance, one might doubt that there is such a thing as human nature, and thus one might doubt that any given human can have a human nature that can be completed or fulfilled. Alternatively, one might accept that there is such a thing as human nature, but one might doubt that completing or fulfilling human nature could constitute a genuine form of value. This doubt could be filled out (a) by pointing to certain nasty human capacities such as selfishness and greed that seem to be central to human nature and then (b) by asking the question "Why should the exercise, development, or actualization of these central but nasty capacities be viewed as a genuine form of value?" Here is my response. If we adopt a nonevaluative conception of human nature, then, yes, nasty human capacities such as selfishness and greed seemingly must be deemed central to human nature. However, in appealing to perfectionist value, we can and should adopt a conception of human nature that is irreducibly evaluative. The idea here, then, is this. Ask the question "What capacities are central to human nature such that the exercise, development, or actualization of them constitutes the well-functioning of the human being as such?" Then answer by saying, "The capacities that should be singled out here are the capacity to deepen or to maintain friendships, the capacity to accomplish worthwhile tasks, the capacity to gain knowledge of oneself and the world in general, and so on." Thus we are led to the view that the basic goods (e.g., friendship, accomplishment, and knowledge) are perfectionist goods; that is, goods that are constitutive of the well-functioning of the human being as such. Of course, in my view, if one functions well as a human being, then that is not enough, on its own, for one's well-being to be advanced. Indeed, for one's well-being to be advanced, one's functioning well as a human being must positively grip one's own individual psychology, that is, by (at least *pro tanto*) satisfying an intrinsic desire that one has. One final point here: if one finds my appeal to perfectionist value too problematic to accept, one might still accept a welfare theory that is a hybrid of objective list theories and desire theories and that is very similar to the desire-perfectionism theory; the idea here is that, instead of conceiving of the basic goods as perfectionist goods, one might conceive of them as goods that are objective in a generic or unspecified manner.

Objection 3

In my view, the most important objection to the desire-perfectionism theory is the missing desires objection. This objection comes from objective list theorists, and it can be put as follows: "The desire-perfectionism theory implies that, if someone lacks the desire for friendship, or health, or accomplishment, etc., then this basic good is not a component of his or her well-being. But that is highly implausible. For, even if someone lacks the desire for friendship, or health, or accomplishment, etc., the fact remains that he or she lives a richer or fuller life—that is, a life higher in well-being—inasmuch as he or she engages in friendship, or attains health, or accomplishes something, etc."

Because I have dealt with this objection at length in previous work (Lauinger, 2012, pp. 84–120; Lauinger, 2013a), I will merely sketch the line of response to it that I favor. The first point to note is that, barring unusual cases such as those involving psychological disorders, people *just do* intrinsically desire the basic goods: friendship, health, accomplishment, and so on. Indeed, it seems that intrinsic desires for the basic goods are simply *built into* the vast majority of people. So, barring unusual cases, the missing desires objection does not arise or apply. With regard to unusual cases, some of these can be left aside because they are fanciful. Others, however, are nonfanciful (i.e., realistic) and therefore must be considered. What, for instance, can be said about cases involving psychological disorders? Do severely depressed humans really have intrinsic desires for accomplishment? And do those with eating disorders really have intrinsic desires for health? I think that, for some cases involving psychological disorders, a careful examination will reveal that, against the initial appearances, the humans in question really do intrinsically desire the basic good in question, in which case the missing desires objection does not arise or apply. For example, I think that, if we thoroughly examine cases of severe depression, then we will conclude that severely depressed people actually do want accomplishment (on this point, see Lauinger, 2012, pp. 94–98). There are, however, other cases involving psychological disorders where I admit that the humans in question lack desires for the basic good in question. For cases of this kind, I must deny that the basic good in question adds to the well-being of the humans in question. Though I am not completely comfortable making this denial, I believe that, in all cases where the humans in question lack desires for the basic good in question, there are actually good reasons to deny that the basic good in question adds to the well-being of the humans in question (e.g., see Lauinger, 2012, pp. 101–105, where I discuss extremely autistic individuals who seem to lack desires for the basic good of friendship).

Objection 4

Earlier I noted that the desire condition of the desire-perfectionism theory entails that, for any given state of affairs that instantiates a basic good for someone, it need not be true that he or she intrinsically desires this state in order for this state to count as an aspect of his or her welfare because it is enough if he or she simply intrinsically desires the basic good that this state instantiates for him or her. Pro-attitude theorists (e.g., desire theorists) and others might object that this kind of psychological fulfillment or connection to a person's pro-attitudes is not substantial enough. But think of the matter this way. It seems too strong to claim that, in order for any given state of affairs to count as an aspect of one's well-being, one must have a pro-attitude toward this state of affairs. There are, after all, plenty of things that intrinsically prudentially benefit us even though we have no pro-attitude toward them (say, because we do not even know about them). So it seems that we need to move to a different, less direct kind of connection between pro-attitudes and the states of affairs that are aspects of well-being. It is this line of thought that has led me to formulate the desire condition of the desire-perfectionism theory in the way that I have. One further point here: I think that, if a state of affairs that is an aspect of one's well-being is actually obtaining and one is consciously aware of its actually obtaining, then one inevitably will form (or else will already have) an intrinsic desire for it. Here we can return to the example involving Bob, who intrinsically desires knowledge but who does not have any antecedent intrinsic desire to know anything about Sidgwick's ethical views (say, because he has never even heard of Sidgwick). If the state of affairs *Bob's gaining knowledge of Sidgwick's ethical views* is actually obtaining, and Bob is consciously aware of its actually obtaining, then I think that it is inevitable that Bob will form an intrinsic desire for this state, where this intrinsic desire is something that flows out of Bob's intrinsic desire for the basic good of knowledge. Granted, it is logically possible for a human to have an intrinsic desire for a basic good and yet to lack an intrinsic desire for a state of affairs (a) that falls under this basic good, (b) that is actually obtaining, and (c) that this human is consciously aware of. Still, I believe that, in all nonfanciful cases, there inevitably will be an overflow of intrinsic desire (i.e., of noninstrumental motivational force) for the basic good in question to the state that falls under this basic good, provided that this state is actually obtaining and that the person in question is consciously aware of this state's actually obtaining. This seems to me to be a matter of psychological necessity for humans in our world (i.e., the actual world) and in metaphysically possible worlds that are close to ours (i.e., ones with the same laws of nature and substantially similar histories).

Objection 5

One might object that, if that we adopt the desire-perfectionism theory, then the task of measuring well-being will be too difficult. So let me here say something about how measurement might proceed on the desire-perfectionism theory. In measuring the amount of well-being contained in any object that is an aspect of one's well-being, we need to consider both (a) the amount of perfectionist value for oneself that this object contains and (b) the strength of one's intrinsic desire for this object (or, if one has no intrinsic desire for this object, we must consider the strength of one's intrinsic desire for the basic good that this object falls under). Or, more simply put, in measuring well-being, we must consider both the objective value factor and the desire factor. Let me take each of these factors in turn.

Regarding the objective value factor, we can do what objective list theorists might do when measuring well-being, except that we can stress that we are here measuring perfectionist value, not well-being. Thus we can use the same measurement procedures that I outlined when discussing measurement on objective list theories at the end of the section "Initial Comments on Objective List Theories," though, again, we would here be measuring perfectionist value, not well-being. The ultimate aim would be to arrive at a measurement for each human that at least somewhat accurately tells us how much perfectionist value he or she is deriving (a) in relation to each basic good and what falls under it for him or her and (b) in overall terms. As I indicated at the end of that section, there are difficulties that attach to measurement within objectivist parameters. Perhaps most notably, there is a question to ask about the weightings for the basic goods. Should we be taking all of the basic goods to be of equal worth (i.e., when measuring how much objective [i.e., perfectionist] value they contain for each human)? The desire-perfectionism theory could be worked out in different ways here, but my own preference here is to assume an equal weighting for each basic good because all of the basic goods (i.e., knowledge, accomplishment, friendship, health, aesthetic experience, and pleasure) seem to me to make equal contributions to the well-functioning of the human being as such.

Turning now to the desire factor, let me note four sets of points. (1) As I indicated earlier, desires matter in tie-breaking cases: if two objects that are aspects of one's well-being have an equal amount of perfectionist value for oneself, and if one has a stronger intrinsic desire for one of these objects, then the more strongly intrinsically desired object contains more welfare value for oneself than the less strongly intrinsically desired object. This tie-breaking point matters for the ordering of the basic goods in one's life. Since I think that all of the basic goods have an equal weighting in terms of the amount of perfectionist value that they contain for oneself, it follows that they will be prudentially ordered for oneself in accordance with the strengths of one's desires for each of them. Thus, if one more strongly intrinsically desires friendship than any other basic good, friendship will have more intrinsic prudential value for oneself than any other basic good. (2) I believe that there are various actual cases of the following sort: out of two states of affairs that are aspects of one's well-being, the first state contains (at least slightly) more perfectionist value for oneself than the second state, and yet the second state contains more welfare value for oneself than the first state, where this is so because one has a much stronger intrinsic desire for the second state than for the first state. (3) I am not sure, as of now, what to say about measurement in relation to the desire factor for cases where (a) one lacks an intrinsic desire for a state of affairs that is an aspect of one's well-being while (b) one has an intrinsic desire for the basic good that this state of affairs falls under for oneself. Obviously, in such cases, we must consider the strength of one's intrinsic desire for the basic good that this state of affairs falls under. But that is a very general claim, and it does not tell us much about how, exactly, to proceed in such cases. (4) Speaking generally, I have to admit that I do not, as of now, have a fully worked out view regarding measurement on the desire-perfectionism theory. While I am confident that human well-being is a function of, and only of, perfectionist value and intrinsic desire, I am not sure, as of now, about the exact proportions that are in play here for perfectionist value and intrinsic desire.

Conclusion

There are two different visions of what human beings are that I have privileged in constructing the desire-perfectionism theory. One vision is a broadly Aristotelian one according to which humans have various capacities that are central to their functioning well as to the kinds of things they are—that is, as human beings. This broadly Aristotelian vision captures something necessary for well-being, but it is, as it were, only half of the story. The other half of the story derives from a vision of human beings as unique individuals with different sets of intrinsic desires, and, importantly, this desire-focused vision of humans is itself informed by a Lacanian view according to which each human self is constituted by a particular and dynamic chains-of-signifiers-plus-desire-flow structure.[28] Whereas the broadly Aristotelian vision stresses our common human nature and the fact that, at some deep level, we are all the same and function well as humans in the same ways, the desire-focused vision stresses the fact that, at some deep level, we are all different and, in particular, have different sets of intrinsic desires. Hopefully this chapter has given us reason to believe that these two different visions can be combined into one coherent whole to produce a true and adequately informative account of human well-being.

Notes

1. I use "well-being," "welfare," and "prudential value" as synonyms.
2. Pro-attitudes are favorable attitudes.
3. Roger Crisp is a well-known proponent of one kind of mental state theory, namely, *welfare hedonism*: the view that well-being consists in, and only in, pleasure (2006, pp. 98–125). If one believes that well-being is necessarily experiential (i.e., such that nothing can prudentially benefit a person unless it enters into his or her experience), then one will be strongly inclined to accept welfare hedonism (on this point, see Bramble, 2016, p. 207). I do not believe that well-being is necessarily experiential. That said, I do believe that each human's well-being must be "strongly tied" to him or her. I have written about this matter in relation to objective list theories (Lauinger, 2013b), and what I say there can be adapted to the hybrid theory of well-being that I am defending in this chapter.
4. John Finnis (1980, pp. 59–99), Mark Murphy (2001, pp. 6–138), Martha Nussbaum (2000, pp. 70–86), Christopher Rice (2013), and Guy Fletcher (2013) are examples of philosophers who are objective list theorists. Also, some eudaimonic theories of well-being in psychology seem to be objective list theories (e.g., see Ryff & Singer, 2008), and some theories of well-being advanced by scholars working in the field of public health are objective list theories (e.g., see VanderWeele, 2017).
5. To my knowledge, Finnis is the only actual objective list theorist who says things that push in the direction of denying (c). Both his comments on pleasure being required for a full participation in a basic good (1980, p. 96) and his comments on subjectively ordering basic goods in one's life (1980, pp. 103–106) push in this direction. However, even in Finnis, I cannot find any clear denial of (c).

6. In psychology and everyday life the word "perfectionism" connotes unreasonable expectations of flawlessness for oneself or others. But in philosophy the word does not have these connotations.

7. Finnis (1998, p. 91) and Murphy (2001, pp. 76–80) are two examples of objective list theorists who accept that well-being (i.e., prudential value) and perfectionist value are metaphysically identical.

8. For some substantiation of this point, see Lauinger (2012, pp. 59–60).

9. In justifying any proposed list of basic goods, there are different methods that one might employ. For instance, following Tyler VanderWeele, one might emphasize that the items on one's proposed list (a) are generally viewed as ends (and so not as merely instrumental goods) and (b) are nearly universally desired by humans (2017, p. 8149). Or again, one might proceed (a) by sifting through the objects of one's own desires until one finds some general items that one judges always to be intrinsically good for oneself and then (b) by asking others, both within one's own culture and outside one's own culture, what they find when they sift through the objects of their own desires, all with the aim of arriving at a duly refined list of basic goods. Though I know that my proposed working list of basic goods is controversial, it seems to pass muster with respect to the two reasonable methods of justification that I have just mentioned (for more discussion of this matter, see Lauinger, 2012, pp. 59–70, 115–120). Also, I say "working" list because I am open to revising my proposed list.

10. These thoughts of mine on self-ratings, interviews with friends and family members, and interviews with experts are adapted from what others have said about life-satisfaction measurements (e.g., see Diener, Lucas, & Oishi, 2009, pp. 64–66).

11. For a discussion of experience sampling and the day reconstruction method, see Kahneman, Krueger, Schkade, Schwarz, and Stone (2004) and for comments concerning brain scanning or, more generally, physiological measures of well-being, see Kahneman and Riis (2005, pp. 298–300).

12. Some present-day objective list theorists hold not only that there is no objective ordering or hierarchy among the basic goods, but, indeed, that there is a thoroughgoing incommensurability among the basic goods and their instances, one that renders the task of measuring well-being largely irrelevant on objective list theories (e.g., Finnis, 1980, pp. 81–133; Murphy, 2001, pp. 182–187).

13. Other philosophers have stressed this point (e.g., Sumner, 1996, pp. 20–25).

14. This claim is sometimes referred to as the *thesis of internalism* about a person's good. For two well-known discussions of this thesis, see Railton (2003, p. 47) and Rosati (1996).

15. For more discussion of this last point, see Lauinger (2012, pp. 82–83).

16. The content of this paragraph is largely based on (a) my reading of Lacan (1992, pp. 311–325) and Bailly (2009) and (b) discussions I have had with Wilfried Ver Eecke.

17. "Metonymy" refers to associative connections among words and chains of words (e.g., if I am thinking of the college where I teach and then I think of my office, that is a metonymic move).

18. Denegation is, as Lionel Bailly notes, "saying the opposite of what you unconsciously mean" (2009, p. 59). Bailly elaborates: "But the experienced analyst knows instantly when she/he hears denegation ('*Of course, he's likeable enough*' nearly always means I don't like him)" (2009, p. 69).

19. Murphy says that inner peace is on the list of basic goods, where inner peace is the good of having no desires that one believes to be unsatisfied (2001, p. 123).

20. In saying "regardless of whether it connects at all to one's pro-attitudes," I am referring to pro-attitudes that are *external to* desire-fulfillment itself. Since desire-fulfillment contains the pro-attitude of desire inside itself, this clarification is worth making.

21. Granted, there might be a way out for objective list theorists here (e.g., they might say that the basic good in question is not desire fulfillment as such, but rather is something narrower, such as *harmless* desire fulfillment). Still, even if a way out exists here, convincingly articulating it would take some work.

22. These other responses do not conflict with (and so might be combined with) the response whereby objective list theorists claim that desire fulfillment is on the list of basic goods.

23. Christopher Woodard (2016, p. 163) has previously discussed criticisms of Fletcher's objective list theory that are similar to the two that I am noting here.

24. For a discussion of other kinds of hybrid theories of well-being (e.g., subjective-subjective hybrids, see Woodard, 2016, pp. 169–170).

25. I have previously used this label, "the desire-perfectionism theory" (Lauinger, 2012).

26. In this example, Bob does not desire to know about Sidgwick's ethical views because Bob has never heard of Sidgwick. But there are cases where people are aware of states of affairs that instantiate basic goods for them and yet where they lack desires for these states of affairs due to erroneous beliefs that they have. This, then, is another reason for formulating the desire condition of the desire-perfectionism theory in the way that I have (on this point, see Lauinger, 2012, p. 85, where I discuss a graduate student who falsely believes that her dissertation is a failure and who in turn has lost the desire to finish her dissertation, when in fact finishing her dissertation is an instance of accomplishment that is prudentially beneficial for her).

27. Here one might ask: "But why do you think that Bob intrinsically desires the basic good of knowledge? Why should we not think, instead, that Bob simply wants *certain kinds* of knowledge?" I believe that, in all cases involving normally functioning humans, people do want knowledge as such, friendship as such, and so on (on this point, see Lauinger, 2012, pp. 87–91).

28. In synthesizing Aristotelian and Lacanian ideas, I have been influenced by discussions with Wilfried Ver Eecke and by reading Alasdair MacIntyre (2004, pp. 1–38).

About the Author

William A. Lauinger is Associate Professor of Philosophy and Coordinator of the Ethics Program at Chestnut Hill College in Philadelphia, Pennsylvania. He is the author of *Well-Being and Theism: Linking Ethics to God* (Continuum, 2012) and various articles in ethics and the philosophy of religion. Most of his research focuses on human well-being: on what it is, on how to attain it, and on how it connects to other important phenomena, such as morality and religion.

Author Note

For helpful comments on this paper, thanks to the editors of this volume: Matthew Lee, Laura Kubzansky, and Tyler VanderWeele. And for helpful discussion, thanks to all participants at the Interdisciplinary Workshop on Happiness, Well-Being, and Measurement at Harvard University in April of 2018. This work was supported in part by a grant from the John Templeton Foundation and by the Lee Kum Sheung Center for Health and Happiness. The views expressed in this chapter represent the perspective of the author and do not reflect the opinions or endorsement of any organization. I have no known conflict of interest to disclose. Correspondence concerning this chapter should be directed to William A. Lauinger, Chestnut Hill College, 14 E Gravers Lane, Philadelphia, PA 19118 (lauingerw@chc.edu).

References

Adams, R. (1999). *Finite and infinite goods.* New York: Oxford University Press.
Bailly, L. (2009). *Lacan: A beginner's guide.* Oxford: Oneworld Publications.
Bramble, B. (2016). The role of pleasure in well-being. In G. Fletcher (Ed.), *The Routledge handbook of the philosophy of well-being* (pp. 199–208). New York: Routledge.
Crisp, R. (2006). *Reasons and the good.* Oxford: Clarendon.
Diener, E., Lucas R., & Oishi S. (2009). Subjective well-being: The science of happiness and life satisfaction. In S. Lopez & C. R. Snyder (Eds.), *The Oxford handbook of positive psychology* (pp. 63–73). New York: Oxford University Press.
Finnis, J. (1980). *Natural law and natural rights.* New York: Oxford University Press.
Finnis, J. (1998). *Aquinas.* New York: Oxford University Press.
Fletcher, G. (2013). A fresh start for the objective-list theory of well-being. *Utilitas, 25*(2), 206–220.
Griffin, J. (1986). *Well-being: Its meaning, measurement and moral importance.* Oxford: Clarendon.
Kagan, S. (2009). Well-being as enjoying the good. *Philosophical Perspectives, 23*(1), 253–272.
Kahneman, D., Krueger, A. B., Schkade, D. A., Schwarz, N., & Stone, A. A. (2004). A survey method for characterizing daily life experience: The day reconstruction method. *Science, 306*(5702), 1776–1780.

Kahneman, D., & Riis, J. (2005). Living, and thinking about it: Two perspective on life. In N. Baylis, F. A. Huppert, & B. Keverne (Eds.), *The science of well-being* (pp. 285–301). New York: Oxford University Press.

Lacan, J. (1992). *The seminar of Jacques Lacan, Book VII: The ethics of psychoanalysis, 1959–1960.* D. Porter (Trans.), J. A. Miller (Ed.). New York: W. W. Norton and Company.

Lauinger, W. (2012). *Well-Being and theism: Linking ethics to God.* New York: Continuum.

Lauinger, W. (2013a). The missing-desires objection to hybrid theories of well-being. *Southern Journal of Philosophy, 51*(2), 270–295.

Lauinger, W. (2013b). The strong-tie requirement and objective-list theories of well-being. *Ethical Theory and Moral Practice, 16*(5), 953–968.

MacIntyre, A. (2004). *The unconscious: A conceptual analysis* (revised ed.). New York: Routledge.

Murphy, M. (2001). *Natural law and practical rationality.* New York: Cambridge University Press.

Nussbaum, M. (2000). *Women and human development: The capabilities approach.* New York: Cambridge University Press.

Railton, P. (2003). *Facts, values, and norms.* New York: Cambridge University Press.

Rice, C. (2013). Defending the objective list theory of well-being. *Ratio, 26*(2), 196–211.

Rosati, C. (1996). Internalism and the good for a person. *Ethics, 106*(2), 297–326.

Ryff, C., & Singer, B. (2008). Know thyself and become what you are: A eudaimonic approach to psychological well-being. *Journal of Happiness Studies, 9,* 13–39.

Sumner, L. W. (1996). *Welfare, happiness, and ethics.* Oxford: Clarendon.

VanderWeele, T. (2017). On the promotion of human flourishing. *Proceedings of the National Academy of Sciences of the United States of America, 114,* 8148–8156.

Woodard, C. (2016). Hybrid theories. In G. Fletcher (Ed.), *The Routledge handbook of the philosophy of well-being* (pp. 161–174). New York: Routledge.

9

The Challenge of Measuring Well-Being as Philosophers Conceive of It

Anne Baril

Abstract

Many philosophers find the prospect of working with researchers in the social and behavioral sciences exciting, in part because they hope that these researchers might be able to measure well-being as the philosopher conceives of it. In this chapter, I consider how the measurement of well-being, as it is conceived of by philosophers, might feasibly be facilitated. I propose that existing scales can be employed to measure well-being as philosophers conceive of it. I support this conclusion through an in-depth discussion of an example. I explain how the scale of psychological well-being developed by Carol Ryff and validated in more than 750 empirical studies (Ryff, 2016, 2018) may be employed to measure the extent to which a person has realized an ostensible basic good. This discussion will be illustrative of the general method that may be employed to bring empirical researchers and philosophers into contact in a way that will facilitate the measurement of well-being as philosophers conceive of it.

Many philosophers find the prospect of working with researchers in the social and behavioral sciences exciting, in part because they hope that these researchers might be able to measure well-being as the philosopher conceives of it. Yet there are challenges of measuring well-being as philosophers conceive of it, challenges serious enough to make one wonder whether such hopes can be fulfilled. In this chapter, I review some of these challenges and consider whether the measurement of well-being as philosophers conceive of it might yet be facilitated. Dovetailing with recent work by Margolis, Schwitzgebel, Ozer, and Lyubomirsky (Chapter 13, in this volume), I propose

Anne Baril, *The Challenge of Measuring Well-Being as Philosophers Conceive of It* In: *Measuring Well-Being*. Edited by: Matthew T. Lee, Laura D. Kubzansky, and Tyler J. VanderWeele, Oxford University Press (2021). © Oxford University Press. DOI: 10.1093/oso/9780197512531.003.0010 that existing scales can be employed to measure well-being as philosophers conceive of it. I support this conclusion through an in-depth discussion of an example. I explain how the Psychological Well-Being Scale (PWBS) developed by Carol Ryff may be employed to measure well-being according to just one philosophical account of well-being (an "objective list theory" of well-being; see later discussion). This discussion will be illustrative of the general method that may be employed to bring measures of well-being developed by empirical researchers—those of psychologists as well as others in the social and behavioral sciences—into contact with philosophical conceptions of well-being in a way that will facilitate the measurement of well-being as philosophers conceive of it.

It is too much to expect that a psychological measure (or a set of such measures) will provide us with an *infallible test* for well-being as philosophers conceive of it.[1] The relevant question, I propose, when it comes to the measurement of well-being as philosophers conceive of it, is not whether a measure will provide us with an infallible test for well-being as philosophers conceive of it, but whether there is something meaningful to be gained by such measurement. I argue that there is.

The chapter proceeds as follows. First, I review some of the main philosophical approaches to well-being and some of the main challenges that arise when attempting to measure well-being as philosophers conceive of it. Through discussion of the example of the PWBS and an objective list theory of well-being, I will show how items from an existing scale may be used to measure the extent to which a person has realized an ostensible basic good. I'll then briefly indicate how this same method might be used in connection with other measures and other basic goods. Finally, I will review some limitations of the proposed method and argue that, despite these limitations, there is good reason to attempt to measure well-being as philosophers conceive of it.

Philosophical Approaches to Well-Being

Philosophers who research well-being are interested in what benefits us or harms us, in what makes our lives go better or worse. Of course, there are many things that benefit us, not all of which are especially interesting to philosophers. Brooms, for example, benefit us by helping us clean the floor; cars benefit us by helping us get where we want to go (or achieve status or express ourselves through quirky bumper stickers). Brooms and cars are examples of things that are frequently of *instrumental value*: they can *benefit us indirectly* in virtue of serving as means to achieving something else that benefits us, such as having clean floors or arriving at our desired destinations. The primary object of philosophical investigations of well-being, however, is not what is of merely instrumental value (nor what is merely indicative of, or correlative with, value), but what is of *final value*: that which *benefits us directly*; that which, in itself, makes us better off.[2] Brooms and cars are instrumentally valuable, but, intuitively, they are not finally valuable. We can see this by engaging in a simple thought experiment: we can ask ourselves whether we can imagine circumstances in which having a broom or a car *doesn't* benefit a person. It seems as though we can. We can, for example, imagine circumstances in which a person doesn't benefit from having a broom: circumstances in which she has another, better way to clean the floor, such as a vacuuming robot, for example, or circumstances in which she doesn't care whether the floor is clean (e.g., because her house is going to be demolished the following day). We can, it seems, imagine circumstances in which having a broom doesn't benefit a person in any way. This little thought experiment gives us evidence that it's not the broom, itself, that benefits a person, but these other things, such as having a clean floor—evidence, in other words, that the broom is only instrumentally valuable, not finally valuable, or valuable in itself: that it doesn't benefit us directly, only indirectly, via its connection to other goods.

Other things, by contrast, are finally valuable: good for us, just in themselves, even when they do not help us secure anything else.[3] Pleasurable experiences, for example, seem to make a person's life go better quite independently of any other effects they may have. Intuitively, the pleasure of basking in the sun or playing a favorite sport makes a person's life go better even if it doesn't help her achieve some further end, such as getting a suntan or lowering her blood pressure. If so, then pleasurable experiences are among what philosophers call *basic goods*: things that benefit us directly; things that are good for us, just in themselves.[4,5]

A central task of philosophers who investigate well-being is to establish what the basic goods are. Some philosophers are monists, arguing that there is just one basic good—that is, one general type of thing that directly benefits a person. *Experientialists*, for example, argue that it is experiences of some specified sort (e.g., pleasurable ones) that directly benefit a person (Feldman, 2004). *Preferentists*, on the other hand, argue that it is having one's preferences or desires satisfied (Brandt, 1979, pp. 126–129; Railton, 1986; Sidgwick, 1907).[6] Other philosophers are pluralists, arguing that there are a plurality of basic goods. *Objective list theorists*, for example, argue that there are a number of things that directly benefit a person.[7] Friendship, knowledge, happiness or pleasure, aesthetic experience, and achievement are a few of the items that frequently appear on pluralistic lists of basic goods (Finnis, 1980/ 2011; Fletcher, 2013; Hooker, 1998; Moore, 2000; Murphy, 2001; Rice, 2013). This tripartite division of theories of well-being is traditional, following Parfit (1984); there are also a number of theories that do not fit neatly into any of these categories, including value fulfillment theories (Raibley, 2010; Tiberius, 2018), hybrid theories (Kagan, 2009; Lauinger, Chapter 8, in this volume), and L. W. Sumner's account of well-being as authentic life satisfaction (Sumner, 1996; see later discussion). This short survey of philosophical accounts of well-being demonstrates the extent of disagreement that exists among philosophers about the essential nature of well-being.[8]

The Challenges of Measuring Well-Being as Philosophers Conceive of It

Philosophers strive to improve our understanding of the fundamental nature of well-being through philosophical reflection, including the use of thought experiments like the one discussed earlier. For the most part, philosophical research does not address questions that can be answered through empirical research—questions like: Who actually *is* well off? Are there things individuals can do to make their lives better? What public policies will best help individuals improve their lives? Yet the interest of most philosophers in well-being is not merely theoretical, but practical. Philosophers who investigate well-being often do so, in part, because we hope that by better understanding the fundamental nature of well-being, we will be better positioned to improve our lives and the lives of others. Many philosophers find the prospect of working with researchers in the social and behavioral sciences exciting, in part because they hope that these researchers, with their expertise at measuring well-being, might be able to measure well-being *as the philosopher conceives of it* and, ultimately, to tell us how we can make people's lives better (again, on the philosopher's conception of "better").

Yet measuring well-being as philosophers conceive of it proves challenging. For one thing, as we have seen, philosophers are interested in identifying the basic goods—the things that directly benefit a person—but there is disagreement among philosophers about what are the basic goods. Accordingly, there are a number of philosophical conceptions of well-being, and a measure of well-being on one philosophical conception cannot be expected to be a measure of well-being on another philosophical conception. For example: a measure comprising items concerning the quantity and quality of a person's positive experience may measure well-being as an experientialist conceives of it; its relationship to well-being as the preferentist or objective list theorist conceives of it will be less clear. Likewise for measures that would satisfy the preferentist or objective list theorist.

Furthermore, each of these general types of theory includes a number of individual theories. For example, historically there have been experientialists who have held that the prudential value of pleasure is a function not only of its intensity and duration but its "quality," while other experientialists have denied this (Bentham, 1789/1907; Mill, 1861/2001). Thus a measure of well-being as one experientialist conceives of it will not necessarily be a measure of well-being as another experientialist conceives of it. Given the diversity of philosophical positions, developing a measure that would satisfy the curiosity of all, or even a majority of, philosophers quickly becomes an unwieldy task. Any manageable measure of well-being can be expected to satisfy the curiosity of defenders of just one or at most a few of the many philosophical accounts of well-being. And since no single theory of well-being has garnered the support of more than a small percentage of the philosophers investigating well-being, it would be only a small percentage of philosophers whose curiosity is satisfied, no matter which theory it is.

Moreover, well-being as philosophers conceive of it is not something that can easily be measured. We may illustrate with just one type of philosophical account, a standard version of preferentism.[9] According to preferentists, what directly benefits a person are not mental states of the person, such as the state of *believing* that her desires are satisfied or the state of *taking pleasure in thinking* that they are satisfied; what directly benefits a person is for her desires to actually *be* satisfied; that is, for the state of affairs she desires to actually obtain, whether the person knows it or not.[10]

An example may help illuminate this point. Imagine a woman who has anonymously given up a child for adoption and now, many years later, desires that the child was placed with a loving family. According to preferentists, this woman is better off if this desire is satisfied—if the child was, as a matter of fact, placed with a loving family—even if the woman never learns that this is the case. In a case like this one, determining whether the desired state of affairs obtains through empirical investigation is at the very least infeasible; in other cases it will be impossible. Imagine, for example, that a person desires a relationship with a Higher Power. It may be possible to determine through empirical investigation whether the person *believes* she has a relationship with a Higher Power, but this is not what, according to preferentists, benefits her: what benefits her is for the state of affairs she desires to *actually* obtain— for her to *actually* have a relationship with a Higher Power. And this is not something that can be established through empirical investigation.[11]

Well-being, then, will be difficult to measure even as conceived by defenders of the simplest form of preferentism. And most philosophical accounts of well-being are far more complex, in ways that make well-being as it is conceived of by defenders of these theories still more difficult to measure. For example, we saw in the previous section that mental states such as desires or pleasurable experiences play an important role in well-being as many philosophers conceive of it. Many of these philosophers do not think that *every* mental state of the relevant sort (or, in the case of preferentists, its realizer[12]) benefits a person, only those that meet certain conditions. A common condition imposed is an epistemic one: it is often held that a mental state of the relevant sort (or its realizer) directly benefits a person only if it is one the person would have were she appropriately epistemically positioned—for example, if she were "fully informed, duly reflective, perfectly rational, free of prejudice and bias" (Kagan, 2009, p. 254) or if she "knew and vividly appreciated all of the non-evaluative facts" (Heathwood, 2015, p. 139). See also Brandt (1979, p. 126–129), Dorsey (2010), Griffin (1986, p. 11), Kauppinen (2012, pp. 366–368), Kraut (1994, p. 40), Raibley (2010, pp. 606–607), and Sumner (1996).

A thought experiment can help us understand why many philosophers believe some such condition exists. Consider a troubling instance of adaptive preferences in which a person has been subjected to abuse and has, over time, internalized the attitudes of her abusers, such that she now desires only to serve them. Intuitively, having *this* desire—the desire to serve her abusers— satisfied does not make this person better off. By restricting the desires, satisfaction of which directly benefit a person, to desires that meet some epistemic condition, preferentists are able to deny that having this kind of adaptive preference satisfied directly benefits a person.[13]

We can see that, in order to accurately measure an individual's well-being as such philosophers conceive of it, it would not be enough to measure the degree to which her desires were satisfied; it would also be necessary to evaluate what we might call the epistemic quality of these desires. This is just one example to illustrate the kinds of condition that some philosophers claim that mental states must meet in order to directly benefit a person, but it is illustrative of how philosophical accounts of well-being can be complex in ways that make well-being, as defenders of these theories conceive of it, difficult to measure. And since we must first measure well-being in order to answer other empirical questions about it, such as how we might promote it, overcoming these difficulties in measurement is a necessary step toward answering these other questions as well.[14]

There are, then, challenges that arise when we attempt to bring together empirical researchers, with their expertise measuring well-being, and philosophers, with their expertise reflecting on well-being. Philosophers can feel frustrated that what empirical researchers wind up measuring is not, in the end, well-being, because their measures can be insensitive to the distinctions that philosophers think are so important. Empirical researchers, in turn, may reason that developing a measure that is sensitive to these distinctions would be infeasible and that it is better to have a measure of well-being we can actually implement, even if in certain cases—such as the case of someone whose well-being is improved by unknowingly having a desire satisfied—the measure will not be perfectly accurate.

A Method for Measuring Well-Being as Philosophers Conceive of It: An Illustration

In light of these challenges, some may conclude that attempts to measure well-being as philosophers conceive of it should be abandoned. However, in light of how much there is to be gained from philosophers and researchers in the social and behavioral sciences working together to measure well-being as philosophers conceive of it, it's well worth proceeding with such attempts so long as we do so with sensitivity to the preceding challenges. This means, first, making every effort to develop a measure that is sensitive to the nuances of the philosophical conception, and, second, in the event that one's measure is less than perfectly accurate, being transparent about the ways in which it falls short. Such transparency is important not only for the sake of honesty, but to help pave the way for future efforts to measure well-being as the philosopher conceives of it more accurately.

This chapter represents one philosopher's attempt to say, a little more clearly, what it would look like to measure well-being as philosophers conceive of it in a way that is sensitive to the preceding challenges. I'll begin with an illustration: I will show how one might use just one existing psychological scale—the PWBS—to measure well-being according to just one philosophical account of well-being—objective list theory. In this section, I focus on making the positive case in support of the conclusion that existing scales may be adapted to measure well-being as it is conceived of by philosophers; then I will consider the particular challenges that confront attempts to measure well-being on this philosophical conception.

Friendship

As noted earlier, objective list theorists are pluralists, often including friendship, knowledge, happiness or pleasure, aesthetic experience, and achievement among the things that directly benefit a person. For the sake of illustration, I will isolate just one item on the list—just one (ostensible) basic good—and explain how the PWBS could be adapted to measure the extent to which a person has realized it in her life.

Consider a kind of deep, rich personal relationship that it is plausible to think is an important part of what makes our lives go well.[15] Philosophers who count some such relationship among the basic goods typically call it "friendship." Here I will offer a characterization of friendship that includes many of the features that philosophers have proposed are characteristic of it (Helm, 2013) and then consider the extent to which the PWBS can serve as an instrument for measuring the extent to which a person has realized friendship on this philosophical conception.

For simplicity, I will refer to friendship on this philosophical conception simply as "friendship." Of course, there are many kinds of relationships we casually call friendships, not all of which are plausible candidates for a basic good. I don't wish to engage in a dispute about whether the kind of relationship I will describe here merits the term "friendship" more than any of these other relationships. The aim here is to give an account of the kind of deep, rich personal relationship that is the best candidate for being a basic good. The term "friendship" is merely a convenient label. As an initial characterization, we may say that friendship is

A distinctively personal relationship that is grounded in a concern on the part of each friend for the welfare of the other, for the other's sake, and that involves some degree of intimacy (Helm, 2013, n.p.).

There are many kinds of personal relationships that can be friendships in the present sense, including familial relationships, romantic relationships and even some working relationships, such as relationships involving extended, intimate collaboration on a creative or research project. Friendships are characterized in large part by deep-seated dispositions of the friends. Friends are disposed to care about each other for their own sakes. They are disposed to consider one another's feelings: to take joy in their successes, share in their disappointments, and so on. Friends are disposed to act on their friends' behalf—to promote their welfare, to support them in their pursuit of their aims, and so on, not for any ulterior motive, but just for the friend's own sake. Friends love each other for who they are, esteem each other for their merits (Stroud, 2006). A friend is committed to reminding her friend "of what's really valuable in life and to foster within her a commitment to these values so as to prevent her from going astray" (Helm, 2013, n.p.; Whiting, 1991). Friends trust one another in a way that makes true intimacy possible, sharing thoughts or experiences they wouldn't share with other more casual acquaintances. Friends take each other seriously, in such a way that their values, interests, reasons, and so on provide one another with *pro tanto* reasons to value and think similarly. Moreover, the relationship is *dynamic*— friends mutually influence each other's sense of value in a way that supports intimacy (Friedman, 1989; Helm, 2013). Friends have a sense of solidarity premised on the sharing of values and a sense of what is important. They feel empathy toward one another, even to the point of sharing in one another's pride and shame (Helm, 2013; Sherman, 1987; Taylor, 1985). Finally, and perhaps most simply, friends spend time together, not only in the sense that they are in one another's presence, but in the sense that they partake in shared activities in an engaged way.[16]

The PWBS

The PWBS is a prominent multidimensional measure of psychological well-being that has been especially influential in elucidating the eudaimonic aspects of this larger construct (Ryff, 1989, see also Ryff et al., Chapter 4, in this volume). At a time when empirical research concerned with well-being focused mainly on reports of happiness, and life satisfaction, the PWBS was developed to probe what it is to be "self-actualized, individuated, fully functioning or optimally developed" (Ryff, 2013, pp. 11–12). The scale distinguishes six key dimensions of what has since been called "eudaimonic" well-being: autonomy, environmental mastery, personal growth, positive relations with others, purpose in life, and self-acceptance. I refer the reader to the chapter by Ryff et al. (Chapter 4, in this volume), and in particular to Box 4.2, "Definitions of Theory-Guided Dimensions of Eudaimonic Well-Being," which gives, for each factor, a description of a high and low scorer and a sample item of measurement.

Friendship and the PWBS

How does friendship, so understood, relate to the PWBS? Can the PWBS serve as a measure of the extent to which a person has realized friendship in her life—as "a measure of friendship"?

When considering the prospects for the PWBS as a measure of friendship, a natural place to begin is with the positive relations with others (PR) factor. Many of the items of measurement that are part of the PR factor seem to correspond, in the relevant way, to friendship (where, to remind the reader, by "friendship" I mean friendship *on the preceding philosophical conception*). For example, consider the following items (from Ryff's 54-item scale, see Ryff (1989), Ryff and Keyes (1995), and Ryff, Boylan, and Kirsch (Chapter 4, in this volume); unless otherwise noted, all items of measurement that I discuss are from this scale):

PR7. People would describe me as a giving person, willing to share my time with others.
PR1. Most people see me as loving and affectionate.
PR9. I know that I can trust my friends, and they know that they can trust me.

Based on the preceding account of friendship, we can say that a friend is one who is willing to spend time with her friend, who is empathetic, and who cares about her friend for her own sake. We can expect this kind of person to be described by others (at least her friends) as "a giving person, willing to share her time with others." Friends love and care for one another; thus they will be—and will be seen as—loving and affectionate (at least, in their capacity *as* friends—a point to which I shall return later). Finally, friends trust one another. Thus we can expect friends to score highly on PR7, PR1, and PR9. (Some readers may have concerns here, e.g., about the limitations of self-reported measures, but—to remind the reader—I am deferring a discussion of limitations to the approach I am outlining here until later in the chapter.)

PR1, PR7, and PR9 relate relatively directly to some of the features of friendship. There are also others that relate less directly. Consider, for example,

PR4. I enjoy personal and mutual conversations with family members or friends.

Based on the preceding account of friendship, friends spend time together, "partake in shared activities in an engaged way." Presumably this includes having conversations. Moreover, since friends esteem one another for their merits and are disposed to share in one another's joys and disappointments, the parties to these conversations will not ignore what the other person says or engage in self-indulgent monologues. Rather, conversations among friends will be characterized by active and empathetic listening; the mutual sharing of thoughts, feelings, experiences; and so on. Thus we can expect friends to score highly on PR4.

Some features of friendship, so understood, are apparently not captured by the items in the PR factor, either individually or taken together. Take, for example, the way friends are committed to reminding one another of what's valuable and to help keep each other from going astray. Friends are willing to challenge one another and, in turn, are receptive to each other's challenges. This element of mutual challenge does not seem to be captured by the items of that are part of the PR factor.

The element of mutual challenge characteristic of friendship may, however, be captured when we broaden our scope to include other factors on the PWBS. Consider, for example, the following items that are part of the autonomy (A) factor:

A1. I am not afraid to voice my opinions, even when they are in opposition to the opinions of most people.

A7. It's difficult for me to voice my own opinions on controversial matters. (rs)
A9. I judge myself by what I think is important, not by the values of what
     others think is important.

A person who scores highly on this factor will presumably be the kind of person who will, in conversation, be willing to speak up and challenge her friend when she seems to be straying from her value commitments.

Being the kind of person who is able to challenge friends when appropriate is just one side of mutual challenge. The other is being the kind of person who will, in conversation, be open to a friend's suggestion that there is room for her to improve. This may be at least partially captured by items such as the following, from the Personal Growth (PG) factor:

PG6. I do not enjoy being in new situations that require me to change my old
     familiar ways of doing things. (rs)
PG7. For me, life has been a continuous process of learning, changing, and
     growth.
PG8. I gave up trying to make big improvements or changes in my life a long
     time ago. (rs)

The upshot, I propose, is that when a person scores highly on the A and PG factors, *in conjunction with* the preceding personal relations factors, it is reasonable to expect that her friendships *are* ones that have the element of mutual challenge that is a part of friendship.

Friendship, on the preceding conception, is—like many ostensible basic goods—a complex entity that is difficult to measure. Given its complexity, no single item taken alone can measure it. Yet the present discussion provides an illustration of the way in which items of measurement, even items from different factors, can, in conjunction, form a system that can provide a measure of, if not all, at least many of the features of friendship.

A Method for Measuring Well-Being as Philosophers Conceive of It: Further Examples

In the previous section, I gave an extended illustration to show how items from an existing scale may, in conjunction, provide a measure of the extent to which a person has realized an ostensible basic good. Here I will give a couple more examples to illustrate the proposed method involving other philosophical accounts of well-being and other measures before turning to a discussion of some of the limitations of the proposed method.

Other Philosophical Accounts of Well-Being

The extended example of the previous section shows how it is possible for items of measurement to be constructed into a web that can serve as a measure of a basic good. While only one such good—friendship—was discussed, the same general formula may be followed, *mutatis mutandis*, to measure other basic goods.

For example, one of the items frequently included on objective list theorists' lists of basic goods is rational agency (though they do not always use this term; e.g., Finnis [1980] includes "practical reasonableness," Griffin [1986] includes "components of human agency," Murphy [2001] includes "excellence in agency," and Parfit [1984] includes "rational activity"). Philosophers give different accounts of what exactly rational agency consists in, but items such as the following, from the environmental mastery (EM) and purpose in life (PL) factors of the PWBS, are promising as partial measures of the extent to which a person has realized the basic good of rational agency:

EM4. I am quite good at managing the many responsibilities of my daily life.
EM6. I generally do a good job of taking care of my personal finances and affairs.
EM8. I have difficulty arranging my life in a way that is satisfying to me. (rs)
PL4. I don't have a good sense of what it is that I am trying to accomplish in my life. (rs)
PL6. I enjoy making plans for the future and working to make them a reality.

As another example, consider L. W. Sumner's theory of well-being, according to which well-being is identified with "authentic life satisfaction" (Sumner, 1996). Life-satisfaction, according to Sumner, has both a cognitive aspect and an affective aspect: the person who is satisfied with her life both has a positive evaluation of the conditions of her life (e.g., judges that it is a good one) and experiences her life in a certain way (e.g., as enriching, rewarding, satisfying, fulfilling). However, intuitively, merely being satisfied with one's life does not make one well off. (Recall the troubling case of adaptive preferences discussed earlier.) Thus Sumner imposes conditions that an individual's satisfaction with her life must meet if it is to represent a genuine benefit to her. One such condition is an autonomy condition: the person's values (at least insofar as they bear on her satisfaction with her life) must be "in some important sense, *her own*" (Sumner, 1996, p. 167). If a person's satisfaction with her life is based on values that she doesn't endorse, or if they were formed by a process that undermined her capacity to critically assess her own values, then, even if she is satisfied with her life, she is not—on Sumner's view—well-off.

A review of the details of Sumner's account is outside the scope of this chapter, but the following items, from the EM and the self-acceptance (SA) factors of the PWBS, appear indicative of the cognitive aspect of life-satisfaction, on Sumner's view.

EM9. I have been able to build a home and a lifestyle for myself that is much to my liking.
EM8. I have difficulty arranging my life in a way that is satisfying to me. (rs)
SA1. When I look at the story of my life, I am pleased with how things have turned out.
SA5. I made some mistakes in the past, but I feel that all in all everything has worked out for the best.
SA8. The past had its ups and downs, but in general, I wouldn't want to change it.

Regarding the autonomy condition on an individual's satisfaction with her life, there are two aspects of autonomy worth mentioning in connection with the measurement of authentic life-satisfaction using items from the PWBS. First, if a person is highly susceptible to social pressures, this can inhibit the formation of values that are truly her own (Sumner, 1996, pp. 168–171). Items like the following, from the A factor of the EBWS, can measure a person's susceptibility to social pressures:

A3. I tend to worry about what other people think of me. (rs)
A6. I have confidence in my opinions, even if they are contrary to the general consensus.

Second, if a person's range of experience is highly curtailed, this can potentially undermine a person's autonomy, in Sumner's sense. If a person has a very limited set of experiences, she will be unlikely to develop the perspective needed to engage in the critical assessment of her values that is necessary if these values are to be truly her own (Sumner, 1996, p. 170). Items like the following, from the PG factor of the EBWS, can measure the degree to which a person is open to having new experiences and enjoys being in novel situations and thus may give an indication of whether she has had the kind of experience in virtue of which she is well-positioned to critically assess her values:

PG1. I am not interested in activities that will expand my horizons. (rs)
PG3. I think it is important to have new experiences that challenge how you think about yourself and the world.
PG6. I do not enjoy being in new situations that require me to change my old familiar ways of doing things. (rs)

The preceding items from the A and PG factors may, then, give an indication of whether a person is autonomous, in Sumner's sense, and thus an indication of whether her satisfaction with her life is authentic. In conjunction with the items measuring a person's satisfaction with life, they can serve as the basis of a measure of the extent to which a person is authentically satisfied with her life. For example: if a person expresses high satisfaction with her life but has a low score on the preceding items from the A and PG factors, we might have reason to doubt she is autonomous, in Sumner's sense; we would then have less reason to think that her satisfaction with her life is authentic and, accordingly, less reason to think that she is well-off, in Sumner's sense, than if she were to score highly on the A and PG factors.

Other Measures

I have illustrated how one might measure well-being as philosophers conceive of it with items from the PWBS, but one might use items from other scales, or even multiple scales in conjunction. For example, the following items from the Satisfaction with Life Scale (Deiner, Emmons, Larsen, & Griffin, 1985) may serve as a measure of life-satisfaction on Sumner's view:

"In most ways my life is close to my ideal."
"I am satisfied with my life."

And the following items from the UCLA Loneliness Scale (Russell, Peplau, & Cutrona, 1980) may be used to measure the extent to which a person has realized (or failed to realize) friendship, in the preceding sense:

> "I have nobody to talk to."
> "I feel as if nobody really understands me."
> "My social relationships are superficial."

These items may be used to measure life-satisfaction and friendship, respectively, either on their own or, conceivably, in combination with items from the PWBS or other scales.

The items that can help us measure well-being as philosophers conceive of it needn't come from measures of well-being or qualitative aspects of life; they can also come from other kinds of measures. Consider the way in which the A and PG factors were used to indicate whether a person is the kind of person to bring an element of challenge to her friendships and to indicate whether a person's life satisfaction is authentic. It may be that there are items from other kinds of measures that can play this role as well. For example, it may be that items from the openness factor of the Five Factor Model of Personality are indicative of the degree to which a person is open to having the kind of aesthetic experiences that, according to some objective list theorists, directly benefit a person (McCrae & Costa, 1987).

These examples are suggestive of the possibilities that exist for adapting existing scales to measure well-being as it is conceived of by philosophers.

Limitations of the Proposed Method

Up to this point I have emphasized the positive case to be made in support of the conclusion that existing scales could be adapted to measure well-being as philosophers conceive of it. Now I will mention a few of the limitations of the proposed method, illustrating with the example discussed (of the PWBS and friendship) before turning to a consideration of the prospects for measuring well-being as philosophers conceive of it.

Items of Measurement Only Evidence the Realization of Basic Goods When They Logically Relate to It in the Right Way

I have argued we could expect friends to score highly on PR7, PR9, PR1, and PR4: that is, *if* a person has realized friendship in her life, *then* we can expect her to score highly on these items. But this doesn't imply that *if* a person scores highly on these items we *then* can expect her to have realized friendship. To illustrate, consider PR7: "People would describe me as a giving person, willing to share my time with others." I argued earlier that if someone is a friend, then we could expect her to score highly on PR7 because, given the above characterization of friendship, one cannot be a friend (on that characterization) without, in at least some contexts, being a giving person, willing to share her time with others.[17] However, the (loose) implication does not work the other way around: one could score highly on PR7 *without* being engaged in friendships. This is because there are many ways of "being a giving person, willing to share our time with others" other than through close personal relationships; one could, for example, share one's time with others by volunteering in ways that don't bring one into personal contact with others, such as collecting litter from a community park or sewing colorful pillowcases to brighten children's hospital rooms.

The upshot is that scoring highly on PR7 should not, in itself, be regarded as evidence of friendship; rather it must be treated as part of a body that, taken together, evidences friendship. For example, there are items on the PWBS that mention personal relationships explicitly. PR2, for example, elicits a response about whether the respondent has close friends with whom to share her concerns. Scoring highly on these items, then, *does* imply that an individual has close personal relationships. When an individual scores highly on these items, we can infer that she does have close personal relationships; when she also scores highly on PR7, we can posit the assumption that she exercises her willingness to share her time with others not only in impersonal ways, but also in the context of these personal relationships and thus that these relationships have at least this one feature characteristic of friendships. (Even this, of course, would only give us evidence that the individual's personal relationships have this one feature of friendship; we would need other measures to determine whether they have the other features characteristic of friendship.)

A *low* score on PR7, by contrast, *may* apparently be regarded as evidence of a lack of friendship: if a person is *not* the kind of person who is willing to share her time with others, this would seem to pretty directly evidence the conclusion that she does not have friendships, in the above sense. (Again, I am assuming the accuracy of self-reports; I'll return to this issue momentarily.)

The general point is that even when we see a link between an item of measurement and an ostensible basic good, we must be clear about what kind of link it is. It will not always be the case that a high score on some item of measurement, taken in isolation, gives us evidence—even *prima facie* evidence—concerning the extent to which the respondent has realized a basic good. Individual items will provide such evidence only when they are logically related to the realization of a basic good in the proper way.

The Limitations of Self-Reported Measures

A feature of many measures of well-being, including the PWBS, that many philosophers will be inclined to see as a serious limitation is the fact that the data generated by such measures are self-report data. Psychologists have developed various strategies for counteracting a number of the biases and limitations to which self-reports can be subject (Crowne & Marlowe, 1960; Hart, Ritchie, Hepper, & Gebauer, 2015; Strahan & Gerbasi, 1972; Wojcik, Hovasapian, Graham, Motyl, & Ditto, 2015), but there is a feature inherent to self-reported measures that will be of concern to philosophers: the fact that, even in the best-case scenario, the data generated by self-reported measures are data about the subject's good-faith representations of states of affairs rather than the states of affairs themselves. Consider, for example, PR7: "People would describe me as a giving person, willing to share my time with others." To score highly on this item, the individual must "strongly agree" with this statement. When she does, the information gleaned from this item is not, strictly speaking, information that the subject *is* "a giving person, willing to share her time with others" or even that people *would in fact* describe her in this way; at best, the information gleaned is that the subject *sincerely believes* that people would describe her in this way. But she could of course be wrong. Indeed, it would seem that any given person in the normal course of events actually has very little evidence about how others would describe her and so, even setting aside the possibility of bias, could quite *easily* be wrong. And a person's *wrongly* believing that people would describe her as "a giving person, willing to share her time with others" is not evidence that she enjoys positive relations with others.

Philosophical Accounts of Well-Being Are Often Fine-Grained in Ways It Would Be Difficult for a Measure to Capture

Finally, as discussed, many philosophical accounts of well-being have nuances that make well-being according to these accounts difficult to measure. Considering objective list theory in relation to the PWBS gives us the opportunity to make this point more concretely. I'll mention two kinds of nuances that raise difficulties for the measurement of friendship.

First, there are nuances of the account of friendship itself: of what, specifically, friendship involves. The preceding characterization of friendship included many features of friendship, but it was only a sketch. Even if two philosophers agree that among the basic goods are personal relationships perfectly fitting that description, there is plenty about which they may yet disagree. For example: according to the preceding characterization of friendship, friends trust one another. But we have not yet said what, more specifically, this trust involves. Does trust among friends extend to helping one another commit immoral acts (Cocking & Kennett, 2000)? Does it require believing the best about one's friend even against the evidence—that she couldn't possibly be guilty of a crime, for example, even if all the evidence points in that direction (Keller, 2004; Stroud, 2006)? These may be details, but they are details that make up a full-blooded philosophical account of the kind of trust that is part of friendship. Without some such details, the claim that friends "trust" one another lacks meaningful content. The PWBS doesn't probe for those details. Indeed, it's hard to see how a measure *could* probe for such details and stay manageable. But, unless it does, we will be limited in how far we can establish whether the individual's relationships *are* characterized by trust and, to that extent, limited in how far we can establish whether the individual has realized friendship.

Second, there are nuances of the account of how friendship contributes to well-being. Any theory of well-being, if it is to be complete, must give an account not only of what the basic goods are, but how these goods contribute to well-being. A hedonist about well-being, for example, must give an account of whether each and every pleasure contributes equally to well-being or if the way in which pleasure contributes to well-being is—to put it one way—subject to a law of diminishing returns, such that the more pleasure one already has, the less any additional instance of pleasure contributes to one's well-being. Likewise for friendship. One might hold that no matter how many friendships a person already has, more friendship always makes her better off. (Call this the maximizing view.) But this is somewhat counterintuitive. Intuitively, even if it benefits a person to have friends, it doesn't follow that it always benefits her to have *more* friends. There may, for example, be a threshold beyond which more friendships don't benefit a person any further. (Call this the threshold view.) Some of the items on the PWBS are worded in such a way that they appear to measure friendship on the maximizing view, rather than the threshold view. For example, PR5 asks about how *many* people the respondent has to listen when she needs to talk.[18] Likewise, PR6 asks whether it seems to the respondent that other people have *more* friends than she does.[19] If what directly benefits a person is having high-quality friendships—even if only a few—then items like PR5 and PR6 will give a false negative, counting respondents as not realizing the basic good of friendship simply because they only have a modest number of friends.

The Prospects for Measuring Well-Being as Philosophers Conceive of It: Conclusion

I have proposed that there are ways in which existing scales might be adapted to measure ostensible basic goods; alternatively, one might develop entirely new scales, tailored to measure well-being on some philosophical conception (see Chapter 8, in this volume, p. 234), or one might do both (see Chapter 13, in this volume). Whether one adapts existing scales to this purpose or develops an entirely new scale, there are a number of challenges to which one must be sensitive. Given that there are in fact a number of philosophical conceptions of well-being and that we cannot expect a measure of well-being on one conception to serve as a measure of well-being on another, I have proposed that ostensible basic goods must be treated individually. The discussion of the preceding examples has shown how this might be done; however, the discussion of the limitations of the proposed method in the previous section suggests that optimism should be tempered. Of all extant scales, the PWBS seems most well-suited to the purpose of measuring friendship; even so, the items on the PWBS do not provide a measure of friendship, as the philosopher conceives of it, that will enable us to identify, with perfect accuracy, who among respondents has realized the basic good of friendship and who has not. The nuances of the philosophical account of friendship and of how it contributes to well-being are difficult to capture with extant items of measurement; the connections between the individual items of measurement and the actual presence of friendship in a person's life are often indirect; and, given the nature of self-reported measures, the data gathered through these items will be, at best, data about the respondent's good-faith representations of states of affairs rather than the states of affairs themselves. And this is not to mention that friendship, according to pluralistic objective list theorists, is just one *element* of well-being; even if we could establish that a person has realized the basic good of friendship, we will only have part of the answer to the question of whether she has realized *well-being*. These are some of the challenges that arise for the measurement of friendship. They may not be exactly the same set of challenges we encounter when we attempt to measure well-being as it is conceived of by other philosophers, but they are indicative of the kind of limitations we may expect to encounter when we engage in such attempts.

In light of these limitations, what conclusions we should draw about the prospects for measuring well-being as philosophers conceive of it?

Let us grant that it will not be possible to develop, for every philosophical account of well-being (what we may call) a perfectly accurate measure: a measure that will identify, with perfect accuracy, subjects' levels of well-being on some philosophical conception. Let us grant, in other words, that for many philosophical accounts of well-being there will inevitably be a cleavage, even a systematic cleavage, between the measure and that which it purports to measure (as illustrated in the example of measuring well-being as it is conceived of by preferentists using self-reported measures—see Note 11). Philosophers who typically conduct their research from the armchair may be inclined to regard any systematic cleavage between a measure and that which it purports to measure as a failure, but this would be a mistake. There is often something to be learned from a measure, even when it is less than perfectly accurate. Return to the example of using self-reporting measures to measure well-being as conceived by preferentists (Note 11). I have noted how such a measure cannot be trusted to give a perfectly accurate measure of each individual's level of well-being, since (for example) a given individual's ignorance or false beliefs can result in a score that is higher or lower than her actual levels of well-being, on this account. It is nevertheless possible, however, that with a large enough sample, we will get meaningful data—data that will help us see a pattern, for example. Philosophers should keep in mind that there are many different kinds of things to be learned from such measures, not all of which are undermined by a cleavage—even a systematic cleavage—between a measure and that which it purports to measure. Evaluating a measure is not something that is properly done, unilaterally, by the philosopher from the armchair; psychologists have well-established methods of evaluating the quality of psychological measures. A degree of interdisciplinary deference is in order in regards to which ways of a measure's falling short of perfection are troubling and which are within an acceptable margin of error.[20,21]

This is one reason why it would be a mistake for philosophers to give up on attempts to measure well-being on philosophical conceptions on the grounds that there will be a cleavage between a measure and that which it purports to measure. There is another, more pragmatic, reason as well: if philosophers are unwilling to accept a degree of such cleavage, it is unlikely that they will be invited to participate in the further development of measures of well-being. Philosophers can learn a lot from such participation even if, at present, the measures of well-being fall short of their hopes for measuring well-being as they conceive of it. Moreover, if philosophers bow out of the discussion now, they forego opportunities to shape the empirical measurement of well-being in ways that make measures more sensitive to the nuances of philosophical accounts of well-being—something in which, as I have said, many philosophers have a vested interest. Consider again the example of using self-reporting measures to measure well-being as conceived by preferentists. It may be impossible to accurately measure each individual's level of well-being, on this conception. (Recall the example of the individual who desires a relationship with a Higher Power.) Yet there are ways of designing measures that can measure a given individual's level of well-being on this conception *more* accurately. The subject's self-reports could, for example, be supplemented with the reports of others (e.g., reports about whether the subject's desires are satisfied or about how trustworthy the subject is concerning whether her desires are satisfied) or with direct measures confirming whether the state of affairs the subject desires really does obtain (e.g., measures that confirm whether the subject who desires to have children, or live in a safe neighborhood, does indeed have children or live in a safe neighborhood, see also Chapter 8, especially pp. 235–236, and Chapter 13, especially p. 401, both in this volume). In some cases, an item of measurement could be made more sensitive to the nuances of some philosophical account of well-being through some simple adjustments in wording. (For example, an item like PR7 could be made into a more accurate measure of friendship by replacing "people" with "my friends.") By participating in research measuring well-being on philosophical conceptions, even when the measure is not as accurate as a philosopher might wish, the philosopher helps create opportunities for philosophers—herself or others who come after—to help shape measures in a way that will make them more sensitive to the nuances of philosophical conceptions of well-being—and, to the extent that these nuances in conceptions of well-being track genuine nuances in well-being, an opportunity to help advance research on what makes our lives go better or worse.

There is much to be gained when researchers from the humanities and the social and behavioral sciences engage in meaningful collaboration with the mutual aim of understanding and measuring well-being. By considering how existing psychological scales may be adapted to measure well-being as philosophers conceive of it and discussing the challenges that confront such attempts—as well as attempts to create new measures designed with philosophical conceptions of well-being in mind—I hope to have helped facilitate such collaboration.

Notes

1. Indeed, psychological measures, like scientific measures generally, do not generally give an *infallible* test for that which they measure. Consider a thermometer: it is easy to imagine a situation in which a thermometer reads 60° when the temperature is not, in fact, 60°. Likewise for psychological measures: it is easy to imagine situations in which an individual's score according to some measure of well-being does not represent her actual level of well-being.

2. By "instrumental value" and "final value," then, I mean what philosophers would call "instrumental prudential value" and "final prudential value (Kauppinen, 2012); likewise, *mutatis mutandis*, for "instrumentally valuable" and "finally valuable."

3. Indeed, if nothing were finally valuable, it would be puzzling how things could be instrumentally valuable: there must, it seems, be something of value to which the item in question relates in virtue of which it is instrumentally valuable (Aristotle, 2000, book I, chapter 2).

4. This way of using the term "basic goods" differs from the way it is used in certain global policy contexts in which the term "basic goods" is sometimes used to refer to goods and services such as clean water, housing, and electricity. These things are unlikely

candidates for "basic goods" in the present terminology. (For example, having electricity is not good in itself; it's good in virtue of the quality of life it facilitates.)

5. Not all philosophers would use the *term* "basic good" to refer to that which directly benefits a person; it is commonly associated with objective list theories. For simplicity's sake, I will use the term to refer to any (ostensible) direct contributor to well-being, such as having one's desires satisfied on certain preferentist accounts.

6. Note that what directly benefits a person, according to preferentism, is not being or feeling satisfied, but having her preferences or desires satisfied (or "fulfilled" as it is sometimes put—see Chapter 13, in this volume); that is, for the state of affairs the person desires or prefers to obtain. I will return to this point later.

7. By "objective list theorists" I will mean *pluralistic* objective list theorists and thus contrast (pluralistic) objective list theory with monistic experientialist theories such as hedonism. This way of organizing philosophical theories of well-being is traditional, following Parfit (1984), but cf. Fletcher (2013).

8. This categorization of philosophical accounts of well-being is similar to that offered by Margolis et al. (Chapter 13, in this volume). Note that I will understand "objective list theorists" as including defenders of what Margolis et al. call "eudaimonic" theories, as well as "non-eudaimonic objective-list" theories; indeed, since items like wealth and beauty are virtually never regarded as basic goods by full-fledged philosophical accounts of well-being, it is so-called eudaimonic theories that will be the paradigm examples of objective list theories in the present terminology.

9. To simplify, I'll hereafter restrict my discussion of preferentism to a version of preferentism according to which what directly benefits a person is the satisfaction of her desires; what I say of this view will also be true, *mutatis mutandis*, for versions of preferentism according to which what directly benefits a person is the satisfaction of preferences.

10. A nonstandard version of preferentism, according to which a person is directly benefited by *believing* that she is getting what she wants, is discussed in Heathwood (2006).

11. Given these points, there will be a systematic cleavage between self-reported measures of well-being as it is conceived of by the preferentist (see Chapter 13, in this volume) and that which it purports to measure: in cases in which a subject believes a desire has been satisfied when it hasn't, her score will be too high, and in cases in which she believes a desire hasn't been satisfied when it has, her score will be too low.

12. To speak carefully, in the case of desires, it's not the mental state—the desire—itself that is held to benefit a person, but its *realizer*: the desired state of affairs.

13. For some other objections to preferentist or experientialist theories of well-being, see Brandt (1982, p. 179), Griffin (1986, pp. 16–17), Lauinger (Chapter 8, in this volume), Nagel (1979, p. 4), and Nozick (1974, pp. 44–45).

14. It may be rejoined that there are other ways in which empirical researchers can measure well-being on philosophical conceptions apart from measuring the extent to which a person has realized an (ostensible) basic good; for example, perhaps there are ways to measure things that do not, according to philosophers, benefit a person directly but which *correlate* to that which *does* benefit a person directly, on all the major

philosophical conceptions. (For example, perhaps having a sense of belonging to a community is pleasurable *and* satisfies a desire we all have, and so on.) This rejoinder, however, only pushes the problem one step back, since to establish a correlation to a basic good one would still need to measure that basic good.

15. Philosophers who suggest that close personal relationships of some sort are among the basic goods include Finnis (1980), Fletcher (2013), Griffin (1986), Lauinger (2013), Murphy (2001), and Rice (2013).

16. "He ought therefore at the same time to perceive the being of his friend, and this will come about in their living together and exchanging words and thoughts; this is what living together would seem to mean in the case of people and not, as in the case of cattle, grazing in the same place" (Aristotle, 2000, p. 1170b).

17. This assumes that the individual's self-reports are accurate, an issue to which I will return momentarily.

18. PR5. I don't have many people who want to listen when I need to talk. (rs)

19. PR6. It seems to me that most other people have more friends than I do. (rs)

20. Philosophers who are reluctant to defer to psychologists in this way should remember the limitations of their own methods of research. All philosophers, for example, construct arguments that include premises which, in turn, rest on assumptions that the philosopher is not in a position to adequately support through argument; we all must take certain things as given. This feature of philosophical practice (and, indeed, inquiry in general) is so entrenched that philosophers may not be inclined to see it as a limitation, but, of course, that's exactly what it is. Without establishing the truth of every background assumption we depend on, we cannot be said to have definitively proved our conclusion. Yet, despite this, we don't conclude that we should give up altogether on giving arguments in support of our conclusions.

21. This isn't to say that psychologists' standards are immune to challenge from outsiders to the discipline. It is rather to say that the role of the philosopher is as a participant in deliberation, including deliberation about the validity of measures. It's only when researchers from different disciplines come to understand the others' standards and the reasons for them that they are in a position to be helpful participants in the kind of collective deliberation that will result in methodological improvement.

About the Author

Anne Baril is Lecturer in Philosophy at Washington University in St. Louis. She has research interests in ethics, epistemology, and their intersection. Her work appears in such journals as *Synthese*, *Episteme*, and the *Southern Journal of Philosophy*. Currently she is writing a book in which she argues that epistemic virtue is integral to the development of moral character and a constitutive contributor to well-being.

Author Note

I would like to thank Alicia Hall, Dan Haybron, Allan Hazlett, Matthew Lee, Seth Margolis, Eric Schwitzgebel, and Alan Wilson for their helpful feedback on this chapter; the editors of this volume; and the participants in the Interdisciplinary Workshop on Happiness, Well-Being, and Measurement, hosted by the Human Flourishing Program in the Institute of Quantitative Social Science and the Lee Kum Sheung Center for Health and Happiness, both at Harvard University. This work was supported in part by a grant from the John Templeton Foundation and by the Lee Kum Sheung Center for Health and Happiness. The views expressed in this chapter represent the perspective of the author and do not reflect the opinions or endorsement of any organization. I have no known conflict of interest to disclose. Correspondence concerning this chapter should be directed to Anne Baril, Washington University in St. Louis, CB 1073, One Brookings Drive, St. Louis, MO, 63130-4899 (anne.m.baril@gmail.com).

References

Aristotle. (2000). *Nicomachean ethics*. R. Crisp (Ed.). Cambridge: Cambridge University Press.

Bentham, J. (1789/1907). *An introduction to the principles of morals and legislation*. Oxford: Clarendon.

Brandt, R. (1979). *A theory of the good and the right*. Oxford: Clarendon.

Brandt, R. (1982). Two concepts of utility. In H. B. Miller & W. H. Williams (Eds.), *The limits of utilitarianism* (pp. 169–185). Minneapolis: University of Minnesota.

Cocking, D., & Kennett, J. (2000). Friendship and moral danger. *The Journal of Philosophy, 97*(5), 278–296.

Crowne, D. P., & Marlowe, D. (1960). A new scale of social desirability independent of psychopathology. *Journal of Consulting Psychology, 24*(4), 349–354.

Deiner, E., Emmons R. A., Larsen R. J., & Griffin, S. (1985). The satisfaction with life scale. *Journal of Personality Assessment, 49*(1), 71–75.

Dorsey, D. (2010). Three arguments for perfectionism. *Noûs, 44*(1), 59–79.

Feldman, F. (2004). *Pleasure and the good life*. Oxford: Oxford University Press.

Finnis, J. (1980/2011). *Natural law and natural rights*. Oxford: Clarendon.

Fletcher, G. (2013). A fresh start for the objective-list theory of well-being. *Utilitas, 25*(2), 206–220.

Friedman, M. (1989). Friendship and moral growth. *Journal of Value Inquiry, 23*, 3–13.

Griffin, J. (1986). *Well-being: Its meaning, measurement, and moral importance*. New York: Clarendon.

Hart, C. M., Ritchie, T. D., Hepper, E. G., & Gebauer, J. E. (2015). The balanced inventory of desirable responding short form (BIDR-16). *SAGE Open*, October–December, 1–9.

Heathwood, C. (2006). Desire satisfactionism and hedonism. *Philosophical Studies, 128*, 539–563.

Heathwood, C. (2015). Desire-fulfillment theory. In G. Fletcher (Ed.), *The Routledge handbook of philosophy of well-being* (pp. 135–147). Abingdon, UK: Routledge.

Helm, B. (2013). Friendship. In E. Zalta (Ed.). *The Stanford encyclopedia of philosophy*. http://plato.stanford.edu/entries/friendship/.

Hooker, B. (1998). Does moral virtue constitute a benefit to the agent? In Crisp, R. (Ed.). *How should one live?: Essays on the virtues* (pp. 141–156). New York: Oxford University Press.

Kagan, S. (2009). Well-being as enjoying the good. *Philosophical Perspectives, 23*(1), 253–272.

Kauppinen, A. (2012). Meaningfulness and time. *Philosophy and Phenomenological Research, 84*(2), 345–377.

Keller, S. (2004). Friendship and belief. *Philosophical Papers, 33*(3), 329–351.

Kraut, R. (1994). Desire and the human good. *Proceedings and Addresses of the American Philosophical Association, 68*, 39–54.

Lauinger, W. (2013). The missing-desires objection to hybrid theories of well-being. *Southern Journal of Philosophy, 51*, 270–295.

McCrae, R. R., & Costa, P. T. (1987). Validation of the five-factor model of personality across instruments and observers. *Journal of Personality and Social Psychology, 52*(1), 81–90.

Mill, J. S. (1861/2001). *Utilitarianism.* G. Sher (Ed.). Cambridge, MA: Hackett.

Moore, A. (2000). Objective human goods. In R. Crisp & B. Hooker (Eds.), *Well-being and morality: Essays in honour of James Griffin* (pp. 75–89). New York: Clarendon.

Murphy, M. (2001). *Natural law and practical rationality.* Cambridge: Cambridge University Press.

Nagel, T. (1979). *Mortal Questions.* Cambridge: Cambridge University Press.

Nozick, R. (1974). *Anarchy, State and Utopia.* New York: Basic Books.

Parfit, D. (1984). *Reasons and Persons.* New York: Clarendon.

Raibley, J. (2010). Well-being and the priority of values. *Social Theory and Practice, 36*(4), 593–620.

Railton, P. (1986). Facts and values. *Philosophical Topics, 14*(2), 5–31.

Rice, C. (2013). Defending the objective list theory of well-being. *Ratio, 26*, 196–211.

Russell, D., Peplau, L. A., & Cutrona, C. E. (1980). The revised UCLA Loneliness Scale: Concurrent and discriminant validity evidence. *Journal of Personality and Social Psychology, 39*(3), 472–480.

Ryff, C. D. (1989). Happiness is everything, or is it? Explorations on the meaning of psychological well-being. *Journal of Personality and Social Psychology, 57*, 1068–1081.

Ryff, C. D. (2013). Psychological well-being revisited: Advances in the science and practice of eudaimonia. *Psychotherapy and Psychosomatics, 83*(1), 10–28.

Ryff, C. D. (2016). Eudaimonic well-being and education: Probing the connections. In D. W. Harward (Ed.), *Well-being and higher education: A strategy for change and the realization of education's greater purposes* (pp. 37–49). Washington DC: Bringing Theory to Practice.

Ryff, C. D. (2018). Well-being with soul: Science in pursuit of human potential. *Perspectives on Psychological Science, 13*(2), 242–248.

Ryff, C. D., & Keyes, C. L. M. (1995). The structure of psychological well-being revisited. *Journal of Personality and Social Psychology, 69*(4), 719–727.

Sherman, N. (1987). Aristotle on friendship and the shared life. *Philosophy and Phenomenological Research, 47*, 589–613.

Sidgwick, H. (1907). *The methods of ethics* (7th ed.). London: MacMillan.

Sumner, L. W. (1996). *Welfare, happiness and ethics.* Oxford: Oxford University Press.

Strahan, R., & Gerbasi, K. C. (1972). Short, homogeneous versions of the Marlow-Crowne Social Desirability Scale. *Journal of Clinical Psychology, 28*, 191–193.

Stroud, S. (2006). Epistemic partiality in friendship. *Ethics, 116,* 498–524.

Taylor, G. (1985). *Pride, shame, and guilt: Emotions of self-assessment.* Oxford: Oxford University Press.

Tiberius, V. (2018). *Well-being as value fulfillment: How we can help each other to live well.* Oxford: Oxford University Press.

Whiting, J. (1991). Impersonal friends. *Monist, 74,* 3–29.

Wojcik, S. P., Hovasapian, A., Graham, J., Motyl, M., & Ditto, P. H. (2015). Conservatives report, but liberals display, greater happiness. *Science, 347* (6227), 1243–1246.

10

Human Flourishing

A Christian Theological Perspective

Neil G. Messer

Abstract

This chapter outlines one Christian theological account of human flourishing, with its roots in the Reformed Protestant tradition, but also drawing
on other Christian traditions and disciplinary perspectives. Human flourishing is understood as the fulfillment of God's good purposes for human
creatures and (following the Reformed theologian Karl Barth) includes
the dimensions of relationship with God, relationships with others, living
a physically embodied and integrated life, and living out a particular vocation in a particular place and time. This theological account of flourishing is brought into dialogue with current social-scientific models of
well-being, particularly hedonic and eudaimonic models, and points of
agreement and critique are identified. Finally, the chapter suggests a few
ways in which this theological account might have practical implications
for the measurement and promotion of well-being or human flourishing.

This chapter outlines one particular Christian theological account of human
flourishing and explores some of its implications for the issues raised and
discussed in this volume. That account has its roots in the Reformed theological tradition—that is, the branch of Protestant Christianity that originated
in sixteenth-century Geneva and the work of reformers such as John Calvin
(Calvin, 1559/1845). However, it has been developed in an ecumenical and
interdisciplinary way, drawing on theological sources from other Christian
traditions (such as the medieval Catholic thinker Thomas Aquinas) and
engaging with a range of disciplines including philosophy and disability
studies.[1]

Neil G. Messer, *Human Flourishing* In: *Measuring Well-Being*. Edited by: Matthew T. Lee, Laura
D. Kubzansky, and Tyler J. VanderWeele, Oxford University Press (2021). © Oxford University Press.
DOI: 10.1093/oso/9780197512531.003.0011

The chapter approaches the discussion of well-being and measurement from a slightly oblique angle. The original context of my account of flourishing was an attempt to understand health and disease theologically, in order to provide an analytical lens through which to examine a range of bio-ethical problems. The result was a theological account of health and disease in the context of human flourishing (Messer, 2013). That account had four stages: first, an understanding of humans as creatures; second, an account of health as an aspect of creaturely flourishing; third, an understanding of disease in relation to evil, sin, and death; fourth, a sketch of some practical implications of this account, particularly in the context of healthcare. The third and fourth stages have less relevance to the present volume, but the first and second can serve as the basis for a theological understanding of flourishing that may be brought into dialogue with current social-scientific accounts of well-being. The next two sections of the chapter summarize those stages of my account of flourishing, after which the following sections explore some of its implications for the understanding and measurement of well-being.

Humans as Creatures

The first stage in this account of flourishing is to recall that the Christian tradition thinks of human beings as God's *creatures* (Messer, 2013, pp. 164–174). Three important insights follow from this.

First, "creature" is a theological category. In Christian theology, to describe humans as creatures is to claim that we, in common with all created things, owe our existence to the good purposes of a loving and sovereign God. If we wish to know what it means to be a human *creature*, we are enquiring about God's purposes. But since God, in the Christian tradition, is infinite and transcendent, how can finite creatures like us gain any understanding of God's purposes? The various Christian traditions will answer that question in different ways. The Reformed tradition, in which this account is rooted, tends to emphasize the limits of our capacity to understand God and God's ways out of our own intellectual and experiential resources. This is because we are both finite creatures and sinners (as discussed later in this section). Therefore, this tradition typically attaches great importance to God's self-revelation to humanity. In this Christian perspective, that divine self-disclosure is seen centrally in the person and work of Jesus Christ, to whom the Scriptures witness (cf. Barth, 1932/1975, ch. 1). That is one reason why the Bible is foundational for Christian theology.

It is worth noting in passing that this theological account is not in competition with evolutionary or other scientific accounts of human nature and has no need to deny or reject these accounts. Science cannot tell us that we are—or that we are not—God's *creatures*. However, those who understand themselves on theological grounds to be God's creatures will find plenty to learn from relevant scientific disciplines about the form taken by our kind of creaturely existence (for a few examples of the voluminous literature on theology and evolution, see Deane-Drummond, 2009; Messer, 2007; Northcott & Berry, 2009).

Second, "creature" is a normative or evaluative as well as descriptive category. To describe ourselves as creatures is to claim that our existence, and its particular form, reflect God's *good* purposes. It is objectively *good* to be a human creature. This kind of theological account, in other words, resists the modern separation of description from evaluation or fact from value.

This is not to say that everything about human life as we experience it is good, or is what God wills. Another central claim of Christian faith is that the world as we know it is profoundly broken and distorted by the presence of evil. This takes various forms, one of which is often referred to as "natural evil": the natural processes of the created world, as we experience them, do not fully reflect God's good purposes. For example, many kinds of natural process may bring about suffering, death, and destruction for both human and non-human creatures, much of which seems hard to reconcile with the loving purposes of a good God (for discussion of one aspect of this, see Messer, 2018; Southgate, 2008). Another form of evil is what the Christian tradition refers to as "sin," a much misunderstood word. "Sin" does not simply mean moral wrongdoing, though there is of course a relationship between the two. Fundamentally, sin is a theological, not simply a moral or ethical, category. It names a basic distortion in our relationship with God, from which spring all kinds of other distortion in our relationships with one another, ourselves, and the created world (see, e.g., McFadyen, 2000). Though it may seem paradoxical to say this, there is good news at the heart of Christian talk of sin and evil, because the heart of Christian faith and theology is the message and doctrine of *salvation*. This refers to the Christian claim that God has acted decisively through the life, death, and resurrection of Jesus Christ to overcome sin and evil. Along with the doctrine of salvation comes *eschatological* hope: the promise of a future age in which evil will finally be a thing of the past, and God's good purposes for human life and all creation will be completely fulfilled.

The ambivalent character of the present world—created good, but also flawed and distorted by evil—is one reason why this theological perspective emphasizes the need for revelation to inform theological and ethical understanding. If we wish to understand God's good purposes for human creatures, we cannot simply read them off our observations or scientific investigations of what human life, as we experience it, is actually like. This is because human life, as we experience it and investigate it in this world, is always already a complex mix of the good and the broken (cf. Bonhoeffer, 1949/2005, pp. 319–320). This is not to deny the value of experience or scientific investigation for informing theological understanding, but insights from these sources will have to be critically appropriated, and their significance interpreted through a theological lens, if they are to do so.

Third, "creature" is a *teleological* category: one that implies purposes, goals, or ends. To be a creature of a particular kind is to be a being whose good consists in the fulfillment of the goals or ends appropriate to this kind of creature. But the goods, goals, and ends of human creaturely being come in various shapes and sizes. To borrow a distinction made by the twentieth-century theologian Dietrich Bonhoeffer (1949/2005, pp. 146–170), we can say that human creatures have "ultimate" and "penultimate" ends. The *ultimate* has to do with the salvation and eschatological hope mentioned earlier: our ultimate end is the complete fulfillment of all that God has created us to be. It is only God, not we, who can bring this about: this hope is available to us simply because of God's free and generous love, or what theologians call God's grace.[2] The *penultimate* refers to the conditions of life in this world, for which humans are called to take responsibility. The penultimate matters because it is in this world, in the here and now, that humans can encounter God's love and the promise of the ultimate. In theological perspective, life in this world has real, great, but not ultimate, importance.

Our ultimate end is eternal life with God. Within that horizon, we have all kinds of penultimate ends: purposes and goals that are good for human lives to be directed toward in this world. I shall say a little more about what this means in the next section. Some of our penultimate ends are universal: goals or purposes that are appropriate to any of us, just by virtue of being creatures of this particular, human, kind. Others are particular: to do with the particular forms that different human lives take in different times and places. And even universally human ends have to be realized in particular ways in each of our lives.

One caveat about this teleological account of human life should be noted. As I have already emphasized, humans are both finite creatures and sinners, and that means we are very easily mistaken about our own and our neighbors' good. Ignorance, self-interest, and prejudice, among other things, may distort our understandings of what it means for a human life to flourish or be fulfilled. So a healthy suspicion is needed about the ways in which our notions of the human good may be wrongheaded, partial, or distorted, and we should welcome critical perspectives that can call attention to these distorted understandings and help to correct them. In the context of a theological discussion of health and human flourishing, for example, important critical perspectives are offered by disability studies and theological reflections on disability (Messer, 2013, pp. 51–101, 151–161).

Health and Creaturely Flourishing

To flourish as a human creature is to fulfill the goods, goals, and ends that belong to this kind of creaturely life. But we need to put a good deal of flesh on that skeletal definition to have a useful or informative account of either health or human flourishing.

The great twentieth-century Reformed theologian Karl Barth offers one way of doing this. He gives an account of Christian ethics in terms of "the command of God the Creator": God's gracious call or summons, which sets us free to be the creatures God has made us to be. Barth identifies four dimensions to this divine summons (Barth, 1951/1961). The first he calls "freedom before God": we have been made for relationship with God, and God's command sets us free for that relationship. The second is "freedom in fellowship": we are relational and social creatures, and God's command sets us free to live in good relationships with one another. The third is "freedom for life": we are called simply to *be* creatures of our kind; physically embodied creatures in whom body and psyche form one integrated whole. The final dimension is "freedom in limitation": we are finite creatures, and our creaturely life must always therefore be lived in particular times, places, and ways.

Barth locates health in the third of these dimensions: he describes it as "strength for human life"; the power to answer God's call and live a life of this kind. For Barth, that power itself is God's gift: health is not something human agency or skill can create, though we can do a good deal to promote and support it (or indeed to damage it). He also describes it as "capability, vigour and freedom . . . the integration of the organs for the exercise of psychophysical functions" (Barth, 1951/1961, p. 356). It is, in other words, the capacity to live the kind of life in which the various physical and other aspects of human creaturely being are integrated into one well-functioning whole.

We might think of health, in short, as the fulfillment of *some* penultimate human goals and ends of life: those that have to do with sustaining our integrated, physically embodied lives. It is a real and great, but penultimate, good: it is not of ultimate importance.[3] Some healthcare practices and aspirations tend to obscure or deny this distinction between ultimate and penultimate goods; in effect they treat health as a goal of overriding importance, to be pursued at all costs by any means necessary. Attaching ultimate importance to a real but penultimate good is a species of what the Christian tradition calls *idolatry*, a destructive kind of mistake for all concerned.

Also, in this perspective, health is *one* aspect of human creaturely flourishing among others—not the whole of it, as the World Health Organization (WHO) definition asserts: "Health is a state of complete physical, mental and social well-being and not merely the absence of disease or infirmity" (World Health Organization, 2014, p. 1). "Health" names one good of embodied creaturely human life. But as Barth's fourfold scheme of "the command of the Creator" suggests, there are other goods that belong to this kind of creaturely life, and to try and subsume them all under the heading of health would strain the understanding of the latter.

Moreover, as noted earlier, this theological tradition understands human life and the world to be "very good" (Genesis 1:31, New Revised Standard Version) yet also "fallen": that is, broken and distorted by human sin and other aspects of evil. In a fallen world, there is the possibility of tragic conflict between human goods, so that some goods can only be realized at the cost of others. This tragic aspect of the human condition is not seen as a permanent state of affairs. Christian theology maintains the eschatological hope of a "new heaven and a new earth" (Revelation 21:1): a promised future age in which the fallenness of the world is overcome, human existence is transformed, and God's good purposes for creation find their ultimate fulfillment. In this eschatological future, there will be no tragic conflict between human goods, and perfect flourishing will be a reality. But that is an eschatological hope: human flourishing in the present age will always be partial at best, subject to limitations, hindrances, and tragic conflicts be-tween genuine goods.

While I have claimed that human goods are diverse and not fully com-mensurable, the boundaries between the different aspects of creaturely flour-ishing are not watertight. Although health is one particular human good, it is of course related to others. For example, it affects and is affected by human relationships; and, as Barth emphasizes, it also has social, political, and economic aspects. "The will for health of the individual," he remarks, "must . . . also take the form of the will to improve, raise and perhaps radically transform the general living conditions of all" (Barth, 1951/1961, p. 363).

Health, Creaturely Flourishing, and Well-Being

The WHO definition of health, quoted earlier, equates health, well-being, and (at least by implication) the whole of human flourishing. It has often been criticized for having too narrow a view of well-being or flourishing, in particular for excluding spiritual well-being (e.g., Chirico, 2016; Larson, 1996; Vader, 2006). In the account of health summarized in the previous two sections, I have offered a different criticism (also made by other authors): that it is too wide a definition of health. It is a mistake to equate health with well-being or flourishing if the latter are understood in such wide-ranging ways. "Health," I have argued, is better understood as naming a narrower domain of the good of human creatures: one aspect of our creaturely flourishing, not the totality of it.[4]

If this is correct, what of the relationship between well-being and flour-ishing? I did not differentiate clearly between them in my earlier account, where my main concern was to mark out the limits of health (Messer, 2013, pp. 174–175). Yet well-being, as it is often conceptualized in current social-scientific literature, is narrower in its scope than the totality of human flour-ishing. For example, the focus tends to be on psychosocial well-being, and this is often differentiated from health, in part so that correlations between the two can be investigated. Yet a complete account of human flourishing will surely include physical and mental health, as VanderWeele (2017, p. 8149) observes.

While there may be good reasons to broaden the ways in which well-being is conceptualized and measured, from the theological perspective outlined in this chapter there is something to be said for maintaining a distinction between well-being and flourishing. In this perspective, "flourishing" must first and foremost be understood theologically. It refers to every aspect of what it means to realize God's good purposes for the kind of creature we are: the fulfillment of our creaturely goals or ends in relationship with God, in human relationship and community, in the integrity of our own physical and mental life, and in our particular contexts and vocations (Barth, 1951/1961). In the nature of the case, the fulfillment of God's purposes for God's creatures is not something that human investigators could ever fully operationalize and measure empirically. Empirical measures of well-being will, at best, only be proxies for certain aspects of this complete theological understanding. (This would be true even if empirical measures of spiritual well-being or religious engagement were added into the mix: these could only ever be partial proxies for a person's relationship with God, which Christian traditions would say can be fully known only to God.) To borrow a phrase from Karl Barth, in this theological perspective, empirical investigations will disclose only "phenomena of the human" (Barth, 1948/1960, p. 122), not the full reality of what it is to be a human creature before God.

Of course, this is not to deny the value of such empirical measures and investigations. Particularly when policy and practice are being considered, there is real value in having proxy measures that can give some degree of insight into what is (or is not) conducive to the flourishing of human creatures. The distinction I have made between flourishing and well-being should simply serve as a reminder of the limits of what can be known empirically about the flourishing of human creatures. Among other things, this should encourage a certain epistemic humility in our assessments of what makes for human flourishing.

Given this theological caveat, what might be said theologically about the various concepts and accounts of well-being found in current social-scientific literature? The following sections outline some brief reflections.

The Structure of Well-Being and the Diversity of Human Goods

Some psychological accounts of well-being, notably Ryff's six-factor model, emphasize that there are diverse aspects of well-being, which are distinct and not fully translatable into one another (e.g., Ryff, 1989; Ryff, Boylan, & Kirsch, Chapter 4, in this volume). The theological account outlined here will support the idea that human goods are diverse and not fully commensurable. It might, however, press more sharply the question of conflicts between these goods. As I argued earlier, a theological understanding of this world as good yet "fallen" will regard complete flourishing as an eschatological hope. In this age, genuine goods may be in tragic conflict with one another.

Therefore, this theological account of flourishing might well agree up to a point that a model such as Ryff's names some genuine human creaturely goods (I emphasize "up to a point": some of the qualifications I have in mind here will be explained in the next two sections). But it will predict that tragic conflicts between these aspects of well-being will be a common and inescapable human experience. It might also predict that there could be situations in which well-being itself (as conceptualized by an account like Ryff's) may be in tension or conflict with other aspects of human flourishing before God. For instance, the fulfillment of some individuals' particular vocations to serve God and their neighbors might come at some cost to aspects of their own psychological well-being.

Indeed, this is not just a theoretical possibility. In their study of human benevolence and the experience of divine love, Lee and his colleagues give diverse examples of individuals whose vocations led them to accept what one described as the "cup of suffering" (including psychological pain and distress).

> The people we interviewed did not escape suffering in responding to a divine call to serve others; their biographical narratives are often filled with pain that accompanied their faith-filled responses and their reliance on supernatural power to persevere. (Lee, Poloma, & Post, 2013, p. 131)

Yet the sense that they were following their vocations enabled them to "[understand] the pain in a different way" (Lee et al., 2013, p. 132), so that the "cup of suffering" was also, paradoxically, a "cup of joy" (Lee et al., 2013, p. 130, citing Baker, 2007). This study offers empirical evidence of Christian believers who understand their own experience in something like the theological way I have outlined: that following a vocation, even at the cost of psychological or other suffering, can be recognized as a form of flourishing.

The Specific Content of Well-Being

An important part of the discussion in the recent literature on well-being has been concerned with hedonic and eudaimonic views and with debates and disagreements between them (e.g., Ryan & Deci, 2001). There have also been attempts at rapprochement between the two, integrating them into holistic accounts combining elements of both, such as the Comprehensive and Basic Inventories of Thriving (Su, Tay, & Diener, 2014). The theological account of flourishing outlined in this chapter may find some resonance with aspects of various accounts, including hedonic and eudaimonic ones. However, its encounter with these accounts will also be critical, raising various questions.

Hedonic accounts focus on subjective well-being, understood as life satisfaction, positive mood, and absence of negative mood (Ryan & Deci, 2001, p. 144). This view is strongly influenced by the utilitarian philosophy of Jeremy Bentham and his successors (Bentham, 1780/2007), and well-being in this perspective is closely associated with pleasure and the satisfaction of desire.

If human beings are understood theologically as embodied creatures, then it might seem that human desires can be seen in some way as indicators of the needs that must be met for our creaturely lives to be sustained and reproduced. At a basic level this need not be denied, yet a well-known biblical text, from that collection of Jesus' teaching known as the Sermon on the Mount, begins to complicate the picture:

> Is not life more than food, and the body more than clothing? . . . Therefore do not worry, saying, "What will we eat?" or "What will we drink?" or "What will we wear?" For it is the Gentiles who strive for all these things; and indeed your heavenly Father knows that you need all these things. But strive first for the kingdom of God and his righteousness, and all these things will be given to you as well. (Matthew 6: 25, 31–33)

The Christian tradition has often been ambivalent, if not downright suspicious, about human desire. At times that suspicion has taken quite extreme forms, but, properly understood, Christian ambivalence about desire springs from the understanding of human creaturely life as both good and "fallen." As the saying of Jesus just quoted suggests, the things we need to sustain our creaturely life can be seen as genuine goods, which God "knows that we need." Yet our desires may be distorted and disordered by that complex condition of alienation from God, one another, ourselves, and the world which the Christian tradition names as sin. The social, political, and structural aspects of sin may also include the co-option or manipulation of human desires to serve unjust or oppressive ends. Desire will therefore be seen as, at best, an unreliable guide to the good of human creatures. Traditions of asceticism in Christianity witness to this insight and to the idea that human desires must be disciplined or educated if they are to be directed more toward genuine flourishing (Gorringe, 2001, ch. 4). Moreover, as noted earlier, human creaturely life in this world is seen against an eschatological horizon. This suggests that the things we need to sustain our lives in this present world should be understood as genuine, but *penultimate* rather than ultimate, goods.

All of this suggests that the theological perspective I have outlined will encourage a rather critical stance toward hedonic accounts of well-being. This theological perspective may seem to have closer kinship with eudaimonic views such as Ryff's, and in some ways this is very likely true. The teleological character of eudaimonic accounts (e.g., Ryff, 2014, p. 11) resonates with the teleological picture of health and flourishing that I have offered (see Messer, 2013, pp. 164–174). Also, the Aristotelian roots of the concept of *eudaimonia* are closely linked to an understanding of virtue that has been influential in Christian theology and ethics.[5]

Nevertheless, while there may be an affinity between this theological account of flourishing and eudaimonic accounts of well-being, the relationship will still be a critical one. Consider for example the six factors in Ryff's eudaimonic account: autonomy, environmental mastery, personal growth, positive relations with others, purpose in life, and self-acceptance (Ryff, 2014, table 1). To a greater or lesser extent, the theological account of flourishing I have set out is likely to respond "Yes, but. . . " to most or all of these factors. I offer a few examples to illustrate areas of broad agreement and others where there will be more questioning and critique.

Positive relations with others: The way Ryff describes this category has much in common with the theological understanding of flourishing that I have outlined. Close, trusting relationships, empathy, affection, intimacy, concern for others' welfare, and so forth should all find their place within that aspect of creaturely flourishing which Barth calls "freedom in fellowship" (Barth, 1951/1961, pp. 116–323). A theological account in which relations with others are summed up by the great commandment to "love your neighbor as yourself" (Leviticus 19:18; Matthew 22: 39; and parallels) may go beyond Ryff's description on the grounds that the meaning of loving one's neighbor is not exhausted by the features she names, but there will be a good deal of agreement nonetheless.

Self-acceptance: The theological perspective I have articulated will doubtless recognize the importance of self-acceptance for a sense of well-being. Yet there is a deep ambiguity about this because Christians know themselves to be forgiven sinners. This would seem at least to complicate the business of feeling positive about one's past life, for example (cf. Ryff, 2014, table 1). The theological vision that informs my account will suggest that self-acceptance becomes a real possibility just because we are loved and accepted by God, without having done anything to deserve God's love. This raises a question about truthfulness in relation to self-acceptance. A truthful form of self-acceptance will be seen as one that is clear-sighted about our flaws, failures, and sins, yet able to rejoice in the love and acceptance of God, which makes possible our transformation into better and more complete human creatures.[6] Could there, by contrast, be forms of self-acceptance that would be better understood as self-deception?[7] Might there be aspects of our past life that we would be right *not* to feel positive about? This theological view of the self-acceptance of forgiven sinners would suggest that there could be .

Autonomy: In some contexts, especially healthcare ethics, autonomy is a problematic concept for many theologians (e.g., Messer, 2011, ch. 8). The concept, and the widely held ethical principle of respect for autonomy, are criticized for presupposing an excessively individualistic and agonistic understanding of what it is to be human, downplaying the importance of relationships and interdependence for a flourishing human life.[8] More fundamentally, the core understanding of autonomy as self-rule or self-determination seems to be called into question by a New Testament text from one of St. Paul's letters: "[D]o you not know . . . that you are not your own? For you were bought with a price; therefore glorify God in your body" (1 Corinthians 6:19–20). In the theological perspective suggested by this text, we are in a sense "owned" by the God who created us, who reconciled us to Godself through the work of Christ, and who promises the transformation and complete fulfillment of our lives in God's good future (Messer, 2011, pp. 216–217). Yet, despite these theological criticisms, some of the concerns articulated in Ryff's description of autonomy would find strong echoes in New Testament depictions of a good life. One early church leader, for example, exhorts his readers to grow into a Christian maturity in which they will no longer be "tossed to and fro and blown about by every wind of doctrine" (Ephesians 4:14). This certainly seems to have something in common with Ryff's description of the high scorer for autonomy who is "able to resist social pressures to think and act in certain ways" (Ryff, 2014, table 1).

In short, these examples suggest that the theological account of human flourishing I have outlined may resonate with various psychological accounts of well-being, particularly eudaimonic views such as Ryff's. But the encounter between these views and this theological perspective is also likely to be a mutually critical one. I would think that the critical questions these views put to one another have the potential to be helpful and illuminating for both.

Basic Visions of the Human Good

This kind of positive but critical response to some of the specific content in different accounts of well-being reflects a more fundamental question about the basic vision of the human good that informs those accounts. Perhaps I can put the point this way. The previous section was concerned with the contrasts between hedonic and eudaimonic understandings of well-being and with positive and critical theological responses to both. Yet in the Sermon on the Mount (Matthew 5–7)—historically one of the most influential biblical texts in shaping Christian visions of the good life—one finds a rather different understanding from either.

To be sure, there is common ground. According to Pennington (2017, pp. 41–68), the Sermon sets out a vision of human flourishing with roots in the Aristotelian virtue tradition as well as the wisdom literature of the Hebrew Bible. In the Sermon, the key word used to denote flourishing is *makarios* (usually, though misleadingly, translated "blessed"), which is close in meaning to *eudaimonia*. However, the Sermon's vision of flourishing is strikingly different from an Aristotelian understanding. It opens with a famous statement of what it means to be *makarios*.

> Blessed [*makarioi*] are the poor in spirit, for theirs is the kingdom
>   of heaven.
> Blessed are those who mourn, for they will be comforted.
> Blessed are the meek, for they will inherit the earth.
> Blessed are those who hunger and thirst for righteousness, for
>   they will be filled.
> Blessed are the merciful, for they will receive mercy.

Blessed are the pure in heart, for they will see God.

Blessed are the peacemakers, for they will be called children of God.

Blessed are those who are persecuted for righteousness' sake, for theirs
    is the kingdom of heaven. (Matthew 5:3–10)

As Pennington (2017, pp. 137–168) observes, this is a dark and paradoxical
vision of a good human life. Flourishing is associated with "poverty of spirit,"
mourning, "meekness" or humility (which Aristotle would have considered a
vice), hungering and thirsting, and persecution. As a vision of human flourishing, it makes sense only because of the eschatological promise expressed
in the second half of each saying: that God will bring about "the kingdom of
heaven," a state of affairs in which God's good purposes for creation are fulfilled, and the broken and disordered world we presently inhabit is healed,
transformed, and fulfilled. The people who truly flourish are those who live
in the light of that eschatological promise, even though doing so will invite
suffering in the present age.

The point of this comparison is that while there may be common ground
between the theological vision of human flourishing articulated in this
chapter and current accounts of well-being, if we dig down far enough we
are likely to find some deep differences in their basic assumptions about the
human good. Moreover, this will not be true only of theological accounts.
Any account of well-being will depend on some basic assumptions about the
human good, whether or not those assumptions are articulated. Different
accounts will be shaped by different basic assumptions, which may in some
respects be incompatible with those that shape other accounts.

Consider for instance the contrasting visions that inform hedonic and
eudaimonic views (Ryan & Deci, 2001, pp. 143–148). As noted earlier, hedonic accounts generally have deep roots in Bentham's utilitarianism, which
makes definite and particular claims about the human good, with pleasure
and the absence of pain at the heart of its conception. Now this view does
not come out of nowhere, but has a particular genealogy, including a complex relationship with Protestant Christianity: in some ways it has roots in a
Protestant Christian past, while also, in Bentham's hands, contributing to a
rejection of that Christian past (cf. McKenny, 1997, pp. 17–20). Hedonic theories of well-being rest in some way or other on this philosophical substructure. Eudaimonic theories, as we have already seen, rest on a different kind
of philosophical substructure, one shaped in part by the thought of Aristotle.
These are not the kind of differences that can be fully resolved empirically.

This suggests we should perhaps be cautious about trying to harmonize or synthesize contrasting accounts. There is a risk that a "holistic" synthesis of rival accounts may be built on a combination of basic assumptions or visions that are in fact incompatible with one another, in which case the resulting account of well-being may turn out to be incoherent to a greater or lesser extent. It might be better to acknowledge that some of the differences between models of well-being simply reflect rival conceptions of the human good.

Practical Implications

This is all very well, but when there is a need to produce usable measures to assess the impact of public policy, healthcare interventions, or other potential determinants of well-being, the theological critiques outlined in the preceding sections may seem like unhelpful theoretical quibbles. So what are the practical implications of my account, and is it likely to help or hinder the assessment of well-being in the various contexts in which current models are used?

The critique itself may have a contribution to make. First, it will serve as a reminder that human flourishing is broader than the aspects often considered in psychological accounts of well-being. Therefore, it will raise the question whether empirical measures of well-being need to be broadened to include other aspects of flourishing. In this respect it may support others who raise questions about broadening the scope of well-being measures and offer proposals for doing so (e.g., VanderWeele, 2017).

Next, this theological perspective will insist that well-being and flourishing must be understood against a transcendent horizon. Recall that in this theological account, a claim about human flourishing is ultimately a claim about the fulfillment of God's good purposes for human creatures. As I argued earlier, this implies among other things that there are limits to what can be measured empirically. So this theological critique will serve as a reminder of the limits of measurement in investigating well-being, a potentially useful cautionary note to sound when constructing studies and interpreting data.

Third, an obvious objection that might be raised about the practical applicability of this theological perspective is this: your theological account is shaped by a particular belief system, so why should it have any relevance to those who do not share that belief system? Yet, as I suggested in the preceding section, the very particularity of my theological account is a reminder that other accounts of well-being also depend on particular philosophical (or even implicitly theological) assumptions about the human good, assumptions that cannot be tested empirically. This suggests that the kind of theological perspective I have offered can encourage a critical self-awareness on the part of those offering and using other models of well-being about the particularity and built-in assumptions of their own models. In turn, this emphasizes the value of interdisciplinary dialogue among social scientists, philosophers, and theologians, which may help to make these built-in assumptions more explicit, subject them to critical examination, and perhaps thereby aid the construction of stronger and more coherent models. As I suggested earlier, however, one effect of such dialogue might be to sharpen, rather than resolve, differences between the various models.

Aside from critiques and cautionary notes, might this theological perspective have more constructive contributions to make to the discussion about measuring well-being and flourishing?

It might seem that one way to make such a contribution would be to try to turn the theological account of flourishing into an alternative model alongside others, such as hedonic and eudaimonic accounts, by operationalizing its various aspects and deriving empirically testable measures from them. I would be cautious about taking this route for reasons that have already been suggested. First, in this theological perspective, flourishing refers first and foremost to the fulfillment of God's good purposes for human creatures. As I have already emphasized, not every aspect of this fulfillment could even in principle be tested empirically, and empirical measures will at best only reflect "phenomena of the human" (Barth, 1948/1960, p. 122), not the reality. For those aspects which could be operationalized, the empirical measures might end up not looking very different from some of those in existing models. A related concern is that some of what is most important and distinctive in the theological account could (so to say) be lost in translation.

However, as I have already suggested, this account could lend theological support to proposals for broadening measures of flourishing, for example by including health and virtue as additional domains (VanderWeele, 2017). Could it also suggest other domains or measures that could be added to models of flourishing? A seemingly obvious example would be the domain of spirituality and/or religious participation; yet, on closer examination, attempting to incorporate this domain in social-scientific studies of health and well-being turns out to be conceptually and theologically fraught (Shuman & Meador, 2003).[9] Further careful consideration would be needed to establish whether there are theologically satisfactory and scientifically workable ways of including religion or spirituality in measures of well-being or flourishing.

Whatever this theological account might or might not add to the measurement of well-being and flourishing, it is likely to have a good deal to say about the conditions that are *conducive* to flourishing. In this way it could very well connect with social-scientific discussions of what VanderWeele (2017) calls "pathways to flourishing." There is a well-established tradition of Christian reflection on this issue, focused particularly on the concept of the *common good*. The language of "the common good" in this sense has its roots in Catholic social teaching, but in recent years has attracted increasing interest from other traditions (McGrail & Sagovsky, 2015).[10] I have argued elsewhere that the Reformed theological tradition on which the present account is based can find important points of contact with common-good thinking of this sort (Messer, 2009).

A standard definition of the common good is "the sum of those conditions of social life which allow social groups and their individual members relatively thorough and ready access to their own fulfillment" (Paul VI, 1965, para. 26). In other words, the common good is the sum total of social conditions that make the *flourishing* of human beings and communities possible. This suggests quite a broad range of concerns: Catholic and other Christian reflection on the common good draws attention to political rights, family life, education, employment, economic well-being, cultural life, peace and security, among other things (e.g., *Catechism of the Catholic Church*, 1997, paras. 1905–1912; McGrail & Sagovsky, 2015). From a different theological angle, the common good tradition once again foregrounds the social, economic, and political concerns touched on earlier in connection with Karl Barth's account of health. If we use this theologically grounded concept to frame our thinking about pathways to human flourishing, it is likely to broaden the focus of our attention and suggest that our talk of flourishing will be incomplete if it neglects these social, economic, and political factors.

Conclusion

This chapter has outlined one particular Christian theological account of human flourishing, with its roots in the Hebrew Bible and New Testament and the Christian tradition's history of reflection on those texts. I have argued that this theological account offers rich possibilities for mutually critical and illuminating dialogue with social-scientific accounts of well-being. I have explored various points of contact, dialogue, and critique in the later sections of this chapter, though other concerns—such as the social, economic, and political aspects mentioned at the end of the previous section—have only been briefly touched on and could usefully be developed in future discussions.

Mine is, of course, by no means the only possible Christian theological account. Different Christian traditions might offer accounts of flourishing that differ in some respects and might approach the dialogue with the social sciences differently from this chapter. There could be a lively intra-Christian debate about human flourishing, well-being, and how they can be studied and measured, to say nothing of the possibilities for dialogue and debate between different faith traditions. I would think that debates both within and between faith traditions about how human flourishing should be understood and promoted might complicate the current discussion of well-being and measurement, but, in the end, can only enrich it.

Notes

1. As such, it is likely to contrast in some ways, but also to have some common ground and points of contact, with other accounts of human flourishing grounded in philosophy, psychology, or biology (e.g., Chapters 6, 8, 9, and 13, all in this volume).
2. This raises a complex question, since the Reformed tradition is particularly associated with a doctrine of predestination in which God has foreordained only the "elect" to be saved (Calvin, 1559/1845, chs. 21–24). On the face of it, this might seem to qualify claims about God's love and generosity, though advocates of the doctrine would vigorously dispute this. Space does not permit a discussion of the centuries-long argument over predestination; suffice it to say that not all major theologians in the Reformed tradition have endorsed this doctrine in anything like Calvin's version (see McCormack, 2000).
3. This understanding is lived out in one way by those who accept risks to their health for the sake of following a vocation to serve God and their neighbors, including some of those interviewed by Lee and colleagues in their major recent study of Christian benevolence (e.g., Heidi Baker: see Lee, Poloma, & Post, 2013, pp. 54–56). In another sense, something like this insight may be at work in anyone (certainly any believer) who sets limits to their own pursuit of health because they recognize that by pursuing it too obsessively they lose sight of other human goods.

4. A similar insight from a different angle can be found in VanderWeele (2017); see also VanderWeele, McNeely, and Koh (2019).

5. There is some ambivalence on both sides of this connection, however. VanderWeele (2017, p. 8149) critiques eudaimonic theories for neglecting virtue, though Ryff (2014, p. 11) explicitly makes the connection between them. On the theological side, an Aristotelian concept of virtue has been particularly influential on Catholic ethics thanks to the work of the medieval philosopher-theologian Thomas Aquinas (e.g., Thomas Aquinas, 1920, *Prima Secundae*, questions 55–67) but has often been regarded with suspicion by Protestants. In recent decades, virtue ethics has enjoyed a revival in Protestant as well as Catholic ethics thanks to the work of authors such as MacIntyre (1981) and Hauerwas (1981), but the language of virtue nonetheless has its stringent theological critics. My own view, in brief, is that virtue does have a place in a theological conception of human creaturely flourishing but must be understood in a somewhat different way from the Aristotelian tradition (see Messer, 2013, pp. 172–174).

6. This finds frequent expression in Christian spiritual and devotional writing. One eloquent example is the seventeenth-century Anglican George Herbert's well-known poem "Love bade me welcome" (Herbert, 1633).

7. This question may find some resonance with some of the concerns explored by Xi and Lee (Chapter 15, in this volume, citing Horney, 1950).

8. Outside the theological arena, concerns similar to these have also been raised by others, including some feminist critics (Mackenzie & Stoljar, 2000).

9. There are well-known conceptual problems even with saying what we mean by "religion" and "spirituality," but, apart from these, one theologically fraught aspect of this discussion, which is the particular target of Shuman and Meador's critique, would be the attempt to show a correlation between religious practice and good health or well-being.

10. However, for some critical comments on the language of "the common good," see Bretherton (2010, pp. 28–29).

About the Author

Neil G. Messer is Professor of Theology at the University of Winchester, UK, and the author of several books including *Theological Neuroethics: Christian Ethics Meets the Science of the Human Brain* (Bloomsbury, 2017) and *Science in Theology: Encounters between Science and the Christian Tradition* (Bloomsbury, 2020). He has been a Guest Professor in the Center for Theology, Science, and Human Flourishing at the University of Notre Dame, and is Co-convener of the joint Theology and Neuroethics Interest Group of the Society of Christian Ethics, Society of Jewish Ethics, and Society for the Study of Muslim Ethics. His research is concerned with the intersections of Christian theology, ethics, healthcare, and the biosciences.

Author Note

This work was supported in part by a grant from the John Templeton Foundation and by the Lee Kum Sheung Center for Health and Happiness. The views expressed in this chapter represent the perspective of the author and do not reflect the opinions or endorsement of any organization. I have no known conflict of interest to disclose. Correspondence concerning this chapter should be directed to Neil G. Messer, Department of Theology, Religion and Philosophy, University of Winchester, Sparkford Road, Winchester, SO22 4NR, UK (Neil.Messer@winchester.ac.uk).

References

Baker, H. (2007). A cup of suffering and joy. www.unitedcaribbean.com/ heidibaker-cupofjoyandsuffering.html

Barth, K. (1932/1975). *Church dogmatics* (*Vol. 1.1*, 2nd ed.). (G. W. Bromiley, Trans.). Edinburgh: T & T Clark.

Barth, K. (1948/1960). *Church dogmatics* (*Vol. 3.2*). (H. Knight, G. W. Bromiley, J. K. S. Reid, & R. H. Fuller, Trans.). Edinburgh: T & T Clark.

Barth, K. (1951/1961). *Church dogmatics* (*Vol 3.4*). (A. T. Mackay, T. H. L. Parker, H. Knight, H. A. Kennedy, & J. Marks, Trans.). Edinburgh: T & T Clark.

Bentham, J. (1780/2007). *An introduction to the principles of morals and legislation*. Mineola, NY: Dover.

Bonhoeffer, D. (1949/2005). *Ethics*. (R. Krauss, C. C. West, & D. W. Stott, Trans.). Minneapolis, MN: Fortress Press.

Bretherton, L. (2010). *Christianity and contemporary politics: The conditions and possibilities of faithful witness*. Chichester, UK: Wiley-Blackwell.

Calvin, J. (1559/1845). Institutes of the Christian religion. (H. Beveridge, Trans.). https://www.ccel.org/ccel/calvin/institutes

Catechism of the Catholic Church (1997). Catechism of the Catholic Church (vatican.va).

Chirico, F. (2016). Spiritual well-being in the 21st century: It is time to review the current WHO's health definition. *Journal of Health and Social Sciences, 1* (1), 11–16.

Deane-Drummond, C. E. (2009). *Christ and evolution: Wonder and wisdom*. London, England: SCM.

Gorringe, T. J. (2001). *The education of desire*. London: SCM.

Hauerwas, S. (1981). *A community of character: Toward a constructive Christian social ethic*. Notre Dame, IN: University of Notre Dame Press.

Herbert, G. (1633). Love (III). In *The temple*. www.ccel.org/h/herbert/ temple/Love3.html

Horney, K. (1950). *Neurosis and human growth: The struggle toward self-realization*. New York: WW Norton.

Larson, J. S. (1996). The World Health Organization's definition of health: Social versus spiritual health. *Social Indicators Research, 38*, 181–192.

Lee, M. T., Poloma, M. M., & Post, S. G. (2013). *The heart of religion: Spiritual empowerment, benevolence, and the experience of God's love*. New York: Oxford University Press.

MacKenzie, C., & Stoljar, N. (Eds.). (2000). *Relational autonomy: Feminist perspectives on autonomy, agency, and the social self*. New York: Oxford University Press.

MacIntyre, A. (1981). *After virtue: A study in moral theory*. London: Duckworth.

McCormack, B. (2000). Grace and being: The role of God's gracious election in Karl Barth's theological ontology. In J. Webster (Ed.), *The Cambridge companion to Karl Barth* (pp. 92–110). Cambridge: Cambridge University Press.

McFadyen, A. (2000). *Bound to sin: Abuse, holocaust and the doctrine of sin.* Cambridge: Cambridge University Press.

McGrail, P., & Sagovsky, N. (Eds.). (2015). *Together for the common good: Towards a national conversation.* London: SCM.

McKenny, G. P. (1997). *To relieve the human condition: Bioethics, technology, and the body.* Albany, NY: State University of New York.

Messer, N. (2007). *Selfish genes and Christian ethics: Theological and ethical reflections on evolutionary biology.* London: SCM.

Messer, N. (2009). Morality, the state and Christian theology. *Crucible* (April–June), 16–23.

Messer, N. (2011). *Respecting life: Theology and bioethics.* London: SCM.

Messer, N. (2013). *Flourishing: Health, disease, and bioethics in theological perspective.* Grand Rapids, MI: Eerdmans.

Messer, N. (2018). Evolution and theodicy: How (not) to do science and theology. *Zygon, 53*(3), 821–835.

Northcott, M. S., & Berry, R. J. (Eds.). (2009). *Theology after Darwin.* Carlisle, UK: Paternoster.

Paul VI. (1965). Pastoral constitution on the Church in the modern world gaudium et spes. www.vatican.va/archive/hist_councils/ii_vatican_council/documents/vat-ii_cons_19651207_gaudium-et-spes_en.html

Pennington, J. T. (2017). *The Sermon on the Mount and human flourishing: A theological commentary.* Grand Rapids, MI: Baker Academic.

Ryan, R. M., & Deci, E. L. (2001). On happiness and human potentials: A review of research on hedonic and eudaimonic well-being. *Annual Review of Psychology, 52,* 141–166.

Ryff, C. D. (1989). Happiness is everything, or is it? Explorations on the meaning of psychological well-being. *Journal of Personality and Social Psychology, 57*(6), 1069–1081.

Ryff, C. D. (2014). Psychological well-being revisited: Advances in the science and practice of eudaimonia. *Psychotherapy and Psychosomatics, 83,* 10–28.

Shuman, J. J., & Meador, K. G. (2003). *Heal thyself: Spirituality, medicine, and the distortion of Christianity.* New York: Oxford University Press.

Southgate, C. (2008). *The groaning of creation: God, evolution, and the problem of evil.* Louisville, KY: Westminster John Knox Press.

Su, R., Tay, L., & Diener, E. (2014). The development and validation of the Comprehensive Inventory of Thriving (CIT) and the Brief Inventory of Thriving (BIT). *Applied Psychology: Health and Well-Being.* doi:10.1111/aphw.12027

Thomas Aquinas (1920). *The summa theologiae of St. Thomas Aquinas* (2nd ed.). (Fathers of the English Dominican Province, Trans.). www.newadvent.org/summa/ index.html

Vader, J. P. (2006). Spiritual health: The next frontier. *European Journal of Public Health, 16*(5), 457.

VanderWeele, T. J. (2017). On the promotion of human flourishing. *Proceedings of the National Academy of Sciences of the United States of America, 114* (31), 8148–8156.

VanderWeele, T. J., McNeely, E., & Koh, H. K. (2019). Reimagining health—flourishing. *Journal of the American Medical Association, 321* (17), 1667–1668.

World Health Organization. (2014). Basic documents (48th ed.). http://apps.who.int/gb/bd/

11

Comparing Empirical and Theological Perspectives on the Relationship Between Hope and Aesthetic Experience

An Approach to the Nature of Spiritual Well-Being

Mark R. Wynn

Abstract

While hope and the experience of beauty both have a claim to be key constituents of the spiritual life, it is not obvious that there is any deep-seated connection between them. Here, I examine three ways of developing the idea that there is some such association. I draw on empirically informed as well as theological perspectives, and, on this basis, I address a further question, one concerning the respective contributions of different kinds of enquiry to our understanding of spiritual well-being.

In this chapter, I shall be concerned with the relationship between two dimensions of spiritual well-being: openness to aesthetic experience, and hope understood as a trait of character. For the most part, the experience of beauty in particular will provide the focus for our discussion, although on occasion our interest will be in aesthetic experience more generally. For present purposes, a spiritual ideal of life can be defined fairly minimally, as a vision of what it is to live well relative to some conception of the human condition and perhaps, in turn, some conception of the fundamental nature of things. The notion of spiritual "well-being" is to be understood similarly; that is, in terms of living successfully by reference to some conception of the human condition. As we shall see, Thomas Aquinas gives one way of filling out this account for a theistic reading of the human condition in particular.

Mark R. Wynn, *Comparing Empirical and Theological Perspectives on the Relationship Between Hope and Aesthetic Experience* In: *Measuring Well-Being.* Edited by: Matthew T. Lee, Laura D. Kubzansky, and Tyler J. VanderWeele, Oxford University Press (2021). © Oxford University Press. DOI: 10.1093/oso/9780197512531.003.0012

In this context, the notion of "hope" is to be taken in a similarly broad way; that is, as a general disposition in life, rather than as pertaining simply to one or more isolated episodes of hopefulness, as when I hope that I will be able to make it to work on time today despite the Headingley traffic. When understood in this way, hope is capable, in principle, of serving as one of the core constituents of a well-lived life. Aquinas's suggestion that hope concerns "a future good, arduous but possible to attain" provides a helpful specification of the target of hope in standard cases (Aquinas, 1947, ST 2a2ae 17. 1).

For present purposes, I shall mostly take for granted that the person whose relationship to the world is infused by hope enjoys to that extent a state of spiritual well-being, while the person who suffers a radical lack of hope is to that extent spiritually impoverished. In defense of this reading of the significance of hope, it is worth recalling that hope is, of course, a central value in traditional religious accounts of the spiritual life: in the Christian context, for example, it is one of the three theological virtues. (The *locus classicus* for this teaching is Paul's first letter to the Corinthians, ch. 13.) And it is not difficult to find secular accounts of spiritual well-being that share this commitment to hope as a key constituent of the well-lived life. See, for instance, Wielenberg's (2005) defense of hope as a secular ideal of life and Cottingham's (2009) theistic response.

Openness to the experience of beauty is also commonly regarded as significant for spiritual well-being. There is, for instance, a long-standing tradition of thinking of the divine or of fundamental reality otherwise conceived as in some sense beautiful and of human beings as able to apprehend, in some degree, that beauty. The single best-known example of this understanding is perhaps the account developed by the character of Diotima in the *Symposium*, a text whose influence on later philosophical theology has been pervasive, but a willingness to conceive of the divine nature in broadly aesthetic terms and to suppose that the divine beauty is revealed in some measure in the material world is also evident in, for example, biblically grounded accounts of the spiritual life (see, e.g., the much-cited words of Psalm 19: "the heavens declare the glory of the Lord"), and, once again, there are secular counterparts for these traditions. Sherry (2002) provides an instructive overview of ideals of beauty in biblical and theological tradition, and Wolterstorff (2004) explores the significance of aesthetic experience for secular forms of spirituality, noting for instance the quasi-religious seriousness that is characteristic of some forms of engagement with "high art."

While hope and the experience of beauty both have some claim to be key constituents of the spiritual life, it is not just obvious, I take it, that there is any deep-seated connection between them, so that the person of hope is more apt to experience beauty by virtue of being hopeful or that the person who is relatively susceptible to the experience of beauty is thereby disposed to be hopeful. In this chapter, I consider three ways of developing the idea that there is some such association between aesthetic experience and hope. If we can show that there is such a connection, then we will have a new appreciation of the significance of each for the spiritual life. For instance, if it turns out that the person who is relatively open to aesthetic experience is, to that extent, more likely to be hopeful, then openness to aesthetic experience will be important for spiritual well-being not only as one of its constituent elements, but also because of its contribution to the formation of hope.

So one aim of this chapter is to clarify the relationship between aesthetic experience and hope considered as constituents of spiritual well-being. In the course of the discussion, I shall draw on a variety of sources, including empirically informed and theological texts. And this diversity will enable us to address a further question concerning the contribution of different kinds of enquiry to the study of spiritual well-being. So, overall, the goal of the discussion is to examine the connection between two major dimensions of spiritual well-being—and in the process to consider the relationship between empirical and theological accounts of what it is to live well.

I begin by reviewing three accounts of the relationship between the experience of beauty and hope. I start by introducing a text from William James, where he considers the relationship between hope—or loss of hope—and the appearance of the everyday world. Then I turn to a recent study in empirical psychology of the relationship between hope and appreciation of beauty. And finally, I sketch a theological perspective on the relationship between hope and aesthetic experience. Having reviewed these methodologically diverse sources, I present some general conclusions about the respective contributions of different forms of enquiry to our understanding of the nature of spiritual well-being—and, in particular, the relationship between hope and sensitivity to beauty.

William James on Hope and Aesthetic Experience

William James's classic text *The Varieties of Religious Experience* (1902) is concerned not simply with experiences which are focally of God or sacred reality otherwise conceived but also with world-directed forms of religious experience. And as we shall see, his discussion of this latter kind of experience bears very directly on the question of how we might conceive of the relationship between aesthetic experience, hope, and spiritual well-being. Let us approach these themes by first of all considering James's presentation of a secular example of the relationship between hope and the appearance of the everyday world. He writes,

> In the practical life of the individual, we know how his whole gloom or glee about any present fact depends on the remoter schemes and hopes with which it stands related. Its significance and framing give it the chief part of its value. Let it be known to lead nowhere, and however agreeable it may be in its immediacy, its glow and gilding vanish. The old man, sick with an insidious internal disease, may laugh and quaff his wine at first as well as ever, but he knows his fate now, for the doctors have revealed it; and the knowledge knocks the satisfaction out of all these functions. They are partners of death and the worm is their brother, and they turn to a mere flatness. The lustre of the present hour is always borrowed from the background of possibilities it goes with. (James, 1902, p. 141)

On the view developed here, our ability to find objects in our environment of interest or significance is tied to our ability to locate them within a future-referenced narrative: these objects have import for us in so far as they form part of our own ongoing story. If that is so, James reasons, then when I learn that my death is imminent, so that there is no future for me, then my environment is liable to be drained of significance. And here he is describing the perceptual counterpart of that condition: as things cease to have practical significance for me because they are no longer folded into my future projects, so their appearance changes, with the result that the everyday perceptual world loses its "lustre."

It is natural to read James's talk of the "glow and gilding" of "present facts" as an allusion to the color or "hue" of the perceptual field. As he notes in the ensuing discussion, if a person is suffering from melancholy, then the world may appear to them as gray and lifeless. For such a person, James (1902, p. 151) comments, "the world now looks remote, strange, sinister, uncanny. Its color is gone, its breath is cold, there is no speculation in the eyes it glares with." (The closing phrase in this remark is of course an echo of Macbeth's address to the ghost in Act 3, Scene 4 of Shakespeare's play.) The experience of the old man in our text seems similarly to be one of the world as drained of color and significance.

We might take James to be referring to a similar but in principle distinguishable phenomenon when he speaks of how this man's relationship to the world has "turned to a mere flatness." In normal experience, the perceptual field is not only colored, rather than gray, but also structured, so that certain items stand out relative to others. And these patterns of salience reflect, of course, our assessment of the varying significance of things in our environment for our practical projects: we will be focally conscious of those things which we take to be in this respect most important, while others will be consigned to the periphery of our awareness. (In some cases, it may be better to say that patterns of salience constitute our assessment of the varying significance of items in our environment rather than reflecting some independently established sense of their import.) But when a person's practical relationship to the world has broken down, as it has for the man in James's text, then there will be no variation in the significance that attaches to the objects of experience because all such objects will then be equally devoid of practical import. And this truth, James seems to be suggesting, can be registered in experience, in the flatness of the perceptual field.

So this passage invites us to suppose that a loss of hope—here, the old man's loss of hope for his own future—can be associated with a change in the appearance of the everyday world, with the result that the world ceases to be an object of perceptual interest—and loses its capacity, therefore, to serve as a focus for aesthetic contemplation. As we might expect, James thinks that this correlation can also run in the other direction, from a renewal of hope to a restoration of the appearance of the everyday world. To understand this possibility, he turns to reports of conversion experience, noting that

> When we come to study the phenomenon of conversion or religious regeneration, we shall see that a not infrequent consequence of the change operated in the subject is a transfiguration of the face of nature in his eyes. A new heaven seems to shine upon a new earth. (James, 1902, p. 151)

In striking contrast to the experience of the old man, in conversion experience, James is suggesting, everyday objects, including objects in the natural world, may appear brighter or more vivid. And we might suppose that in the convert's experience, these objects will also appear as more boldly defined so that the perceptual field is contoured rather than "flat."

For our purposes, we want to know, of course, whether this transformation in the appearance of the everyday world has an aesthetic dimension and whether it is significantly related to a change in hope in rather the way that the experience of the sick man was, on James's account of the matter, a consequence of his loss of hope. Let's take these questions in turn.

When James speaks in this text of a "transfiguration in the face of nature" and of "a new heaven shining on a new earth," it is already at least implied that this renewal in the appearance of the everyday world is to be understood in aesthetic terms. He cites various reports of conversion experience that confirm this reading. One convert comments: "Natural objects were glorified, my spiritual vision was so clarified that I saw beauty in every material object in the universe" (James, 1902, p. 250). Another source writes: "Not for a moment only, but all day and night, floods of light and glory seemed to pour through my soul, and oh, how I was changed, and everything became new. My horses and hogs and even everybody seemed changed" (James, 1902, p. 250). And in a similar vein, the puritan theologian Jonathan Edwards, as cited by James, describes his conversion experience in these terms:

> The appearance of everything was altered; there seemed to be, as it were, a calm, sweet cast, or appearance of divine glory, in almost everything. God's excellency, his wisdom, his purity and love, seemed to appear in everything; in the sun, moon, and stars; in the clouds and blue sky; in the grass, flowers, and trees; in the water and all nature; which used greatly to fix my mind. (pp. 248–249)

These texts speak of the everyday world, including "horses and hogs," and especially of the natural order, as newly glorified or infused with a kind of light following conversion. Of course, brightness or clarity has long been regarded as one of the defining qualities of beauty. See, for instance, Thomas Aquinas's suggestion that beauty consists in "brightness," *claritas*, together with "integrity" and "proportion" (1947, ST 1a 39. 8). And, among the divine attributes, it is perhaps the idea of divine "glory" which above all sustains the thought that the divine goodness has an aesthetic dimension. (Of course, believers also talk of divine beauty but this usage is, I take it, less common in, for example, biblically informed traditions.) It is significant, therefore, that these sources all speak of the world as newly glorified. It is also evident that what is being described is a change not in the world's intrinsic character but in its appearance to the convert. (See, e.g., Edwards's insistent use of the word "appear" and its cognates.) So these texts are concerned with the presentation of the world in perceptual terms to the properly appreciative viewer, and aesthetic experience involves, of course, this same mode of engagement with sensory things.

Let's consider next whether James's discussion of conversion experience has some bearing on the connection between hope and aesthetic experience. In his account of the sick man, James invites us to suppose that hope, or lack of hope, can leak into the appearance of the everyday world. As he says, the man now knows that his present circumstances "lead nowhere." In short, this is a man who has ceased to find any practical significance in his environment and who is, to that extent, devoid of hope. In Aquinas's terms, for this man, it is no longer possible to attain the future good. And this hopelessness, James is suggesting, finds expression in his experience of the world, which now appears as flat and gray and can no longer serve, therefore, as an object of aesthetic contemplation. Might we consider conversion experience as the converse of this case, not only in so far as it involves a renewal in the appearance of the world, but also in so far as that change is driven by a restoration—rather than loss—of hope?

James gives us some reason to endorse this view. As we have seen, when discussing the case of the sick man, he notes that the "chief part" of the value of a "present fact" depends on its "framing." And he goes on to suggest that a person's framing or contextualizing of their experience of the everyday world can derive not only from their assessment of their worldly prospects, in medical or other terms, but also from their religious commitments. He develops the point in these remarks:

> Let our common experiences be enveloped in an eternal moral order; let our suffering have an immortal significance; let Heaven smile upon the earth, and deities pay their visits; let faith and hope be the atmosphere which man breathes in;—and his days pass by with zest; they stir with prospects, they thrill with remoter values. Place round them on the contrary the curdling cold and gloom and absence of all permanent meaning which for pure naturalism and the popular science evolutionism of our time are all that is visible ultimately, and the thrill stops short, or turns rather to an anxious trembling. (1902, p. 141)

When set alongside James's discussion of the sick man, this passage suggests the following picture of the relationship between hope and aesthetic experience. A person's experience of the everyday world is framed by their "remoter schemes and hopes"—and these schemes and hopes can enter into the appearance of the world through their contribution to the patterns of salience and hue of the perceptual field. Hence the sick man who no longer sees any enduring point in his current projects—and who is suffering, therefore, from a radical loss of hope—may find that the world has been drained of significance, where this change is registered in a loss of color and structure in the perceptual field. Conversely, the religiously committed person who breathes in an "atmosphere" of "faith and hope" and who takes their current endeavors to have a "permanent meaning" may find that their everyday environment acquires thereby a deepened significance. And, by analogy with the case of the sick man, we might suppose that this significance can also be registered directly in perceptual terms—only now, the world will appear as vivid rather than gray and as deeply contoured rather than flat. Arguably, this is exactly the sort of perceptual change that James's converts are reporting when they take the world, post conversion, to be brighter and even newly "glorified."

So James offers us one way of thinking of the relationship between hope and aesthetic experience and of the contribution of each to spiritual well-being. In general, the spiritual life requires, we might say, taking up some sort of practical stance in the world. And James's discussion suggests that adopting any such stance depends on our capacity to live with at least a modicum of hope since hope is a condition of being practically oriented in our dealings with a given sensory context. And when we are so oriented, then the world will be perceptually engaging and, accordingly, at least potentially an object of aesthetic contemplation; when we are not, then the world is apt to appear flat and unsatisfactory. This account contrasts rather strikingly with the traditional emphasis in aesthetic theory on the idea that the object of aesthetic experience should be appreciated simply for itself and independently of any reference to its practical import. A classic account of this sort can be found in Clive Bell's (1913) text *Art*. The implication of James's discussion seems to be that even if the immediate object of aesthetic experience is not appreciated as an object of use, it is still necessary that the perceiver's relation to the wider world should not be drained of practical significance.

In the *Varieties*, James is mostly interested in experiences of conversion which are not directly under the person's control. But elsewhere—notably in his 1896 essay "The Will to Believe"—he allows that religious commitments can be chosen, whether directly or indirectly. And if we combine these accounts, then we might suppose that religious commitments can play an important therapeutic role in human life: on this view, by choosing to frame our experience in the terms provided by a religious narrative, we may be able to gain access to an enlivened perceptual world. And if that is so, then we may have a good practical reason so to choose. However, these matters lie beyond the scope of our present discussion.

An Empirical Approach to Beauty Experience, Hope, and Well-Being

I shall return to James's discussion of the relationship between hope and the experience of beauty at various points in the remaining discussion. But first of all, let's consider a modern empirical study of the relationship between hope and aesthetic experience. Rhett Diessner and his colleagues have addressed these matters using what they call the Engagement with Beauty Scale (EBS)—an instrument for measuring beauty experience of their own devising. Let us begin by taking note of some key features of this instrument.

When completing the EBS, subjects are asked to score their responses to various observations concerning three kinds of beauty: what Diessner calls natural, moral, and artistic beauty (Diessner, Solom, Frost, Parsons, & Davidson, 2008). These scores are recorded on a 7-point scale, running from "very unlike me" to "very much like me." For each of the three varieties of beauty, there are standardly four observations of the following form. (Here I have taken the case of natural beauty as representative of the general approach.)

1. I *notice beauty* in one or more aspects of nature.
2. When *perceiving beauty* in nature, *I feel* changes in my body, such as a lump in my throat, an expansion in my chest, faster heart beat, or other bodily responses.
3. When *perceiving beauty* in nature, *I feel* emotional, it "moves me," such as feeling a sense of awe, or wonder or excitement or admiration or upliftment.
4. When *perceiving beauty* in nature *I feel* something like a spiritual experience, perhaps a sense of oneness, or being united with the universe, or a love of the entire world (Diessner et al., 2008, p. 329, emphasis in the original).

It is clear, then, that the EBS is intended to track both a person's propensity to notice beauty and their tendency to respond to the experience of beauty with feeling. Hence, as its name indicates, the scale aims to record "engagement" with (and not simply perception of) beauty: the higher a person's scores across these four observations, the more deeply they will have engaged with the relevant kind of beauty. It is notable that the experience of beauty is here tied to "spiritual experience," which in turn is related to a conception of the fundamental nature of things: see, for example, the idea that beauty experience may be connected to or involve "a sense of being united to the universe." So, in this respect, Dissener's notion of the "spiritual" is broadly comparable to the one that we have been using in our earlier discussion. Having introduced the EBS, let us now return to the question of how we are to understand the relationship between hope and the experience of beauty.

In a 2006 paper, Diessner and his co-investigators describe how they used the EBS to study this relationship. Twenty-nine students were invited to complete the EBS and then to keep a weekly log of their experiences of beauty over a 12-week period. For each week of the study, the students were asked to complete this task: "Describe something you *felt* was beautiful . . . " (Diessner, Rust, Solon, Frost, & Parsons, 2006, p. 309, emphasis in the original) and to write between three sentences and three paragraphs in their log for each of the cases of natural, artistic, and moral/behavioral beauty. At each of the weekly meetings of the class, the instructor would invite three students to read aloud from their log entry for that week, so the class would hear, each week, a description of one example of beauty experience for each of the categories of natural, artistic, and behavioral beauty. Finally, at the close of the semester, 1 week after the submission of their concluding log, the students completed the EBS once again.

At the beginning and end of the study, the students also completed the Adult Dispositional (Trait) Hope Scale (Snyder et al., 1991). Diessner notes that this measure aims to capture hope along two dimensions: "goal directed determination (agency) and the ability to plan ways for meeting one's goals (pathways)" (Diessner et al., 2006, p. 308). (Hence the aim of the scale is to record both attachment to ends and the capacity to identify appropriate means for the achievement of those ends. Clearly, hope is being understood here as a general disposition, or trait of character, in keeping with the perspective that we have adopted in this discussion.) Finally, in addition to the experiment group, there was a comparison group, comprising 23 students, who did not participate in the log exercise but did complete the EBS and Hope Scale at the same times as the first cohort.

Diessner and his colleagues note that their study aimed to test these three hypotheses:

(1) College students who experience 12 weekly activities for engaging with natural, artistic and moral beauty will experience a significant increase in their trait hope; (2) Trait hope will significantly correlate with college students' levels of engagement with natural, artistic and moral beauty, as measured by the total score on the Engagement with Beauty Scale . . . (3) College students who experience 12 weekly activities for engaging with natural, artistic and moral beauty will develop higher levels of engagement with natural, artistic and moral beauty. (Diessner et al., 2006, p. 307)

With respect to (1), the research team concluded that participation in the weekly activities was correlated with an increase in hope, as measured on Snyder's scale: there was a significant rise in that trait in the intervention but not in the comparison group (Diessner et al., 2006, p. 311). Regarding (2), they found that there was a significant correlation between agential (rather than pathways) hope and engagement with moral beauty and beauty overall as measured by the EBS (Diessner et al., 2006, p. 311). This reflects, they surmise, the mostly conative character of agential hope, as compared with the more cognitive nature of pathways hope. (The distinction between these two dimensions of hope is grounded, I take it, in a distinction between means and ends, where grasping the necessary means involves knowledge of the relevant cause–effect relations and is, to that extent, cognitive, whereas grasping the end as an end requires only that one be attracted to it and is, to that extent, primarily conative.) Last, with respect to the third hypothesis, the team found that participating in the weekly exercises was significantly correlated with increased engagement with moral beauty but not with natural or artistic beauty.

While the investigators declined to make any causal claims on the basis of their study, it would be natural to take these findings to show that participation in the weekly exercise was not just correlated with an increase in hope and in engagement with moral beauty—see the first and third findings—but also, whether directly or indirectly, the cause of these changes. After all, the experimental setup was designed to ensure that any difference between the experimental and comparison groups, other than the first group's participation in the weekly exercises, would be irrelevant to any change in their relative hopefulness or relative engagement with beauty across the course of the study. (If these changes could be explained by reference to the demographic of the groups, then the study would cease to be of interest, of course, as a measure of the relationship between participation in the weekly exercises and the tendency to be hopeful or engaged by beauty.) So if the increase in hope and engagement with moral beauty in the experimental but not the comparison group is to be explained at all, then, *prima facie*, it seems that there is only one difference to which we can appeal: namely, participation in the weekly exercises. The experimenters note that they feel unable to represent the connection with increased engagement with beauty and increased hope as causal because the students were not assigned to the experimental and comparison groups on a random basis. (The experimental and control groups were simply drawn from different classes of the same course; see Diessner et al., 2006, p. 307.) However, they do allow that the study "lends credence to" the idea that engaging in the log exercise produces an increase in hope (p. 311).

More speculatively, we might suppose that there is an explanatory link running from participation in the exercises to increased engagement with moral beauty and from there to increased agential hope. There is some reason to think in these terms because the students participating in the exercises were, after all, required to attend to moral beauty on a weekly basis over a period of some 3 months and there would be no cause for surprise if repeatedly attending to moral beauty in this regular, focused way, even if only for a short time each week, should produce, by the close of the study, an increased disposition to notice and respond to moral beauty even if this change were to prove relatively short-lived. It is not too difficult, then, to see how participation in the log exercise might produce an increase in sensitivity to beauty, given that attending to beauty in this structured way may be in some measure habit-forming, at least in the short run.

Moreover, given the form of the EBS questionnaire, it is relatively easy to see why increased sensitivity to, say, moral beauty may in turn involve (rather than cause) an increase in hope. The first four observations on the EBS regarding the experience of moral beauty read as follows:

9. I *notice moral beauty* in human beings.
10. When *perceiving* an act of *moral beauty I feel* changes in my body, such as a lump in my throat, an expansion in my chest, faster heart beat, or other bodily responses.

11. When *perceiving* an act of *moral beauty I feel* emotional, it "moves me," such as feeling a sense of awe, or wonder or excitement or admiration or upliftment.

12. When *perceiving* an act of *moral beauty I feel* something like a spiritual experience, perhaps a sense of oneness, or being united with the universe, or a love of the entire world. (Diessner et al., 2006, p. 329, emphasis in the original)

So the person who scores highly for sensitivity to moral beauty is to that extent likely to register a relatively high score for these observations. That is, they are relatively likely to notice moral beauty, and, when noticing moral beauty, they are in turn relatively likely to experience positive emotions such as "wonder" and "upliftment" and to enjoy a felt sense of identification with the world, or a felt sense of the goodness of the world, and to experience correlative bodily changes. But if one person is in general more likely than another to experience such emotions and associated bodily responses—whether because they are more likely to notice moral beauty, or because when they notice moral beauty they are more likely to have such experiences, or for some combinations of these reasons—then, other things being equal, should we not think of this first person as the more hopeful of the two given simply what we mean by "hope" in this context?

It is worth recalling here that for the purposes of this enquiry, "hope" signifies not simply an occasional or localized attitude, but a generalized demeanor in life, one which is broadly positive about how events will turn out—or, at least, broadly positive about the spirit in which events may be received, however they turn out. And, if that is so, then the connection between increased sensitivity to moral beauty, as understood on the EBS, and increased hope will turn out to be at least in part analytic (i.e., true by virtue of the definition of relevant terms) given that a high score for engagement with moral beauty on the EBS will typically involve a high score for traits that in part comprise generalized hope of this kind: namely, traits such as the propensity to feel "love of the entire world," or "awe" and "upliftment."

In these ways, we can construct a narrative that goes beyond the relationship of succession that Diessner et al. report: there is reason to suppose not simply that participation in the weekly exercises is followed by an increase in hope and an increase in engagement with moral beauty, but also that it is the cause of the increased engagement with moral beauty, which in turn helps to explain, analytically rather than simply causally, the increase in hope. In this way, we can also understand the second of Diessner's findings concerning the correlation between hope and engagement with beauty overall as measured by the EBS. In brief, the connection between engagement with beauty, as measured by the EBS, and hope should be seen, once again, as at least in part analytic: since this study takes "engagement" with beauty to be realized in experiences of "awe," "wonder," and so on, there is some reason to expect an association between such engagement and the conative dimension of hope in particular, by virtue simply of what we mean by hope in this context.

Allowing for all of this, it is natural to wonder why participation in the weekly exercises correlates with a higher score for engagement with moral beauty but not a higher score for engagement with natural or artistic beauty. There are, no doubt, various ways in which we might try to account for this discrepancy, and, for present purposes, we do not need to reach a view on the matter. Most simply, we might wonder if participants in the study had more of an opportunity to observe moral rather than natural or artistic beauty. If even simple actions like holding open a door for someone can count as instances of moral beauty, then in a campus environment (as elsewhere), there should be an abundance of opportunities in everyday life to observe moral beauty. By contrast, if the campus is relatively built-up or if students spend much of their time indoors, then a university environment may afford relatively little opportunity to observe natural beauty. And if paintings or other works of art are not much in evidence on the campus, then they may have similarly limited opportunity to engage with artistic beauty. If there is any such difference in the relative incidence of moral, natural, and artistic beauty in the university environment, that would help to explain why the process of habituation we postulated earlier may operate more readily for moral rather than natural or artistic beauty, so that participation in the study results in an increase in engagement with moral beauty but not with natural or artistic beauty. In thinking about why participation in the log exercise should be correlated with an increased engagement with moral but not natural or artistic, beauty, it may also be relevant to note that, for the case of moral beauty, but not natural or artistic beauty, the EBS contains two additional observations along with the four standard observations we noted above, namely:

13. When perceiving an act of moral beauty I find that I desire to become a better person.
14. When perceiving an act of moral beauty I find that I desire to do good deeds and increase my service to others (Diessner et al., 2006, p. 329).

But again, these matters are not our immediate concern, so let us return to the main thread of our account.

As we have seen, in his discussion of the old man, William James presents a narrative that runs from the experience of loss of hope, to a state of practical disorientation, to an impoverishment of the perceptual world. And, conversely, in his discussion of religious experience, he points to the possibility of a narrative that runs from a restoration of hope (including here religiously grounded hope) to a revivification of the perceptual world, where this change in the world's appearance may have a strongly aesthetic character. In their discussion, Diessner and his colleagues are moving, I have been suggesting, in the opposite direction. Their study invites us to suppose that attending to beauty and reflecting on the experience of beauty in a regular, disciplined way may result in a greater propensity to engage with beauty (in particular, with moral beauty), which may in turn be associated with an increase in hope.

James and Diessner agree that hope is important for human well-being. For James, as we have seen, it is closely tied to the capacity to orient oneself in the world in practical terms. And, at the beginning of their paper, Diessner (2006, p. 301) and his colleagues remark that: "Hope correlates with, and may be necessary for, academic success, athletic achievement, various forms of social development, as well as the development of optimism and general happiness." Hence on this view, hope appears to be integral to the well-lived human life across a wide range of domains. And for both James and Diessner, it follows that an understanding of the nature and preconditions of hope can guide therapeutic interventions aimed at improving human well-being. For James, it seems that such interventions should start with the attempt to engender hope, which may in turn lead to an enhancement of the person's lifeworld. As we have seen, Diessner's account invites a movement in the other direction. (His paper is aptly entitled: "Beauty and Hope: A Moral Beauty Intervention.") On this approach, the person who undertakes the necessary practical exercises can become more fully engaged with beauty, and, in turn, they may then be more hopeful—and in so far as we take this connection between beauty engagement and hope to be analytic, then we should say that this increased disposition to engage with beauty involves of itself an increase in hope.

I shall develop a fuller account of the relationship between James's and Diessner's discussions at the close of this chapter. But first let us examine one further way of understanding the relationship between hope and aesthetic experience and the significance of both for spiritual well-being. Here I turn to a theological perspective.

A Theological Approach

I am going to begin this review of the relevance of theological sources for our theme by presenting one theologically informed account of the nature of spiritual well-being. For this purpose, I shall draw on the work of Thomas Aquinas, but it is not difficult, I suggest, to find close counterparts for his approach in a range of other religious traditions, including non-Christian traditions. So this discussion of the structure of the spiritual life, from the vantage point of religious traditions, is intended to be of general import. Having introduced this understanding of the nature of spiritual goods, we can then develop a further, theologically informed account of the relationship between aesthetic experience and hope to set alongside the two accounts we have already discussed.

At the core of any Christian account of the nature of the good or worthwhile human life will stand a conception of neighbor love and, accordingly, a consideration of Aquinas's understanding of the structure of the spiritual life might very naturally start here, with his account of neighbor love. Of course, Christians have thought of neighbor love as good and indeed, for themselves, as obligatory for a variety of reasons. Most simply, Christians are bound to think of this way of life as required, for them, because it is after all mandated by Jesus (see, e.g., Mark 12:31). While he accepts, naturally, that neighbor love is binding upon Christians for this reason, Aquinas provides a further rationale for its status—as obligatory—in the Christian understanding of the good life when speaking of neighbor love as a theological virtue.

In *Summa Theologiae* 2a2ae 25. 4, Aquinas puts to himself a question about the scope of neighbor love by asking whether it extends to our enemies, to ourselves, our bodies, the angels, and so on. In general terms, his answer is that I am to treat as my neighbor any creature who will share in the beatific vision. Here, for example, is his answer to the question of whether the angels properly fall within the scope of neighbor love. While this question may not seem to be of any very pressing importance from the perspective of our own time, Aquinas's answer is representative of what he says when determining the proper limits of neighbor love in other cases and is worth considering at least for that reason.

As stated above (Question [23], Article [1]), the friendship of charity is founded upon the fellowship of everlasting happiness, in which men share in common with the angels. For it is written (Mt. 22:30) that "in the resurrection . . . men shall be as the angels of God in heaven." It is therefore evident that the friendship of charity extends also to the angels. (ST 2a2ae 25. 10, ellipsis in the original)

We are all familiar with the idea that truths about the history of our relationship to another person can shape the character of our moral relations with them in the present. (To take a simple example, if I have wronged someone, say, by breaking a promise, then, *prima facie*, I have a reason to make good that wrong in the present if there is an opportunity to do so at least by offering an apology and perhaps by other means.) In this passage, Aquinas seems to be envisaging another, less familiar kind of connection. Perhaps future-referenced, or eschatological, truths concerning our relationship with others can also shape the character of our moral relations with them in the present. Here, Aquinas's suggestion seems to be that if, in the eschatological future, the angels will share with us in a "fellowship of everlasting happiness," then that establishes the appropriateness of a certain attitude toward them here and now. The same kind of reasoning will apply to our dealings with our fellow human beings, he thinks—and accordingly, we have a duty to extend the love of neighbor to them as well as to the angels.

There are obvious practical reasons why future-referenced truths do not in fact play much of a role in shaping our sense of our moral relations to others since the future is, of course, from our human vantage point, very often uncertain. But the considerations that make it appropriate for me to apologize in the present for being the source of a past wrong would presumably make it appropriate for me to apologize in the present for being the source of a future wrong were I to know of that wrong in the present. For instance, if I were to know here and now that I will culpably harm another person, then it seems that, other things being equal, I have a reason to apologize to them here and now, if there is an opportunity to do so. (Of course, there is an air of paradox in the idea that I might in the present disavow an action that I will myself freely perform at a later time. But let us bracket that point.)

The case that concerns Aquinas is not quite so straightforward as that of harm, but it is not too difficult to think of parallels between his example of eschatological friendship and morally significant truths concerning the past. If I once had a close friendship with someone, one that involved sharing in fundamental goods, then there is ready moral sense in the idea that I can be called upon to act in certain ways in the present as a condition of honoring that friendship. And we might suppose that this is so even if the friendship has now lapsed. Analogously, Aquinas seems to be proposing that a future truth concerning my friendship with another rational creature, where that friendship involves sharing in a uniquely profound good, namely the vision of God or participation in the divine life, in a further, postmortem state, can also call for practical acknowledgment in the present. Neighbor love, he suggests, is itself a form of friendship (ST 2a2ae 23.1) and its appropriateness is grounded in a prospective and perfected friendship that we will enjoy in our relations with others in the beatific vision.

The relationship between truths concerning my friendship with another person, whether in the past or the future, and the kind of conduct that I am called to exhibit in my relations with them in the present seems to be broadly one of existential congruence. If I know that a person has been or will be my friend, then my conduct toward them in the present is in principle open to assessment as being more or less adequate, more or less fitting—more or less congruent—relative to those truths about our friendship. These considerations need not, of course, be overriding, but they can form part of the mix of reasons that are relevant to the question of how I should relate myself to another person in the present. It is also worth being clear that, on this account of the matter, my treatment of my neighbor counts as appropriate not by virtue of making certain outcomes more likely (not, for instance, by making it more likely that I will attain the beatific vision or that my neighbor will do so), but because in this way I am able to give due acknowledgment to the truth that I will one day share with other human beings, and the angels, in the fundamental good of the vision of God. In this sense, the appropriateness of my action is more existential than causal: existential and causal ways of determining the appropriateness of a course of action are alike tied to an assessment of the future, but only the second case is concerned with bringing about a particular future.

While Aquinas's discussion of neighbor love turns on the idea of the beatific vision in particular, what matters for our purposes is the structure of his account, especially in so far as it involves the notion of existential congruence—a notion which could be employed by a spiritual tradition with very different metaphysical commitments. It is worth adding that, for Aquinas himself, the ideal of neighbor love can be grounded, it seems, not only in the claim that we will one day share with others in the beatific vision, but also in the more modest proposal that it is possible that we will do so. In the article that follows the passage I have quoted here, Aquinas (ST 2a2ae 25. 11 ad 2) writes: "In this life, men who are in sin retain the possibility of obtaining everlasting happiness: not so those who are lost in hell, who, in this respect, are in the same case as the demons." And, in the same article, he notes that for a person to be entitled to neighbor love, it is enough for them to "retain the possibility" of sharing in the beatific vision. Accordingly, if we take this text as our starting point, then we may wish to say that the relevant theological teaching against which we are to measure our relations to others in the present is not the claim that we will one day share with them in the beatific vision, but the claim that it is possible, metaphysically, that we will do so. The case I develop here could also be formulated in these terms.

Aquinas's discussion of neighbor love falls within his wider account of the nature of the well-lived human life. Following Aristotle, Aquinas supposed, of course, that there are acquired moral virtues, produced by a process of habituation, where the measure of success in our dealings with the world is provided by our human nature. And in keeping with theological tradition, he thought that there are, in addition, theological virtues, which relate the person directly to God. Finally, alongside these two categories of virtue, he is proposing that there are also virtues which relate a person to God indirectly, that is, via their relation to the created world. Distinguishing between the latter two cases, he writes that the theological virtues

. . . are enough to shape us to our supernatural end as a start, that is, to God himself immediately and to none other. Yet the soul needs also to be equipped by infused virtues in regard to created things, though as subordinate to God. (Aquinas, ST 1a2ae 63.3 ad.2)

Let us call these further virtues that enable the person to relate to created things "as subordinate to God" *infused moral virtues*. While Aquinas does not classify neighbor love as an infused moral virtue, it is clear that neighbor love resembles these virtues in being directed at goods which have a hybrid character when compared with the goods of the acquired moral and the theological virtues: that is to say, the goods of the infused moral virtues are like the goods of the acquired moral virtues in so far as they concern the person's relation to the created order, but, at the same time, they are grounded in a God-directed teleology and in this respect resemble the goods of the theological virtues.

So, in brief, the goods of the infused moral virtues and of neighbor love considered as an infused moral virtue are realized in so far as a person succeeds in their relations to the created order (here like the acquired moral virtues), where the measure of success in those relations is provided by relationship to God (here like the theological virtues). The notion of infused moral virtue serves, then, as a conceptual hinge, allowing Aquinas to bring together Aristotle's account of the well-lived human life and the account of the theological virtues that he had inherited from his theological forebears. Let us refer to the goods of the infused moral virtues, therefore, as "hybrid goods" to mark the fact that they concern our relations to created things, where the measure of appropriateness in our dealings with these things is provided by our theological context as disclosed in revelation. As we have seen, appropriateness in this context can be understood in terms of existential congruence rather than causal efficacy. In sum, at the core of the Christian ideal of the spiritual life stands the practice of neighbor love, which is directed at various hybrid goods in so far as it is concerned with our relations to other human beings, here and now, where the measure of success in those relations is provided by the narrative of the beatific vision and, in turn, therefore, by relationship to God.

We have been considering a theological account of spiritual well-being that turns on the idea of hybrid goods and the associated idea that our relations to the world can be more or less appropriate relative to our theological context. Let us consider next the relevance of this general approach for an appreciation of the contribution of aesthetic goods to the spiritual life. Aquinas's account of neighbor love invites us to suppose that a person's thoughts, feelings, attitudes, desires, and behavior are all open to assessment as more or less adequate relative to theological context. But his discussion and standard treatments of the idea of neighbor love do not, so far as I can see, touch on the idea that the quality of a person's perception of the world can also be assessed in these terms. If our perceptual experience can be deemed more or less appropriate on theological grounds, then we will have a further sphere of life in addition to those provided by our behavior, attitudes, and so on within which hybrid goods can in principle be realized. Let us think further about this possibility.

As we have seen in our earlier discussion, in our everyday dealings with the world, some objects stand out as relatively salient while others are consigned to the margins of our awareness. Implied in a given ordering of the perceptual field of this kind is a judgment about what is properly deserving of attention. And accordingly, we can assess patterns of salience in moral and theological terms: a given pattern will be morally appropriate in so far as it affords most prominence to those objects that for moral reasons are most deserving of attention and will be theologically fitting in so far as the salience of objects tracks their importance relative to the relevant theological narrative.

It may be that we can understand the experiences reported by James's converts in these terms. As we have seen, these experiences are not directly of God, so they are capable, in principle, of realizing hybrid goods. For instance, we might suppose that in the convert's experience, the patterns of salience that inform the perceptual field conform to a divinely ordered hierarchy of values, so that what stands out in the perceptual field is what is deserving of attention given the relevant theological truths. To the extent that the world's appearance is so structured, then it will hold up a kind of mirror to the divine mind: the relative significance of objects, as is recorded in the patterns of salience that inform the perceptual field, will match the importance those objects hold from the divine vantage point. This is one way of understanding Jonathan Edwards's comment that, following his conversion, God's wisdom "seemed to appear in everything." Perhaps we can make sense of this remark, at least in part, by supposing that the patterns of salience that are inscribed in the perceptual field can track the relative importance of objects in the divine conception of the world. In such a case, the world as it appears would indeed present a kind of image of the divine wisdom.

In the same sort of way, we might suppose that the perceptual field can more fully image a divine scale of values when the patterns of salience by which it is structured become, in general, bolder or more sharply defined. After all, if the perceptual field is relatively flat, then it will fail to register any significant variation in the importance of objects. And this, we might suppose, must contrast with the divine perspective on the world, which involves, surely, a profound sense of the differentiated significance of things. Accordingly, we might suppose that, in relevant cases, the convert's experience will involve a generalized deepening in the patterns of salience that inform the perceptual field and that, in this way, too, it is possible for the divine wisdom to shine through the appearance of the everyday world.

Perhaps we can give a similar account when thinking about the change in hue that seems to be a recurring feature of conversion reports. As we have seen, these reports speak of the world as seeming brighter following conversion, or as newly "glorified." In this respect, too, it seems that we can assess the appearance of the world as more or less fitting relative to our theological context. For if the world is divinely created, and if it bears in some degree the vestiges of its divine origins, then it might be said that it is, to that extent, only appropriate that it should appear to us as bright or vivid rather than as dull or lacking in lustre.

In these various ways, we can give some content to the idea that a person's experience of the everyday world can, in principle, be judged as more or less adequate relative to their theological context. And if that is right, then hybrid goods can be realized not only in our world-directed thoughts, behavior, and attitudes, but also with respect to the quality of our perception of the sensory world. Moreover, as we have seen, it seems clear that the new appearance of the world following conversion typically has a strongly aesthetic dimension: converts report that the world seems newly beautiful, or newly glorified, or, as James puts the point in his summation of such reports, as "transfigured" or such that "a new heaven seems to shine upon a new earth." In such cases, the alignment between the person's perception of the world and the relevant theological narrative will have an aesthetic dimension. Let us think a little more closely about the nature of the aesthetic goods that arise in such cases.

The newly brightened appearance of the world, as described by converts, could be regarded as beautiful, no doubt, from a purely secular point of view. Similarly, we might think of the bolder, more vivid definition of the contents of the perceptual field as aesthetically pleasing independently of reference to theological considerations. But it is also clear that at least some converts see the world in its post-conversion guise as beautiful because of its participation in the divine beauty or divine glory. Hence Edwards writes that "there seemed to be, as it were, a calm, sweet cast, or appearance of divine glory, in almost everything." And as we have seen, James remarks that the experience can be represented in terms of a new heaven seeming to shine upon a new earth. The language of "glory" also invites the thought that the new-found beauty of the world involves in some way a breaking in of the divine beauty. If we take these reports at face value, as a record of the phenomenology of the relevant experiences, then there is some reason to say that, in the experience of the convert, the world is found to be beautiful because of its perceived relation to a primordial divine beauty. To the extent that these experiences are to be read in these terms, then we should say that this new-found beauty has inherently a theological structure: this experience of beauty consists, at least in part, in material objects appearing as translucent to their divine source. Conceived in these terms, the aesthetic goods that arise in conversion cannot be adequately identified using a purely secular vocabulary since the beauty that is disclosed in such experiences has inherently, from the vantage point of the experiencer, a theological structure.

Once again, we can try to make sense of this possibility by reference to the notions of salience and hue. For instance, as we have seen, we might understand the convert's report that the sensory world appears as diaphanous to the beauty of the divine nature by supposing that their perceptual field now conforms to a divinely ordered scale of values, so that the world as it appears to them images the divine vantage point on the world. If that conformity of the world's appearance to the divine mind is at least a possibility, then we can make some sense of the idea that the divine nature might in some way be disclosed in or, to use a language that is closer to our sources, shine through the appearance of the everyday world. In this way, we can understand how the convert's experience is capable of realizing an aesthetically charged hybrid good: their world-directed experience is now congruent with their theological context because aligned with a divinely ordered scale of values, and, as a result, the divine nature—and the divine beauty—can now shine through the appearance of the everyday world.

It is worth noting that these theologically constituted aesthetic goods are, potentially, both pervasive and deep—pervasive because they can be realized, in principle, whenever we perceive the world, which is to say in much of our experience, and deep because they concern the appropriateness of our lives as perceivers not simply in relation to some finite good or localized context, but with respect to the divine good and our ultimate context. Accordingly, there is some reason to suppose that if they arise at all, then these perceptual hybrid goods will be of fundamental importance for spiritual well-being.

Drawing on the ideal of neighbor love, we have been considering Aquinas's account of the structure of hybrid goods and, in turn, the nature of spiritual well-being, and the ways in which aesthetic experience may contribute to human well-being so conceived. We have yet to examine the implications of this approach for an account of the relationship between hope and aesthetic experience. A full treatment of these matters would require a detailed discussion of Aquinas's conception of faith. We can note at least the main outlines of that conception here. Aquinas is clear that faith (or at least, the right kind of faith: what he calls "formed" faith) is voluntary. (For the distinction between formed and unformed faith, see *Summa Theologiae* 2a2ae 4.3.) And accordingly, belief in the articles of faith, such as the life of the resurrection, is voluntary, rather than the product of a compelling argument of some sort. So the person who orders their life around the realization of those hybrid goods that will be possible if there is a beatific vision is to that extent motivated by hope, rather than by simple belief as conventionally understood. After all, belief as ordinarily understood (for instance, my belief that there is a computer before me now or that Brisbane is the capital of Queensland) cannot be produced at will. So, on this picture, we should say that the Christian— with the aid, of course, of God's grace—chooses to commit themselves to the truth of the doctrine of the beatific vision in a spirit of hope. And accordingly their pursuit of those hybrid goods that will be realizable should the doctrine prove to be true is also grounded in theological hope.

Here, then, is another way of understanding the relationship between hope, the experience of beauty, and spiritual well-being. In brief, for Aquinas, the Christian accepts the idea of the beatific vision and the other elements of the Christian story in a spirit of hope. And this commitment in turn grounds their pursuit of those hybrid goods that will be realizable should the Christian story hold true. And these goods, I have been suggesting (here extending Aquinas's own account), include, in principle, not only behavioral and attitudinal but also perceptual and aesthetic goods, which arise in so far as the appearance of the everyday world is congruent with the relevant theological narrative. In the case of conversion experience, we can bring these themes together by supposing that when the believer takes the sensory world to be transparent to the divine beauty, they commit themselves thereby, in a spirit of hope, to the truth of the idea of divine glory.

We have been examining three methodologically diverse accounts of the relationship between hope, the experience of beauty, and spiritual well-being. In conclusion, let us consider more closely how these approaches compare with one another and what the contribution of each might be.

Comparing Empirical and Theological Perspectives on Hope, the Experience of Beauty, and Spiritual Well-Being

Let us begin by considering the nature of spiritual well-being, starting with the perspective of William James. In the *Varieties* as more generally, James is writing most fundamentally as a psychologist. And the values and disvalues which he discusses in the *Varieties* can all be identified, I suggest, in psychological terms. The sick man suffers from a state of practical disorientation and an impoverishment of his perceptual world. And, conversely, the person who enjoys a state of well-being is practically oriented and experiences the world as colored rather than gray and contoured rather than flat. These accounts of well-being or lack of well-being do not depend on any metaphysical story: a psychological vocabulary and reference to what is manifest directly in experience will suffice to pick out the relevant goods and bads.

Of course, James does allow that the holding of a religious worldview can make a difference to well-being, but for him the role of a worldview seems to be simply to provide a way of framing our relationship to the world, which in turn will enable our practical and perceptual engagement with our sensory environment: on this view, therefore, religious states of affairs do not feature as constituents of well-being. Instead beliefs about such states of affairs can serve as enablers of well-being, and those beliefs can play this role whether or not they are true. So while he is concerned with the contribution of religious commitment to spiritual well-being, James's approach is to this extent psychological: his interest is in the connection between a person's framing beliefs and the way the world appears to them, and for this purpose it is of no consequence whether or not those beliefs are true.

By contrast, on the Thomistic view of spiritual well-being, we cannot specify the relevant goods—what I have been calling hybrid goods—independently of reference to the appropriate theological narrative. Why not? Because here the goods consist in the alignment between the person's world-directed thoughts, activity, and (to take the case that has been of particular concern to us) perception of the everyday world, on the one side, and a given theological narrative, on the other. So, on this account, it matters that the relevant theological narrative should be true. For example, in our account of the ways in which perceptual states may in part constitute hybrid goods, we have appealed to theological claims such as these: the world is created; from the divine perspective, creatures carry a clearly differentiated significance; and the divine nature is glorious. And hybrid goods will arise in so far as a person's world-directed thought, activity, and so on are congruent with the states of affairs recorded in these and other doctrinal claims. And in turn, therefore, these goods cannot be identified, at least not in terms of their fundamental nature, independently of reference to theological context.

For some perceptual hybrid goods, the person's experience need not extend to any item picked out in the relevant theological narrative. Suppose, for instance, that a person's experience of the world is contoured rather than flat. Even if that experience has no religious content, then it will to that extent realize a hybrid good since it will then conform to the divine assessment of the significance of creatures for the reasons we have discussed. The kind of experience described by, among others, Jonathan Edwards is rather different in this respect: here, it seems to the subject of the experience that the divine wisdom is presented to them in perceptual terms. So in this case, it is not just that the appearance of the world is theologically appropriate: in addition, the congruence between the world's appearance and the relevant theological truth is revealed directly to the person in experience. (Here I simply presuppose that the presentation of a theological truth in experience is reason enough for thinking of the experience as congruent with that truth.)

In sum, the practical and perceptual benefits that provide the focus for James's account of spiritual well-being may perhaps be induced by adopting a religious worldview, but they can obtain independently of the truth of any such worldview and can be identified independently of reference to any such worldview. By contrast, on Aquinas's view, spiritual well-being involves in large part hybrid goods. So on this approach, spiritual well-being requires, to this extent, the truth of the relevant theological narratives and cannot be identified independently of such narratives. Naturally, Diessner's understanding of well-being shares the psychological focus of James's account. As we have seen from his discussion of hope, he thinks of well-being as including "academic success, athletic achievement, various forms of social development, as well as the development of optimism and general happiness." Diessner does not include religious commitments in this list but, from his perspective, they could presumably play a Jamesian kind of role in contributing to well-being so understood.

So, in general terms, our discussion points to a basic distinction between empirical and theological approaches to the nature of well-being. As described here, both are concerned with well-being that is realized here and now in our relations to the everyday world, but, by contrast with empirical approaches, the theological perspective that we have been sketching is committed to the transcendent dimension of some of the relevant goods. It is worth emphasizing that these accounts are not in competition with one another to the extent that one and the same state of affairs may realize both kinds of good. On the Thomistic view that we have been considering here, the goods that are the province of psychology can be conceptualized in broadly Aristotelian terms, and hybrid goods do not disrupt those Aristotelian goods since they are concerned with a further kind of significance that can attach to our everyday activities, in addition to Aristotelian kinds of significance.

Hence, for example, a brightened perceptual field can count as good both as a psychological state and because of its contribution to a hybrid good. To put the point in the form of a general principle—here borrowing a remark from Aquinas (ST 1a 1.8 ad 2)—we may say that on this approach "grace does not destroy nature but perfects it."

So far, we have been considering empirical and theological perspectives on the nature of well-being. To conclude, let us note how these different kinds of source understand the relationship between the two constituents of well-being with which we have been concerned here, namely, hope and aesthetic experience.

As we have seen, Diessner's paper investigates the possibility that beauty experience and hope are correlated. Since this is an empirical study, the underlying assumption seems to be that any connection between the two will not turn out to be simply analytic. I have suggested that there is some reason to think that the connection that emerges in the study reflects at least in part an analytic connection between the tendency to engage with moral beauty, as understood here, and hope, but. bracketing that point, Diessner's kind of enquiry invites us to proceed on the assumption that while hope and beauty experience may be correlated, and one may be the cause of the other, each can be understood without reference to the other. By contrast, on James's view, as we have developed it here, there is a tighter connection between hope and the appearance of the everyday world. If I am to have the kind of practical hope that James describes, then I must have some sense of the differentiated significance of the objects in my environment, where this sense is realized in the perceptual field in so far as it is structured and colored. In the absence of such hope, there will be no such differentiation. So, on this view, hope of a certain kind seems to be a prerequisite for the world appearing as other than flat and gray, and hope is therefore a prerequisite for beauty experience, even if it is not of itself sufficient for beauty experience.

On the Thomistic account that we have been developing, there is again a broadly conceptual connection between some kinds of beauty experience and hope. Some hybrid goods can be realized even if the person does not recognize as much: for instance, if the perceptual field is contoured rather than flat, then it will to that extent realize a hybrid good—it will to that extent be theologically appropriate—whether or not the subject of the experience subscribes to or even has any knowledge of the relevant theological narrative. However, as we have seen, the conversion experiences that are cited by James seem to have a different character. Here, key elements of the relevant theological narrative are presented to the person in their experience of the world: for instance, it may seem to the person that the divine glory is made manifest in their experience of the world. If we adopt a Thomistic reading of these cases, then we should say that a theological narrative is the object of the person's hope and at the same time presented to them in the world's appearance. And as we have seen, in such cases, the aesthetic dimension of the person's experience has inherently a theological structure: the experience is one of the divine wisdom or glory shining through the appearance of the everyday world. Given this Thomistic approach, we could say that in such cases, the person's hope in the truth of the relevant theological narrative takes perceptual form in an experience of the beauty of the world. That is, the person's hopeful commitment to the truth of the relevant theological narrative is realized not only in a purely mental attitude of assent to the narrative, but also in their taking their experience of the world to be a manifestation of the divine glory, divine wisdom, or some other divine attribute.

So our three accounts furnish three perspectives on the nature of the connection between hope and beauty experience. Diessner's social psychological account invites us to think of beauty experience and hope as extrinsically related. On this approach, it is for empirical study to uncover any association between the two. James's account suggests that beauty experience, in so far as it depends on our finding the world perceptually engaging, is rooted in the state of being practically hopeful in our relationship with the world, where that state is realized, at least in part, in the color and structure of the perceptual field. Here, the relationship between hopefulness and beauty experience is, we might say, existential: to find the world practically or existentially meaningful is to take the objects in our environment to bear a differentiated significance, where that sense of variation in significance is inscribed in the perceptual field, which in turn makes it possible for the world to stand as an object of aesthetic appreciation. Last, on the Thomistic approach we have been considering, the connection between beauty experience and hope will sometimes reflect their common object: here, the theological narrative that is the object of the person's hope is presented in experience so that hope takes on a perceptual form. In this case, the connection between hope and beauty experience is tighter still than in James's account: beauty experience is now a mode of hopeful engagement with the world.

Finally, it is notable that these three perspectives also carry different therapeutic implications. Diessner takes his study to support the idea of "beauty intervention" as a way of building up a person's hope. James's account appears to run in the other direction: it is only the person of hope who can experience the world as practically and perceptually meaningful and who is open therefore to encountering it as an object of aesthetic appreciation. On this view, therapeutic intervention might most naturally begin with the question of how to shape the framing assumptions that a person brings to experience. Finally, on a Thomistic perspective, it is less clear that there is any kind of priority. For instance, it may be that the convert's newly hopeful attitude toward the world and newly hopeful attitude toward the relevant theological narrative are realized, at least in part, in their new experience of the world as beautiful. But equally on this approach, there may be some sense in following James in trying to cultivate the relevant kinds of hope or in following Diessner and seeking to develop the requisite kinds of perceptual sensitivity.

In sum, what we might term the social-psychological, existential-psychological, and theological perspectives can each speak to the question of the nature of spiritual well-being and the question of how the constituent elements of well-being—such as hope and openness to beauty—may be related to one another. These various accounts need not be in competition with one another. In particular, we might reasonably regard the Jamesian and Thomistic perspectives as proposing a deepening of the kinds of insight that are available in social psychological studies by moving beyond the idea that the relationship between the constituent elements of spiritual well-being is simply extrinsic and showing how that connection can be grounded in existential and theological kinds of significance. And, in the same way, we might think of the Thomistic perspective as offering, in conceptual terms, a deepening of the Jamesian approach in so far as it represents beauty experience of the relevant kind as a case of hopeful engagement with the world rather than seeing hopeful engagement as simply one of the background conditions for beauty experience.

About the Author

Mark R. Wynn is the Nolloth Professor of the Philosophy of the Christian Religion at the University of Oxford. He is the author of *Spiritual Traditions and the Virtues: Living Between Heaven and Earth* (Oxford University Press, 2020) and *Renewing the Senses: A Study of the Philosophy and Theology of the Spiritual Life* (Oxford University Press, 2013).

Author Note

I am grateful to the Editors for their most helpful comments on a draft of this chapter. I would also like to thank the John Templeton Foundation and St. Louis University for providing a grant to support the research for the paper as part of the project Happiness and Well-Being: Integrating Research Across the Disciplines, which ran from 2015 to 2018. Additional support was provided by the John Templeton Foundation and by the Lee Kum Sheung Center for Health and Happiness. The views expressed in this chapter represent the perspective of the author and do not reflect the opinions or endorsement of any organization. I have no known conflict of interest to disclose. Correspondence concerning this chapter should be directed to Mark Wynn, mark.wynn@oriel.ox.ac.uk.

References

Aquinas, T. (1947). *Summa theologica*. (Fathers of the English Dominican Province Tr.). New York: Benziger Brothers.

Bell, C. (1913). *Art*. New York: F. A. Stokes.

Cottingham, J. (2009). *Why believe?* London: Continuum.

Diessner, R., Solom, R., Frost, N., Parsons, L., & Davidson, J. (2008). Engagement with beauty: Appreciating natural, artistic and moral beauty. *Journal of Psychology, 142*(3), 303–329.

Diessner, R., Rust, T., Solom, R. C., Frost, N., & Parsons, L. (2006). Beauty and hope: A moral beauty intervention. *Journal of Moral Education, 35*(3), 301–317.

James, W. (1896/1948). The will to believe. In James, W. (Ed.), *Essays in pragmatism* (pp. 88–109). New York: Hafner Press.

James, W. (1902). *The varieties of religious experience: A study in human nature*. London: Longman, Green & Co.

Sherry, P. (2002). *Spirit and beauty: An introduction to theological aesthetics*. London: SCM.

Snyder, C. R., Harris, C., Anderson, J. R., Holleran, S. A., Irving, L. M., Sigmon, S. T., . . . Harney, P. (1991). The will and the ways: Development and validation of an individual differences measure of hope. *Journal of Personality and Social Psychology, 60*(4), 570–585.

Wielenberg, E. (2005). *Value and virtue in a Godless universe*. Cambridge: Cambridge University Press.

Wolterstorff, N. (2004). Art and the aesthetic: The religious dimension. In Kivy, P. (Ed.), *The Blackwell guide to aesthetics* (chapter 18). Oxford: Blackwell.

PART 3

ADVANCING
THE CONVERSATION
ABOUT MEASUREMENT

12

The Comprehensive Measure of Meaning

Psychological and Philosophical Foundations

Jeffrey A. Hanson and Tyler J. VanderWeele

Abstract

The topic of meaning has been of interest both in philosophy and psychology. The psychology research community has put forward a number of instruments to measure meaning. Considerable debate has taken place within philosophy on the objective versus subjective status of meaning in life and on the global versus individual or personal aspects of meaning. Here, we make use of an emerging consensus in the psychology literature concerning a tripartite structure of meaning as cognitive *coherence*, affective *significance*, and motivational *direction*. However, we enrich this understanding with important distinctions drawn from the philosophical literature to distinguish subdomains within this tripartite understanding. We use the relevant philosophical distinctions to classify existing measurement items into a seven-fold structure intended to more comprehensively assess an individual's sense of meaning. The proposed measure, with three items in each subdomain drawn from previous scales, constitutes what we put forward as the Comprehensive Measure of Meaning. We hope that this measure will enrich the empirical research on the assessment of, and on the causes and effects of, having a sense of meaning.

Meaning is now widely recognized as essential to human well-being, and numerous studies have documented the association between perceived meaningfulness and a host of improved psychological benefits. Meaning in life might be understood as *having a sense of the greater context of the importance or value of one's life and actions and of life in general.* Baumeister (1991) has argued that a meaningful life may be compatible in significant ways with

Jeffrey A. Hanson and Tyler J. VanderWeele, *The Comprehensive Measure of Meaning* In: *Measuring Well-Being.* Edited by: Matthew T. Lee, Laura D. Kubzansky, and Tyler J. VanderWeele, Oxford University Press (2021). © Oxford University Press. DOI: 10.1093/oso/9780197512531.003.0013 being unhappy, but a happy life is impossible without meaning. He shows at some length how a sense of meaning supports happiness, with considerable evidence drawn from contemporary psychological research (pp. 214–218). Similarly, Steger (2009) provides a thorough catalogue of studies that have shown that "people who believe their lives have meaning or purpose appear to be better off," including by being happier; enjoying greater overall well-being; and reporting higher life satisfaction, control over their lives, and work satisfaction. They also experience less negative affect, depression (see also Chen, Kim, Koh, Frazier, & VanderWeele, 2019; Mascaro & Rosen, 2005; and, for depression and posttraumatic stress see Owens, Steger, Whitesell, & Herrera, 2009), anxiety, workaholism, suicidal ideation (see also Heisel & Flett, 2004), substance abuse, and need for therapy. These benefits are also relatively stable and independent from other forms of well-being when tracked over the course of a year (p. 680). Finally, Heintzelman and King (2014a) canvass additional evidence that "self-reports of meaning in life are associated with higher quality of life, especially with age, superior self-reported health, and decreased mortality" (p. 561) with yet further evidence from a recent meta-analysis that a sense of purpose in life is associated with better physical health and greater longevity (Cohen, Bavishi, & Rozanski, 2016).

The importance of meaning in life is no longer in dispute in psychological research. As the topic has gained traction, thanks in part to the advent of positive psychology as a transformative movement within the discipline, the question of meaning in life as a matter of philosophic research and investigation has undergone a parallel revival in analytic, Anglo-American discourse after decades of neglect (Adams, 2002; Hepburn, 1966; Metz, 2002; Wiggins, 1976). That neglect is largely attributable to the dominance of *logical positivism*, according to which the very question of the meaning of life is incoherent, as meaning was conceived as a strictly semantic phenomenon. With the collapse of logical positivism's hegemony, the question of the meaning of life has migrated into new terrain. Most English-speaking philosophers writing on the subject today do so under the conviction that meaning is not merely a feature of sentences but a feature of the sort of value human lives can have (Cottingham, 2003; Landau, 2017; Metz, 2002, 2013; Thomson, 2003; Wolf, 2010, 2015). This feature of value is widely agreed to be irreducible to either happiness (which is often conceived hedonically) or moral worth (which is conceived in a variety of ways that are compatible with a life also being called meaningful). Given the broad consensus shared in both psychological and philosophical discourses on the value and importance of meaning, one urgent challenge to psychological research on meaning is how to measure it.

The philosophical discussion may be able to lend yet further assistance to psychological research. Because the issue of meaning is being rediscovered in a discourse that prizes analytical precision, rigorous distinctions, and clarity of terms, philosophical categorizations can bring some valuable clarity to social science investigation. Past and persistent conceptual ambiguities and conflations of terms have already been decried in a number of important studies (George & Park, 2016; Heintzelman & King, 2014a; Martela & Steger, 2016), and in this chapter we draw on philosophical distinctions to resolve some of these problems, at least when it comes to measuring meaning. This volume is concerned with measuring well-being, one element of which is meaning (Ryff, 1989; Su, Tay, & Diener, 2014; VanderWeele, 2017). Our proposed measure, the Comprehensive Measure of Meaning (CMM), is primarily intended to incorporate the results of philosophical discussion into an established framework coming to predominate the psychological literature on measuring meaning. Future work will assess the psychometric properties of the measure. The CMM principally makes use of a wide variety of items, or their adaptation, already employed in previous scales, but it categorizes these in ways consistent with important distinctions derived from the philosophical literature. We proceed in three parts. In the first section, we discuss shortcomings in previous measures of meaning devised by psychological methods. A reader interested only in the CMM itself could skip to the second part, where we explain the emerging consensus that is forming in the psychological literature around a tripartite conception of meaning measurement comprising coherence, significance, and direction. In the third part, we exposit the CMM, showing how it uses this emerging consensus but introduces new and more discriminating distinctions within it inspired by philosophical discussions to make our instrument the most comprehensive and targeted yet devised.

Existing Measures of Meaning

The attempt to measure meaningfulness has its own history, to which we now turn. The earliest instruments currently regarded as relevant to measuring meaning were in fact restricted in scope to investigations of purpose, a target widely regarded in contemporary psychological literature and research as merely one component of meaningfulness as a whole. Most frequently used in empirical research among these early surveys is the Purpose in Life (PIL) test (Bronk, 2014, p. 22; Crumbaugh & Maholick, 1964). The PIL test, while widely used and critically studied (Crumbaugh, 1968; Pinquart, 2002, p. 96), has also received sustained and repeated criticisms, often in the context of justifications for the implementation of new measures. Many of the items on the PIL seem to have more to do with life satisfaction or enthusiasm levels than purposefulness (e.g., "My life is: empty, filled only with despair/running over with exciting things"; "I am usually: bored/enthusiastic"). Steger, Frazier, Oishi, and Kaler (2006) point out that items like these, as well as "I feel really good about my life," "could tap any number of constructs aside from meaning, such as mood" (p. 81). A comparable concern is raised by Damon, Menon, and Bronk (2003), who also question the PIL's treatment of "meaning" and "purpose" as synonyms (p. 122), a distinction the CMM, like some recent others (George & Park, 2017), seeks to uphold because purpose is now viewed as just one subconstruct belonging to meaning, with purpose being more end-directed and meaning concerning an understanding of the greater context. Likewise the PIL's inclusion of an item concerning the attractiveness of suicide seems distracting and at best tangential to the issue of purpose (Steger et al., 2006, p. 81). Yalom (1980) in particular lodged a criticism against the PIL (despite its use in more than 50 PhD dissertations by that time) to this effect: "Although, for example, life satisfaction or consideration of suicide may be related to meaning in life, they are even more obviously related to other psychological states—most notably depression" (p. 456). Yalom argued that the PIL suffered from "substantial, indeed devastating" conceptual confusion, lack of methodological explanation, and ambiguity in item terminology (pp. 456–457), yet he reluctantly conceded that the instrument was (then) "the only game in town" (p. 457).

Ebersole and Quiring claimed (1989) to have confirmed a modest social desirability correlation with PIL scores alleged in a much earlier unpublished study as well as suspected by reviewers of the PIL (Domino, 1972; Yalom, 1980, p. 456), while remaining agnostic as to whether this correlation should be regarded as confounding the results of the PIL (Ebersole & Quiring, p. 306). Dyck (1987) raised a potential objection to the PIL on the grounds that it was fashioned with two sets of criteria in view: existential relevance and patient discriminability. These criteria depended, somewhat vaguely, on what Crumbaugh and Maholick called a "background in the literature of existentialism, particularly in *logotherapy*, and a guess as to what type of material would discriminate patients from nonpatients" (1964, p. 201), but the criteria sets' independence from or dependence upon one another was unknown (Dyck, 1987, p. 441). Moreover, Dyck pointed out that the PIL does not convincingly pick out a distinct pathology but rather seems to correlate significantly with absence of depression (p. 442; Frazier, Oishi, & Steger, 2003, p. 257). This confusion is a particular problem for the precepts of the logotherapeutic approach relied upon by the PIL's authors, according to which lack of purpose is a pathology in its own right referred to as "noogenic neurosis" (Crumbaugh & Maholick, 1964; Garfield, 1973). Additional studies designed to ascertain whether depression and low purpose in life as measured by the PIL were indistinguishable from each other seemed to indicate that the two are not factorially independent (Dyck, 1987; Reker & Cousins, 1979). As early as 1972, Braun questioned the discriminant validity of the PIL, and, as recently as 2004, Schulenberg (2004) found a −0.70 correlation between PIL scores and Outcome Questionnaire (OQ) Symptomatic Functioning subscale scores, which are meant to assess symptomatic problems relating to anxiety, depression, and substance abuse. In sum, multiple studies finding "different, multiple factor structures" have left unclear "the underlying structure of the PIL," which the authors never specified in the first place (Frazier et al., 2003, p. 258; see also Chamberlain & Zika, 1988; McGregor & Little, 1998; Reker & Cousins, 1979). Furthermore, while the PIL aspires to value-neutrality, qualitative research undertaken by C. A. Garfield (1973) caused him to lodge an objection against the PIL that its core concepts were perceived in radically different ways by different groups within a diverse sampling of test-takers. While it was apparent to him that the PIL measured differences in perceived purpose, the way to understand purpose was so different in different demographics that the results were not entirely reliable. "Cultural contamination," Garfield contended, was high (p. 403), leading him to conclude that "there is reasonable doubt as to the consistency of the meanings of test items across subcultural groups" (p. 405). Finally, since the PIL uses different words or phrases for anchors across each of its different items, confusion on the part of respondents seems almost unavoidable (Bronk, 2014, p. 25; Schulenberg, 2004, p. 480). Whether the scale anchors (which vary from item to item) were truly bipolar has also been questioned. For instance, the PIL posits that "wanting to have 'nine more lives just like this one'" is the opposite of "prefer[ring] never to have been born," an odd dichotomy (Edwards, 2007, p. 49). Because we are convinced that purpose is a subset of meaning and further persuaded that the PIL suffers from significant problems despite its apparently generally acceptable psychometric properties (Bronk, 2014, p. 24; Schulenberg, 2004, pp. 479–480) we largely avoided using PIL items for the CMM.

In the almost 40 years since Yalom sharply critiqued the PIL, not only have his concerns been echoed, but a variety of instruments with similar aims to the PIL also have been introduced. Crumbaugh himself devised a companion instrument to the PIL, the Seeking of Noetic Goals (SONG) test, which was meant to assess the search for meaning or perceived absence of it rather than the presence of achieved meaning. SONG scores however were not shown to be reliably inversely proportional to PIL scores (Bronk, 2014, p. 27), and the test was accused of conceptual inconsistency and compounding rather than reducing the problem of overlap between the pathological noogenic neurosis that PIL was meant to diagnose versus depression (Dyck, 1987, p. 445). Finally, in the decades since the introduction of the SONG, it has become apparent on the basis of numerous studies that the relationship between perceived presence of meaning and perceived absence is considerably more complex than Crumbaugh theorized (Schulenberg, Baczwaski, & Buchanan, 2014, p. 695). Of particular importance here is Heintzelman and King's conclusion that if the need for meaning is a fundamental one for human beings, then it would stand to reason that searching for meaning would be compatible with perceived meaning being already present in the subject. "If meaning in life is a central human motivation," they suggest, "then even in the presence of meaning, the desire for meaning might persist" (Heintzelman & King, 2014a, p. 570). Despite some early enthusiasm for the potential of combining the PIL and SONG in research and clinical settings (Reker & Cousins, 1979), serious objections have been raised, and the SONG test has rarely been used for research (Steger et al., 2006; p. 81); only one of its items appears in the CMM.

G. T. Reker (Reker & Peacock, 1981) claimed to have confirmed the complementary nature of the PIL and SONG (p. 264) and, on the basis of the judgment that together these two instruments provided evidence for a multidimensional life attitude construct (consisting in fact of "10 interpretable independent dimensions" [p. 264]), sought to consolidate the two measures into one "single reliable and valid instrument that would measure the multidimensional nature of attitudes toward life" (p. 264). The result was the Life Attitude Profile (LAP), which originally encompassed 56 items and was later slightly abbreviated to a still arguably cumbersome 48 items (Bronk, pp. 27–28; Erci, 2008; Reker & Peacock, 1981). The LAP is therefore like the PIL and SONG in being inspired by Frankl's conception of existential meaning (Frankl, 1984), and it aimed to consolidate rather than challenge this basic inspiration. The most serious defect in the LAP is shared by its predecessors: namely, that these instruments assess a number of constructs perhaps related to meaning but not perceived meaning as such. "The LAP would appear to have inherited these problems along with the PIL items it incorporated" (Frazier et al., 2003, p. 260). The LAP also repeats SONG items like "I feel the need for adventure and 'new worlds to conquer'" and "I hope for something exciting in the future," sentiments that seem more like indications of present dissatisfaction or escapist impulses rather than a search for meaning per se. As Frazier et al. (2003) point out, "a theoretical basis for incorporating death concerns was not explicated," (p. 258) other than a breezy declaration by the instrument authors that "death concerns are a part of life" (Reker & Peacock, 1981, p. 264). The LAP also betrays a distaste for boredom, featuring reverse-coded items like "Life to me seems boring and uneventful." Again, a question could be raised here as to whether an item like this truly targets perceived meaning. Heintzelman and King (2014b) have shown for example that "natural regularity and routines and patterns" as well as "mundane habits" constitute an underappreciated source of meaning in many people's lives (p. 157). These recent findings correct a long-standing bias in the philosophical and psychological literature toward excitement, novelty, and stimulus, as if meaning can only be found in "profound events" (p. 158) or "highly vivid" (p. 157) moments rather than ordinary ones. Many early measures of meaning share in this bias, disfavoring ordinary and routine activities as if these were an impediment rather than an aid to meaningful living.

The Life Regard Index (LRI) was created in large part to address concerns that the PIL (and by implication the LAP) is too value-loaded. The authors raise for particular concern the fact that "the PIL implies that the more someone sees himself as responsible and the more he perceives his life to be under his own control, the greater his degree of positive life regard" (Battista & Almond, 1973, p. 411). On the basis of this observation, they conclude that "Although these are interesting hypotheses to be tested, it is not clear *a priori* that the experience of one's life as meaningful is related to these beliefs" (p. 411). While Battista and Almond distinguish what they call positive life regard from perceived meaningfulness, and they intend to measure the former rather than the latter, the point that the PIL is biased toward responsibility, control, and autonomy as ingredients of perceived meaning or purpose is one worth considering. Eschewing what they called "philosophical" theories about the meaning of life, the authors tried to develop what they view as a value-free or relativistic approach, one that would allow for greater latitude in respondents' thinking about what constitutes meaningful living. In furtherance of that end, Battista and Almond end up jettisoning the term "meaningful life" in favor of "positive life regard," in their words "to avoid any confusion and conflicting definitions" (p. 410). The LRI then is meant to be agnostic about which systems of beliefs can serve as a potentially fulfilling framework and open to the fact that many such systems are capable of potentially providing such fulfillment (p. 414).

Debats, van der Lubbe, and Wezeman (1993) confirmed that these intentions for the LRI are successfully attained in their study (p. 344), and they document other studies with positive results for clinical use of the LRI (p. 338). Chamberlain and Zika (1988), however, were more skeptical about whether the purported structure of the LRI, which the authors intended to comprise two factors—framework and fulfillment—actually holds up under second-order analysis (p. 595). Reker and Wong (1988) also raised concerns that positive life-regard is in fact not reducible to meaning but is instead closely related to self-esteem (p. 235) ("Other people seem to feel better about their lives than I do"). This is a serious concern given that previously devised instruments have also been repeatedly criticized for failing to target a specific construct of meaningfulness rather than positive affect or some other closely related construct of a similar sort, like absence of depression. Edwards (2007) also registers a drawback, to the effect that the LRI's items are repetitive (p. 52) and no explanation was given about their derivation or selection (p. 51). Suspicions that positive life regard has more to do with affect or self-esteem rather than meaning per se remain though. Morgan and Farsides (2009) mention that the LRI's "multi-dimensionality at the second-order level implies that it may also tap content that is peripheral to the meaning in life construct" (p. 199). In a largely appreciative revisiting of the LRI, Debats (1998) nevertheless concluded that "several studies showed that LRI scores correlated most significantly with scores on various well-being measures," a point that counts in favor of the clinical relevance of perceived meaning (p. 256). However, predictably, this means that the direction of causality cannot be determined without longitudinal study (p. 256). Furthermore, Debats draws attention to evidence suggesting that subjects from different cultural backgrounds score differently than predicted on the LRI, again implying a possible bias (pp. 255–256).

In the end though, we agree with Battista and Almond that empirical testing should discriminate between formulae of a single, "philosophical" meaning of life and relativistic, plural conceptions. While they prefer the latter, and we agree that this is bound to be the preferred approach for social science research, they concede that "the contention of philosophical theories that there is a 'higher' or 'ultimate' meaning to life is especially challenging to the relativistic perspective," and they call for further critical examination of the assumptions underlying both positions (p. 425). Similarly, Debats makes the crucial point that "the conceptual framework from which the LRI was derived views personal meaning as essentially a subjective, personal experience" (p. 256). This could stand in fact as a critique of all the measures canvassed so far. Continuing with Debats's important point, "there is as yet no final resolution to the debate about the relative weight that *objective* (moral) and *subjective* (experiential) criteria should have in determining what essentially constitutes 'personal meaning'" (p. 256). It may be objected that social scientific investigation cannot resolve this debate, and we take the point. However, the question of objective versus subjective sources of meaning in life is one that is very much alive in contemporary philosophical discussions (Metz, 2013; Wolf, 2010, 2015), and we think it crucial to investigate at least people's perceptions of the objective value of their endeavors as a potential source of perceived meaning. Our measure cannot provide evidence for the strength of any one philosophical theory of the meaning of life or for the genuine objective value of the sources of people's perceived meaning in life (no measure could), but it does seek to document respondents' perception that such philosophical theories have an influence on their lives and that their activities are objectively valuable. We will return to the impact that this view had on our shaping of the CMM in the final section of this chapter.

Further refinements that the CMM employs were derived from insights provided by Morgan and Farsides (2009) in their development of the Meaningful Life Measure (MLM). Speaking of the PIL, LRI, and Ryff's Psychological Well-Being scales, they write that "an additional problem with all three scales is that they variously include items with multiple content domains or potentially confounding clauses (e.g. 'I have some goals or aims that would personally give me a great deal of satisfaction if I could accomplish them'; 'If I should die today, I would feel that life has been very worthwhile'; 'I feel good when I think of what I've done in the past, and what I hope to do in the future')" (p. 199) or, similarly from Ryff (1989), the negatively worded item, "I live life one day at a time and don't really think about the future." We have sought likewise to abstain from using items with this level of potentially confusing complexity. Similarly, we follow Morgan and Farsides in their observation that many items in common use assess a sense of life's meaning as being contingent on some other factor like acceptance of death, and so we have foregone items that seem to depend on some other factor. That being said, the MLM still largely draws on PIL and LRI for its items, and thus once more potential problems persist. In addition to the reservations already surveyed, MacDonald, Wong, and Gingras (2012) point out that the MLM is too narrow to be a comprehensive measure of the meaning construct because it is focused almost entirely on purpose. As we will soon see, purpose is indeed a vital component of the meaning construct, but it is only a component according to the emerging consensus around measuring meaningfulness. Some of the more recent scales (e.g. Krause, 2004; George & Park, 2017; Steger et al., 2006), discussed further later, arguably do accurately target meaningfulness. However, as will be argued in the third part of this chapter, none yet does so with the precision, finer distinctions, and breadth that will be possible in the CMM (George & Park, 2017, p. 615).

Emerging Consensus

In the past several years, broad agreement has been achieved in the conceptualization of perceived meaning. It is now widely considered essential to capture cognitive, affective, and motivational aspects of perceived meaning. The first subconstruct, sometimes called *coherence*, refers to *the intellectual perception that one's life, values, and relation to the world express an intelligible pattern and are part of a context or narrative that makes sense of one's existence or existence in general.* The second subconstruct, sometimes called *significance*, refers to *a sense of importance or value in one's having existed and/or in one's activities and pursuits.* Finally, the third subconstruct, which we will call *direction*, refers to *having objectives that help direct, prioritize, and make sense of choices, goals, and actions.* This third subconstruct is often referred to as "purpose," but for reasons we describe later, we prefer "direction." These components were hammered out in their present shape at least as early as Reker and Wong's 1988 article "Aging as an Individual Process." There the authors describe first a "*cognitive component* [that] has to do with making sense of one's experiences in life;" second a "*motivational component* . . . [that]

refers to the value system constructed by each individual [where] values are essentially guides for living, dictating what goals we pursue and how we live our lives"; and third, an "*affective component*" that captures the "feelings of satisfaction and fulfillment" that accompany "the realization of personal meaning" (pp. 220–221). This threefold schema builds on an earlier definition of meaning as "cognizance of order, coherence and purpose in one's existence, the pursuit and attainment of worthwhile goals, and an accompanying sense of fulfillment" (p. 357; Reker & Wong, 1988, p. 221).

Hicks and King (2009) note that motivational and cognitive components have been taken into account by previous psychological definitions of meaning in life. Expanding on this base and moving in the direction of a tripartite understanding of meaning, the authors offer what they call an "expansive conceptual definition: 'Lives may be experienced as meaningful when they are felt to have significance beyond the trivial or momentary, to have purpose, or to have a coherence that transcends chaos'" (p. 641). Here again we find a broad conceptual definition that seeks to account for an affective component to do with felt significance, a motivational sense of purpose, and a cognitive grasp on coherence. Concentrating on what they take to have been the least explored of these three subconstructs, affective significance, they show how perceptions of meaning are distinguishable from positive affect or happiness (p. 646), with which the affective subconstruct of meaning might otherwise be confused.

Steger (2012a) by contrast focuses attention on cognitive coherence and motivational purpose, speaking of the former as a source for generating the latter, a defensible interpretation that has some support in the literature (see Wong, 1998, p. 405, fig. 19.1). On Steger's analysis, the cognitive component of meaning grounds us in our life experiences, coalescing memories into a continuous narrative, articulating theories about how the world around us operates, and testing theories about how we are perceived by others. The cognitive component thus facilitates integrating new experiences into a web of extant associations, increasing a sense of integration and unified coherence across the self and its wide-ranging experiences. This cognitive basis provides a foundation for assigning value to desirable pursuits and aspirations, which in turn give rise to goals and plans to accomplish in service of larger aims. In this way, he explains how the meaning construct differs from related phenomena. By uniting the cognitive and motivational domains, meaning controls a number of other important subsidiary processes of assigning value and shaping decision-making (p. 166). Steger's work thoroughly documents the many positive correlations between high meaning in life and various other markers of psychological and sociological well-being (pp. 167–175).

Heintzelman and King (2014b) explore in some depth the cognitive component, but they affirm the threefold distinction as comprehensive and clear as well as being increasingly employed in the literature. The three common themes they identify are "purpose (i.e., goal direction), significance (i.e., mattering), and coherence (i.e., the presence of reliable connections)" (p. 154). Citing the earlier definition offered by Steger (2012a), they highlight with underlining and parenthetical italicized insertions the terminology he chooses as picking out the same three themes that they argue form the core of an increasingly popular exhaustive understanding of meaning: "Meaning is the web of *connections, understandings,* and *interpretations* that help us *comprehend* our experience (*coherence*) and *formulate plans directing our energies* to the achievement of our *desired future* (*purpose*). Meaning provides us with the sense that *our lives matter* (*significance*), that they *make sense* (*coherence*), and *that they are more than the sum* of our seconds, days, and years (*significance*)" (p. 154, quoted from Steger, 2012a, p. 165).

Martela and Steger (2016) undertake a similar act of editorializing when they quote from King, Hicks, Krull, and Del Gaiso (2006) and add numerals to pick out what they take to be the implicit tripartite structure of King et al.'s definition: "Lives may be experienced as meaningful when [1] they are felt to have significance beyond the trivial or momentary, [2] to have purpose, or [3] to have a coherence that transcends chaos" (p. 531, quoted from King et al., 2006, p. 180). The only further modification that might be desirable in this particular quote is that the word "or" before the numeral "3" might be changed to "and," a grammatical move that would more nearly reflect the current thinking on meaning as a threefold structure. In Martela and Steger's judgment, "We thus seem to be moving toward understanding meaning in life as having three facets: one's life having value and significance, having a broader purpose in life, and one's life being coherent and making sense" (p. 531).

King, Heintzelman, and Ward (2016) also recapitulate the King, Hicks, Krull, and De Gaiso definition and identify therein

> three central components of meaning [that] are highlighted in this definition and throughout the literature on this topic: purpose, significance, and coherence. *Purpose* refers to having goals and direction in life. *Significance* entails the degree to which a person believes his or her life has value, worth,

and importance. *Coherence*, characterized by some modicum of predicta-bility and routine, allows life to makes sense to the person living it (p. 212).

Finally, George and Park (2016) also conclude that "recently, a tripartite view of MIL [meaning in life] as composed of three distinct subconstructs—comprehension, purpose, and mattering—has been gaining momentum" (p. 205). George and Park also account for what they take to be the advantages of this growing momentum behind a consensus view. First, they are optimistic that this agreement will furnish further much-needed concep-tual clarity in research into meaning in life (p. 205), a development hailed as progress by Martela and Steger (2016) as well (p. 531). George and Park (2016) also see an advantage to the tripartite schema inasmuch as they take it that this will facilitate integration of research on meaning in life into a larger body of research on meaning in general, such as the work that is being done on meaning-making for instance (pp. 205, 206). Their definition of meaning in life parallels to a large extent the formulas we have already considered. For them meaning in life can be understood as "*the extent to which one's life is experienced as making sense, as being directed and motivated by valued goals, and as mattering in the world*" (p. 206, emphasis in original). At the same time as they wittingly corroborate a basic structure common to other current researchers, they call for future work to be done on establishing the relationships between the three subconstructs and how these in turn relate to broader questions of meaning (p. 206). Martela and Steger (2016) agree that there is more work yet to be done on this front. They urge that "even though scholars have pointed toward this distinction, thus far the characteristics of and differences between these three facets of meaning have not been prop-erly fleshed out," (p. 531) and furthermore, "no research up to date has prop-erly examined all three proposed facets of meaning in life simultaneously" (p. 532). George and Park (2016) hypothesize that the three domains could very well interact, such that low levels in one might be reflected in the others, and high levels would likely be seen across the board (p. 214).

The philosophical literature also provides reasons to draw further rel-evant distinctions within the meaning construct. A leading expert like Metz (2013) clarifies at the beginning of his magnum opus that despite philosophy's ostensible interest in "*the* meaning *of* life" his work is not ded-icated to this topic. Some philosophers, he admits, "might also or instead be interested in considerations of whether the universe has a meaning or of whether the human species does. However, I do not address these 'holist' or 'cosmic' questions in this book" (p. 3). Instead, he pursues the "individualist construal," according to which the philosopher is concerned only to clarify "how, if at all, the existence of individual human beings can be significant" (p. 3). On this emphasis, the title of his book, *Meaning in Life*, could just as easily have been rendered as *Meaning in a Life*. What this important example proves is that while some psychologists especially write about global coherence as if it were exclusively the province of philosophy, even significant philosophers of meaning in life disavow global coherence as a subject for research. Not all, however, do so. Another leading theorist, Seachris (2013), holds the view that inquiry into *the* meaning *of* life is rational and warranted. Seachris and Metz, though, agree that there is an important difference here. Again, terminology varies, but the point stands. The point is that even if there is substantive divergence in interest among philosophers as to which set of questions is most interesting or important, there is unanimous agreement that there is a relevant distinction here worth preserving, and the CMM seeks to do just that by distinguishing between a global and individual level of perceived meaning as coherence. Similar terminological issues of course arise in the psychology literature. Haidt (2006), for example, contrasts questions about the "purpose *of* life," which he considers on a grand cosmic scale, with questions about "purpose *within* life," which pertain to what one should do to have a fulfilling and meaningful life. He argues that the two may be related, but one may be able to answer the latter without having answers to the former.

Out of respect for a distinction now well-entrenched in both philosophical and psychological terminologies, we will continue to refer to the overall construct targeted by the CMM as "meaning in life." However, we admit that a component of what we are calling "meaning in life," namely, global coherence, is indeed what philosophers have come to call "meaning of life." We reiterate that the CMM cannot address the viability of any theory of the "meaning of life," but we also recognize that for many people "meaning in life" is precisely supported by a theory of the "meaning of life" as one of its component parts. Like many philosophers and psychologists, therefore, we have crafted the CMM to remain formally agnostic as to the "meaning of life" but open to the prospect that respondents' personal sense of "meaning in life" may very well be sustained to some degree by an intellectual appreciation for what they take to be the "meaning of life" as a whole. We thus retain the term "meaning in life" for the construct in question, and we proceed, in what follows, with the use of the subconstruct terms "coherence," "significance," and "purpose/

direction," which are more commonly employed in the writings on this tri-partite consensus.

Consequent upon this growing realization that meaning is best thought of as structured around these three domains has been an immediate recognition that prior measures of meaning in life were not adequate. Martela and Steger (2016), speaking of the three domains of meaning in life, register a concern that "empirical research has thus far proceeded without differentiating them from each other" (p. 533). Without these distinctions being carefully drawn, items from measures like the Meaning in Life Questionnaire, Life Attitude Profile, Sense of Coherence Scale, and PIL test tap into coherence and purpose, for example, but these distinct subconstructs are ambiguously run together by summing scores, and some measures compound the ambiguity further by packing in additional domains to these three that do not have nearly the same credible grounds for inclusion in the construct of meaning (p. 533). In a similar spirit George and Park (2017) praise the tripartite schema for avoiding the pitfall of combining "three potentially distinct dimensions into a singular, more diffuse concept" (p. 614) while condemning previous measures for deriving a single, unidimensional score, thereby aggregating different domains and precluding examination of how each subconstruct interacts with relevant variables, thus yielding simplistic and distorted conclusions (pp. 614–615). In their judgment, even existing measures like the Life Regard Index, Life Attitude Profile, and MLM that have subscales roughly corresponding to one or more of the three agreed-upon domains of meaning still do not specifically target a single subconstruct and often have items that conflate the subconstructs (p. 615; see also George & Park, 2016, pp. 215–216).

Introducing the Comprehensive Measure of Meaning

With increased conceptual clarity it is now possible to devise a measure that more successfully captures key aspects of meaning. As King et al. (2016) point out, although the tripartite definition, or indeed any definition "may not capture every possible nuance of meaning in life, it is an approximation that allows us to view this experience through the lens of science. It is a workable conceptual definition that permits measurement" (p. 212). So far only one measure of meaning has been devised in direct response to the tri-partite schema, the Multidimensional Existential Meaning Scale (MEMS), introduced by George and Park (2017). In devising the CMM, we found the most common ground with George and Park's MEMS, appreciated all the items they use, and have no serious objection to it or its use in empirical research. However, we are convinced that measures of meaning need further refinement along lines derived from philosophical argument and from hints within the existing psychological literature that have not been taken into account by any prior measure. The primary goal of designing the CMM was to incorporate yet further distinctions within the tripartite division, so we broke down each subconstruct into further subdivisions in order to capture still more nuance and specificity in the way respondents are asked to think about their experience of coherence, significance, and direction (our preferred terminology for the three major subconstructs).

Selection of Items

In devising the CMM we were strongly committed to using existing items if at all possible. We compiled a master list of items from the PIL test (Crumbaugh & Maholick, 1964), the SONG test (Crumbaugh, 1977), the Life Attitude Profile-Revised (Erci, 2008), the Life Regard Index (Debats, van der Lubbe, & Wezeman, 1993), the Sense of Purpose Inventory-Revised (Sharma, 2015), the Satisfaction with Life Scale (Pavot & Diener, 2009), the Sense of Coherence Scale (Antonovsky, 1993), Carol Ryff's Purpose in Life Subscale (Ryff, 1989), the MLM (Morgan & Farsides, 2009), the Personal Meaning Profile (PMP; MacDonald et al., 2012), Neal Krause's Meaning in Life Subscale (Krause, 2004), the Spiritual Meaning Scale (Mascaro, Rosen, & Morey, 2004), the Meaning in Life Questionnaire (Steger et al., 2006), the MEMS (George & Park, 2017), the Life Purpose Questionnaire (Hutzell, 1989), the Purpose-in-Life Scale (Robbins & Francis, 2000), the Comprehensive Inventory of Thriving (Su et al., 2014), the Logo-Test (Thege, Martos, Bachner, & Kushnir, 2010), the Self-Transcendence Scale (Haugan, Rannestad, Garasen, Hammervold, & Espnes, 2012), the Life Evaluation Questionnaire (Salmon, Manzi, & Valori, 1996), the Meaning in Life Scale (Jim, Purnell, Richardson, Golden-Kreutz, & Andersen, 2006), the Functional Assessment of Chronic Illness Therapy-Spiritual Well-Being Scale (Peterman, Fitchett, Brady, Hernandez, & Cella, 2002), the Meaning in Suffering Test (Starck, 1985), the Revised Youth Purpose Survey (Bronk & Finch, 2010), and the Inventory of Positive Psychological Attitudes (Kass et al., 1991). Altogether almost 700 items were compiled, many of which appeared on more than one measure.

The items were then sorted by keyword, with a view to identifying what common themes were most prevalent. As expected, items referring to meaning, purpose, significance, goals, coherence, control, satisfaction, understanding, accomplishment, worthwhileness, and fulfillment accounted for a sizeable portion of the items. Idiosyncratic items or outliers ("I take initiative," "Life has treated me fairly," "If I could choose, I would prefer never to have been born") received less attention when it came time to select which to keep.

We began to exclude items that we judged irrelevant to meaning per se or its three constitutive subconstructs. As outlined in our criticisms of previous measures in the first section of this chapter, we discounted items that had to do with confidence in the face of death, aversion to suicide, or willingness to hypothetically live the same life over again. Similarly we excluded items that appealed to mood or positive affect, many of which privileged exuberance, enthusiasm, or passion, all feelings that seem to us distinct from the construct of meaning. For similar reasons and again in light of recent evidence alluded to earlier, we did not use items that privileged novelty, difference, variety, or excitement and those that downgraded boredom, routine, or habit. Many items prized responsibility, consistency, stability, and control, and many also emphasized the importance of altruism; all such items were set aside as again being off the subject. We agree with Morgan and Farsides (2009) that "certain items appear to measure specific beliefs and value-outlooks such as a sense of responsibility, control, and productivity" (p. 199) and that this is reason enough to reject them. We also judged items that place a high priority on autonomy or being in strict control as culturally contextual and not immediately relevant. The same was the case for items that stressed an orientation toward the future and those that called for respondents to reject perceived maltreatment at the hands of others, perceived subjection to fate or bad fortune, or perceived unfairness, aimlessness, flightiness, restlessness, indifference, or unrealized potential. These items may test positive and healthy attitudes, and those attitudes may be conducive to meaning, but they are not intrinsically related to meaningfulness per se.

Avowedly religious content or items asking respondents to reflect on sectarian theological ideas or principles were discarded as being too particular and culturally bound. Negatively coded items we also did not employ on procedural grounds as they can give rise to errors in responses, and, moreover, the positive interpretation of the negation of these negatively worded items is often ambiguous (Baumgartner, Weijters, & Pieters, 2018; Weijters & Baumgartner, 2012).

Further Distinctions from the Philosophical Literature

Of those that remained, items were then chosen for their fitness in capturing the nuanced domains of meaning we sought to assess, shaped by distinctions in the philosophical literature that we outline here. Within the cognitive coherence subconstruct (1), we make a distinction between global (1.A) and individual (1.B) coherence. The former (1.A) is *having a comprehensive theory or account of the value, importance, origin, and end of life as a whole, at a universal scale, and pertaining to humankind in general*. We would expect persons to score highly here if they have an expansive theoretical view (more or less worked out in detail) as to the meaning of human existence and the world as such. The latter (1.B) involves *having an understanding of who one is, what one values, and how this relates to one's understanding of the world*. In the philosophical literature, this distinction is sometimes referred to as "meaning *of* life" (1.A), which maps on to what we are calling global coherence, versus "meaning *of my* life" (1.B), or what we are calling individual coherence.

For example, Seachris separates questions directed toward "the *cosmic* or *global* dimension of the question of life's meaning, whereby some sort of explanation (perhaps even *narrative* explanation) is sought that will render the universe and our lives within it intelligible" and "the *individualist* or *local* dimension of the meaning-of-life question" (p. 4). With regard to the content of the coherence construct, we do agree with Martela and Steger (2016, p. 532) and Debats et al. (1995, p. 359) in affirming that a definitive answer to the meaning of life is out of the reach of scientific methodology. No measure can adjudicate an answer as to *the* meaning *of* life, but what we are assessing is whether respondents have such an answer in their own minds (global coherence) and also whether there is a more personal-level conviction that their own lives have meaning (individual coherence). In this respect the CMM is somewhat more ambitious than other measures. The PMP for example constrains itself only to questions about meaning *in* life, by design, though its authors recognize that there is a distinction here: "the Personal Meaning Profile (PMP) represents a comprehensive assessment of one's meaning in life rather than a global subjective assessment of life as meaningful" (MacDonald et al., 2012, p. 359). The CMM differs from the PMP therefore in including a three-item assessment of whether respondents do in fact have "a global subjective assessment of life as meaningful" as well as a three-item assessment of perceived meaningfulness at the individual (or what the PMP calls "personal") level.

In this respect the CMM aims to accomplish a purpose similar to that envisioned by the creators of the Spiritual Meaning Scale (Mascaro et al., 2004). They sought to complement existing measures like the Life Regard Index and the PMP with a measure that would target what they call spiritual meaning as opposed to personal and implicit meaning (p. 846). "Positive life regard," as they rightly note, "involves viewing one's individual life, but not necessarily life itself, as having meaning" (p. 847). The former, meaning in life, or what Yalom called "terrestrial meaning" is distinct from what he called "cosmic" meaning or the meaning of life, and the CMM looks to uphold this distinction. The creators of the Spiritual Meaning Scale also urge preservation of this distinction. They write, "We conceive of spiritual meaning as a capital 'M' Meaning around which one can form a small 'm,' personal meaning" (p. 847). This expresses well the distinction we are making between global and individual coherence. This aspect of the CMM's design is directly responsive to a challenge for future research laid out by King et al. (2016), who observe that while "relations among and potential distinctiveness of these three facets of meaning remain an important area for research, psychometric studies have suggested that these facets of meaning in life may occupy a lower level in a hierarchy, with 'global meaning' at the top" (p. 212).

As to the subconstruct concerned with significance (2), the CMM distinguishes between subjective significance (2.A) and objective significance (2.B). This distinction reflects a major debate in the philosophical literature, one to which we hope empirical research with the CMM will contribute. A taxonomy proposed and developed by Metz (2002) has become widely accepted. According to this classification, theories of meaning in life can be grouped by whether they are subjectivist or objectivist in orientation. Subjectivist theories are those that contend that what makes a life meaningful depends largely on the subject of that life and the favorable attitude they bear toward their life and its perceived value or desirability. On the most extreme subjectivist understanding, someone who collected matchboxes and intrinsically found this meaningful could not be contradicted if the person genuinely felt it were a meaningful activity. A range of possible attitudes are appealed to by different subjectivists, but what is essential to the position is that it suffices for a life to be meaningful that the one living that life bear an approving disposition toward it (Metz, 2002, pp. 792–793).

Objectivists, by contrast, insist that a life being meaningful depends essentially on some positive quality of that life, independently of what a person living such a life might or might not think or believe or feel about it. Under the most extreme objectivist understanding, a pediatrician providing care for children who engaged in the work only for money and found no intrinsic interest or value in it would still be doing meaningful work, independent of their attitude toward the work. Again, a range of possible forms of objective value are referred to by different objectivists as being the essential characteristics that a meaningful life must bear, but objectivist positions are united by their requirement that objective features of a life are what makes that life meaningful, and no life is meaningful merely in virtue of any positive mental orientation that a person might have toward it (p. 796; see also Seachris, 2013, pp. 11–13). Items, then, in the significance subconstruct are designed to test respondents' reliance on either subjective or objective bases for the perceived meaningfulness of their lives. Whereas subjective significance (2.A) corresponds to *subjectively finding one's activities worthwhile,* objective significance (2.B) corresponds to *having achievements, contributions, or activities that are objectively valuable* or (depending on one's theory of value) perhaps at least perceived as valuable by the consensus of others in a relevant community of judges (Brogaard & Smith, 2005; Darwall, 1983). Similar to the discussion of global coherence, self-report of objective significance, of course, does not and cannot establish the existence of objective values. Rather the items capture the extent to which the individual responding has the perception that there is objective significance in their activities and contributions.

Some theories of meaning in life, called "hybrid" by some (Evers & van Smeden, 2016), though we prefer the term "integrated," maintain that meaning in life depends on a suitable concatenation of subjective attitudes with objective values. The most important spokesperson for such a view is Wolf (2010, 2015), who, in one of her pithier formulations of her influential view writes, "A meaningful life must satisfy two criteria, suitably linked. First, there must be active engagement, and second, it must be engagement in (or with) projects of worth. A life is meaningless if it lacks active engagement with anything. A person who is bored or alienated from most of what she spends her life doing is one whose life can be said to lack meaning. Note that she may in fact be performing functions of worth. . . . At the same time, someone who *is* actively engaged may also live a meaningless life, if the objects of her involvement are utterly worthless" (Wolf, 2015, pp. 111–112). According to integrated theories, part of what makes meaningfulness a distinctive form of value is that it depends on an appropriate linking of both subjective and objective aspects of life (Wolf, 2010). This theory, while intuitively appealing and theoretically promising, poses a dilemma for empirical assessment. It is challenging to identify existing items that specifically tap into perceptions of meaningfulness that require a relationship of subjective approval corresponding to objective value. Several candidate items from existing scales that most closely correspond to this hybrid or integrated approach are proposed in the Appendix. The CMM keeps the objective and subjective items separate. This allows the possibility of assessing the extent of alignment between subjective and objective bases of perceived meaning. It also allows for assessing correlation with the proposed hybrid/integrated items to assess, to some extent, whether there are reasons for believing that at least some respondents who score highly on both subjective and objective significance may think of their lives as meaningful because they take it that suitably linked subjective and objective reasons are both available to them.

Finally, in the third motivational subconstruct having to do with purpose or direction (3), we distinguish between three possible levels of goal direction: mission (3.A), purposes (3.B), and goals (3.C). Whereas goals (3.C) are generally understood as essentially *anything one desires to accomplish,* purposes (3.B), in contrast, are *larger life aims that generate and organize goals* (McKnight & Kashdan, 2009). The highest level of the hierarchy, mission (3.A), is effectively *a unified understanding of what one's life should be that generates and guides all of one's activities, goals, and purposes and adjudicates between them when they come into conflict.* Because, under this conceptual scheme, "purposes" is itself the middle level of the hierarchy, we prefer to refer to this entire broader domain as "direction."

There is wide agreement now in the literature that purpose should be distinguished from meaning (the two were previously conflated) (George & Park, 2013, p. 365; Martela & Steger, 2016, pp. 531, 534; Steger, 2012b, p. 382) and that the former is actually best conceived as a component of the latter. Yet the CMM goes further than this in distinguishing between the scope of our various purposes, which range from daily and small objectives to potentially one unifying vision of what one's life as a whole should be or accomplish, a calling or vocation or mission. Conceiving of human action as a set of nested, purposive goals is at least as old as Aristotle. Theological perspectives often focus on the highest level of this hierarchy—vocation, calling, or mission (John Paul II, 1981; Wingren, 1957)—and distinguish it from goals and purposes. Current social science research also supports this basic outlook. McKnight and Kashdan (2009) argue for a distinction between goals as precise and proximate, while "purpose provides a broader motivational component that stimulates goals and influences behavior" (p. 243). They also recognize that a person may have multiple purposes in different areas of life (p. 244), a reality that the CMM accommodates in the purposes (3.B) items. At the same time, the CMM also acknowledges the possibility that people think of their lives as meaningful to the extent that they are even more fully integrated around one single sense of personal mission or calling, a sense that would unify and synthesize all their major projects and the daily tasks undertaken in the furtherance thereof (Emmons, 1999; Rudd, 2012).

Even some theorists who are skeptical of there being a single unifying story of any particular individual's life admit that the way identity generally tends is toward "a more or less unifying and purpose-giving whole" (McAdams, 2001, p. 116). McAdams insists "it would certainly be wrong to maintain that such integration in identity is fully and unproblematically captured in one large story for each life" (pp. 116–117), but again we are interested not in the reality of the self's situation but in people's perception of the meaningfulness of their lives. The CMM therefore assesses the extent to which respondents' sense of meaning is bound up with the impression that they are called to a major unifying life goal. So, Steger (2012a) for one recognizes "the value of finding an overarching goal or mission to which one's life can be dedicated" (p. 166) such that it merits inclusion in empirical measures like the CMM. In his work with Martela, Steger reaffirms the intelligibility of distinguishing a "short-term and perhaps even mundane" sense of purpose and "a more broad and over-arching level" (Martela & Steger, 2016, p. 534). Similarly, Mascaro et al. (2004) show that spiritual meaning of the global sort can link to a sense of "calling, or of feeling called by Life (or Tao, God, Being, or whatever Force it is in which one believes oneself to be a participant) to proceed in a certain direction" (p. 847). Finally, George and Park (2016) muster a wealth of evidence in support of a hierarchical view of goals according to which "abstract high-level goals give rise to more concrete goals below them, which give rise to even more concrete goals below them" (p. 211). The higher level goals are those that lie closest to the heart of our identity and generate the mundane activities that we undertake in pursuit of our highest priorities. To use their example, "the abstract goal of being a good parent gives rise to the goal of providing the child a good education, which in turn gives rise to the more concrete goal of driving the child to school" (p. 211). This threefold hierarchy is precisely what the CMM tries to capture.

The Comprehensive Measure of Meaning

The CMM includes three items in each of the seven subdomains just described. In selecting three items within each subdomain, an attempt was made to select items that had some breadth and were distinct from one another in an attempt to at least crudely capture the conceptualization of each subdomain laid out earlier. As noted, existing items were used whenever possible because many of these had already been subjected to various degrees of cognitive testing. Occasionally, when necessary, modifications to existing items were made when there were ambiguities in the items or when suitable items for the specific subdomains were not found.

The proposed 21 items across the seven subdomains are as follows. References to the articles and scales from which the items were drawn are given in the footnotes along with an indication of the modification of any item, when applicable.

1. Coherence
   A. Global
      i. I have a clear understanding of the ultimate meaning of life.[1]
      ii. The meaning of life in the world around us is evident to me [modified].[2]
      iii. I have a framework that allows me to understand or make sense of human life [modified].[3]

   B. Individual
      i. I understand my life's meaning.[4]
      ii. I can make sense of the things that happen in my life.[5]
      iii. I have a philosophy of life that helps me understand who I am.[6]

2. Significance
   A. Subjective
      i. I am living the kind of meaningful life I want to live [modified].[7]
      ii. Living is deeply fulfilling.[8]
      iii. I feel like I have found a really significant meaning in my life.[9]

    B. Objective
        i. The things I do are important to other people [modified].[10]
        ii. I have accomplished much in life as a whole [modified].[11]
        iii. I make a significant contribution to society.[12]

3. Direction
    A. Mission
        i. I have been aware of an all-encompassing and consuming purpose toward which my life has been directed [modified].[13]
        ii. I have a sense of mission or calling.[14]
        iii. I have a mission in life that gives me a sense of direction.[15]
    B. Purposes
        i. I have a sense of direction and purpose in life.[16]
        ii. I can describe my life's purposes [modified].[17]
        iii. My current aims match with my future aspirations.[18]

    C. Goals
        i. In my life I have very clear goals and aims.[19]
        ii. I have goals in life that are very important to me.[20]
        iii. I have definite ideas of things I want to do.[21]

The three items in the global coherence subdomain assess a sense of the world generally, of human life specifically, and of the ultimate meaning of life. The three items in the individual coherence domain assess the meaning of one's own life, the capacity to understand the meaning of life events, and a philosophy that helps one understand one's identity. The three items in the subjective significance subdomain express a perceived subjective sense of the significance of one's life as a whole, the process of living, and the kind of life one has. The three items in the objective significance subdomain assess the things that one does, one's life as a whole, and one's contributions as being important or significant, either in what the actions are in and of themselves or to society. The three items of the mission subdomain express having a mission or calling, an awareness of that mission, and that mission giving one direction in life. The three items in the purposes subdomain express having a sense of direction or purpose, one's awareness of one's purposes, and one's more immediate goals being aligned with those purposes. Finally, the three items in the goals subdomain express having goals, the importance of those goals, and an awareness of those goals.

Certainly each of the subdomains could be supplemented with additional items. However, for a brief 21-item measure with coverage across the seven subdomains, constrained principally by the availability of existing items, these are the items we would suggest and that form the CMM.

In some cases, it was difficult to distinguish the subdomain of a specific item, and, in the case of certain existing items, ambiguities were often present. Some principles used to categorize various items when the distinctions across subdomains were less clear are as follows. In distinguishing between global versus individual coherence, reference to "my life" rather than "life" in general or "human life" or "the universe" indicated individual coherence, whereas the latter expressions were generally categorized as relating to global coherence. In distinguishing coherence from objective significance, if some aspect of value was found in the action or activity or in accomplishing something, these items were classified as objective significance, whereas if value was derived simply from one's being, then these were classified as concerning coherence. However, as noted earlier, with many such coherence items, the items themselves often entailed particularist philosophical or religious views and so were not specifically considered for the CMM. In distinguishing individual coherence from the various levels of the direction domain, items that indicated "having" goals or an "awareness" of goals and purposes were placed in the direction domain, whereas those that related to "understanding" or purposes being derived from a "philosophy" were placed in the individual coherence subdomain. In distinguishing individual coherence from subjective significance, items that made reference to "values" or "systems of belief" were placed in the individual coherence subdomain, whereas items that could be affirmed without a philosophy were placed in the subjective significance subdomain. In distinguishing objective and subjective significance, reference to "accomplishments" and "achievements" were often placed in the objective significance subdomain, but when reference was made to one's feelings toward these, then this was taken as the more important consideration and the items were placed in the subjective significance domain; whether the item could be affirmed with respect to a trivial activity like "counting pieces of string" or "collecting matchboxes" was often a useful test case as to whether the item pertained to the subjective subdomain. In distinguishing the mission, purpose, and goals subdomains, the use of the singular "a calling" or even "a life purpose" was often taken as an indication of the mission subdomain; items that made reference to "purpose" or "purposes" or "life aim" were generally placed in the purposes subdomain, especially when the item indicated or allowed for a plurality of such purposes; items that made reference to goals or tasks or daily activities were generally placed in the goals subdomain. In some cases, language was ambiguous, such as the use of "life goal," which makes use of the "goal" terminology, but being prefaced by "life" in fact suggests a purpose. Whether the item would be affirmed by simply aiming to pass an exam was often a useful test case to distinguish goals from purposes. The preceding principles are not intended to be comprehensive but merely to indicate some of the considerations that went into the selection of the items and that might be used in the further distinguishing of items if the seven-fold structure of the CMM is also eventually used in other contexts.

It is important to note that the CMM is intended to assess the presence of meaning in one's life. It is not intended to assess related but also important constructs such as seeking to find meaning or the quest for meaning (Crumbaugh, 1968; Steger et al., 2006) or striving for, making progress toward, or achieving goals and purposes. These things can certainly be causes of meaning but are arguably conceptually distinct from meaning itself. Achieving a goal may be a source of meaning, but it may also lead to loss of meaning if, for example, its attainment results in there being nothing further for which one is striving.

Conclusion

The main contribution that we seek to make with the CMM is to clarify the different ways that meaning can be perceived as part of a human life. As crucial as meaning is to well-being, it is a welcome development in the current state of scholarship that a promising means of measuring meaning is becoming clearer and better supported. There is now solid agreement that meaning is multidimensional and that it can be measured by focusing on three subconstructs tapping cognitive coherence, affective significance, and motivational direction. Within these subconstructs, though, it has become apparent from philosophical reflection (which so far has been happening largely in tandem with, but not in conversation with, psychological analysis) that yet finer distinctions can be made. The CMM intends to clarify and codify these distinctions, delineating refinements concerning global and individual "levels" of felt coherence, subjective and objective bases for perceived significance, and varying scopes of felt direction across a range of activities and levels from quotidian to all-encompassing.

We would hope that research applications of the CMM will provide yet greater conceptual clarity around meaning and what it entails, as well as further insight into how the subdomains relate to one another. Understanding how these three domains relate, whether there are predictable correlations among them, and to what extent each domain targets a distinct psychological reality are tasks for immediate future research.

With the further distinctions or subdomains within the CMM, the work of understanding their relations becomes yet more complex. However, we believe that these distinctions may be of importance both in psychology and in potentially using data to inform philosophical discussions and to more adequately assess potential relations between coherence, significance, and direction. Without the further distinctions of the CMM, it may be the case that specific measures, even those employing the tripartite structure, may unwittingly only encompass specific subdomains of meaning. To illustrate this, in Table 12.1 we examine several recent measures of meaning (George & Park, 2017; Krause, 2004; Ryff, 1989; Steger et al., 2006) including one that explicitly employs the tripartite model (George & Park, 2017) to evaluate which of the seven subdomains of the CMM these measures evaluate.

None of these other measures captures all seven subdomains. Each measure tends to favor either objective or subjective significance without inclusion of items related to the other. When examining coherence, each has,

Table 12.1 A mapping of several existing meaning measures to the subdomains of the Comprehensive Measure of Meaning (CMM)

	Global coherence	Individual coherence	Subjective significance	Objective significance	Mission	Purposes	Goals
Ryff (1989)			x			x	x
Krause (2004)	x	x			x	x	x
Steger (2006)	x				x	x	
George and Park (2017)	x			x		x	x

at best, individual coherence and neglects global coherence. Each contains items related to the purposes subdomain but generally only additionally has either the goals or the mission subdomain but not the other, with only the Krause (2004) measure arguably having items corresponding to each of the three levels of the hierarchy of the direction domain. Even the George and Park (2017) measure, which employs the tripartite model and does, of course, have items related to coherence, significance, and direction, focuses for each of the subconstructs only on one or another of the subdomains that the CMM delineates; it has individual but not global significance, objective but not subjective significance, and goals and purposes but nothing on mission or calling. We believe the CMM thus helps better fill out the various domains of the construct of meaning.

Of course, it may turn out that some of these subdomains are more important than others in their effects on various outcomes or that further empirical work suggests that, for certain uses, assessing only a subset of subdomains is adequate. However, on conceptual grounds we think that these distinctions are important, and it will be of interest to see whether that bears out in empirical work. Further work, of course, remains to be done on assessing the psychometric properties of the CMM, work which we likewise plan to undertake in the years ahead, with data collection already currently under way.

We conclude then with some preliminary hypotheses about what we might expect the CMM to reveal in actual use among diverse populations.

We recognize that global coherence (1.A) and individual coherence (1.B) are independent of each other, such that a person might quite consistently believe that their own life makes sense for any number of reasons while being agnostic about whether life as such is coherent or even perhaps denying that it is. By the same token, though we would hypothesize that this would be the more unusual scenario, a person could be convinced that life in general is coherent but regard their own lives as being deficient in coherence. In such cases, which again we would assume would be comparatively rare, it is imagined that an individual would feel themselves to be in the situation of having a strong theoretical view of how human life *should* attain its intended meaning while sensing that their own personal existence was failing to achieve this standard or ideal of what it ought to be, or that one's life seemed difficult to understand within the broader global context. Which scenario will prove more commonplace, the extent to which the two subdomains are correlated, and which scores of the two subdomains are higher, are all open questions.

Recall that with respect to significance, much of the philosophical literature has divided along two different camps: the subjectivist accounts of meaning in life and the objectivist. In view of this distinction, which admits of a spectrum of possible variations, we separate subjective significance (2.A) and objective significance (2.B). The items in the former category are meant to assess the degree to which a person's own self-appraisal or estimation of the worth of their life comes from inward subjective judgment, while the items in the latter category are meant to assess the degree to which a person's judgment about the worth of their life rests on what they take to be the objective value of their projects, activities, or achievements, either in an absolute sense or at least considered important by the consensus of a broader community. A third sort of philosophical theory about meaning in life insists that meaning requires a connection between objectively valuable activities or contributions and a subjective endorsement of those activities or contributions. For measuring purposes, we found it difficult to identify items that clearly targeted both elements in concert in the way that such theories demand. Nevertheless, we have included in a supplemental Appendix three items that we feel at least implicitly assess the degree to which a person might sense that their life is meaningful on grounds simultaneously subjective and objective (Appendix 12.1). We are interested therefore, in the first place, to discover to what extent scores on the subjective significance (2.A) items and objective significance items (2.B) tend to correlate and also how often scores in one of the two subdomains are relatively high and in the other relatively low. Should one or the other of the subdomains be consistently higher, that would not necessarily lend greater credibility or explanatory power to one philosophical theory or another, but it would certainly provide information on how people experience the meaning of their lives, whether they feel that it is bound up more with a subjective sense of fulfillment or with the objective quality of their activities or contributions. Should the three "hybrid/integrated" items in the Appendix be used, it would be of further interest to discover the extent to which high scores on these items correlate or not with high scores on the subjective significance (2.A) or objective significance (2.B) items or both. In this last case, this would again provide at least some additional evidence to help inform the third, hybrid or integrated, theory of meaning in life circulating in the philosophical debate.

Finally, with respect to direction, we again acknowledge that the three "levels" of scope, ranging from mission (3.A), to purposes (3.B), to goals (3.C) are in principle independent. A person, we hypothesize, could score highly on purposes while not necessarily being directed by a strong sense of mission; alternately, a person might score highly on purposes while feeling that their daily goals were not well aligned at present with those purposes. We presume that a person who scores highly on mission (3.A) will generally also score highly on purposes (3.B) and goals (3.C), but we also can see how this might not necessarily be the case. In such an instance, we would imagine that the person has a strong and clear overall plan for their life but feels that, at the present time, their daily activities do not contribute to such a plan. Perhaps someone biding their time through a period of unemployment and awaiting an opportunity to pursue their true calling in the future would fit such a profile. Alternately, we would imagine that it could be quite commonplace for a person to score highly on purposes (3.B) and goals (3.C) while not necessarily feeling themselves to be guided by any great overarching ambition that they would be willing to describe as a mission or calling (3.A). Again, the relations here should prove interesting to answering future research questions.

It would also be of interest to see how the three domains or subconstructs relate to one another, both cross-sectionally or descriptively and also over time, in an attempt to assess causal relations. There is broad agreement that purpose is essential to meaning, but how important is it for that sense of purpose to be all-encompassing in scope? Is it sufficient for people to have a sense of purpose in our more narrow definition ("purposes," 3.B) for individuals to score highly in meaning, or alternatively, is having a more singular sense of mission important? If data were available on these measures over time, might it be possible to provide evidence for the relative causal effects of each of these subconstructs on the others? Might it be the case that coherence most profoundly shapes direction and that direction itself most powerfully affects a subsequent sense of significance? All of these questions would require at least two waves of data collection with the CMM, along with rich data on potentially confounding variables.

One final way of further attempting to understand what for many constitutes "meaning" is our inclusion of a final four items that we are calling "general" in tone (Appendix 12.2) for which there may be some ambiguity as to which subconstruct they pertain or which may pertain to all three (coherence, significance, and direction). These items ask for respondents to gauge their overall impression of how meaningful is their life. Should these items be included, it would be possible to assess correlations between scores in the subdomains with overall assessments of the general meaningfulness that people perceive in their lives. This, too, we would hope could provide further insight into any strong associations between one domain, or even subdomain, and an overall sense of meaningfulness, which in turn might indicate which of the subconstructs is more influential on an overall assessment of meaningfulness.

We welcome the use of the CMM in varied settings and hope it will prove useful for empirical research to facilitate a deeper understanding of the relations between the different domains and subdomains and provide useful information for how people actually experience meaning in life and with what frequency they do so across these subdomains. We also recognize that the CMM builds on other recently proposed measures that also are based on the tripartite model; it is thus our hope that mapping existing measures, identifying what they include or not, and where they overlap or not will be an easier task given the greater specificity of the subdomains deployed here and the selectivity used in assembling the 21 items that constitute the CMM.

Notes

1. Item 38 on the Life Attitude Profile-Revised Scale (Erci, 2008). See also "I think about the ultimate meaning of life," Item 1 on the Seeking of Noetic Goals Test (Reker & Cousins, 1979). See also "I believe that life has an ultimate purpose and meaning," Item 5 on the Personal Meaning Profile (Wong, 1998).
2. Item 7 on the Life Attitude Profile-Revised Scale, originally phrased as "The meaning of life is evident in the world around us" (Erci, 2008).
3. Item 29 on the Life Attitude Profile-Revised Scale, originally phrased as "I have a framework that allows me to understand or make sense of my life" (Erci, 2008). See also "I have a system or framework that allows me to truly understand my being alive," Item 11 on the Meaningful Life Measure (Morgan & Farsides, 2009). Item appears verbatim as Item 28 on the Life Regard Index (Debats et al., 1993).
4. Item 1 on the Meaning in Life Questionnaire (Steger et al., 2006).
5. Item 8 on the MEMS (George & Park, 2017).
6. Item 4A2 (Krause, 2004).
7. Item 18 on the Life Attitude Profile-Revised Scale, originally phrased as "Basically, I am living the kind of life I want to live" (Erci, 2008).
8. Item 2 on the Life Regard Index (Debats et al., 1993).

9. Item 3B (Krause, 2004).
10. Item 3 under "Self-Worth" on the Comprehensive Inventory of Thriving, originally phrased as "The work I do is important for other people" (Su et al., 2014).
11. Item 9 on the Meaningful Life Measure, originally reverse coded as "I have failed to accomplish much in life" (Morgan & Farsides, 2009).
12. Item 49 on the Personal Meaning Profile (Wong, 1998). See also "The things I do contribute to society," Item 2 under "Self-Worth" on the Comprehensive Inventory of Thriving (Su et al., 2014).
13. Item 18 on the SONG test, originally phrased as "I have been aware of an all-powerful and consuming purpose toward which my life has been directed" (Reker & Cousins, 1979).
14. Item 19 on the Personal Meaning Profile (Wong, 1998).
15. Item 37 on the Life Attitude Profile-Revised (Erci, 2008).
16. Item 4 on the Purpose in Life Subscale (Ryff, 1989). Item appears verbatim as Item 4C2 (Krause, 2004).
17. Item 28 on the Sense of Purpose Inventory, originally phrased as "I can describe my life's purpose" (Sharma, 2015).
18. Item 12 on the Sense of Purpose Inventory (Sharma, 2015).
19. Item 2 on the Life Attitude Profile-Revised Scale (Erci, 2008). See also "In life, I have: (7) clear goals and aims," Item 3 on the PIL Test (Crumbaugh & Maholick, 1964).
20. Item 9 from the MEMS (George & Park, 2017).
21. Item 3 on the Life Purpose Questionnaire (Hutzell, 1989).
22. Item 6 on the Meaningful Life Measure (Morgan & Farsides, 2009). Item appears verbatim as 13 on the Purpose in Life Subscale (Ryff, 1989). Item appears verbatim as Item 4D2 (Krause, 2004).
23. Item 11 on the Inventory of Positive Psychological Attitudes (Kass et al., 1991).
24. Item 3 on the Logo-Test Revised (Thege et al., 2010).
25. Item 7 on the Spiritual Meaning Scale (Mascaro et al., 2004).
26. Item 6 (VanderWeele, 2017).
27. Item 2 on the UK's Annual Population Survey's Four-Question Survey of Subjective Wellbeing (Allin & Hand, 2017).
28. Item 2 on the Purpose-in-Life Scale (Robbins & Francis, 2000).

About the Authors

Jeffrey A. Hanson is Senior Philosopher at the Human Flourishing Program in the Institute for Quantitative Science at Harvard University. He is the author of *Kierkegaard and the Life of Faith: The Aesthetic, the Ethical, and the Religious in "Fear and Trembling"* (Indiana University Press, 2017), editor of *Kierkegaard as Phenomenologist: An Experiment* (Northwestern University Press, 2010), and co-editor with Michael R. Kelly of

Michel Henry: The Affects of Thought (Bloomsbury, 2012). His research focuses on issues in philosophy of religion, phenomenology, aesthetics, and ethics.

Tyler J. VanderWeele is John L. Loeb and Frances Lehman Loeb Professor of Epidemiology in the Departments of Epidemiology and Biostatistics at the Harvard T. H. Chan School of Public Health, Director of the Human Flourishing Program, and Co-Director of the Initiative on Health, Religion and Spirituality at Harvard University. His research concerns methodology for distinguishing between association and causation in observational studies, and his empirical research spans psychiatric, perinatal, and social epidemiology; the science of happiness and flourishing; and the study of religion and health, including both religion and population health and the role of religion and spirituality in end-of-life care. He has published more than 300 papers in peer-reviewed journals and is author of the book *Explanation in Causal Inference* (Oxford University Press, 2015).

Author Note

This work was supported in part by a grant from the John Templeton Foundation and by the Lee Kum Sheung Center for Health and Happiness. The views expressed in this chapter represent the perspectives of the authors and do not reflect the opinions or endorsement of any organization. We have no known conflict of interest to disclose. Correspondence concerning this chapter should be directed to Jeffrey Hanson, Human Flourishing Program, Harvard University, 129 Mt. Auburn St. (Suite 1), Cambridge, MA, 02138 (jhanson@fas.harvard.edu).

References

Adams, E. M. (2002). The meaning of life. *International Journal for Philosophy of Religion, 51*, 71–81.

Allin, P., & Hand, D. J. (2017). New statistics for old?—Measuring the wellbeing of the UK. *Journal of the Royal Statistical Society Series A: Statistics in Society, 180*(1), 3–43.

Antonovsky, A. (1993). The structure and properties of the Sense of Coherence Scale. *Social Science and Medicine, 36*(6), 725–733.

Battista, J., & Almond, R. (1973). The development of meaning in life. *Psychiatry, 36*(4), 409–427.

Baumeister, R. F. (1991). *Meanings of life.* New York: Guilford.

Baumgartner, H., Weijters, B., & Pieters, R. (2018). Misresponse to survey questions: A conceptual framework and empirical test of the effects of reversals, negations, and polar opposite core concepts. *Journal of Marketing Research, 55*(6), 869–883.

Braun, J. R. (1972). The Purpose in Life test. In O. K. Buros (Ed.), *The seventh mental measurements yearbook* (p. 531). Lincoln, NE: Buros Center for Testing.

Brogaard, B., & Smith, B. (2005). On luck, responsibility and the meaning of life. *Philosophical Papers, 34*(3), 443–458.

Bronk, K. C. (2014). *Purpose in life: A critical component of optimal youth development.* Dordrecht: Springer Science+Business Media.

Bronk, K. C., & Finch, W. H. (2010). Adolescent characteristics by type of long-term aim in life. *Applied Developmental Science, 14*(1), 35–44.

Chamberlain, K., & Zika, S. (1988). Religiosity, life meaning, and well-being: Some relationships in a sample of women. *Journal for the Scientific Study of Religion, 27,* 411–420.

Cohen, R., Bavishi, C., & Rozanski, A. (2016). Purpose in life and its relationship to all-cause mortality and cardiovascular events: A meta-analysis. *Psychosomatic Medicine, 78*(2), 122–133.

Chen, Y., Kim, E. S., Koh, H. K., Frazier, A. L., & VanderWeele, T. J. (2019). Sense of mission and subsequent health and well-being among young adults: An outcome-wide analysis. *American Journal of Epidemiology, 188*(4): 664–673.

Cottingham, J. (2003). *On the meaning of life.* London: Routledge.

Crumbaugh, J. C. (1968). Cross-validation of Purpose in Life test based on Frankl's concepts. *Journal of Individual Psychology, 24,* 74–81.

Crumbaugh, J. C. (1977). The Seeking of Noetic Goals test (SONG): A complementary scale to the Purpose in Life test (PIL). *Journal of Clinical Psychology, 33*(3), 900–907.

Crumbaugh, J. C., & Maholick, L. T. (1964). An experimental study in existentialism: The psychometric approach to Frankl's concept of noogenic neurosis. *Journal of Clinical Psychology, 20*(2), 200–207.

Damon, W., Menon, J., & Bronk, K. C. (2003). The development of purpose during adolescence. *Applied Developmental Science, 7*(3), 119–128.

Darwall, S. (1983). *Impartial reason.* Ithaca, NY: Cornell University Press.

Debats, D. L. (1998). Measurement of personal meaning: The psychometric properties of the Life Regard Index. In P. T. P. Wong & P. S. Fry (Eds.), *The human quest for meaning: A handbook of psychological research and clinical application* (pp. 237–259). Mahwah, NJ: Erlbaum.

Debats, D. L., van der Lubbe, P. M., & Wezeman, F. R. A. (1993). On the psychometric properties of the Life Regard Index (LRI): A measure of meaningful life. *Personality and Individual Differences, 14*(2), 337–345.

Domino, G. (1972). The Purpose in Life test. In O. K. Buros (Ed.), *The seventh mental measurements yearbook* (pp. 531–532). Lincoln, NE: Buros Center for Testing.

Dyck, M. J. (1987). Assessing logotherapeutic constructs: Conceptual and psychometric status of the Purpose in Life and Seeking of Noetic Goals tests. *Clinical Psychology Review, 7*(4), 439–447.

Ebersole, P., & Quiring, G. (1989). Social desirability in the Purpose-in-Life test. *Journal of Psychology, 123*(3), 305–307.

Edwards. M. J. (2007). *The dimensionality and construct valid measurement of life meaning* (Unpublished doctoral dissertation). Queen's University, Kingston, Ontario.

Emmons, R. (1999). *The psychology of ultimate concerns: Motivation and spirituality in personality.* New York: Guilford.

Erci, B. (2008). Meaning in life for patients with cancer: Validation of the Life Attitude Profile-Revised Scale. *Journal of Advanced Nursing, 62*(6), 704–711.

Evers, D., & van Smeden, G. E. (2016). Meaning in life: In defense of the hybrid view. *Southern Journal of Philosophy, 54*(3), 355–371.

Frankl, V. E. (1984). *Man's search for meaning: An introduction to logotherapy.* New York: Simon and Schuster.

Frazier, P., Oishi, S., & Steger, M. (2003). Assessing optimal human functioning. In W. B. Walsh (Ed.), *Counseling psychology and optimal human functioning* (pp. 171–197). Mahwah, NJ: Erlbaum.

Garfield, C. (1973). A psychometric and clinical investigation of Frankl's concept of existential vacuum and anomie. *Psychiatry, 36,* 396–408.

George, L. S., & Park, C. L. (2016). Meaning in life as comprehension, purpose, and mattering: Toward integration and new research questions. *Review of General Psychology, 20*(3), 205–220.

George, L. S., & Park, C. L. (2017). The Multidimensional Existential Meaning Scale: A tripartite approach to measuring meaning in life, *The Journal of Positive Psychology, 12*(6), 613–627.

Haidt, J. (2006). *The happiness hypothesis.* New York: Basic.

Haugan, G., Rannestad, T., Garasen, H., Hammervold, R., & Espnes, G. A. (2012). The Self-Transcendence Scale: An investigation of the factor structure among nursing home patients. *Journal of Holistic Nursing, 30*(3), 147–159.

Heintzelman, S. J., & King, L. A. (2014a). Life is pretty meaningful. *American Psychologist, 69*(6), 561–574.

Heintzelman, S. J., & King, L. A. (2014b). (The feeling of) meaning-as-information. *Personality and Social Psychology Review, 18*(2), 153–167.

Heisel, M. J., & Flett, G. L. (2004). Purpose in life, satisfaction with life, and suicide ideation in a clinical sample. *Journal of Psychopathology and Behavioral Assessment, 26,* 127–135.

Hepburn, R. W. (1966). Questions about the meaning of life. *Religious Studies, 1*(2), 125–140.

Hicks, J., & King, L. (2009). Meaning in life as a subjective judgment and a lived experience. *Social and Personality Psychology Compass, 3*(4), 638–653.

Hutzell, R. R. (1989). Life Purpose Questionnaire. Institute of Logotherapy Press. In Jeffries, L. L. (1995) *Adolescence and meaning in life.* (Doctoral dissertation). Proquest Dissertations Publishing (9542604). University of Houston, Houston, TX.

Jim, H. S., Purnell, J. Q., Richardson, S. A., Golden-Kreutz, D., & Andersen, B. L. (2006). Measuring meaning in life following cancer. *Quality of Life Research, 15,* 1355–1371.

John Paul II. (1981). *On human work: Laborem exercens.* Washington, DC: USCCB.

Kass, J. D., Friedman, R., Leserman, J., Caudill, M., Zuttermeister, P. C., & Benson, H. (1991). An inventory of positive psychological attitudes with potential relevance to health outcomes: Validation and preliminary testing. *Behavioral Medicine, 17*(3), 121–129.

King, L. A., Heintzelman, S. J., & Ward, S. J. (2016). Beyond the search for meaning: A contemporary science of the experience of meaning in life. *Current Directions in Psychological Science, 25*(4), 211–216.

King, L. A., Hicks, J. A., Krull, J. L., & Del Gaiso, A. K. (2006). Positive affect and the experience of meaning in life. *Journal of Personality and Social Psychology, 90*(1), 179–196.

Krause, N. (2004). Stressors arising in highly valued roles, meaning in life, and the physical health status of older adults. *Journal of Gerontology Series B: Psychological Sciences and Social Sciences, 59*(5), S287–S297.

Landau, I. (2017). *Finding meaning in an imperfect world.* Oxford: Oxford University Press.

MacDonald, M. J., Wong, P. T. P., & Gingras, D. T. (2012). Meaning-in-life measures and development of a brief version of the Personal Meaning Profile. In P. T. P. Wong (Ed.), *The human quest for meaning: Theories, research, and applications* (2nd ed.) (pp. 357–382). New York: Routledge.

Martela, F., & Steger, M. F. (2016). The three meanings of meaning in life: Distinguishing coherence, purpose, and significance. *The Journal of Positive Psychology, 11*(5), 531–545.

Mascaro, N., & Rosen, D. H. (2005). Existential meaning's role in the enhancement of hope and prevention of depressive symptoms. *Journal of Personality, 73*(4), 985–1014.

Mascaro, N., Rosen, D. H., & Morey, L. C. (2004). The development, construct validity, and clinical utility of the Spiritual Meaning Scale. *Personality and Individual Differences, 37*, 845–860.

McAdams, D. P. (2001). The psychology of life stories. *Review of General Psychology, 5*(2), 100–122.

McGregor, I., & Little, B. R. (1998). Personal projects, happiness, and meaning: On doing well and being yourself. *Journal of Personality and Social Psychology, 74*, 494–512.

McKnight, P. E., & Kashdan, T. B. (2009). Purpose in life as a system that creates and sustains health and well-being: An integrative, testable theory. *Review of General Psychology, 13*(3), 242–251.

Metz, T. (2002). Recent work on the meaning of life. *Ethics, 112*, 781–814.

Metz, T. (2013). *Meaning in life: An analytic account.* Oxford: Oxford University Press.

Morgan, J., & Farsides, T. (2009). Measuring meaning in life. *Journal of Happiness Studies, 10*, 197–214.

Owens, G. P., Steger, M. F., Whitesell, A. A., & Herrera, C. J. (2009). Posttraumatic stress disorder, guilt, depression, and meaning in life among military veterans. *Journal of Traumatic Stress, 22*(6), 654–657.

Pavot, W., & Diener, E. (2009). Review of the Satisfaction with Life Scale. In E. Diener (Ed.), *Assessing well-being: The collected works of Ed Diener* (pp. 101–118). Dordrecht: Springer Science+Business Media.

Peterman, A. H., Fitchett, G., Brady, M. J., Hernandez, L., & Cella, D. (2002). Measuring spiritual well-being in people with cancer: The Functional Assessment of Chronic Illness Therapy—Spiritual Well-Being Scale (FACIT-Sp). *Annals of Behavioral Medicine, 24*(1), 49–58.

Pinquart, M. (2002). Creating and maintaining purpose in life in old age: A meta-analysis. *Ageing International, 27*(2), 90–114.

Reker, G. T., & Cousins, J. B. (1979). Factor structure, construct validity and reliability of the Seeking of Noetic Goals (SONG) and Purpose in Life (PIL) tests. *Journal of Clinical Psychology, 35*(1), 85–91.

Reker, G. T., & Peacock, E. J. (1981). The Life Attitude Profile (LAP): A multidimensional instrument for assessing attitudes toward life. *Canadian Journal of Behavioral Science, 13*, 64–73.

Reker, G. T., & Wong, P. T. P. (1988). Aging as an individual process. In J. E. Birren & V. L. Bengtson (Eds.), *Emergent theories of aging* (pp. 214–246). New York: Springer.

Robbins, M., & Francis, L. J. (2000). Religion, personality, and well-being: The relationship between church attendance and purpose in life. *Journal of Research on Christian Education, 9*(2), 223–238.

Rudd, A. (2012). *Self, value, & narrative: A Kierkegaardian approach.* Oxford: Oxford University Press.

Ryff, C. D. (1989). Happiness is everything, or is it? Explorations on the meaning of psychological well-being. *Journal of Personality and Social Psychology, 57*, 1069–1081.

Salmon, P., Manzi, F., & Valori, R. M. (1996). Measuring the meaning of life for patients with incurable cancer: The Life Evaluation Questionnaire (LEQ). *European Journal of Cancer, 32A*(5), 755–760.

Schulenberg, S. E. (2004). A psychometric investigation of logotherapy measures and the Outcome Questionnaire (OQ-45.2). *North American Journal of Psychology, 6*(3), 477–492.

Schulenberg, S. E., Baczwaski, B. J., & Buchanan, E. M. (2014). Measuring search for meaning: A factor-analytic evaluation of the Seeking of Noetic Goals Test (SONG). *Journal of Happiness Studies, 15*, 693–715.

Seachris, J. (Ed.). (2013). *Exploring the meaning of life: An anthology and guide*. Chichester, UK: Wiley-Blackwell.

Sharma, G. (2015). *Sense of Purpose Inventory: Development, psychometric examination, and construct validation*. (Doctoral dissertation). Proquest Dissertations Publishing (3715563). Pennsylvania State University, State Park, PA.

Starck, P. L. (1985). *Guidelines—Meaning in Suffering Test*. Abilene, TX: Viktor Frankl Institute of Logotherapy.

Steger, M. F. (2006). The Meaning in Life Questionnaire: Assessing the presence of and search for meaning in life. *Journal of Counseling Psychology, 53*(1), 80–93.

Steger, M. F. (2009). Meaning in life. In S. J. Lopez & C. R. Snyder (Eds.), *The Oxford handbook of positive psychology* (2nd ed.) (pp. 679–687). Oxford: Oxford University Press.

Steger, M. F. (2012a). Experiencing meaning in life: Optimal functioning at the nexus of well-being, psychopathology, and spirituality. In P. T. P. Wong (Ed.), *The human quest for meaning: Theories, research, and applications* (2nd ed.) (pp. 165–184). New York: Routledge.

Steger, M. F. (2012b). Making meaning in life. *Psychological Inquiry, 23*(4), 381–385.

Steger, M. F., Frazier, P., Oishi, S., & Kaler, M. (2006). The Meaning in Life Questionnaire: Assessing the presence of and search for meaning in life. *Journal of Counseling Psychology, 53*(1), 80–93.

Su, R., Tay, L., Diener, E. (2014). The development and validation of the comprehensive inventory of thriving (CIT) and the brief inventory of thriving (BIT). *Applied Psychology: Health and Well-Being, 6*, 251–279.

Thege, B. K., Martos, T., Bachner, Y. G., & Kushnir, T. (2010). Development and psychometric evaluation of a revised measure of meaning in life: The Logo-Test-R. *Studia Psychologica, 52*, 133–145.

Thomson, G. (2003). *On the meaning of life*. London: Wadsworth.

VanderWeele, T. J. (2017). On the promotion of human flourishing. *Proceedings of the National Academy of Sciences, 114*(31), 8148–8156.

Weijters, B., & Baumgartner, H. (2012). Misresponse to reversed and negated items in surveys: A review. *Journal of Marketing Research, 49*(5), 737–747.

Wiggins, D. (1976). Truth, invention, and the meaning of life. *Proceedings of the British Academy, 62*, 331–378.

Wingren, G. (1957). *Luther on vocation*. Philadelphia: Muhlenberg.

Wolf, S. (2010). *Meaning in life and why it matters*. Princeton, NJ: Princeton University Press.

Wolf, S. (2015). *The variety of values: Essays on morality, meaning, and love*. Oxford: Oxford University Press.

Wong, P. T. P. (1998). Implicit theories of meaningful life and the development of the Personal Meaning Profile. In P. T. P. Wong & P. S. Fry (Eds.), *The human quest for meaning: A handbook of psychological research and clinical applications* (pp. 111–140). Mahwah, NJ: Erlbaum.
Yalom, I. (1980). *Existential psychotherapy*. New York: Basic.

Appendix 12.1 Integrated Significance Items

i. I find it satisfying to think about what I have accomplished in life.[22]
ii. When I think about what I have done with my life I feel worthwhile.[23]
iii. I find fulfillment in the work I am engaged in or for which I am preparing myself.[24]

Appendix 12.2 General Meaning Items

i. My life is meaningful.[25]
ii. I understand my purpose in life.[26]
iii. Overall, to what extent do you feel that the things you do in your life are worthwhile?[27]
iv. I feel my life has a sense of meaning.[28]

13

Empirical Relationships Among Five Types of Well-Being

*Seth Margolis, Eric Schwitzgebel, Daniel J. Ozer,
and Sonja Lyubomirsky*

Abstract

Philosophers, psychologists, economists, and other social scientists continue to debate the nature of human well-being. We argue that this debate centers around five main conceptualizations of well-being: hedonic well-being, life satisfaction, desire fulfillment, eudaimonia, and non-eudaimonic objective list well-being. Each type of well-being is conceptually different, but are they empirically distinguishable? To address this question, we first developed and validated a measure of desire fulfillment and then examined associations between this new measure and several other well-being measures. In addition, we explored associations among all five types of well-being. We found high correlations among all measures of well-being, but generally correlations did not approach unity even when correcting for unreliability. Furthermore, correlations between well-being and related constructs (e.g., demographics, personality) depended on the type of well-being measured. We conclude that empirical findings based on one type of well-being measure may not generalize to all types of well-being.

What, if anything, is inherently good—or universally valuable—for all people, such that every person should value it noninstrumentally insofar as they care about their own well-being or "happiness"? This question is among the most important that human beings ask, and, after thousands of years of contemplation, consensus still eludes us. Philosophers disagree (Alexandrova, 2017; Crisp, 2001/2017; Parfit 1984), as do psychologists (McMahan & Estes, 2011;

Seth Margolis, Eric Schwitzgebel, Daniel J. Ozer, and Sonja Lyubomirsky, *Empirical Relationships Among Five Types of Well-Being* In: *Measuring Well-Being*. Edited by: Matthew T. Lee, Laura D. Kubzansky, and Tyler J. VanderWeele, Oxford University Press (2021). © Oxford University Press. DOI: 10.1093/oso/9780197512531.003.0014

Ryan & Deci, 2001), economists (MacGregor & Pouw, 2017), and ordinary research participants (Pflug, 2009).

Types of Well-Being

Philosophers standardly define well-being, in the most general sense, as what is inherently, ultimately, or noninstrumentally good for a person for that person's own sake. Although any classification of views of well-being will elide some nuances and exclude or fit poorly with some unusual or hybrid views (e.g., the hybrid view of Lauinger, Chapter 8, in this volume), we recognize five main approaches that are conceptually and might be empirically distinguishable: (1) hedonic well-being, (2) life satisfaction, (3) desire fulfillment, (4) eudaimonia, and (5) non-eudaimonic objective list well-being.

According to hedonic approaches to well-being, only pleasure and pain—or, more broadly, positively or negatively valenced emotional states—have intrinsic value (Bentham, 1780/2007; Crisp, 2006; Feldman, 2004; Mill, 1861/2003; Plato, 4th c. BCE/1961). Two other approaches emphasize the satisfaction of desires. According to life satisfaction approaches, what matters is the extent to which one is (authentically) satisfied with one's life as a whole (Neugarten, Havighurst, & Tobin 1961; Sumner, 1996). According to desire fulfillment approaches, what matters is the extent to which one's specific desires, goals, or values are fulfilled—or, alternatively, the extent to which one judges them to be fulfilled—perhaps subject to certain idealizing conditions (Brandt, 1979/1998; Dorsey, 2012; Harsanyi, 1977; Hildenbrand & Sonnenschein, 1991). Two final broad approaches emphasize the attainment of objective goods. According to eudaimonic theories, well-being is a matter of flourishing as a person, especially with respect to the types of psychological goods frequently valued by philosophers, like virtue, friendship, intelligence, and creativity (Aristotle, 4th c. BCE/2002; Kraut, 2007; Mengzi, 4th c. BCE/2008; Nussbaum, 2011). Philosophers usually describe such eudaimonic theories as "objective list" theories because in such theories well-being consists of objectively possessing such goods. In contrast, non-eudaimonic objective list approaches emphasize goods like wealth, beauty, fame, career success, long life, and having children (e.g., as expressed in Homer [8th c. BCE/1951], ancient Chinese Yangism [Knoblock & Riegel, trans., 3rd c. BCE/2000], and popular culture [The LOX, 1998]).

Thus, we recognize three conceptually distinct "subjective" approaches to well-being—hedonic, life satisfaction, and desire satisfaction—which emphasize emotional states or satisfaction of one's desires, and two more "objective" approaches—eudaimonic and non-eudaimonic—which emphasize the attainment of particular lists of goods or types of flourishing. However, because positive emotions and personal satisfaction are among the goods that plausibly belong on objective lists of well-being, and because desire-fulfillment accounts often emphasize the objective fulfillment of one's desires (rather than the subjective judgment that one's desires are fulfilled), the subjective-objective distinction is not quite as sharp as suggested by this simple portrayal.

At least in principle, these five types of well-being could diverge in individual cases. An underachieving sitcom enthusiast might have an overwhelmingly positive balance of positive to negative hedonic states but very little in way of friendship or creative productivity. A self-flagellating monk might be completely satisfied with a hedonically unpleasant, outwardly unproductive life. A universally beloved creative genius might feel painfully dissatisfied that she still falls far short of her envisioned potential. Such people might have high well-being according to one conception but low well-being according to another conception. In principle, some of the five types of well-being might even correlate negatively in some societies or for some groups of people. For example, some people who achieve substantial early fame, creative success, or desire satisfaction may experience less hedonic pleasure on average than do people with only average fame and career success or who attain their life goals more gradually.

Philosophically and conceptually, these types of well-being are distinct. Are they also empirically distinguishable?

One Well-Being or Many Well-Beings?

The variety of approaches to well-being complicates its empirical study. How can scientists investigate well-being without knowing exactly what it is? Researchers typically focus on one or a few types of well-being. For example, a large body of research (see Diener, Lucas, & Oishi, 2018, for a review) has used Diener's (1984) definition of subjective well-being, which combines hedonic well-being and life satisfaction. However, other researchers focus on eudaimonic well-being (e.g., Ryff, 2014; Ryan & Deci, 2001). Does current knowledge about one type of well-being apply equally to other types of well-being? If yes, then the correlations among types of well-being should be roughly equal to the reliabilities of the well-being measures (i.e., the disattenuated correlations being near unity), suggesting that the different types of well-being are best conceptualized as one construct. For example, some argue that hedonic well-being and eudaimonia are empirically indistinguishable for this reason (Disaboto, Goodman, Kashdan, Short, & Jarden, 2016). Or are the types of well-being different enough that they have unique correlates? The higher the correlations between the different types of well-being, the less potential for divergent empirical results, depending on the type of measure used.

Previous research has examined these possibilities with regard to hedonic well-being, life satisfaction, and various conceptualizations of eudaimonia, but not desire fulfillment or non-eudaimonic objective list well-being. This research typically finds correlations that are moderately high, yet low enough to suggest the possibility of notably different underlying phenomena. For example, several studies have produced correlations of less than 0.6 between life satisfaction and positive or negative affect (Arthaud-Day, Rode, Mooney, & Near, 2005; Lucas, Diener, & Suh, 1996). Similarly, the six subscales of the Psychological Well-Being Scale (a common measure of eudaimonia) show only moderate correlations with hedonic well-being and life satisfaction (Ryff & Keyes, 1995), and the Questionnaire for Eudaimonic Well-Being shows correlations of around 0.5 with the Satisfaction with Life Scale and of around 0.6 with the Psychological Well-Being Scale (Waterman et al., 2010). One recent study reported correlations ranging approximately from 0.5 to 0.9 between various measures of affect, satisfaction, and well-being, including a correlation of 0.76 between the Oxford Happiness Questionnaire and the Satisfaction with Life Scale (Medvedev & Landhuis, 2018). Other investigators have found correlations from 0.48 to 0.62 among several theoretically distinct measures of psychological and social flourishing (Hone, Jarden, Schofield, & Duncan, 2014). In sum, it would seem possible to find discriminant validity among measures of hedonic well-being, life satisfaction, psychological flourishing, and eudaimonia.

Even if well-being measures show discriminant validity, it is still possible for most correlates of each type of well-being to be very similar. For example, subjective happiness (typically considered relatively hedonic) and psychological well-being (as measured by the Psychological Well-Being Scale and often considered eudaimonic) show quite similar patterns of correlations with social reputation, clinician judgments of personality, and social behaviors (Nave, Sherman, & Funder, 2008). However, other research has found that correlations between elements of forgiveness and well-being are different for hedonic versus other measures (Maltby, Day, & Barber, 2005). Similarly, perceived job control appears to be related to eudaimonic feelings such as engagement but not to hedonic well-being (Kopperud & Vitters, 2008).

To determine whether different types of well-being can be treated as one or whether they show important empirical differences, we conducted three studies that assess correlations between the five types of well-being and the extent to which correlations between these types of well-being and other constructs depend on the type of well-being measured. Although previous studies have compared two or three types of well-being (usually involving hedonic well-being, eudaimonia, and life satisfaction), none has compared all five types of well-being, and previous studies' choices of measures have often mapped poorly onto the philosophical conceptions.

To assess desire fulfillment, we developed a new measure (described in Study 1). For the remaining four types of well-being, we selected those measures that we judged to most accurately reflect the philosophical conceptions. We measured hedonic well-being with a modified version of the Affect-Adjective Scale, which captures positive and negative affect states (Diener & Emmons, 1984). We measured eudaimonia and life satisfaction with the Riverside Eudaimonia Scale and the Riverside Life Satisfaction Scale, respectively—measures that were developed to match philosophical definitions of these concepts, as well as to have other psychometrically desirable properties (Margolis, Schwitzgebel, Ozer, & Lyubomirsky, 2018, 2019). To assess non-eudaimonic objective list well-being, we used a measure designed to contrast conceptually with the "high-brow" objective goods that are often emphasized in eudaimonic conceptions of well-being. This was the Rich and Sexy Well-Being Scale, which measures "low-brow" lifestyle goods: wealth, sex, beauty, and social status (Margolis et al., 2019).

We also included other well-being measures that cut across the conceptual boundaries of the five views of well-being. In particular, we included a popular measure of general happiness, which does not define happiness for participants but rather lets them use their own definition (Lyubomirsky & Lepper, 1999). We also included the Psychological Well-Being Scale, which, despite sometimes being interpreted as a measure of eudaimonic well-being, appears to measure psychological well-being in general rather than specifically the attainment of objective goods like wisdom and accomplishment (Ryff & Keyes, 1995). The Psychological Well-Being Scale is designed to measure aspects of positive functioning identified throughout the history of psychological science. Thus, those who endorse a certain type of eudaimonic perspective as it has been developed by psychologists may view these six factors as well-being itself (or a close approximation). Other thinkers who view eudaimonic flourishing in terms of an objective list of important human goods may regard the items of the Psychological Well-Being Scale as too focused on self-ratings of subjective states (such as moods and feelings of satisfaction or disappointment) rather than self-ratings of objective attainments. Furthermore, non-eudaimonic well-being theorists may view the six factors of this scale as potential causes of well-being. Last, in addition to our desire fulfillment measure, we developed a measure of desire satisfaction that blends desire fulfillment and life satisfaction.

We assessed participants using these well-being measures and typical correlates of well-being, including demographics, the Big Five, the dark triad, values, and response biases (Studies 2–4). All materials, data, and R code for this project can be accessed at osf.io/48fex.

Developing a Measure of Desire Fulfillment and Desire Satisfaction

Method

Participants

We recruited participants (N = 252) from Prolific Academic, a service based in the United Kingdom that connects online participants with researchers. Participants from around the world create a Prolific Academic account and can then complete surveys posted by researchers, assuming they meet the eligibility requirements. In this study, participants were eligible to participate if they spoke English as their first language. They were 18–66 years old (mean [M] = 31.1, standard deviation [SD] = 10.6) and 33% female. A majority (68%) of our participants were from the United States, 15% were from the UK, and 71% were Caucasian. A plurality (40%) of participants were employed full-time and another 27% were employed part-time.

Procedure

After reading a short description of our study and consenting, participants responded to the following prompt: "What are the 6 most important things you want in life? Take a few moments and think about these things. List these desires below."

Desire Fulfillment Score. On the next page, participants were told: "Now, for each of your desires, please rate the extent to which you believe you are fulfilling it." At this point, participants' previously listed desires were displayed, and they were instructed to rate the fulfillment of each desire on a 7-point Likert scale from "Not at all" to "Extremely." The overall "desire fulfillment" score was the average of these six ratings.

Desire Satisfaction Score. Below these ratings, participants were instructed to "please scroll up and briefly review how fulfilled your desires are." They were then asked to rate, "How satisfied are you with how fulfilled your desires are?" (from 1 = "Completely dissatisfied" to 7 = "Completely satisfied"). This constituted the "desire satisfaction" score.

Two weeks later, participants were recontacted through Prolific Academic and asked to complete the same survey again. Of the 252 participants of the initial survey, 188 (75%) completed the follow-up survey. They were compensated for each survey they completed.

Results

Reliability

The desire fulfillment ratings during the initial survey featured a McDonald's ω_t (an estimate of reliability based on the magnitude of factor loadings relative to error variances) of 0.85. When these ratings were averaged within each timepoint, the test-retest correlation was 0.78. The desire satisfaction item had a test-retest correlation of 0.75.

Correlations with Dropout

Desire fulfillment and desire satisfaction were correlated at $r = 0.77$ (95% confidence interval [CI] [0.72, 0.82], $p < 0.001$). Participants who did not return for the follow-up scored higher in initial desire fulfillment and desire satisfaction. Desire fulfillment was significantly and positively correlated with dropout ($r = 0.13$, 95% CI [.01, 0.25], $p = 0.04$), but the correlation between desire satisfaction and dropout was not significant. ($r = 0.07$, 95% CI [$-.05, 0.20$], $p = 0.25$).

In an informal, post-hoc analysis of the free response fields where people listed their desires, we found that the most commonly mentioned desires involved family, happiness, health, love, money, and educational and career goals. Because spiritual goals were rarely listed, this measure likely does not tap spiritual desires or spiritual well-being (a limitation it shares with many other well-being measures: see Chapters 10, 11, and 16, all in this volume).

Brief Discussion

Both desire fulfillment and desire satisfaction scores from our measure demonstrated acceptable levels of reliability. In addition, we believe the items of each measure have face validity with respect to the targeted philosophical conceptions. With this newly developed measure of desire fulfillment, we were positioned to conduct the next set of studies, which required measures of each of the five types of well-being. Accordingly, Studies 2 through 4 examined the empirical relationships among the five types of well-being, including comparing correlations between different types of well-being and other measures. Finally, these three studies provided data on the construct validity of our desire fulfillment and desire satisfaction measures.

Studies 2–4: Empirical Comparison of Five Types of Well-Being

Method

Participants
For each of the three studies, we recruited participants from Prolific Academic. See Table 13.1 for demographic information about the participants in each study.

Procedure
In each study, participants viewed a short description of the study and consented. They then completed questionnaires and received compensation for their participation.

Table 13.1 Demographic information for participants in Studies 2–4

	Study 2	Study 3	Study 4
Sample size	504	303	406
Age	$M = 35.1$, $SD = 12.0$	$M = 31.9$, $SD = 11.6$	$M = 36.3$, $SD = 11.8$
Female	51%	45%	58%
From United Kingdom	79%	20%	57%
From United States	1%	69%	14%
Caucasian	82%	73%	78%
Nonreligious	46%	44%	42%
Christian	29%	31%	35%
Median education level	Undergraduate degree	Undergraduate degree	College / A Levels
Median personal income	£10,000–19,999	£10,000–19,999	£10,000–19,999
Median household income	£30,000–39,999	£40,000–49,999	£30,000–39,999
In a relationship	52%	37%	62%
Employed full-time	49%	37%	42%
Employed part-time	24%	30%	23%

Measures

Table 13.2 indicates the constructs that were measured in each study, and Table 13.3 provides reliability coefficients. See later discussion for descriptions of the measures used to assess each construct. The proportion of missing responses on these measures was very low (less than 0.5% in each study). We imputed missing data using predictive mean matching.

Five Types of Well-Being

Hedonic Well-Being. Participants completed the Affect-Adjective Scale (Diener & Emmons, 1984), which assesses positive and negative affect. The measure asks participants to rate the extent to which they typically feel specific emotions (e.g., "pleased" and "worried/anxious") on a 7-point Likert scale. The original scale had nine items, but we added three low-arousal items ("peaceful/serene," "dull/bored," and "relaxed/calm") to ensure that the scale had low arousal as well as high arousal emotions, which is important for most

Table 13.2 Constructs measured in Studies 2–4

		Study 2	Study 3	Study 4
Five types of well-being	Hedonic well-being	X	X	X
	Life satisfaction	X	X	X
	Desire fulfillment		X	X
	Eudaimonia	X	X	X
	Rich and Sexy Well-Being	X	X	X
Other types of well-being	Desire satisfaction		X	X
	Psychological well-being	X	X	
	Happiness	X	X	
Personality	Big Five traits	X	X	X
	Big Five facets	X	X	
	Dark Triad	X	X	
	Values			X
Response biases	Socially desirable responding		X	X
	Experimenter demand		X	

accounts of hedonic well-being. We computed hedonic well-being scores by reverse scoring negative affect items and then averaging all affect items.

Life Satisfaction. We measured life satisfaction with the Riverside Life Satisfaction Scale, which reflects a broader philosophical conception of life satisfaction than does the more commonly used Satisfaction with Life Scale, although the two measures are highly correlated (Margolis et al., 2018). This measure asks participants to indicate their agreement with three statements that directly endorse life satisfaction (e.g., "I like how my life is going") and three reverse-coded statements that endorse life dissatisfaction (e.g., "If I could live my life over, I would change many things"). Participants rated these items on a 7-point Likert scale.

Desire Fulfillment and Desire Satisfaction. Participants were given the measure described in Study 1.

Eudaimonia. We assessed eudaimonia with the Riverside Eudaimonia Scale, as this measure was designed to match philosophical conceptualizations of eudaimonia or objective flourishing, drawn from a review of the

Table 13.3 Reliability (McDonald's ω_t) of measures in Studies 2–4

		Study 2	Study 3	Study 4
Five types of well-being	Hedonic well-being	0.93	0.96	0.92
	Life satisfaction	0.93	0.93	0.91
	Desire fulfillment		0.85	0.83
	Eudaimonia	0.77	0.78	0.79
	Rich and Sexy well-being	0.88	0.90	0.90
Other types of well-being	Psychological well-being	0.85	0.84	
	Happiness	0.90	0.90	
Personality	Extraversion	0.87	0.88	0.60
	-Sociability	0.84	0.87	
	-Assertiveness	0.80	0.81	
	-Energy Level	0.73	0.75	
	Agreeableness	0.82	0.84	0.58
	-Compassion	0.70	0.72	
	-Respectfulness	0.71	0.73	
	-Trust	0.72	0.74	
	Conscientiousness	0.88	0.89	0.66
	-Organization	0.85	0.80	
	-Productiveness	0.78	0.77	
	-Responsibility	0.71	0.80	
	Negative emotionality	0.92	0.93	0.80
	-Anxiety	0.82	0.84	
	-Depression	0.85	0.87	
	-Emotional volatility	0.82	0.88	
	Open-mindedness	0.85	0.87	0.65
	-Aesthetic sensitivity	0.80	0.83	
	-Intellectual curiosity	0.70	0.74	
	-Creative imagination	0.75	0.78	
Dark Triad	Machiavellianism	0.80	0.82	
	Psychopathy	0.78	0.82	
	Narcissism	0.81	0.81	

(*continued*)

Table 13.3 *Continued*

		Study 2	Study 3	Study 4
Values	Conformity			0.38
	Tradition			0.41
	Benevolence			0.51
	Universalism			0.56
	Self-direction			0.42
	Stimulation			0.31
	Hedonism			0.40
	Achievement			0.36
	Power			0.57
	Security			0.37
Response biases	Socially desirable responding		0.82	0.83
	Experimenter demand		0.92	

recent philosophical literature on the topic (e.g., Hurka, 2011; Kraut, 2007; Nussbaum, 2011; Rice, 2013; see also Baril, Chapter 9, in this volume, on the difficulty of measuring eudaimonic well-being as philosophers conceive of it) and has favorable psychometric properties (Margolis et al., 2019). This measure contains five items rated on a 7-point Likert scale (e.g., "I have realized my creative, artistic, intellectual, or athletic potential").

Non-Eudaimonic Objective List Well-Being. We administered the Rich and Sexy Well-Being Scale (Margolis et al., 2019), which measures the frequency and quality of sex, personal wealth, personal beauty, and social status (e.g., "When I'm in the room, people listen to me"). The 16-item scale is rated using 7-point Likert scales.

Other Measures of Well-Being

Psychological Well-Being. Participants completed an 18-item version of the Psychological Well-Being Scale (Ryff & Keyes, 1995), which assesses six aspects of psychological flourishing (autonomy, environmental mastery, personal growth, positive relations with others, purpose in life, and self-acceptance). Items (e.g., "In general, I feel I am in charge of the situation in which I live") were rated on a 6-point Likert scale. Although this measure is often interpreted as a measure of eudaimonic well-being, we have argued that its content is a mix of items that are eudaimonic in the standard philosophical "objective list" sense of eudaimonia, combined with items that reflect subjective goods that may not correlate with objective flourishing (Margolis et al., 2019). For example, some of the items seem to measure life satisfaction ("When I look at the story of my life, I am pleased with how things have turned out") or negative emotion ("The demands of everyday life often get me down"). In addition, the Psychological Well-Being Scale lacks ratings of constructs often deemed important to eudaimonia (e.g., creative achievement).

Happiness. We measured self-described global happiness with the Subjective Happiness Scale (Lyubomirsky & Lepper, 1999). This measure asks participants to rate their happiness, without providing an explicit definition (e.g., that happiness is hedonic or eudaimonic), thereby allowing participants to use their own definition of happiness. For example, one item asks, "In general, I consider myself" with anchors of "not a very happy person" and "a very happy person." This 4-item measure used 7-point Likert scales. Recent evidence suggests that participants might differ in whether they construe "happiness" entirely subjectively or instead as also having an objective component (Kneer & Haybron, 2019).

Personality

Big Five Traits and Facets. In Studies 2 and 3, participants completed the Big Five Inventory–2 (i.e., BFI-2; Soto & John, 2017a). This 60-item scale measures each Big Five trait with three facets. In Study 4, we measured Big Five traits with the Big Five Inventory–2 Extra-Short (i.e., BFI-2-XS; Soto & John, 2017b), which measures each trait with three items and does not include facet subscales. Both the BFI-2 and BFI-2-XS use 5-point Likert scales and ask participants to rate the extent to which statements apply to them (e.g., "I am someone who is outgoing, sociable").

Dark Triad. In Studies 2 and 3, participants completed The Dirty Dozen (Jonason & Webster, 2010), which measures Machiavellianism, psychopathy, and narcissism, each with four items. Participants rated their agreement with statements such as "I have used deceit or lied to get my way" (for Machiavellianism) on a 7-point Likert scale.

Values. In Study 4, participants completed the 58-item Schwartz Values Survey (Schwartz, 1992), which asked them to rate the extent to which each value is "a guiding principle in [their lives]" on a scale ranging from -1 (opposed to my values) to 7 (of supreme importance). Items included "politeness (courtesy, good manners)" and "wealth (material positions, money)." The values were scored into 10 subscales, as described by Schwartz (1992).

The reliabilities of these subscales were generally poor (see Table 13.3). Thus, results with these values should be interpreted with caution.

Response Biases. These measures were included to verify that the scores on scales were not solely a result of socially desirable responding or experimenter demand.

Socially Desirable Responding. In Studies 3 and 4, we administered the 16-item version of the Balanced Inventory of Desirable Responding (Hart, Ritchie, Hepper, & Gebauer, 2015). Items such as "I always know why I like things" and "I am very confident of my judgments" were rated on a 7-point Likert scale with anchors of strongly disagree, disagree, slightly disagree, neither agree nor disagree, slightly agree, agree, and strongly disagree.

Experimenter Demand. In Study 3, participants completed the Perceived Awareness of the Research Hypothesis Scale (Rubin, 2016), which asks participants to rate how confident they are that they have determined the research hypotheses, with items such as "I knew what the researchers were investigating in this research." This 4-item scale uses a 7-point Likert scale.

Demographic Characteristics. Demographic information was provided by Prolific Academic. We used the following variables: age (continuous), gender (dichotomous), education (ordinal, 6 levels), relationship status (dichotomous), personal income (ordinal, 12 levels), and household income (ordinal, 12 levels). The relationship status question included several categorical responses, but we converted this variable into a dichotomous variable by scoring participants who responded "in a relationship" or "married" as a 1, and scoring those who responded as "divorced," "never married," "separated," "single," or "widowed" as a 0.

Analytic Approach

Most of our correlational analyses examine the eight measures of well-being discussed earlier. For our correlational analyses, we first correlated the relevant variables in each study. We then disattenuated those correlation matrices using McDonald's ω_t. Because our desire satisfaction measure is one item, we set its reliability coefficient to the test-retest correlation. It was important to disattenuate the correlations so that differences between correlations were not due to differences in reliability. After the correlation matrices for each study were disattenuated, we meta-analyzed the correlation matrices using a fixed-effects approach and inverse variance weighting for pooling. The disattenuated correlations were meta-analyzed over all studies that included the measures. Thus, some disattenuated correlations are meta-analyzed over two, rather than three studies.

Results and Discussion

Relationships Between Types of Well-Being

Table 13.4 displays the meta-analytic disattenuated correlations among the eight measures of well-being. Four of these measures were included in all three studies and the other four measures were included in two studies (see Table 13.2).

Some disattenuated correlations approached 1, suggesting that the constructs were nearly indistinguishable empirically. In this case, future studies would not benefit from measuring both constructs. Instead, they could choose one measure, and results should not substantially depend on which measure is selected.

Desire satisfaction was nearly identical to desire fulfillment and life satisfaction. The correlation between desire satisfaction and desire fulfillment may have been upwardly biased because the desire satisfaction item had participants examine their responses to the desire fulfillment measure. However, the two constructs may simply be extremely similar. Likewise,

Table 13.4 Meta-analytic disattenuated correlation matrix of well-being measures[a]

		1	2	3	4	5	6	7
Five types of well-being	1. Hedonic well-being	—						
	2. Life satisfaction	0.79	—					
	3. Desire fulfillment	0.71	0.77	—				
	4. Eudaimonia	0.62	0.72	0.66	—			
	5. Rich and Sexy well-being	0.50	0.54	0.58	0.56	—		
Other types of well-being	6. Desire satisfaction	0.81	0.93	0.98	0.74	0.56	—	
	7. Psychological well-being	0.76	0.85	0.72	0.89	0.59	0.77	—
	8. Happiness	0.82	0.78	0.75	0.64	0.57	0.83	0.79

[a]All correlations are significant at $p < 0.05$.

desire satisfaction and life satisfaction may be very highly correlated because the cognitive evaluation of life satisfaction may involve assessing desire fulfillment. For example, if the life satisfaction measure prompts participants to evaluate their satisfaction with domains of their life (e.g., work, family, social), in response, participants may be examining their fulfillment of desires such as "to succeed at work" and "to have strong familial bonds." The very high correlation between desire satisfaction and life satisfaction is consistent with this cognitive process of evaluating life satisfaction.

Two of the eight measures, eudaimonia and Rich and Sexy well-being, showed relatively low correlations with other types of well-being. Eudaimonia and Rich and Sexy well-being are both more "objective" forms of well-being, with each being a potential list of objectively attained goods. Although we measured these types of well-being with subjective assessments of objective attainment, their relative objectivity might explain their relative separation from the other types of well-being. Objective attainments and subjective experience can separate for a variety of reasons, such as emotional resilience, hedonic adaptation, the relative psychological unimportance of some or all of the putative objective goods, or the adoption of "adaptive preferences" (Elster, 1983) that match what is realistically attainable. One exception to this general trend is that eudaimonia and psychological well-being were also very highly correlated, likely because they are both attempts to measure eudaimonia and contain both objective and subjective elements.

Although Rich and Sexy well-being showed relatively low correlations with other forms of well-being, these correlations were nonetheless higher than some people might expect. One possibility is that sex life, wealth, beauty, and social status are more closely related to overall life satisfaction, happiness, or other forms of well-being than people with "high-brow" views of human flourishing tend to think. Another possibility is that a generally upbeat or optimistic person may respond to both the Rich and Sexy Well-Being Scale and other measures of well-being in a relatively positive manner, inflating correlations between Rich and Sexy well-being and other well-being measures. Alternatively but not incompatibly, someone low in Rich and Sexy well-being (i.e., relatively low-status, unattractive, poor, and alone) may be dissatisfied with their life, feel that their desires are unfulfilled, lack frequent positive emotions, and be more focused on obtaining those resources than on achieving such ends as virtue or productive creativity (cf. Maslow, 1943).

Relationships Between Types of Well-Being and Other Measures

Correlations between types of well-being and demographic factors were generally similar across types of well-being (see Table 13.5). For example, age was weakly and positively correlated with all forms of well-being except Rich and Sexy well-being. Women scored higher than men on all types of well-being, again with Rich and Sexy well-being as the exception. As one might expect, educational attainment related most strongly to the more objective forms of well-being (i.e., eudaimonia and Rich and Sexy well-being). Being in a relationship was positively and relatively moderately correlated with all forms of well-being, but it was especially important for life satisfaction and Rich and Sexy well-being. When evaluating life satisfaction, one may assess different life domains, and romantic relationships are likely to be an important domain for many people. Thus, it is not surprising that having a partner would particularly affect life satisfaction. Similarly, high wealth, beauty, and

Table 13.5 Meta-analytic disattenuated correlations between demographics and types of well-being[a]

		Age	Female status	Education	Relationship status	Personal income	Household income
Five types of well-being	Hedonic well-being	0.12*	0.01	0.05	0.17*	0.16*	0.10*
	Life satisfaction	0.07*	0.10*	0.11*	0.29*	0.18*	0.17*
	Desire fulfillment	0.07	0.05	0.10*	0.24*	0.19*	0.18*
	Eudaimonia	0.11*	0.13*	0.16*	0.19*	0.12*	0.07*
	Rich and Sexy well-being	0.01	−0.07*	0.20*	0.30*	0.26*	0.27*
Other types of well-being	Desire satisfaction	0.12*	0.11*	0.08*	0.23*	0.20*	0.19*
	Psychological well-being	0.10*	0.09*	0.15*	0.25*	0.19*	0.16*
	Happiness	0.09*	0.03	0.07*	0.20*	0.19*	0.13*

[a] * = $p < 0.05$. Demographic variables were treated as having a reliability of 1.

status may all increase the likelihood of being in a relationship, and having a partner likely makes sexual behavior more available. Personal and household incomes were also moderately and positively correlated with well-being. However, income was especially important for Rich and Sexy well-being and relatively weakly associated with eudaimonia. We would expect income to be particularly important for Rich and Sexy well-being, given its items measuring wealth.

Mirroring previous research (Steel, Schmidt, & Shultz, 2008), the Big Five personality traits were generally highly correlated to well-being, with open-mindedness being an exception (see Table 13.6). However, these associations depended on the type of well-being. For example, although extraversion is sometimes thought to be particularly associated with hedonic well-being, extraversion showed higher correlations with eudaimonia, psychological well-being, Rich and Sexy well-being, and happiness than the other types of well-being. Eudaimonia, psychological well-being, and Rich and Sexy well-being each has a social component, which may explain their particularly high correlations with extraversion. The high correlation between extraversion and happiness suggests participants' own conceptions of happiness may include social interaction and high-arousal positive emotions. Agreeableness was moderately and positively correlated with all forms of well-being except with Rich and Sexy well-being, which was correlated to agreeableness to a lesser extent, as one might expect. Conscientiousness was particularly highly correlated with psychological well-being and relatively less correlated with Rich and Sexy well-being compared to other forms of well-being, perhaps because conscientiousness secures markers of success that are less outwardly noticed than those comprising Rich and Sexy well-being. Negative emotionality was strongly and negatively correlated with all forms of well-being, but these associations were weaker with eudaimonia and Rich and Sexy well-being perhaps due to the relative subjectivity of negative emotionality. Interestingly, open-mindedness was particularly associated with eudaimonia and psychological well-being. Previous research has suggested that open-mindedness is relatively unimportant for happiness compared to other Big Five traits. However, this finding does not extend to eudaimonic well-being. Open-mindedness may be particularly related to eudaimonia as open-mindedness could help people achieve their creative potential and even enhance feelings of meaning in life.

Table 13.6 Meta-analytic disattenuated correlations between Big Five traits and types of well-being[a]

	Five types of well-being					Other types of well-being		
	Hedonic well-being	Life Satisfaction	Desire fulfillment	Eudaimonia	Rich and Sexy well-being	Desire Satisfaction	Psychological well-being	Happiness
Extraversion	**0.48***	**0.46***	**0.44***	**0.61***	**0.63***	**0.43***	**0.68***	**0.62***
-Sociability	0.34*	0.35*	0.36*	0.45*	0.47*	0.37*	0.47*	0.48*
-Assertiveness	0.29*	0.32*	0.35*	0.44*	0.53*	0.28*	0.51*	0.36*
-Energy Level	0.61*	0.60*	0.52*	0.68*	0.56*	0.57*	0.78*	0.76*
Agreeableness	**0.43***	**0.34***	**0.31***	**0.43***	**0.14***	**0.37***	**0.50***	**0.47***
-Compassion	0.24*	0.20*	0.18*	0.40*	0.08*	0.25*	0.42*	0.30*
-Respectfulness	0.33*	0.21*	0.15*	0.29*	-0.01	0.18*	0.39*	0.32*
-Trust	0.51*	0.41*	0.41*	0.46*	0.28*	0.47*	0.49*	0.57*
Conscientiousness	**0.40***	**0.41***	**0.37***	**0.47***	**0.24***	**0.42***	**0.56***	**0.32***
-Organization	0.21*	0.23*	0.22*	0.29*	0.09*	0.25*	0.35*	0.15*
-Productiveness	0.40*	0.41*	0.29*	0.55*	0.29*	0.32*	0.63*	0.40*
-Responsibility	0.39*	0.42*	0.32*	0.41*	0.15*	0.36*	0.55*	0.35*
Negative emotionality	**-0.79***	**-0.62***	**-0.53***	**-0.47***	**-0.45***	**-0.59***	**-0.71***	**-0.79***
-Anxiety	-0.74*	-0.59*	-0.55*	-0.39*	-0.38*	-0.63*	-0.59*	-0.71*
-Depression	-0.86*	-0.79*	-0.68*	-0.61*	-0.57*	-0.79*	-0.83*	-0.90*
-Emotional Volatility	-0.55*	-0.45*	-0.42*	-0.34*	-0.27*	-0.44*	-0.55*	-0.58*
Open-mindedness	**0.12***	**0.07***	**0.07***	**0.45***	**0.21***	**0.01**	**0.36***	**0.19***
-Aesthetic sensitivity	0.05	0.04	0.01	0.34*	0.10*	0.00	0.19*	0.12*
-Intellectual curiosity	0.05	0.05	0.05	0.38*	0.17*	-0.03	0.33*	0.12*
-Creative imagination	0.23*	0.22*	0.20*	0.57*	0.29*	0.18*	0.45*	0.27*

[a] * = $p < 0.05$.

Table 13.7 Meta-analytic disattenuated correlations between Dark Triad traits and types of well-being[a]

		Machiavellianism	Psychopathy	Narcissism
Five types of well-being	Hedonic well-being	−0.13*	−0.28*	−0.17*
	Life satisfaction	−0.09*	−0.26*	−0.09*
	Desire fulfillment	−0.03	−0.26*	−0.05
	Eudaimonia	−0.11*	−0.40*	−0.02
	Rich and Sexy well-being	0.20*	−0.01	0.23*
Other types of well-being	Desire satisfaction	−0.08	−0.30*	−0.09
	Psychological well-being	−0.14*	−0.40*	−0.15*
	Happiness	−0.10*	−0.35*	−0.08*

[a] * = $p < 0.05$.

Unsurprisingly, the Dark Triad traits were negatively associated with well-being (see Table 13.7). Psychopathy was particularly detrimental for most types of well-being but, interestingly, unrelated to Rich and Sexy well-being. Perhaps the generally negative correlations between psychopathy and well-being were reduced when measuring Rich and Sexy well-being because people with psychopathic traits achieve Rich and Sexy well-being. Furthermore, Rich and Sexy well-being correlated *positively* with Machiavellianism and narcissism, while the other seven measures were either unrelated or correlated negatively. Again, possession of Dark Triad traits might be useful in obtaining wealth, beauty, sex, or the more superficial forms of social esteem. Alternatively, Machiavellian or narcissistic individuals might tend to rate themselves highly in Rich and Sexy well-being despite lacking the actual underlying traits.

Table 13.8 presents the disattenuated correlations between Schwartz Values Survey values and well-being in Study 3. Conformity, tradition, and achievement were correlated most with well-being. Interestingly, "hedonism" or "affective autonomy" (e.g., pleasure, self-indulgence, leisure) was not statistically associated with hedonic well-being. Valuing something does not ensure that one has it, and this might be especially true for positive emotions (Gilbert, 2005). Most correlations were somewhat consistent across types of well-being. However, Rich and Sexy well-being, compared to other forms of well-being, was particularly correlated with valuing stimulation, power, and

Table 13.8 Disattenuated correlations between values and types of well-being in Study 4[a]

	Five types of well-being					Other type of well-being	
	Hedonic well-being	Life satisfaction	Desire fulfillment	Eudaimonia	Rich and Sexy well-being	Desire satisfaction	
Conformity	0.44*	0.36*	0.40*	0.40*	0.33*	0.43*	
Tradition	0.40*	0.27*	0.38*	0.32*	0.20	0.42*	
Benevolence	0.25*	0.14	0.19	0.28*	0.15	0.16	
Universalism	0.20	0.08	0.19	0.27*	0.12	0.18	
Self-direction	0.16	0.03	0.12	0.11	0.20	0.09	
Stimulation	0.24	0.14	0.10	0.24	0.38*	0.11	
Hedonism	0.07	-0.10	0.07	-0.05	0.21	-0.03	
Achievement	0.35*	0.20	0.33*	0.42*	0.40*	0.24	
Power	0.12	0.07	0.15	0.09	0.34*	0.14	
Security	0.26	0.17	0.28	0.17	0.32*	0.21	

[a] * = p < 0.05.

security. It is not surprising that people who value stimulation, power, and security would successfully seek out sex, wealth, beauty, and status—that is, the goods of Rich and Sexy well-being. Also, unlike the other types of well-being, eudaimonia was correlated with both benevolence and universalism.

Table 13.9 displays the disattenuated correlations between response biases (i.e., socially desirable responding and experimenter demand) and types of well-being. All forms of well-being seem to be associated with socially desirable responding, suggesting that socially desirable responding may be unavoidable in well-being research. Of the eight types of well-being, Rich and Sexy well-being was least correlated with socially desirable responding, perhaps because participants felt that asserting oneself as sexy, wealthy, beautiful, and high status was tawdry or boastful. Experimenter demand was weakly associated with all types of well-being, except Rich and Sexy well-being, with which it was moderately correlated.

The Structure of Well-Being

To evaluate the structure of well-being, we examined the meta-analytic disattenuated correlations between the five types of well-being. We extracted eigenvalues of this correlation matrix, which suggested one factor (eigenvalues = 3.6, 0.6, 0.4, 0.3, 0.2). An exploratory factor analysis with oblimin rotation and two factors separated Rich and Sexy well-being, as a singleton, from the other four types of well-being. We also examined the

Table 13.9 Meta-analytic disattenuated correlations between response biases and types of well-being[a]

		Socially desirable responding	Experimenter demand
Five types of well-being	Hedonic well-being	0.49*	0.04
	Life satisfaction	0.42*	0.04
	Desire fulfillment	0.37*	0.15*
	Eudaimonia	0.48*	0.08
	Rich and Sexy well-being	0.25*	0.25*
Other types of well-being	Desire satisfaction	0.38*	0.13*
	Psychological well-being	0.50*	0.07
	Happiness	0.37*	0.06

[a] * = $p < 0.05$. Correlations with experimenter demand are not meta-analytic because this construct was only measured in Study 3.

correlations between the items of the five types of well-being. The eigenvalues of this matrix also suggested one factor (first eight eigenvalues = 15.4, 3.8, 2.2, 2.1, 1.9, 1.6, 1.3, 1.1). Exploratory factor analyses could categorize items in a systematic manner. For example, an eight-factor exploratory factor analyses with oblimin rotation formed factors with the following items: (1) desire fulfillment, (2) eudaimonia and status, (3) wealth, (4) beauty, (5) sex, (6) negative affect, (7) life satisfaction, and (8) positive affect. An exploratory bifactor analysis arranged items into the same groups. A nine-factor model did not divide the eudaimonia and status items, but a two-factor exploratory factor analysis with just those items did divide the items by the measure. However, although exploratory factor analyses can divide the well-being items systematically, the eigenvalues suggest one general well-being factor.

General Discussion

The Empirical Distinctness of the Five Types of Well-Being

Although the five types of well-being—hedonic, life satisfaction, desire fulfillment, eudaimonic, and non-eudaimonic objective list—are characterized by important conceptual differences, it is reasonable to wonder whether these types of well-being differ empirically. Previous research has only examined this question tangentially. Often types of well-being are compared within a single domain, and only a few types are considered. By contrast, we compared five types of well-being and examined correlations both between these types of well-being and between the types of well-being and several other constructs. We found that even when the correlations among the five types of well-being were disattenuated, they mostly did not approach 1. Undoubtedly, the types of well-being are highly correlated. However, the correlations are not so high as to prevent the possibility that researchers could obtain different results depending on the type of well-being measured. Indeed, we found that the typical correlates of well-being displayed different patterns of association with different types of well-being. These differences were large enough to substantially affect conclusions that one might draw about well-being based on the different measures. For example, the Big Five personality trait of open-mindedness correlated at $r = 0.01$ with desire satisfaction well-being but at $r = 0.45$ with eudaimonic well-being.

Due to the pattern of eigenvalues we found (suggesting a 1-factor model of well-being), one might wonder why different types of well-being show different patterns of association with other constructs. We think the bifactor model provides a reasonable answer. The bifactor model includes a general well-being factor but also specific factors for each type of well-being. With this structure, one would expect the pattern of eigenvalues we observed, as well as the different patterns of association we found for each type of well-being.

Because results will differ when different measures of well-being are used, research findings using one type of well-being will not necessarily hold true for other types of well-being. This possibility will need to be examined empirically. We suggest that future investigators be mindful of the similarities and differences among the different types of well-being. Discovering something new about one type of well-being provides an opportunity to extend or replicate with other types of well-being. For example, if pet ownership is found to predict hedonic well-being, researchers might examine whether there is a similar association between pet ownership and life satisfaction or eudaimonia.

Well-being scientists should consider whether their general theories of well-being (e.g., Diener & Biswas-Diener, 2008; Emmons, 1986; Lyubomirsky & Layous, 2013; Ryan & Deci, 2000; Sheldon & Elliot, 1999) apply equally to all of the types of well-being that we have identified or whether they require adjustment or clarification in light of these different conceptualizations.

A New Desire Fulfillment Measure

One separate but related research program involves desire fulfillment. Some social scientists may prefer to study this type of well-being because it theoretically reflects the types of goal pursuit in which economists and other social scientists are often interested. Accordingly, we developed a brief measure of desire fulfillment and present construct validity evidence for this measure. At least in its surface content, this measure is more directly connected than other types of well-being measures to people's specific behavioral choices and priorities and to their self-evaluated progress toward their top-priority life goals. The extent to which one's highest priority desires are fulfilled is notably distinct from the extent to which one experiences hedonic well-being and overall life satisfaction (e.g., in cases where attainment of one's goals leaves one still unhappy and dissatisfied). It is also distinct from attaining the objective goods that society values, whether those goods are eudaimonic or non-eudaimonic. In sum, our new desire fulfillment measure aims to capture well-being in the specific sense of an individual's success in obtaining what they think they want, whether that is career, family, education, travel, living situation, wealth, personal ethical development, creative success, or anything else.

Choosing a Well-Being Measure

No one measure of well-being appears to be psychometrically superior to all the rest. Therefore, researchers' choice of well-being measure should reflect their theoretical aims. For example, because open-mindedness is particularly related to eudaimonia, an experiment that seeks to bolster open-mindedness might benefit by including a measure of eudaimonia as an outcome. Investigators interested in the antecedents and consequences of materialism may wish to focus on Rich and Sexy well-being. Other investigators might be interested in finding situations or populations where the measures diverge, such as groups with substantial eudaimonic or Rich and Sexy well-being but low hedonic well-being.

A great deal of well-being research has focused on the composite construct of subjective well-being (see Diener et al., 2018, for a review). Prioritizing a certain form of well-being can accelerate progress because all findings using the same construct can be integrated. However, research using well-being composites—whether they represent subjective or other forms of well-being—may miss important differences among the constituent types of well-being. Researchers may need to unpack their composites to examine the different types of well-being separately. Indeed, research on hedonic well-being often examines positive and negative affect separately (e.g., Larsen & Ketelaar, 1991; McNiel & Fleeson, 2006; Steel et al., 2008) because the two are not opposite ends of the same spectrum (Diener & Emmons, 1984).

Limitations and Future Directions

Our studies were limited by the exclusive use of online samples, which constrains the generalizability of our findings, and the use of subjective self-report measures. Such measures seem uniquely appropriate for assessing life satisfaction and possibly desire fulfillment, to the extent that these constructs involve cognitive evaluations. We look forward to the development of improved measures of hedonic, eudaimonic, and objective list well-being. For example, experience sampling methods (ESM) may provide the best measure of hedonic well-being. By capturing affect in the moment, ESM is less impacted by memory biases than self-report measures that require participants to recall and aggregate their feelings over days, weeks, or longer. With novel tools such as smartwatches, smarthomes, and wearable technologies, hedonic well-being may soon be measured continuously, more objectively, and without input from the participant. Relatively objective measures are also superior to subjective measures for assessing eudaimonic and objective list well-being as these types of well-being involve the objective properties of one's life. For example, knowledgeable informants could rate whether an individual has reached her creative or intellectual potential (eudaimonic well-being) or is attractive and high-status (Rich and Sexy well-being). However, such quasi-objective measures will often be either unavailable or too expensive in many research contexts. In addition, our results may have been different if we used a different conceptualization of non-eudaimonic objective list well-being (see, e.g., Fletcher, 2013).

Philosophical Implications

To endorse a measure of well-being is to take a philosophical stand. If a researcher claims to measure "well-being" *in general* by means of an instrument that measures life satisfaction *specifically*, that researcher is implicitly treating life satisfaction as the best available index of what constitutes a human life that is going well. However, as Haybron (2007) has argued, a person with low expectations or who has the virtues of gratitude or fortitude might feel entirely satisfied with a life that is not in fact going well by the standards of a different philosophical theory of human well-being. To the extent that different types of well-being fail to correlate, such concerns are not merely in-principle or limited to a few marginal cases. Different conclusions drawn from different measures of well-being can lead to major differences in recommended public policy and major differences in the assessment of people's lives.

A central aim of positive psychology is the empirical study of how to promote human well-being. But unless investigators know what human well-being is, they do not know what they are studying. Scientists might attempt to duck the philosophical issue by hoping for tight correlations between all of types of well-being, such that it matters little which type is measured, but that hope is ill-founded. As a fallback approach, a scientist might create a composite measure that blends all types of well-being into a single construct, but to do so means to adopt a different sort of philosophical commitment, to a kind of even-handed pluralism (for some thoughtful defenses of well-being pluralism, see Bishop, 2015; Diener, 1984; Seligman, 2011; VanderWeele, 2017). There is no such thing as a value-free measure of human flourishing. We are all philosophers.

To conclude, if social scientists seek to study and promote human well-being, they should illuminate the philosophical value commitments that are implicit in the choice to measure it one way rather than another, and they should vigorously debate which measure or measures are best for which empirical and policy purposes.

About the Authors

Seth Margolis recently completed his Ph.D. in Psychology at the University of California, Riverside. He worked with Dr. Sonja Lyubomirsky in her Positive Activities and Well-Being Laboratory. His research focuses on well-being measurement, quantitative methodology, and personality interventions that boost well-being.

Eric Schwitzgebel is Professor of Philosophy at University of California, Riverside. His books include *Describing Inner Experience? Proponent Meets Skeptic* (with Russell T. Hurlburt; MIT Press, 2007), *Perplexities of Consciousness* (MIT Press, 2011), and *A Theory of Jerks and Other Philosophical Misadventures* (MIT Press, 2019). His research explores the limits of self-knowledge, the nature of attitudes, moral psychology, methodological limitations in the study of consciousness, and the relationship between intellectual moral reflection and real-world moral choice.

Daniel J. Ozer is Professor of Psychology at the University of California, Riverside. He is a past President of the Association for Research in Personality and the author of *Consistency in Personality: A Methodological Framework* (Springer, 1986). His research in personality assessment, structure, and scale construction includes the study of personality traits, personal goals, and daily behavior.

Sonja Lyubomirsky is Distinguished Professor and Vice Chair in the Department of Psychology at the University of California, Riverside, where she has been recognized with the Faculty of the Year (twice) and Faculty Mentor of the Year Awards. Dr. Lyubomirsky's research focuses on how to increase happiness and positive emotions, with a focus on expressing gratitude, practicing kindness, and boosting connection as interventions. She is the author of *The How of Happiness* (Penguin, 2008) and *The Myths of Happiness* (Penguin, 2013), translated in 36 countries. She has received many honors, including the Diener Award for Outstanding Midcareer Contributions in Personality Psychology, the Christopher J. Peterson Gold Medal, the Distinguished Research Lecturer Award, and a Positive Psychology Prize.

Author Note

This research was supported by a grant from Happiness and Well-Being: Integrating Research Across the Disciplines, Saint Louis University. Additional support was provided by the John Templeton Foundation and by the Lee Kum Sheung Center for Health and Happiness. The views expressed in this chapter represent the perspectives of the authors and do not reflect the opinions or endorsement of any organization. We have no known conflict of interest to disclose. Correspondence concerning this chapter should be directed to Seth Margolis, Department of Psychology, 900 University Ave., Riverside, CA, 92521 (sethmmargolis@gmail.com).

References

Alexandrova, A. (2017). *A philosophy for the science of well-being*. New York: Oxford University Press.

Aristotle (4th century BCE/2002). *Nicomachean ethics*. (C. J. Rowe & S. Broadie, Trans.). New York: Oxford University Press.

Arthaud-Day, M. L., Rode, J. C., Mooney, C. H., & Near, J. P. (2005). The subjective well-being construct: A test of its convergent, discriminant, and factorial validity. *Social Indicators Research, 74*, 445–476.

Bentham, J. (1780/2007). *Introduction to the principles of morals and legislation*. Minelo, NY: Dover.

Bishop, M. A. (2015). *The good life*. Oxford: Oxford University Press.

Brandt, R. B. (1979/1998). *A theory of the good and the right*. Amherst, NY: Prometheus.

Crisp, R. (2001/2017). Well-being. *Stanford encyclopedia of philosophy* (Fall 2017 Edition). https://plato.stanford.edu/archives/fall2017/entries/well-being.

Crisp, R. (2006). *Reasons and the good*. Oxford: Oxford University Press.

Diener, E. (1984). Subjective well-being. *Psychological Bulletin, 95*, 542–575.

Diener, E., & Biswas-Diener, R. (2008). *Happiness: Unlocking the mysteries of psychological wealth*. Hoboken, NJ: Blackwell Publishing.

Diener, E., & Emmons, R. A. (1984). The independence of positive and negative affect. *Journal of Personality and Social Psychology, 47*, 1105–1117.

Diener, E., Lucas, R. E., & Oishi, S. (2018). Advances and open questions in the science of subjective well-being. *Collabra: Psychology, 4*, 15.

Disabato, D. J., Goodman, F. R., Kashdan, T. B., Short, J. L., & Jarden, A. (2016). Different types of well-being? A cross-cultural examination of hedonic and eudaimonic well-being. *Psychological Assessment, 28,* 471–482.

Dorsey, D. (2012). Subjectivism without desire. *Philosophical Review, 121,* 407–442.

Elster, J. (1983). *Sour grapes.* Cambridge: Cambridge University Press.

Emmons, R. A. (1986). Personal strivings: An approach to personality and subjective well-being. *Journal of Personality and Social Psychology, 51,* 1058–1068.

Feldman, F. (2004). *Pleasure and the good life: Concerning the nature, varieties, and plausibility of hedonism.* Oxford: Oxford University Press.

Fletcher, G. (2013). A fresh start for the objective-list theory of well-being. *Utilitas, 25,* 206–220.

Gilbert, D. (2005). *Stumbling on happiness.* New York: Random House.

Harsanyi, J. (1977). Morality and the theory of rational behavior. *Social Research, 44,* 623–656.

Hart, C. M., Ritchie, T. D., Hepper, E. G., & Gebauer, J. E. (2015). The Balanced Inventory of Desirable Responding Short Form (BIDR-16). *Sage Open, 5,* 1–9.

Haybron, D. (2007). Life satisfaction, ethical reflection, and the science of happiness. *Journal of Happiness Studies, 8,* 99–138.

Hildenbrand, W., & Sonnenschein, H. (Eds.). (1991). *Handbook of mathematical economics.* Amsterdam: North-Holland.

Homer (8th century BCE/1951). *The Iliad* (R. Lattimore, Trans.). Chicago: University of Chicago.

Hone, L. C., Jarden, A., Schofield, G. M., & Duncan, S. (2014). Measuring flourishing: The impact of operational definitions on the prevalence of high levels of wellbeing. *International Journal of Wellbeing, 4,* 62–90.

Hurka, T. (2011). *The best things in life.* Oxford: Oxford University Press.

Jonason, P. K., & Webster, G. D. (2010). The Dirty Dozen: A concise measure of the dark triad. *Psychological Assessment, 22,* 420–432.

Kneer, M., & Haybron, D. M. (2019). Happiness and well-being: Is it all in your head? Evidence from the folk. www.researchgate.net/publication/ 337494445_Happiness_and_Well-Being_Is_It_All_in_Your_Head_Evidence_from_the_Folk

Knoblock, J., & Riegel, J. K. (3rd century BCE/2000). "Yangist" chapters. In *The annals of Lü Buwei.* Stanford, CA: Stanford University Press.

Kopperud, K. H., & Vitters, J. (2008). Distinctions between hedonic and eudaimonic well-being: Results from a day reconstruction study among Norwegian jobholders. *Journal of Positive Psychology, 3,* 174–181.

Kraut, R. (2007). *What is good and why.* Cambridge, MA: Harvard University Press.

Larsen, R. J., & Ketelaar, T. (1991). Personality and susceptibility to positive and negative emotional states. *Journal of Personality and Social Psychology, 61,* 132–140.

LOX, The. (1998). *Money, power & respect.* New York: Bad Boy Records.

Lucas, R. E., Diener, E., & Suh, E. (1996). Discriminant validity of well-being measures. *Journal of Personality and Social Psychology, 71,* 616–628.

Lyubomirsky, S., & Layous, K. (2013). How do simple positive activities increase well-being? *Current Directions in Psychological Science, 22,* 57–62.

Lyubomirsky, S., & Lepper, H. S. (1999). A measure of subjective happiness: Preliminary reliability and construct validation. *Social Indicators Research, 46,* 137–155.

Maltby, J., Day, L., & Barber, L. (2005). Forgiveness and happiness. The differing contexts of forgiveness using the distinction between hedonic and eudaimonic happiness. *Journal of Happiness Studies, 6*, 1–13.

Margolis, S., Schwitzgebel, E., Ozer, D. J., & Lyubomirsky, S. (2019). A new measure of life satisfaction: The Riverside Life Satisfaction Scale. *Journal of Personality Assessment, 101*, 621–630.

Margolis, S., Schwitzgebel, E., Ozer, D. J., & Lyubomirsky, S. (2020). *Developing measures of "objective" well-being.* Manuscript submitted for publication.

Maslow, A. H. (1943). A theory of human motivation. *Psychological Review, 50*, 370–396.

McGregor, J. A., & Pouw, N. (2017). Towards an economics of well-being. *Cambridge Journal of Economics, 41*, 1123–1142.

McMahan, E. A., & Estes, D. (2011). Hedonic versus eudaimonic conceptions of well-being: Evidence of differential associations with self-reported well-being. *Social Indicators Research, 103*, 93–108.

McNiel, J. M., & Fleeson, W. (2006). The causal effects of extraversion on positive affect and neuroticism on negative affect: Manipulating state extraversion and state neuroticism in an experimental approach. *Journal of Research in Personality, 40*, 529–550.

Medvedev, O. N., & Landhuis, C. E. (2018). Exploring constructs of well-being, happiness and quality of life. *Peer Journal, 6* (E4903). doi:10.7717/peerj.4903.

Mengzi (4th century BCE/2008). *Mengzi.* (B. W. Van Norden, Trans.). Indianapolis, IN: Hackett.

Mill, J. S. (1861/2003). *Utilitarianism.* In M. Warnock (Ed.), *Utilitarianism and on liberty* (pp. 181–235). Malden, MA: Blackwell.

Nave, C. S., Sherman, R. A., & Funder, D. C. (2008). Beyond self-report in the study of hedonic and eudaimonic well-being: Correlations with acquaintance reports, clinician judgments and directly observed social behavior. *Journal of Research in Personality, 42*, 643–659.

Neugarten, B. L., Havighurst, R. J., & Tobin, S. S. (1961). The measurement of life satisfaction. *Journal of Gerontology, 16*, 134–143.

Nussbaum, M. (2011). *Creating capabilities: The human development approach.* Cambridge, MA: Harvard University Press.

Parfit, D. (1984). *Reasons and persons.* Oxford: Oxford University Press.

Pflug, J. (2009). Folk theories of happiness: A cross-cultural comparison of conceptions of happiness in Germany and South Africa. *Social Indicators Research, 92*, 551–563.

Plato (4th century BCE/1961). Protagoras. In E. Hamilton & H. Cairns (Eds.), *The collected dialogues of Plato* (W. K. C. Guthrie, Trans.). Princeton, NJ: Princeton University Press.

Rice, C. M. (2013). Defending the objective list theory of well-being. *Ratio, 26*, 196–211.

Rubin, M. (2016). The Perceived Awareness of the Research Hypothesis Scale: Assessing the influence of demand characteristics. *Figshare.* https://doi.org/10.6084/m9.figshare.4315778.v2.

Ryan, R. M., & Deci, E. L. (2000). Self-determination theory and the facilitation of intrinsic motivation, social development, and well-being. *American Psychologist, 55*, 68–78.

Ryan, R. M., & Deci, E. L. (2001). On happiness and human potentials: A review of research on hedonic and eudaimonic well-being. *Annual Review of Psychology, 52*, 141–166.

Ryff, C. D. (2014). Psychological well-being revisited: Advances in the science and practice of eudaimonia. *Psychotherapy and Psychosomatics, 83*, 10–28.

Ryff, C. D., & Keyes, C. L. M. (1995). The structure of psychological well-being revisited. *Journal of Personality and Social Psychology, 69*, 719–727.

Schwartz, S. H. (1992). Universals in the content and structure of values: Theoretical advances and empirical tests in 20 countries. *Advances in Experimental Social Psychology, 25*, 1–65.

Seligman, M. E. (2011). *Flourish*. New York: Free Press.

Sheldon, K. M., & Elliot, A. J. (1999). Goal striving, need satisfaction, and longitudinal well-being: The self-concordance model. *Journal of Personality and Social Psychology, 76*, 482–497.

Soto, C. J., & John, O. P. (2017a). The next Big Five Inventory (BFI-2): Developing and assessing a hierarchical model with 15 facets to enhance bandwidth, fidelity, and predictive power. *Journal of Personality and Social Psychology, 113*, 117–143.

Soto, C. J., & John, O. P. (2017b). Short and extra-short forms of the Big Five Inventory-2: The BFI-2-S and BFI-2-XS. *Journal of Research in Personality, 68*, 69–81.

Steel, P., Schmidt, J., & Shultz, J. (2008). Refining the relationship between personality and subjective well-being. *Psychological Bulletin, 134*, 138–161.

Sumner, L. W. (1996). *Welfare, happiness, and ethics*. Oxford: Oxford University Press.

VanderWeele, T. J. (2017). On the promotion of human flourishing. *Proceedings of the National Academy of Sciences of the United States of America, 114*, 8148–8156.

Waterman, A. S., Schwartz, S. J., Zamboanga, B. L., Ravert, R. D., Williams, M. K., Bede Agocha, V., . . . Brent Donnellan, M. (2010). The Questionnaire for Eudaimonic Well-Being: Psychometric properties, demographic comparisons, and evidence of validity. *Journal of Positive Psychology, 5*, 41–61.

14

Measures of Community Well-Being

A Template

Tyler J. VanderWeele

Abstract

A proposal is put forward for a measure of community well-being that can be adapted to numerous specific contexts. The community well-being measure extends beyond simple measures of community satisfaction that are often currently employed. The proposed measure includes items in six domains relevant to community well-being: flourishing individuals, good relationships, proficient leadership, healthy practices, satisfying community, and strong mission. Adaptation of the measure for a variety of contexts is provided so that the proposed approach can be used in nations, cities, neighborhoods, families, workplaces, schools, and religious communities. The chapter discusses the complex relationships between individual and community well-being and how measures of community well-being may be useful for tracking and assessment or for reflection purposes and how it might ultimately be used for the improvement of community well-being.

Interest in well-being research and promotion has expanded dramatically in past decades. Much of the progress with respect to the measurement of well-being concerns individual-level measures. Numerous instruments and scales have been developed, have been validated for use in various settings, and are being employed in research and in government and nongovernmental tracking (Allin & Hand, 2017; National Research Council, 2013; OECD, 2013; VanderWeele, 2017). There has also been considerable interest in community well-being (Phillips & Wong, 2017). Although this has not expanded as quickly or dramatically as individual-level research and measures, there

Tyler J. VanderWeele, *Measures of Community Well-Being* In: *Measuring Well-Being.* Edited by: Matthew T. Lee, Laura D. Kubzansky, and Tyler J. VanderWeele, Oxford University Press (2021). © Oxford University Press.
DOI: 10.1093/oso/9780197512531.003.0015

has been a rich set of conceptualizations and discussions concerning community well-being also (cf. Chanan, 2002; Cox, Frere, West, & Wiseman, 2010; Hay, 1996; Lee & Kim, 2016; McHardy & O'Sullivan, 2004; Phillips & Wong, 2017; Prilleltensky & Prilleltensky, 2006). National government and international organizations also track various individual-level objective measures including education, access to healthcare, political participation, crime and safety, life expectancy, literacy, etc., which, when aggregated, are arguably also constitutive components of communal well-being. Environmental assessments, cultural offerings, infrastructure, and national debt, which can only be defined at the aggregate level, are also often tracked. While there is still tremendous scope for improvement in assessing both individual and community objective measures as well as individual subjective well-being measures, the tracking of community-related subjective well-being is arguably yet further behind in its development.

This chapter proposes a general framework to assess subjective community well-being. The proposed conceptualization will be relevant at the national level, but relevant also at the level of more local communities including, for example, neighborhoods, cities, families, workplaces, schools, and religious communities. These distinct community contexts, in spite of their differences, also have much in common, including the centrality of relationships, the need for good leadership, the importance of practices and structures that allow the community to function well, and a strong sense of mission, all hopefully leading to a satisfying experience of the community itself. A template for community well-being will be proposed and then adapted to fit these various national, city, neighborhood, workplace, family, school, and religious community contexts, and the template could be extended also to still more settings. There is of course likely some loss in attempting a general template for community well-being. The concerns of a family are different from those of a workplace or nation. However, as will be discussed, much of what is distinct across these settings in terms of community well-being arguably concerns the objective measures that are relevant in each context. Much of what is subjective—for example, the community seeming to function well and providing a sense of belonging—is arguably similar. In all of these settings, a thriving community will require flourishing individuals, good relationships, proficient leadership, healthy practices, a strong mission, and satisfying community. The material developed here is exploratory in nature and is intended to help clarify the domains and possible items that might be used to more holistically assess community subjective well-being.

Future work will connect the proposed conceptualization to other theoretical constructs and examine the psychometric properties of the proposed measure.

Conceptual Background

A community's flourishing might be understood as a state in which all aspects of the community's life are good. This includes both objective and subjective aspects, at both at individual and aggregate or communal levels (see Figure 14.1) (Lee & Kim, 2016). As noted earlier, numerous individual and communal objective measures have been developed and are routinely being tracked, and considerable progress has been made on the measurement of individual subjective well-being (Allin & Hand, 2017; National Research Council, 2013; OECD, 2013). What is underdeveloped are community subjective well-being measures. A review by Kim and Lee (2014) of 53 community measures concluded that, despite efforts to include objective and subjective elements, there are still far more objective indicators than

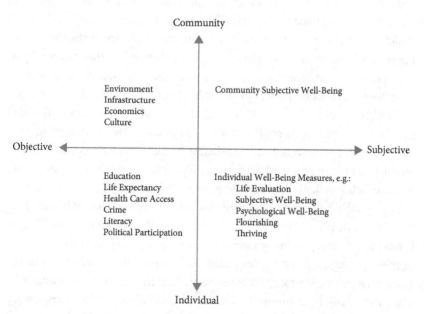

Figure 14.1 Joint dimensions of communal versus individual, and objective versus subjective measures of well-being.

subjective. It is the communal subjective measures that will be the focus here. We refer to this as "community subjective well-being" (or occasionally "community well-being" for short[1]) and distinguish it from the broader concept of communal flourishing encompassing both objective and subjective dimensions (i.e., "all aspects").

Much of what is available with regard to measures of subjective community well-being concerns satisfaction with the community (Lee & Kim, 2016; Sirgy, Widgery, Lee, & Yu, 2010). Sample items include, for example (if the area around the city of Flint, Michigan, were under consideration as the community) (cf. Sirgy et al., 2010): "Overall how satisfied are you with the quality of life in the Flint area?" or "To what extent do you enjoy living in the Flint area?" or "How would you rate the Flint area as a desirable place to live?" Alternatively, other items might assess satisfaction with aspects of a community's culture, community life, administration, or infrastructure (Lee & Kim, 2016). But we may ask whether this is sufficient? Satisfaction is no doubt an important part of community well-being, but relying on satisfaction alone to assess community well-being seems problematic for several reasons. First, satisfaction may be high if someone is simply able to get what they want, rather than because the community is good or well-functioning. An employee may be satisfied with their workplace not because of a well-functioning company with good working relationships contributing to the well-being of the world but simply because they are well paid and get to do what they like to do each day. The concept of community well-being would include, but seems to extend beyond, satisfaction. Second, satisfaction with the community may, in many contexts, be a "lagging indicator," with declines in community well-being causing declines in satisfaction in the long-run but potentially taking time to set in. The community's well-being may decline for some time without substantially affecting satisfaction due to past memories, loyalties, a slowness to change perceptions, or again because it takes time for declines in community well-being to substantially adversely affect the experience of the individual. Third, at a conceptual level, satisfaction alone does not tell us what *constitutes* a good community, only whether individuals are satisfied with it. Satisfaction with a community is undoubtedly important, but the notion of community well-being seems to extend beyond simply being satisfied with the community.

The measure of community subjective well-being proposed here is based around six distinct domains that include, but extend beyond, satisfaction with the community. These domains are flourishing individuals, good relationships, proficient leadership, healthy practices, satisfying community, and strong mission. The first domain, flourishing individuals, concerns the individual members of the community themselves; the second domain concerns relations between these individuals; the third domain concerns relations specifically with those in authority; the fourth domain concerns the structures and practices governing these various relations; the fifth domain concerns the extent to which these relations and structures give rise to a satisfying community; and the sixth domain concerns the extent to which these relations and structures relate to some further mission or end. Before we introduce the measures and its proposed items, we will briefly consider the motivation for each domain and the various items in turn.

At the heart of every community are the individuals of which it is composed. Communal well-being requires, to some extent at least, the well-being of its members. Communal well-being extends beyond just the aggregate of individual well-being, but it is arguably not independent of this. It would be odd to say that a community is thriving if its individual members are not. We will return, in a later discussion, to the conceptual and causal relations between individual and communal well-being, but, at the very least, the well-being of a community is made up in part by the well-being of its members. Good community is constituted in part by *flourishing individuals*.

Perhaps even more central to the notion of communal well-being is the importance of good relationships. There should be close relationships in the community; each person in the community should be respected as a person and trusted. A thriving community will be one in which each person contributes to the well-being of others in the community. Good community is constituted in part by *good relationships*.

For a community to thrive and to do so long-term it will also be important to have good leadership. Those in positions of power and authority should care about the well-being of everyone in the community and of the community itself. The leaders should have the skill and understanding that is needed to lead the community well and should be of sufficient character and consistency that they can be relied on to do what is right. They should be able to inspire others with their vision for the community's well-being. Good community is thus constituted in part by *proficient leadership*.

A well-functioning community will also have healthy practices. There should be structures and practices in place that allow relationships to develop and strengthen, allow the community to sustain itself, allow for the appropriate handling of conflicts and disputes, and allow the community to attain its primary goals. Good community is thus constituted in part by *healthy practices*.

The community itself should ideally be satisfying to be a part of. In most cases, the absence of this will indicate that something is wrong. Each person should have a sense of welcome and belonging in the community, and it should be possible for each person to become more integrated over time. The community should be such that each person thinks that it is a good community to be a part of. Good community is thus constituted in part by *satisfying community*.

Finally, a good community should be fulfilling its purpose or function, whatever that may be. A good community will be one that somehow contributes to the world to make it a better place. The community's purpose or mission would ideally be clear to everyone. Moreover, the community is thriving, as a community, if the community is able to do more together than the sum of what each could accomplish individually and if everyone is needed for the community to fulfill its goals and purposes. Good community is thus constituted in part by *a strong mission*.[2]

The six domains that the measure will attempt to assess are thus flourishing individuals, good relationships, proficient leadership, healthy practices, satisfying community, and strong mission. See Figure 14.2 for a diagrammatic representation. In each of these domains participants will be asked to evaluate the community itself, not simply their own satisfaction with it. Even in the "satisfying community" domain, participants will be asked to assess whether *everyone* is satisfied rather than simply whether the person responding is satisfied. Lee and Kim (2016) refer to these more general assessments pertaining to the entire community as "intersubjective community well-being," a point to which we will return in the discussion.

In the next section, we will use these characteristics of a well-functioning or thriving community to propose a series of items to capture community subjective well-being.

A Template for Community Well-Being

In this section, we present a template for community well-being. As noted, the conceptualization of community well-being here is intended to be sufficiently abstract and broad that the items could be used in a variety of

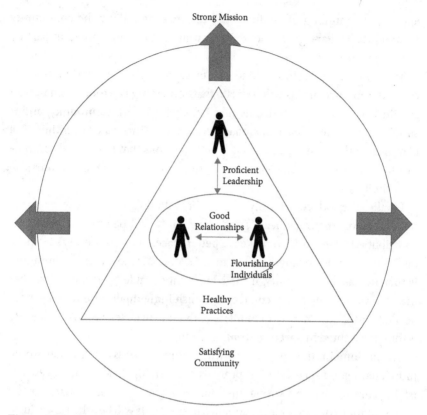

Figure 14.2 Conceptualization of community well-being involving the six domains of flourishing: individuals, good relationships, proficient leadership, healthy practices, satisfying community, and strong mission.

different community settings (e.g., nations, cities, neighborhoods, families, workplaces, schools, religious communities, etc.). The items here make reference to "the community." When used in practice with a specific community (e.g., workplace or family), the generic reference to "the community" could be replaced with "the workplace" or "the family" and other appropriate modifications could also be made (e.g., replacing "those in authority" with "parents"). In the generic items given in this section, the expression "the community," which would be replaced in more specific settings, is underlined. In Appendix 14.1, the various adaptions of the general template for community well-being to specific contexts (city, family, school, etc.) are provided and the changes that were made to the general community subjective well-being template are likewise underlined. Further modification could also be made to the specific versions in the Appendix such as specifying the name of the city (for the city community well-being measure) or simplifying the language of the school community well-being measure if it is to be used for middle-school students.

As noted earlier, the proposed measure is structured around six domains: flourishing individuals, good relationships, proficient leadership, healthy practices, satisfying community, and strong mission. In each of these domains, except the first (the "flourishing individuals" domain), four items, based on the conceptual considerations described earlier, are proposed to assess the domain. This results in 20 items across the final five domains. Preliminary empirical results suggest that consistency of item responses is high within domains and across all items. Five-hundred and fifty-five students ($\alpha = 0.97$) and 184 staff ($\alpha = 0.95$) completed this measure at a private high school in the mid-Atlantic region of the United States during November and December 2019; 1,724 residents of Columubus, Ohio ($\alpha = 0.94$) also completed the measure between October 2019 and January 2020. For the "flourishing individuals" category, various existing individual-level measures of subjective well-being could be used since the literature on individual subjective well-being measures is well-developed (Allin & Hand, 2017; National Research Council, 2013; OECD, 2013; VanderWeele, 2017). An example of an individual subjective well-being measure capturing flourishing individuals by using 12 self-report items and that could be used at the individual level is given in Appendix 14.2 and described in greater detail in VanderWeele (2017). Psychometric properties for the measure ($\alpha = 0.86$) are available elsewhere (Węziak-Białowolska, McNeely, & VanderWeele, 2019a, 2019b). However, other individual-level well-being measures could also be used instead.

Each of the items is given a brief descriptive title, but these could be omitted in the actual administration of the items. The items could be scored 0–10 and anchored only at the end-points (e.g., 0 = Strongly Disagree, 10 = Strongly Agree). Alternatively, a smaller number of response options could be used (e.g., 0–6) with each of the responses anchored so that 0 = Strongly Disagree, 1 = Disagree, 2 = Slightly Disagree, 3 = Neither Agree or Disagree, 4 = Slightly Agree, 5 = Agree, 6 = Strongly Agree.

The proposed items are as follows:

Flourishing Individuals:

Average of individual flourishing measures (see individual flourishing measures in Appendix 14.2)

Good Relationships:
Close Relationships: Everyone has close relationships within the community.
Respect: Everyone is respected within the community.
Trust: Everyone in the community trusts one another.
Mutuality: Everyone contributes to the well-being of others in the community.
Proficient Leadership:
Beneficence: Those in authority truly care about the well-being of everyone in the community.
Integrity: Those in authority in the community can be relied on to do what is right.
Competence: Those in authority have the skills and understanding they need to lead the community well.
Vision: Those in authority are able to inspire the community with their vision.
Healthy Practices:
Relational Growth: There are structures and practices in the community that allow relationships to become closer.
Fairness: There are structures and practices in place that allow the community to deal with conflicts so that everyone is treated fairly.
Sustenance: The community has structures and practices so as to be able to sustain itself.
Achievement: The community has structures and practices that allow it to accomplish its goals.
Satisfying Community:
Satisfaction: Everyone is satisfied with the way things are in our community.
Value: Everyone thinks that this community is a good community to be a part of.

Belonging: Each person has a sense of belonging in the <u>community.</u>

Welcome: There is a sense of welcome in the <u>community</u> so that it is possible for each person to become more integrated over time.

Strong Mission:

Purpose: Our <u>community's</u> shared purpose or mission is clear to everyone.

Contribution: Our <u>community</u> contributes to the world to make it a better place.

Interconnectedness: Everyone is needed for the <u>community</u> to fulfill its goals and purposes.

Synergy: Our <u>community</u> is able to do more with everyone together than we could individually.

Discussion: Open Questions and Future Directions

The proposal provides a broad conceptualization of community subjective well-being that is applicable across different contexts and assesses six domains of community well-being: flourishing individuals, good relationships, proficient leadership, healthy practices, satisfying community, and strong mission. For reasons already given, this conceptualization is arguably more adequate than simply relying on measures of satisfaction with the community alone. We noted above that, in each of these community well-being domains, participants are asked to evaluate the community itself, not simply their satisfaction with it. Even in the "satisfying community" domain, participants are asked to assess whether *everyone* is satisfied rather than simply whether the person responding is satisfied. These more general assessments pertaining to the entire community, Lee and Kim (2016) refer to as "intersubjective community well-being" and distinguish this from what they refer to, in their work, as "community subjective well-being" which are the particular respondent's individual level of satisfaction with, for example, air quality, infrastructure, etc. In the conceptualization given in this chapter, these individual assessments of individual satisfaction would fall under and could be assessed within the "flourishing individuals" domain. These are, however, simply different ways of categorizing the various relevant constructs. Certainly both are worth examining.

In some settings, one might in principle expect close numeric relations between aggregates of individual level measures as compared with
aggregates of "intersubjective" measures. For example, one might hope
for rough equality between means of individuals' self-report of their own
belonging when averaged over the community with means of individuals'
self-report about everyone in the community having a sense of belonging.
However, such approximate equality need not always be the case. It may
be that the vast majority of a community (perhaps more than 80%) does
feel a sense of belonging but that everyone is likewise aware that a minority do not have this experience, so that the mean of the intersubjective assessments is comparatively low. A simple average of individual
perceptions of one's own life or satisfaction may disguise an underlying
communal problem; the intersubjective assessment may help uncover
this. For example, the vast majority may be dissatisfied with Congress but
happy with their own representative (Mendes, 2013). The vast majority
may be satisfied with their own healthcare while acknowledging major
problems in the healthcare system itself. For these reasons, the communal
or intersubjective measures are thus also worth assessing. They are not
necessarily more important than the aggregate of individual perceptions
concerning one's own life, but they do convey additional information.
Once again, both individual assessment and community or intersubjective assessments are worth examining.

As noted earlier, for a community to be flourishing—for all aspects of the
community's life to be good—both the subjective and objective indicators
of high well-being, at both the communal and individual levels, should be
present (see Figure 14.1). The proposal here is not to neglect the objective
aspects such as literacy, crime, or pollution, but rather to supplement them
with both individual- and community-level measures of subjective well-
being. Because measures of community subjective well-being beyond community satisfaction seemed underdeveloped, the contribution of this chapter
is to propose a new template to assess such community subjective well-being.

The template proposed is intended to be sufficiently broad and abstract to
be potentially applicable to different types of communities including nations,
cities, neighborhoods, workplaces, families, schools, and religious communities. Its adequacy in each of these settings and the psychometric properties
of the measure in these different settings remain to be assessed. It may turn
out to be the case that the measure performs more adequately in certain of
these community settings than in others.

One might also reasonably wonder whether a measure intended to assess community well-being in these various diverse settings (including nations, cities, neighborhoods, workplaces, families, schools and religious communities) will be adequate. Might different items be required to assess community subjective well-being in these very different settings? Certainly, the concerns of a family are very different from those of a city. While this is indeed so, it may be that those aspects of well-being that are most disparate across settings are, in fact, the objective measures. The relevant objective measures will likely differ, but, arguably, all communities, to be truly flourishing, need flourishing individuals, good relationships, proficient leadership, healthy practices, satisfying community, and strong mission. Again, it is arguably the relevant objective measures that will be more variable. Political participation, cultural offerings, and roadway infrastructure may be appropriate to nations, cities, and neighborhoods but perhaps less relevant to schools or to children in families. Other objective indicators such as student–teacher ratios or family dinners, will be applicable to schools or families, but not to workplaces, etc. Certain objective aspects of well-being such as health, crime and safety, environment, literacy and education, and economic indicators may be applicable across the different community settings, though the appropriate measures used to operationalize these objective constructs will likely vary across contexts. In any case, a different collection of objective indicators to assess objective well-being will certainly be desirable in different settings, and, ideally, objective and subjective aspects of well-being should both be assessed.

An interesting open question for further research and consideration is whether it is indeed the case that the more general abstract domains of community subjective well-being, in conjunction with an appropriate set of objective measures, are adequate to get a reasonable assessment of communal flourishing or whether more specific aspects of subjective well-being, tailored and unique to each of the contexts (city, family, workplace, etc.) is needed. An advantage of using a common set of items for these six domains of community subjective well-being across contexts is the possibility of establishing in which contexts each domain of subjective well-being is potentially particularly difficult or easy to establish.

Considerable work remains in establishing the psychometric properties of the proposed measure in different contexts and on assessing the conceptual adequacy and item consistency of the six domains. Establishing psychometric properties with a community construct may also present challenges since the construct, "community subjective well-being," although assessed through individual responses, is meant to pertain to the entire community, and so the score for a community would in principle be obtained only through an average of a random sample of the relevant community. It may be considerably easier to collect data on numerous distinct communities in certain settings (e.g., families) than in others (e.g., cities or nations).

The use of the measure may be helpful for tracking and assessment purposes and for identifying aspects of community life that may be most in need of improvement. The use of the measure may also be helpful in assessing whether a community seems, to its members, to be improving or declining over time. The measures are, of course, of interest in aggregate, but it might also be of interest to examine how assessments of a community vary by age, gender, or race/ethnicity. It might also be of interest to examine how and whether assessments differ by the total length of time someone has spent in the community. In communities with high turnover, particular attention may be needed with regard to how to handle newcomers to a community. They may be particularly able to assess whether there is a sense of welcome but may find it more difficult to assess the general levels of satisfaction of the other members of the community. In principle, the community subjective well-being of a particular community could also be assessed by those who are not in fact members of a community, though, in most cases, their knowledge of the community is likely to be more limited. It may also be of interest, and important, to evaluate how assessments of community well-being may differ by whether respondents are or are not leaders within the community.

Another interesting and important direction for future research is the study of the determinants of these various aspects of community well-being in different contexts. With data collected over time, it might be possible to examine which objective indicators seem to contribute most to subjective community well-being and whether this varies across the proposed domains of community subjective well-being and across different contexts such as nations, cities, neighborhoods, workplaces, families, schools, and religious communities. Such studies will be important in focusing policy efforts to bring about a greater sense of community well-being. However, to draw reliable causal conclusions, data on community subjective well-being collected repeatedly over time would be needed (VanderWeele, 2008; VanderWeele, Jackson, & Li, 2016), and in many contexts this may be difficult to obtain.

Another important direction of future research and consideration is the relation between individual well-being and community well-being. As noted earlier, there are difficult conceptual questions concerning these relations. The two are certainly interrelated, both conceptually and causally. A community is arguably not flourishing if its constituent members are not flourishing. The relation is conceptual. Likewise, for at least certain persons, they may not say that "all aspects of my life are good" if their community is not thriving. Here, too, the relation is conceptual: the community's well-being is a constituent component of the individual's subjective well-being. However, there are also causal relations governing the dynamics between individual and community subjective well-being. A well-functioning community will often be causally relevant to (e.g., causally improve) an individual's subjective well-being in the form of pleasant interactions, cleanliness of spaces, or availability of jobs, or opportunities to advance. Likewise individual well-being will often have a causal impact on communal well-being. An individual's sense of purpose or pursuit of the good, for example, may alter the extent to which she or he contributes to the community, tries to make it a better place, or helps others.

Similar issues concerning causal relationships likewise pertain also to objective measures of community well-being. An individual's subjective well-being may lead to greater contributions to a country's educational system, economic progress, or the prevention of air pollution. However, likewise, a community's educational or economic opportunities will in turn enhance an individual's subjective well-being as well as objective individual measures such as their actual educational attainment, income, or longevity. In much of the research on social capital (Berkman, Kawachi, & Glymour, 2014; Gilbert, Quinn, Goodman, Butler, & Wallace, 2013; Kawachi, Subramanian, & Kim, 2008; Portes, 1998), the communal or social relations are viewed principally as a means to economic, health, or other individual goods or ends. Indeed the very term "social capital" suggests that it is conceived of as a means. However, community well-being is arguably not simply a means but also an end in and of itself. While it certainly can be a means to other ends, it is also something that is to be sought for its own sake. The notion and language of "social cohesion" (Berkman et al., 2014; Friedkin, 2004) perhaps comes closer to the broader concept of community subjective well-being. An extensive literature has likewise examined its effects on individual health and well-being outcomes (Berkman et al., 2014; Meijer, Röhl, Bloomfield, & Grittner,

2012). However, social cohesion is arguably more narrowly focused on certain aspects of community well-being pertaining to relationships, similarity, and belonging, with perhaps often less focus on authority and leadership, structures and practices, and a sense of mission. The notion of "collective efficacy" (Bandura, 2000; Goddard, Hoy, & Hoy, 2004; Sampson, Raudenbush, & Earls, 1997) perhaps better captures some of these latter aspects. In any case, it would be of interest also in future research to examine how the various aspects of community well-being relate to different individual-level outcomes and vice versa.

The extent of these causal and conceptual relations may vary across individuals and across communities. The conceptual relations concerning the extent to which communal well-being is a constitutive component of individual well-being might well be stronger in collectivist societies than in individualist societies (Suh, Diener, Oishi, & Triandis, 1998). The ways in which a community's well-being causally affects an individual's well-being may be stronger for someone who is disadvantaged or needy than for someone who is relatively wealthy and seemingly less dependent on the community. Likewise, the extent to which an individual's subjective well-being causally alters the community's thriving may vary across settings. Someone with a strong sense of purpose may be more likely to substantially causally alter a community's well-being in a democracy than in a dictatorship. The relations between communal well-being and individual well-being are both causal and conceptual, and the extent of these relations will vary across settings and individuals.

However, when community well-being is treated as an outcome for a community, it is important, conceptually, to include within this as well measures of individual well-being. A community is not fully thriving if its members are not. The proposed measure thus includes as one of several domains "flourishing individuals," with the understanding that previously developed individual level measures of subjective well-being could be used for these. It would, of course, be possible to make use of the measures while excluding the aggregate of these individual-level measures of subjective well-being. In assessing causal relations and effects of community versus individual well-being on other (perhaps objective) outcomes, it may be of interest to treat individual and community subjective well-being separately. However, again, when the goal is an aggregate measure of community well-being as an outcome, it is arguably reasonable to treat aggregate summaries of individual well-being as one of the categories of community well-being.

The hope for the proposed community subjective well-being measure is that it will be useful in tracking community well-being over time, in assessment and reflection, and, ultimately, in identifying determinants of community well-being and appropriately intervening to improve it. The success of this approach will depend in part on measure validation for these various uses and in different community contexts, on obtaining appropriate data over time, and on appropriately relating objective and subjective measures and meeting challenges present in subjective well-being research more generally. White (2010) has argued that although subjective well-being approaches have tremendous potential to transform policy considerations, there are potential dangers inherent in the approach that must be navigated as well. These include blaming individuals for their condition or the way they feel; ignoring the concept of well-being until basic needs are met; dismissing it because subjective well-being can sometimes be high even if material conditions are poor; or dismissing it on the grounds of its being too broad to be relevant for policy. Progress on better measures and a better understanding of subjective well-being, at both the individual and community levels, will be useful in helping to meet and navigate these challenges. With time, data collection on appropriate measures, and research, we will hopefully come to a better understanding of the determinants of community well-being itself, what might be most lacking in different contexts, and how to improve it.

Notes

1. The shorthand "community well-being" for "community subjective well-being" is perhaps somewhat an abuse of language. The terms "well-being" and "flourishing" are themselves often used almost interchangeably and "community well-being" might thus itself be understood as "a state in which all aspects of the community's life are good." However, because of the rise of the positive psychology movement and its use of the term "well-being," expressions employing "well-being" now carry a strong subjective connotation and thus the slight abuse of language inherent in the shorthand "community well-being" is perhaps somewhat justified.
2. This sixth domain of a community having a strong mission may be more controversial than the others. However, it is arguably the case that any partnership or community is established for some purpose, or aims at some good or end (Aristotle, 4th c. BCE/1995,

I.1.1252a1–7). This in essence is its mission, implicit or explicit. It may be difficult to precisely articulate what the relevant end is across different community contexts. In the case of a city-state, Aristotle took that end to be the making of its citizens good, the promotion of their flourishing (Aristotle, 4th c. BCE/1995).

3. In school or family settings in which individual flourishing is being assessed for adolescents (age 12–18) rather than adults, it will be desirable to modify some of these items due to developmental stage. It is proposed that item 2 be replaced with "In general I consider myself a happy person" (0 = Strongly Disagree, 10 = Strongly Agree); item 6 may be replaced with "I am doing things now that will help me achieve my goals in life" (0 = Strongly Disagree, 10 = Strongly Agree); item 10 may be replaced with "I have people in my life I can talk to about things that really matter" (0 = Strongly Disagree, 10 = Strongly Agree); and item 11 may be replaced with "My family has enough money to live a truly decent life" (0 = Strongly Disagree, 10 = Strongly Agree). These new items were adapted from other measures (Item 2: Lyubomirsky & Lepper, 1999; Items 6 and 10: Carle et al., 2014; Item 11: Patrick, Edwards, & Topolski, 2002). Five-hundred and fifty-five students completed this modified measure at a private high school in the mid-Atlantic region of the United States during November and December 2019 ($\alpha = 0.89$).

About the Author

Tyler J. VanderWeele is the John L. Loeb and Frances Lehman Loeb Professor of Epidemiology in the Departments of Epidemiology and Biostatistics at the Harvard T. H. Chan School of Public Health, Director of the Human Flourishing Program, and Co-Director of the Initiative on Health, Religion and Spirituality at Harvard University. His research concerns methodology for distinguishing between association and causation in observational studies, and his empirical research spans psychiatric, perinatal, and social epidemiology; the science of happiness and flourishing; and the study of religion and health, including both religion and population health and the role of religion and spirituality in end-of-life care. He has published more than 300 papers in peer-reviewed journals and is author of the book *Explanation in Causal Inference* (Oxford University Press, 2015).

Author Note

The author thanks the participants of the workshop on "Health and Happiness in Policy and Practice Across the Globe: The Role of Science and Evidence" hosted by the Lee Kum Sheung Center for Health and Happiness at Harvard University, April 12, 2019, for helpful feedback on the proposed measure; Matthew Lee, Eileen McNeely, Michael Balboni, and members of the Human Flourishing Program at Harvard University for helpful discussions on the conceptualization of community well-being; and members of the Columbus Foundation for further feedback on the specific items employed in the measure. This chapter is a slightly edited reprint of VanderWeele, T. J. (2019). Measures of community well-being: a template. *International Journal of Community Well-Being*, 2, 253–275, https://doi.org/10.1007/s42413-019-00036-8. This work was supported in part by a grant from the John Templeton Foundation (Grant 61075) and by the Lee Kum Sheung Center for Health and Happiness. The views expressed in this chapter represent the perspective of the author and do not reflect the opinions or endorsement of any organization. I have no known conflict of interest to disclose. Correspondence concerning this chapter should be directed to Tyler J. VanderWeele, Harvard T. H. Chan School of Public Health, Departments of Epidemiology and Biostatistics, 677 Huntington Avenue, Boston, MA 02115 (tvanderw@hsph.harvard.edu).

References

Allin, P., & Hand, D. J. (2017). New statistics for old? Measuring the wellbeing of the UK. *Journal of the Royal Statistical Society, Series A, 180*, 1–22.

Aristotle. (4th c. BCE/1995). *The politics of Aristotle*. Barker, E. (Trans.). Oxford: Oxford University Press.

Bandura, A. (2000). Exercise of human agency through collective efficacy. *Current directions in psychological science, 9*(3), 75–78.

Berkman, L. F., Kawachi, I., & Glymour, M. M. (2014). *Social epidemiology*. New York: Oxford University Press.

Carle, A., McIntosh, H., Moore, K. A., Lippman, L., Guzman, L., Ramos, M. F., . . . Caal, S. (2014). *Flourishing children: Defining and testing indicators of positive development*. New York: Springer.

Chanan, G. (2002). *Community development foundation measure of community: A study for the active community unit and research*. London: Development and Statistics Unit of the Home Office.

Cox, D., Frere, M., West, S., & Wiseman, J. (2010). Developing and using local community wellbeing indicators: Learning from the experiences of Community Indicators Victoria. *Australian Journal of Social Issues, 45*, 71–89.

Friedkin, N. E. (2004). Social cohesion. *Annual Review of Sociology, 30*, 409–425.

Gilbert, K. L., Quinn, S. C., Goodman, R. M., Butler, J., & Wallace, J. (2013). A meta-analysis of social capital and health: A case for needed research. *Journal of Health Psychology, 18*(11), 1385–1399.

Goddard, R. D., Hoy, W. K., & Hoy, A. W. (2004). Collective efficacy beliefs: Theoretical developments, empirical evidence, and future directions. *Educational Researcher, 33*(3), 3–13.

Hay, D. I. (1996). *Keep it grounded and keep it simple: Measuring community well-being*. Vancouver, BC: Social Planning and Research Council of British Columbia.

Kawachi, I., Subramanian, S. V., & Kim, D. (2008). *Social capital and health*. New York: Springer.

Kim, Y., & Lee S. J. (2014). The development and application of a community wellbeing index in Korean metropolitan cities. *Social Indicators Research, 119*, 533–558.

Lee, S. J., & Kim, Y. (2016). Structure of well-being: An exploratory study of the distinction between individual well-being and community well-being and the importance of intersubjective community well-being. In Y. Kee, S. J. Lee, and R. Phillips (Eds.), *Social factors and community well-being* (pp. 13–37). Geneva: Springer.

Lyubomirsky, S., & Lepper, H. (1999). A measure of subjective happiness: Preliminary reliability and construct validation. *Social Indicators Research, 46*, 137–155.

McHardy, M., & O'Sullivan, E. (2004). *Five nations community well-being in Canada: The Community Well-Being Index (CWB), 2001.* Indian and Northern Affairs Canada: Strategic Research and Analysis Directorate.

Meijer, M., Röhl, J., Bloomfield, K., & Grittner U. (2012). Do neighborhoods affect individual mortality? A systematic review and meta-analysis of multilevel studies. *Social Science and Medicine, 74*(8), 1204–1212.

Mendes, E. (2013). Americans Down on Congress, OK With Own Representative. Gallup Poll Report, 2013. https://news.gallup.com/poll/162362/americans-down-congress-own-representative.aspx

National Research Council. (2013). *Subjective well-being.* Washington, DC: National Academies Press.

OECD. (2013). *OECD guidelines on measuring subjective well-being.* Paris: OECD.

Patrick, D. L., Edwards, T. C., & Topolski, T. D. (2002). Adolescent quality of life, part II: Initial validation of a new instrument. *Journal of Adolescence, 25*, 287–300.

Phillips, R., & Wong, C. (2017). *Handbook of community well-being research.* Dordrecht: Springer.

Portes, A. (1998). Social capital: Its origins and applications in modern sociology. *Annual Review of Sociology, 24*(1), 1–24.

Prilleltensky, I., & Prilleltensky, O. (2006). *Promoting well-being: Linking personal, organizational, and community change.* Hoboken, NJ: Wiley.

Sampson, R. J., Raudenbush, S. W., & Earls, F. (1997). Neighborhoods and violent crime: A multilevel study of collective efficacy. *Science, 277*(5328), 918–924.

Sirgy, M. J., Widgery, R. N., Lee, D. J., & Yu, G. B. (2010). Developing a measure of community well-being based on perceptions of impact in various life domains. *Social Indicators Research, 96*, 295–311.

Suh, E., Diener, E., Oishi, S., & Triandis, H. C. (1998). The shifting basis of life satisfaction judgments across cultures: Emotions versus norms. *Journal of Personality and Social Psychology, 74*(2), 482–493.

VanderWeele, T. J. (2008). Ignorability and stability assumptions in neighborhood effects research. *Statistics in Medicine, 27*, 1934–1943.

VanderWeele, T. J. (2017). On the promotion of human flourishing. *Proceedings of the National Academy of Sciences of the United States of America, 31*, 8148–8156.

VanderWeele, T. J., Jackson, J. W., & Li, S. (2016). Causal inference and longitudinal data: A case study of religion and mental health. *Social Psychiatry and Psychiatric Epidemiology, 51*, 1457–1466.

VanderWeele, T. J., McNeely, E., & Koh, H. K. (2019). Reimagining health—flourishing. *JAMA, 321*(17), 1667–1668.

Węziak-Białowolska, D., McNeely, E., & VanderWeele, T. J. (2019a). Flourish index and secure flourish index—validation in workplace settings. *Cogent Psychology, 6*, 1598926.

Węziak-Białowolska, D., McNeely, E., & VanderWeele, T. J. (2019b). Human flourishing in cross cultural settings: Evidence from the US, China, Sri Lanka, Cambodia and Mexico. *Frontiers in Psychology, 10*, 1269, https://doi.org/10.3389/fpsyg.2019.01269.

White, S. C. (2010). Analysing wellbeing: A framework for development practice. *Development in Practice, 20*, 158–172.

Appendix 14.1 Communal Well-Being Measures Adapted for National, City, Neighborhood, Workplace, Family, School, and Religious Community Contexts

National Community Well-Being

Flourishing Individuals:
Average of individual flourishing measures (see individual flourishing measures)

Good Relationships:
Close Relationships: Everyone in the nation has close relationships.
Respect: Everyone in the nation is respected.
Trust: Everyone in the nation trusts one another.
Mutuality: Everyone in the nation contributes to the well-being of others.

Proficient Leadership:
Beneficence: Those in authority truly care about the well-being of everyone in the nation.
Integrity: Those in authority in the nation can be relied on to do what is right.
Competence: Those in authority have the skills and understanding they need to lead the nation well.
Vision: Those in authority are able to inspire the nation with their vision.

Healthy Practices:
Relational Growth: There are national structures and practices that allow relationships to become closer.
Fairness: There are structures and practices in place that allow the nation to deal with conflicts so that everyone is treated fairly.
Sustenance: The nation has structures and practices so as to be able to sustain itself.
Achievement: The nation has structures and practices that allow it to accomplish its goals.

Satisfying Community:
Satisfaction: Everyone is satisfied with the way things are in our nation.
Value: Everyone thinks that this nation is a good community to be a part of.
Belonging: Each person in the nation has a sense of belonging.
Welcome: There is a sense of welcome in the nation so that it is possible for each person to become more integrated over time.

Strong Mission:
Purpose: Our nation's shared purpose to enhance the well-being of all and of our country is clear to everyone.
Contribution: Our nation contributes to the world to make it a better place.
Interconnectedness: Everyone is needed for the nation to fulfill its goals and purposes.
Synergy: Our nation is able to do more with everyone together than we could individually.

City Community Well-Being

Flourishing Individuals:
Average of individual flourishing measures (see individual flourishing measures)

Good Relationships:
Close Relationships: Everyone has close relationships within the <u>city</u>.
Respect: Everyone is respected within the <u>city</u>.
Trust: Everyone in the <u>city</u> trusts one another.
Mutuality: Everyone contributes to the well-being of others in the <u>city</u>.

Proficient Leadership:
Beneficence: Those in authority truly care about the well-being of everyone in the <u>city</u>.
Integrity: Those in authority in the <u>city</u> can be relied on to do what is right.
Competence: Those in authority have the skills and understanding they need to lead the <u>city</u> well.
Vision: Those in authority are able to inspire the <u>city</u> with their vision.

Healthy Practices:
Relational Growth: There are structures and practices in the <u>city</u> that allow relationships to become closer.
Fairness: There are structures and practices in place that allow the <u>city</u> to deal with conflicts so that everyone is treated fairly.
Sustenance: The <u>city</u> has structures and practices so as to be able to sustain itself.
Achievement: The <u>city</u> has structures and practices that allow it to accomplish its goals.

Satisfying Community:
Satisfaction: Everyone is satisfied with the way things are in our <u>city</u>.
Value: Everyone thinks that this <u>city</u> is a good community to be a part of.
Belonging: Each person has a sense of belonging in the <u>city</u>.
Welcome: There is a sense of welcome in the <u>city</u> so that it is possible for each person to become more integrated over time.

Strong Mission:
Purpose: Our <u>city's</u> shared purpose <u>to be a good place to live</u> is clear to everyone.
Contribution: Our <u>city</u> contributes to the world to make it a better place.
Interconnectedness: Everyone is needed for the <u>city</u> to fulfill its goals and purposes.
Synergy: Our <u>city</u> is able to do more with everyone together than we could individually.

Neighborhood Community Well-Being

Flourishing Individuals:
Average of individual flourishing measures (see individual flourishing measures)

Good Relationships:
Close Relationships: Everyone has close relationships within the <u>neighborhood.</u>
Respect: Everyone is respected within the <u>neighborhood.</u>
Trust: Everyone in the <u>neighborhood</u> trusts one another.
Mutuality: Everyone contributes to the well-being of others in the <u>neighborhood.</u>

Proficient Leadership:
Beneficence: Those in authority truly care about the well-being of everyone in the neighborhood.
Integrity: Those in authority in the neighborhood can be relied on to do what is right.
Competence: Those in authority have the skills and understanding they need to lead the neighborhood well.
Vision: Those in authority are able to inspire the neighborhood with their vision.

Healthy Practices:
Relational Growth: There are structures and practices in the neighborhood that allow relationships to become closer.
Fairness: There are structures and practices in place that allow the neighborhood to deal with conflicts so that everyone is treated fairly.
Sustenance: The neighborhood has structures and practices so as to be able to sustain itself.
Achievement: The neighborhood has structures and practices that allow it to accomplish its goals.

Satisfying Community:
Satisfaction: Everyone is satisfied with the way things are in our neighborhood.
Value: Everyone thinks that this neighborhood is a good community to be a part of.
Belonging: Each person has a sense of belonging in the neighborhood.
Welcome: There is a sense of welcome in the neighborhood so that it is possible for each person to become more integrated over time.

Strong Mission:
Purpose: Our neighborhood's shared purpose to be a good place to live is clear to everyone.
Contribution: Our neighborhood contributes to the world to make it a better place.
Interconnectedness: Everyone is needed for the neighborhood to fulfill its goals and purposes.
Synergy: Our neighborhood is able to do more with everyone together than we could individually.

Workplace Community Well-Being

Flourishing Individuals:
Average of individual flourishing measures (see individual flourishing measures)

Good Relationships:
Close Relationships: Everyone has close relationships within the workplace.
Respect: Everyone is respected at work.
Trust: Everyone at work trusts one another.
Mutuality: Everyone contributes to the well-being of others at work.

Proficient Leadership:
Beneficence: Management truly cares about the well-being of everyone at work.
Integrity: Management can be relied on to do what is right.

Competence: Those in <u>management</u> have the skills and understanding they need to lead well.

Vision: Those in <u>management</u> are able to inspire <u>employees</u> with their vision.

Healthy Practices:

Relational Growth: There are structures and practices in the <u>workplace</u> that allow relationships to become closer.

Fairness: There are structures and practices in place that allow <u>employees</u> to deal with conflicts so that everyone is treated fairly.

Sustenance: The <u>workplace</u> has structures and practices so that <u>it is not in danger of closure</u>.

Achievement: The <u>workplace</u> has structures and practices that allow <u>employees</u> to achieve their goals.

Satisfying Community:

Satisfaction: Everyone is satisfied with the way things are in our <u>workplace</u>.

Value: Everyone thinks that this <u>workplace</u> is a good community to be a part of.

Belonging: Each person has a sense of belonging in the <u>workplace</u>.

Welcome: There is a sense of welcome in the <u>workplace</u> so that it is possible for each person to become more integrated over time.

Strong Mission:

Purpose: The mission of our <u>company</u> is clear to everyone.

Contribution: Our <u>company</u> contributes to the world to make it a better place.

Interconnectedness: Everyone is needed for the <u>company</u> to fulfill its goals and purposes.

Synergy: Our <u>company</u> is able to do more with everyone together than we could individually.

Family Community Well-Being

Flourishing Individuals:

Average of individual flourishing measures (see individual flourishing measures)

Good Relationships:

Close Relationships: Everyone has close relationships within the <u>family</u>.

Respect: Everyone is respected within the <u>family</u>.

Trust: Everyone in the <u>family</u> trusts one another.

Mutuality: Everyone contributes to the well-being of others in the <u>family</u>.

Proficient Leadership:

Beneficence: <u>The parents</u> truly care about the well-being of everyone in the <u>family</u>.

Integrity: <u>The parents</u> can be relied on to do what is right.

Competence: <u>The parents</u> have the skills and understanding they need to lead the <u>family</u> well.

Vision: <u>The parents</u> are able to inspire the <u>members of the family</u>.

Healthy Practices:

Relational Growth: There are <u>family practices</u> that allow relationships to become closer.

Fairness: There are family practices in place that allow the community to deal with conflicts so that everyone is treated fairly.

Sustenance: The family has structures and practices so as to be able to sustain itself.

Achievement: The family has structures and practices that allow each person to accomplish their goals.

Satisfying Community:

Satisfaction: Everyone is satisfied with the way things are in our family.

Value: Everyone thinks that this family is a good community to be a part of.

Belonging: Each person has a sense of belonging in the family.

Welcome: There is a sense of welcome in the family so that it is possible for each person to become more integrated over time.

Strong Mission:

Purpose: The family's shared purpose of nurturing relationships and each person is clear to everyone.

Contribution: Our family contributes to the world to make it a better place.

Interconnectedness: Everyone is needed for the family to fulfill its goals and purposes.

Synergy: Our family is able to do more with everyone together than we could individually.

School Community Well-Being

Flourishing Individuals:

Average of individual flourishing measures (see individual flourishing measures)

Good Relationships:

Close Relationships: Everyone has close relationships within the school.

Respect: Everyone is respected within the school.

Trust: Everyone in the school trusts one another.

Mutuality: Everyone contributes to the well-being of others in the school.

Proficient Leadership:

Beneficence: Those in leadership truly care about the well-being of everyone in the school.

Integrity: Those in leadership can be relied on to do what is right.

Competence: Those in leadership have the skills and understanding they need to lead the school well.

Vision: Those in leadership are able to inspire the school with their vision.

Healthy Practices:

Relational Growth: There are structures and practices in the school that allow relationships to become closer.

Fairness: There are structures and practices in place that allow the school to deal with conflicts so that everyone is treated fairly.

Sustenance: The school has structures and practices so as to be able to sustain itself.

Achievement: The school has structures and practices that allow it to accomplish its goals.

Satisfying Community:
Satisfaction: Everyone is satisfied with the way things are in our <u>school</u>.
Value: Everyone thinks that this <u>school</u> is a good community to be a part of.
Belonging: Each person has a sense of belonging in the <u>school</u>.
Welcome: There is a sense of welcome in the <u>school</u> so that it is possible for each person to become more integrated over time.

Strong Mission:
Purpose: Our <u>school's</u> shared purpose or mission is clear to everyone.
Contribution: Our <u>school</u> contributes to the world to make it a better place.
Interconnectedness: Everyone is needed for the <u>school</u> to fulfill its goals and purposes.
Synergy: Our <u>school</u> is able to do more with everyone together than we could individually.

Religious Community Well-Being

Note: The items below are phrased specifically with regard to a "church," but when used in other settings, "church" could be replaced by, for example, "synagogue," "mosque," etc.

Flourishing Individuals:
Average of individual flourishing measures (see individual flourishing measures)

Good Relationships:
Close Relationships: Everyone has close relationships within the <u>church</u>.
Respect: Everyone is respected within the <u>church</u>.
Trust: Everyone in the <u>church</u> trusts one another.
Mutuality: Everyone contributes to the well-being of others in the <u>church</u>.

Proficient Leadership:
Beneficence: Those in authority truly care about the well-being of everyone in the <u>church</u>.
Integrity: Those in authority in the <u>church</u> can be relied on to do what is right.
Competence: Those in authority have the skills and understanding they need to lead the <u>church</u> well.
Vision: Those in authority are able to inspire the <u>church</u> with their vision.

Healthy Practices:
Relational Growth: There are structures and practices in the <u>church</u> that allow relationships to become closer.
Fairness: There are structures and practices in place that allow the <u>church</u> to deal with conflicts so that everyone is treated fairly.
Sustenance: The <u>church</u> has structures and practices so as to be able to sustain itself.
Achievement: The <u>church</u> has structures and practices that allow it to accomplish its goals.

Satisfying Community:
Satisfaction: Everyone is satisfied with the way things are in our <u>church community</u>.
Value: Everyone thinks that this <u>church</u> is a good community to be a part of.
Belonging: Each person has a sense of belonging in the community.

Welcome: There is a sense of welcome in the community so that it is possible for each person to become more integrated over time.

Strong Mission:
Purpose: Our church's shared mission is clear to everyone.
Contribution: Our church contributes to the world to make it a better place.
Interconnectedness: Everyone is needed for the church to fulfill its goals and purposes.
Synergy: Our church is able to do more with everyone together than we could individually.

Appendix 14.2 An Individual-Level Subjective Measure of Flourishing That Can Be Included in Assessing Communal Well-Being

The following 12 items (VanderWeele, 2017; VanderWeele, McNeely, & Koh, 2019) could be used as an assessment for individual-level flourishing, for the "flourishing individuals" domain of the community well-being assessment. The 12 items assess several important domains of individual flourishing, including Happiness and Life Satisfaction (Items 1–2), Mental and Physical Health (3–4), Meaning and Purpose (5–6), Character and Virtue (7–8), and Close Social Relationships (9–10). A sixth domain, Financial and Material Stability (11–12) is an important means in sustaining the other domains over time. The background and motivation for these items and the flourishing domains can be found in VanderWeele (2017) and VanderWeele et al. (2019).[3]

Please respond to the following questions on a scale from 0 to 10:

1. Overall, how satisfied are you with life as a whole these days?

    0 = Not Satisfied at All, 10 = Completely Satisfied

2. In general, how happy or unhappy do you usually feel?

    0 = Extremely Unhappy, 10 = Extremely Happy

3. In general, how would you rate your physical health?

    0 = Poor, 10 = Excellent

4. How would you rate your overall mental health?

    0 = Poor, 10 = Excellent

5. Overall, to what extent do you feel the things you do in your life are worthwhile?

    0 = Not at All Worthwhile, 10 = Completely Worthwhile

6. I understand my purpose in life.

    0 = Strongly Disagree, 10 = Strongly Agree

7. I always act to promote good in all circumstances, even in difficult and challenging situations.

    0 = Not True of Me, 10 = Completely True of Me

8. I am always able to give up some happiness now for greater happiness later.

0 = Not True of Me, 10 = Completely True of Me

9. I am content with my friendships and relationships.

0 = Strongly Disagree, 10 = Strongly Agree

10. My relationships are as satisfying as I would want them to be.

0 = Strongly Disagree, 10 = Strongly Agree

11. How often do you worry about being able to meet normal monthly living expenses?

0 = Worry All of the Time, 10 = Do Not Ever Worry

12. How often do you worry about safety, food, or housing?
0 = Worry All of the Time, 10 = Do Not Ever Worry

15

Inner Peace as a Contribution to Human Flourishing

A New Scale Developed from Ancient Wisdom

Juan Xi and Matthew T. Lee

Abstract

Although philosophers and theologians have emphasized the centrality of inner peace for the good life, this concept has not generally been included in research on human flourishing. We argue that inner peace contributes to a more complete form of flourishing for both religious and secular people. We then propose a new instrument, the Inner Peace Scale, to measure inner peace and we provide an initial psychometric evaluation of the instrument based on five empirical studies. We distinguish our scale from related measures, such as contentment, serenity, or tranquility. Our engagement with literature from the social sciences and the humanities, along with our research findings, suggests that inner peace is comprised of three dimensions: acceptance of loss; transcendence of hedonism and materialism; and inner balance and calmness. Greater attention to the dimension of transcending hedonism and materialism may prove especially helpful in advancing the field, particularly in consumeristic societies.

The past two decades witnessed a rapid expansion of social scientific interest in understanding components, conditions, and pathways to human flourishing and well-being, with 14,000 publications mentioning one aspect—subjective well-being—in a single year (Diener et al., 2017). Yet despite the proliferation, progress seems to be limited by conceptual disagreement with regard to the meaning of flourishing. Does this refer to a life without disorders or disturbance, a life full of pleasure and happiness, or a life that

Juan Xi and Matthew T. Lee, *Inner Peace as a Contribution to Human Flourishing* In: *Measuring Well-Being*. Edited by: Matthew T. Lee, Laura D. Kubzansky, and Tyler J. VanderWeele, Oxford University Press (2021). © Oxford University Press. DOI: 10.1093/oso/9780197512531.003.0016 is meaningful and serving a higher purpose but fraught with suffering? Or perhaps a life that is characterized by a profound peace which is beyond the dichotomies of pleasure or sorrow, passion or boredom, honor or dishonor, and living in opulence or poverty? In searching for the answer, many studies have investigated mental disorders, often viewed as the opposite of mental well-being. Studies on happiness and life satisfaction are also plentiful. Research interest on meaning in life and personal growth also well-established (Keyes, 2011; Ryff, 2014). But there has been little research attention paid to *inner peace*, a fundamentally balanced mental state that has been sought after throughout human history (Delle Fave et al., 2016). As a result, there are few discussions in the social science literature on the conceptualization and measurement of inner peace (Kjell, Daukantaite, Hefferon, & Sikström, 2016). The purpose of this chapter is to propose a new instrument, the Inner Peace Scale, to measure inner peace and provide an initial psychometric evaluation of the instrument.

But what is inner peace? There is a metaphor that has often been used to describe deep inner peace: the inner world of the mind is like a calm, quiet, and clear lake (Philippe, 2002, p. 5). It is a quiet that does not imply eventless or emptiness of inner experiences. But it does imply a different mode of inner experience which is always clear, gentle, and grounded no matter the nature of the outer events it is associated with. Just as a quiet lake clearly mirrors clouds, birds, and other happenings passing over it, people with deep inner peace experience their life happenings with great clarity. But just as a perfectly calm lake becomes disturbed during storms, so, too, is the experience of inner peace often transitory. Craving for what one does not have and worrying about losing what one does have can easily disrupt inner balance. However, unlike a natural lake, the calmness of which is not under its own control, people can cultivate and develop their inner peace by learning to experience life circumstances with healthy acceptance and avoid automatic (or "mindless") grasping. Drawing on cross-cultural insights from philosophy, theology, and the social sciences, we define inner peace as a calm and balanced mental state and disposition, one characterized by an attitude of healthy acceptance and an absence of unhealthy grasping.

The state of inner peace may be present in all life circumstances, including challenging or disturbing situations. Our definition is comprised of three distinct dimensions: *acceptance of loss*, *transcendence of hedonism and materialism*, and *inner balance and calmness*. A skillful ability to accept the inevitable losses that are an inherent part of the human condition, along with an avoidance of undue fixation on transitory pleasures and things, fosters a calm and balanced mind. But the latter should not be seen only as an "outcome" because mental balance may also increase the ability to both accept and transcend. All three dimensions are likely related in a dynamic way. It might be helpful to understand the more general outcome of the three dimensions of inner peace in terms of the metaphor of habitually keeping one's "heart free of hatred" while accepting life as it is but *without* becoming complacent about wrongness or injustice (Baldwin, quoted in Hernandez, 2019). Indeed, empirical research reveals that a harmonious approach to life does not necessarily involve conflict avoidance or deflation of self, but in fact is associated with increased personal growth and a strong sense of purpose in a manner that integrates independent and interdependent conceptions of self (Kjell et al., 2016; see also Vallerand, 2008 on harmonious as opposed to obsessive passions). Such self-integration is helpful for working to transform conflict with more self-awareness and interpersonal skill.

A peaceful mental condition can be transitory, but it can also be developed into a stable mental disposition. It requires effort and understanding to develop and maintain this mental condition. As such, it can also be considered a mental process. By framing inner peace as a verb and a noun, we mean to suggest that it is possible to engage in accepting, transcending, and balancing practices; it is also possible to attain these states to a greater or lesser degree. However, measuring inner peace as a transitory mental state, a dynamic process, or a stable mental disposition would require different considerations and different instruments. The new measure introduced in this chapter focuses on inner peace as a relatively stable mental trait—a disposition or habit of mind that can be cultivated and is likely to vary over time—as a first step toward developing measures of mental states and processes. The development of a measure of inner peace as a trait might be especially important if, as some wisdom literature seems to indicate, the flourishing life is built on stable mental condition that is cultivated over a lifetime of philosophic, humanistic, or spiritual practice (Aurelius, 180/2006; Fleischman, 2004; Philippe, 2002). It is also plausible to hypothesize that those who have developed the stable disposition of inner peace will be more likely than others to become effective peace-builders in the world. We also expect that a trait-based measure of inner peace will show stronger relationships to peace-building and flourishing than a more transitory state-based measure.

The three dimensions (acceptance, transcendence, calmness) in our conceptualization may not represent an exhaustive list of all of the possible elements that characterize inner peace. For example, an ability to perceive present reality in terms of the long range, the eternal, or the "big picture" might also be a dimension of inner peace. But we suggest that our three dimensions do address fundamental aspects of the human condition that tend to characterize inner peace and that they are grounded in rich philosophic and theological traditions, both East and West. They are applicable to theistic and non-theistic religious orientations as well as secular ones. As a result, this new measure may be useful across a broad range of cultural contexts. It could also inspire future measurement development and refinement.

Inner Peace as a Cultural Universal

Inner peace has been known by many names across virtually all cultures, both as a desirable *end state of being* and as a *virtuous disposition* worthy of life-long cultivation through specific practices. It has been called the virtue of *good temper* by Aristotle (a disposition aimed at the balance point between excessive anger and indifference) and the highly sought state of mind known to ancient Greeks as *apatheia* (literally, "without passion" or "without suffering," but not indifferent). This Greek term is given somewhat different meanings by Orthodox Christians and Stoic philosophers, but the underlying experience seems to have analogs in other traditions, including one of the four "sublime" meditative states (*upekkhā*) mentioned in the Pali Canon of Buddhism (or *upekṣā* in Sanskrit, both generally rendered as *equanimity* in English). Similarly, Judaism posits *menuchat hanefesh* (peace of mind, resting of the soul) as an important foundation for moral and spiritual development. Hindus associate inner peace with transcending the illusory world of appearances in order to access *Brahman*: absolute reality beyond the distractions of ego. In Christianity, peace, as one of the nine fruits of the Spirit (Galatians 5:22), has been conceived as a necessary virtue developed through contemplation in order to reach union with divine love, as in the *Ladder of Divine Ascent* described by St. John Climacus in the seventh century. Cultivating a peaceful disposition, or alternatively receiving a gift of divine grace, might lead to an overall state of being that St. Paul described as the "peace of God" which "transcends all understanding" (Philippians 4:7). A sense of inner peace is captured by his celebrated words, "Love is patient, love is kind . . . it is not self-seeking . . . it keeps no record of wrongs" (1

Corinthians 13:4–5), and also by his exalted way of engaging with life: "I have learned the secret of being content in any and every situation, whether well fed or hungry, whether living in plenty or in want" (Philippians 4:12).

Inner peace has been understood as making important contributions to human flourishing in both religious and secular settings. In *The Mountain of Silence*, a study of Greek Orthodox Christianity as practiced by the contemporary monks who reside the isolated monasteries of Mount Athos, Kyriacos Markides (2002, p. 81) explains the theological significance of contemplative practices that cultivate inner peace.

> According to Athonite spiritual tradition, when a human being eradicates personal desires completely and reaches the state of *apathia* [liberation from egotistical passions], they become a "vessel of the Holy Spirit." Then whatever that person wishes is given because it is what God actually wishes. The consciousness of the saint is fully attuned with the spirit of God.

Despite their vastly different theologies, there is a strong resonance between this conception of the life of the Christian saint and the pious obedience to "the providential order of the Stoic cosmos" (Kapstein, 2013, p. 110) counseled in ancient Greece, as well as the "secular spirituality" (Lee, 2015, p. 275) evident in the contemporary mindfulness meditation movement and in 12-Step therapeutic groups. These paths all involve overcoming instinctual, hedonistic desires and developing a capacity to accept with equanimity the one's role as a servant of the transcendent, however that is defined. For example, a chapter on "Equanimity" in a nineteenth-century guidebook subtitled *Means of Moral Discipline to the Christian* warns against the dangers of "agitation" caused by "every trivial circumstance of life" to the "humbled heart," whose response to God should always be: "Thy will be done" (Seeley & Burnside, 1838, p. 53).

The 12 steps, originally pioneered by Alcoholics Anonymous (AA) and now applied to many forms of addiction, cultivate a deep humility and a sense of spiritual *reliance* on a higher power rather than an overarching attitude of *defiance* (Lee et al., 2017). Such reliance reflects the notion of becoming a "vessel of the Holy Spirit" that animated the founders of AA. But they sought to make this process of connecting to a higher power and thus becoming more peaceful and giving available to the religious and non-religious alike. According to AA, defiance is "the outstanding characteristic of many an alcoholic" (Alcoholics Anonymous [AA], 1953, p. 31), because alcoholics tend to exhibit a "baseline subjective sense of restlessness, irritability, and discontent" (Sussman, 2010, p. 28)—the opposite of inner peace. The AA "Big Book" frames this lack of peace in terms of egocentrism: "Above everything, we alcoholics must be rid of this selfishness. We must, or it kills us" (AA, 2001, p. 62). Such a state is not limited to those addicted to substances, as the downward trajectory in well-being in the United States in recent years may be partly a function of "a mass-addiction society" that includes many behavioral addictions (Sachs, 2019, p. 124; Sussman, Lisha, & Griffiths, 2011). For 12-step groups, the path to recovery and well-being involves reliance on a higher power of one's own understanding, whether that might be a theistic conception of God or the non-theistic good orderly discipline (G.O.D.) of the 12 steps. AA would generally concur with Bateson (1971, p. 3) that a "spiritual experience" involves "the myth of self-power" being "broken by the demonstration of a greater power" and, therefore, that a sense of flourishing or deprivation may follow depending on the degree to which the disposition of inner peace is present during such experiences or is fostered by them. The decisive shift is from a self-centered, aggressive opposition to the world toward a "complementarity" (Bateson, 1971, p. 16) or "ontological interconnectedness" (Delle Fave et al., 2016, p. 1; Kjell et al., 2016) that manifests in benevolent service to others (Lee et al., 2017; Lee, Poloma, & Post, 2013).

This spirit of complementarity with the world—whether arrived at through religious or secular means—might be a bedrock foundation for flourishing that could help overcome the myriad conceptualizations and sometimes contradictory findings that seem to indicate a high level of disorganization in the field. After all, grounding *complete well-being*—also labeled *flourishing*, which includes physical health and social relationships (VanderWeele, 2017)—in hedonistic factors such as the balance of positive and negative affect has proved challenging (King, 2001). Some cultural traditions normalize negative affect while others do not (Myers & Diener, 1995), and well-established social scientific traditions eschew hedonistic markers of well-being (Schneider, 2011). There is much more to flourishing than positive affect, and some are pushing back against what they describe as the "tyranny of the positive attitude" (McDonald & O'Callaghan, 2008, p. 128), despite the demonstrated value of such attitudes. And although often overlapping, the meaningful life is not always a happy one (Baumeister, Vohs, Aaker, & Garbinsky, 2013; King, 2001; Lee et al., 2013).

By including transcendence of hedonism and materialism, a common religious and philosophic theme, our conception of inner peace provides a different approach to well-being which may serve as an antidote to dominant pleasure-seeking cultural trends. Some of the markers of flourishing could serve as psychological defense mechanisms and "adaptive preferences" (Elster, 1983/2016), thus enabling acceptance of degrading conditions of various kinds. This includes the positive affect that some experience when viewing violent media, as well as the acceptance of inequities that increase mortality in some groups while providing others with a comfortable life of privilege. Such harmful effects are fundamentally inconsistent with inner peace because this is based on the thoughtful understanding of difficult life situations rather than automatic reactions of fear or avoidance. Existentialist philosophy and depth psychology have both explored the self-alienation that results from the conditioned acceptance of adaptive preferences and their attendant psychological defense mechanisms. Although it may be "a source of never-ending astonishment" to witness "how comparatively well a person can function with the core of himself not participating" (Horney, 1950, p. 161), this would hardly be a model of the flourishing life. In sum, our review of the world's great wisdom traditions and social science research suggests that attainment of inner peace may be a cultural universal that could provide a deeper principle to guide the development of the science of flourishing. However, inner peace is not generally included in social scientific studies on the topic, perhaps because a suitable measure has not yet been developed.

Inner Peace and Well-Being in Social Science Research

Although inner peace has historically been considered an important indicator of well-being in both Western and Eastern cultures, it is rarely mentioned in modern social sciences. For example, psychological and mental health research have long focused on negative emotions and mental disorders (Fredrickson, 1998). This is to some degree due to the substantial array of problems imposed by such emotions and disorders on individuals and for society. However, the marginalization of positive mental experiences in theoretical development and empirical studies has been challenged by researchers arguing that the eradication of symptoms does not automatically lead to mental health and well-being (Keyes, 2005; Payton, 2009). Being well is more than just being free from problems. And people grow from dealing with their problems and achieve higher levels of well-being (Frankl, 1963;

Ryff, 2014). Indeed, the cultivation of positive mental functioning can be used as treatments of or prevention for mental health disorders and emotion problems. This has been evident in the success of the 12-step therapeutic approaches for different types of addictive behaviors and mindfulness-based interventions for a variety of mental disorders.

As researchers turn their attention toward the positive side of human experiences, a major focus has been on pursuing happiness and other high-arousal positive emotions such as joy and amusement. Hedonic happiness, defined as maximizing the pleasure in life, has become "the mascot for most of what is good and meaningful in life" (Cordaro, Glass, & Anderson, 2016, p. 221). The neglect of theoretical concepts describing human experience deeper than "feeling good" has been criticized as a "narrow band" investigation of well-being and flourishing (Schneider, 2011, p. 32). Moreover, researchers argue that the striving for happiness can be harmful because if well-being is reducible to feeling good, "drug abusers would be the happiest people on the planet" (Hayes, 2008, p. ix). Challenging the focus on pleasure-seeking hedonism, a purpose/growth-seeking eudaimonism has inspired further theory building and measurement developing of well-being. Drawn from Greek philosophy and multiple Western psychological traditions, Ryff's well-known psychological well-being model considers six dimensions of well-being: purpose in life, personal growth, environmental mastery, positive relationship, autonomy, and self-acceptance. However, inner peace was not a part of this influential conceptualization and operationalization of psychological well-being. Other frameworks of flourishing also omit a robust measure of this aspect (Delle Fave et al., 2016; Hone, Jarden, Schofield, & Duncan, 2014).

Very recently, research on low-arousal positive mental states which are similar to inner peace, such as contentment, tranquility, harmony, and serenity, started to emerge but in a very limited number and often with inconsistent conceptualization (Berenbaum et al., 2018; Cordaro et al., 2016; Kjell et al., 2016). There are also emerging discussions recently in the psychological literature on interesting new concepts such as "innate mental health" (Kelly, Pransky, & Lambert, 2015, p. 269), where the mind is at its natural healthy state without the contamination of egoistic feelings or thoughts, a state that can be considered to some degree similar to inner peace. However, inner peace, which is central to human experience of well-being, has not drawn much direct research attention. Delle Fave (2016, p. 8) and colleagues note that most research on the psychology of happiness imposes a Western-biased, high-arousal, affect-based definition conceived a priori by scholars, whereas "harmony"—comprised of inner peace, balance, contentment, and psychophysical well-being—is preferred by laypersons from all countries (except Croatia). "Well-being," a broader category that includes happiness, has similarly been framed in self-centered ways in scientific research that orients survey respondents toward self-gratification and atomistic, individual notions of growth and self-actualization (Kjell et al., 2016). If given the option, the majority of the world's population seems to reject this selfish and individualistic construal of happiness, life satisfaction, and well-being. Laypersons—even those living in Western, individualistic, and non-traditional societies—instead prefer an inner harmony with self and outer harmony with others that speaks to the fundamental interconnectedness of all of life (Delle Fave et al., 2016). Although consistent with our synthesis of the literature, the conceptualization of harmony as inclusive of psychophysical well-being (Delle Fave et al., 2016) is perhaps too broad, while the five-item measure of harmony developed by Kjell et al. (2016) is perhaps too narrow to encompass all of the domains of inner peace. Nevertheless, the work of these scholars has helped reveal significant limitations in the extant literature and provides a helpful foundation for the development of our multidimensional measure.

Inner Balance, Acceptance, and Transcendence

Although known by different names, an *engaged balance* or *equanimity* as perhaps the core characteristic of inner peace is shared by different cultural traditions and approaches. "Engaged balance" means that inner peace is an active mental state as a person actively participates in life situations in the manner described by St. Paul and others reviewed earlier. It is not avoidance or indifference (Philippe, 2002). Individuals make efforts to find and maintain inner balance or equanimity rather than passively follow the default mental model, which tends to produce automatic reactions to stimuli in the environment (e.g., perceive a threat, feel the fear, and react with avoidance) (Farb et al., 2007; Fredrickson, 1998; Horney, 1950; Singer, 2007; Williams & Penman, 2011). In a reactive mode of living, we are "tossed to and fro" by life, with limited freedom, awareness of mental processes, and ability to make conscious choices (Oldfather, quoted in Kapstein, 2013, p. 106). Engagement means that we do not have to react with anger and revenge after an insult, or, when enticed by a commercial, we can choose not to crave and go shopping. Instead, we can consciously maintain inner balance which facilitates reflection on the most constructive response. A person with deep inner peace lives life fully without shunning unpleasant experiences, the opposite of experiential avoidance or spiritual bypass (Fox, Cashwell, & Picciotto, 2017) or purposely pursuing pleasant experiences as do modern Western materialists (Belk, 1988; Richins & Dawson, 1992). As such, inner peace belongs to a free person who bears the gifts and losses of fortune with equanimity (Spinoza, 1677/1996). In the Catholic tradition, for example, inner peace "has nothing to do with any type of impassivity, extinction of sensitivity, cold indifference or being wrapped up in oneself" (Philippe, 2002, p. 7). Instead,

> [i]t is the necessary corollary of love, of true sensitivity to the sufferings of others and of an authentic compassion. Because only this peace of heart truly liberates us from ourselves. . . [and] only one who possesses this interior peace can efficaciously help his neighbor. (Philippe, 2002, p. 7)

It takes a lot of effort and practice to understand and overcome the automatic mental model. According to both Eastern and Western traditions, freedom from the rule of the habitual mental and behavior patterns is developed from an understanding of the transitory nature of all phenomena, all life circumstances—pleasant or unpleasant—and the necessity of changes. This understanding of the ephemeral, transitory nature of the world of appearance enables one to transcend one's self-identification with specific people, things, and life situations, and the associated inner experiences, including sensations, emotions, and thoughts constructed by one's ego (Kabat-Zinn, 2010; Safran & Segal, 1990; Segal, Williams, & Teasdale, 2013). "Sadness over some good which has perished is lessened as soon as the man who has lost it realizes that this good could not, in any way, have been kept" (Spinoza, as cited by Nadler, 2016). Because of the impermanent nature of all things, life is like a constant flow, and a wise person who lives in equanimity enjoys life without falling into either avoidance or clinging (Hart, 1987). This is reflected in the idea of Confucianism that when there are no stirrings of pleasure, anger, sorrow, or joy, the mind is centered in equilibrium (Feng, 1948).

Engaged inner balance as the essential component of inner peace can be considered as the unique feature to distinguish inner peace from similar low-arousal positive mental states and other indicators of well-being that have been documented in the literature. Inner peace is different from tranquility because it is not an absence of movement or activity (Ellsworth & Smith, 1988). One can deal with challenging life situations with inner peace. It is also different from contentment, which has been described as a mental state associated with a "perceived wholeness" (Cordaro et al., 2016) because one can experience a sense of incompleteness and still maintain a peaceful mind. However, tranquility and contentment could foster inner peace. Finally, inner peace is also different from the emptiness of emotion because one fully experiences emotions while also being free from the stirring/disturbance that accompanies such emotions. A person with inner peace experiences his or her emotions in a balanced way.

According to multiple wisdom traditions, this inner balance or equanimity exists in the absence of stirring or disturbance from two opposite directions: (1) feelings and actions against undesirable or unpleasant experiences and (2) feelings and actions toward the acquisition of desirable or pleasant experiences. The absence of aversion, in a practical sense, means encountering undesirable or unpleasant experiences with complete acceptance (Boyd-Wilson & Walkey, 2015). With unconditional acceptance, one can engage with difficult life situations without reacting with negative emotions and actions (Kabat-Zinn, 2010; Segal et al., 2013). It is helpful to note that prayer, religious ritual, mindfulness meditation (including secular versions), and many other practices can help to cultivate such acceptance, but our interest is in developing a measure of the trait of inner peace, rather than exploring the pathways that might cultivate it. Of course, due to the impermanent nature of life, losses in different aspects of life are constantly encountered by individuals, such as losing a valued thing, a relationship, a status, a nice feeling, a good job, etc. It is therefore not surprising that many religious and secular teachings are focused on acceptance of loss. A person with inner peace would accept these losses and treat them similarly to other changes in life. Because the sense of inner balance or equanimity can be maintained in all situations, inner peace is not just the absence of disturbance but also can be considered as beyond disturbance from any life circumstances (De Rivera & Paez, 2007).

The equilibrium of the inner world can be broken from another direction—desires and actions directed to the acquisition of pleasant experiences. This viewpoint is shared by Greek philosophers who see egoistic passion as a threat to inner peace (Markides, 2001), by teachers of world major religions who see material possession and sensory pleasure as hindrance to spiritual growth, and by members of Eastern cultures who tend to value balance and harmony more than excitements and pleasures (Lee, Poloma, et al., 2013; Tsai, Knutson, & Fung, 2006). Dangers associated with clinging to or craving for pleasant experiences are especially emphasized by Buddhism. As stated in the *Platform Sutra of the Six Patriarch*, all sufferings are developed from egoistic pleasure-seeking. Embodied in the Buddha's four noble paths, true well-being can only emerge when one completely quiets all one's desires and stays in the natural peaceful mind (Kornfield, 2011). Similar ideas were stated repeatedly among Stoics and Western philosophers. For example, Spinoza considers too much love for things that are doomed to perish as a kind of sickness of mind. To him, positive affects, such as passionate love and joy, restrict our autonomy and threaten our well-being just as do negative ones (Spinoza, 1677/1996).

This idea has also been emphasized by modern positive psychologists, who have found in empirical research that pleasant feelings are short-lived, and, in most cases, people don't get happier in the long run (Diener, Lucas, & Scollon, 2006; Myers, 1992). The reason is simple: "every desirable experience—passionate love, a spiritual high, the pleasure of a new possession, the exhilaration of success—is transitory" (Myers, 1992, p. 53). However, for members of consumeristic cultures (Belk, 1988), it may be hard to conceive that a mind seeking after pleasure is at risk of losing its balance. In the culture of materialism, where a large proportion of a society desires to consume goods for pleasure and happiness (Belk, 1988; Sointu, 2005), there is a danger that questions such as the sustainability of hedonic happiness, whether or not pleasure-seeking would harm long-term well-being, or how the taken-for-granted lifestyle such pleasure-seeking requires might impact the broader ecology, are not consciously evaluated. To live in inner peace does not mean one must eliminate sensory pleasure and happiness. Peaceful people enjoy pleasure and happiness with an engaged balance and without craving for unhealthy levels. When maximizing pleasure in life is exalted as the culturally desired goal, and people seek their happiness "fix" (Hayes, 2008, p. ix) with more achievements, social relationships, wealth, power, spiritual rapture, etc., inner peace recedes to the background and is seldom used as an indicator for inner health. In the face of the hedonistic and materialistic culture spreading across the globe, finding inner peace may require awakening from and transcending such pleasure-seeking and consumer-driven cultural norms.

Based on the preceding discussion, we conceptualize inner peace as an engaged inner balance, acceptance of loss, and transcendence of hedonism

and materialism. In the next section, we present five studies on the construction and evaluation of a new and brief instrument for inner peace based
on our conceptualization. All original data collection was approved by the
University of Akron's Institutional Review Board.

Study 1: Scale Construction and Factor Structure of the Inner Peace Scale (IPS)

Method

Participants and Procedures

Although a nationally representative sample would be ideal for studying
inner peace, we used a sample of college students as a reasonable place to
start the scale construction. Data were obtained from a sample of students
enrolled in introduction to sociology courses and research methods courses
in the spring semester of 2018 at a large, Midwestern US university (Sample
A). All students in these courses received a link to take the survey online
through the Qualtrics platform. All participating students received extra
course credit in return for their participation.

Sample descriptive statistics are reported in Table 15.1. Sample A ($n = 557$)
was composed of 332 females (59.6%) and 225 males (40.4%), with a mean
age of 20.23 (standard deviation [SD] = 4.98). About two-thirds of the sample
were white (65.0%), 23% were black, about 6% were Asian, and another 6%
were of other races. Forty-one percent of respondents were self-identified
as Christian, 19% self-identified as Catholic, 17% as other religions such as
Muslim or Buddhist, and about 23% considered themselves nonreligious.

Measure

As mentioned in the previous section, we defined inner peace as a fundamentally balanced mental condition that is beyond the influence of
one's particular life experiences and their affective valence (pleasant, unpleasant, neutral). We further divided the concept of inner peace into three
dimensions: (1) free from being depressed or troubled by undesirable life
conditions, (2) free from craving for or clinging to desirable life conditions,
and (3) maintaining a mind with calmness and inner balance. As suggested
in the literature, understanding the transitory nature of life situations is critical for inner balance, transcendence, and acceptance. Accordingly, when

Table 15.1 Descriptive statistics for samples

	Sample A (n = 557)		Sample B (n = 46)		Sample C (n = 81)		Sample D (n = 106)	
	Mean(sd)/ Proportion	n	Mean(sd)/ Proportion	n	Mean(sd)/ Proportion	n	Mean(sd)/ Proportion	n
Age	20.2(5.0)	553	21.8(5.9)	46	21.0 (4.8)	81	22.8(2.4)	106
Gender								
Female	59.6	332	58.7	27	70.4	57	75.47	80
Male	40.4	225	41.3	19	29.6	24	24.53	26
Race								
White	65	362	80.4	37	69.2	56		
African American	22.8	127	6.5	3	16.5	13		
Asian	5.6	31	8.7	4	4.9	4	100	106
Native American	1.1	8	0	0	1.23	1		
Other races	5.6	31	4.4	2	8.64	7		
Hispanic origin								
Yes	3.8	21	8.7	4	2.47	2		
No	96.2	536	91.3	42	97.53	79	100	106
Religious background								
Christian	40.8	225	23.9	11	37	30		
Catholic	19.1	105	17.3	8	11.1	9		
Other religion	17.2	95	17.3	8	12.3	10		
None or nothing specific	22.9	126	41.3	19	39.5	32		

we chose the wording of the questions, we emphasized the understanding of the impermanent nature of life. Guided by this conceptualization, we developed a pool of 22 items covering all three dimensions (Table 15.2). The 22 items were included in the online survey administered to the 557 college students (Sample A). Response choices followed a 5-point Likert-style scale with 1 = Almost never and 5 = Almost always. We reverse-coded items that measured inner peace from a negative direction. Stata 15.1 was used for the analysis. There were only a few cases with missing values. Listwise deletion was used for missing values.

Results

Exploratory Factor Analysis

As the initial effort for scale development for inner peace, we intentionally included a larger number of items than desired. Exploratory factor analysis (EFA) was utilized to clarify factor structure and identify a set of best indicators for the concept. In doing so, Sample A was randomly split into two halves, with one half serving as the calibration sample and the other half as the validation sample. Using the calibration sample ($n = 278$), we started with an EFA on the 22 items using the principal factor method to extract factors. The first three factors extracted accounted for 90% of total common variances. Although the third eigenvalue (0.89) was relatively smaller, it accounted for 11% of the total common variances and the Scree plot showed a clear three-factor pattern. After we reran the analysis by restricting the number of factors to 3, there were quite a few items which had low loadings on all three factors. With a careful study of the correlation matrix, we found that there were six items that had near zero or weak correlations ($r < 0.30$) with all other variables. Not surprisingly, the six items had high uniqueness in the EFA, which means a large proportion of their variance was not shared by other items or accounted for by the three factors. We deleted these 6 items. There were still three items in the EFA with uniqueness greater than 0.75. We excluded these three items also.

In the next round of EFA with the remaining 13 items, our goal was to further clarify the factor structure and interpret the factors. For this purpose, promax rotation was utilized for its ability to account for correlations among latent factors (Fabrigar, Wegener, MacCallum, & Strahan, 1999). This analysis revealed a three-factor model with seven items loaded on factor 1, three

Table 15.2 Inner Peace Scale item-factor structure and loadings from the results of confirmatory factor analysis on the validation portion of Sample A ($n = 279$)

	Standardized	Unstandardized (SE)	Scale Reliability	ITC	Item Mean	Item SD	Missing
Factor 1: Acceptance of loss			0.72				
1. I find myself in a prolonged sadness when I lose something I really like. (reverse coded)	0.7	1.00 (0.00)		0.64	2.88	1.17	1
2. I find myself worried about losing something or someone. (reverse coded)	0.64	0.88 (0.11)		0.63	2.35	1.12	1
3. I am troubled by the thought that nothing lasts forever. (reverse coded)	0.7	1.11 (0.13)		0.63	3.06	1.28	2
Factor 2: Inner balance and calmness			0.78				
4. I find that my mind is very calm and quiet.	0.74	1.00 (0.00)		0.59	2.74	1.22	1
5. I feel a profound sense of peace in my mind.	0.86	1.10 (0.10)		0.59	3.03	1.16	4
6. I maintain a balanced mind when bad things happen to me.	0.59	0.69 (0.09)		0.57	3.13	1.07	3
Factor 3: Transcending hedonism and materialism			0.63				
7. When I am in a very positive situation, I wish that it would last forever. (reverse coded)	0.49	1.00 (0.00)		0.43	1.78	0.95	1
8. I am happiest when I get what I want. (reverse coded)	0.59	1.21 (0.22)		0.41	2.38	0.94	1
9. I find myself craving for things or pleasant feelings. (reverse coded)	0.7	1.47 (0.29)		0.55	2.27	0.97	1

Items excluded after the second round of EFA

When I experience an unpleasant situation, it is hard for me to stay calm.

When things are not going my way, I become irritated.

I am easily frustrated.

I find my mind is disturbed by things that happen to me.

Items excluded after the first round of EFA

When I am in a very pleasant situation, I remind myself that it can change.

I try to push away or avoid things that I do not like.

When I stuck in a bad traffic jam, I remind myself that I will not be

stuck there forever.

When I am upset, I remind myself that things will change.

When I encounter an unexpected problem such as a flat

tire, I can

smile at the situation.

I maintain a balanced mind when good things happen to me.

I easily accept changes in my life.

I feel peaceful even when bad things happen to good people.

I feel an urge to fix the situations that I do not like.

on factor 2, and three on factor 3. The three items loaded on factor 3 were clearly measuring craving for or clinging to hedonistic experiences or material gratification. We labeled this factor as "Transcending hedonism and materialism." The three items loaded on factor 2 were quite obviously centered on a balanced and peaceful mind. We labeled this factor "Inner balance and calmness." However, the items loaded on factor 1 were not easy to interpret. Three of the seven items were focused on mental experiences associated with loss. The other four items were about different negative emotions such as the feeling of irritation and frustration, but lacked a clear, conceptual focus. Guided by our conceptualization of inner peace, and also to keep a balanced factor structure, the three items focusing on the acceptance of loss were retained and the other four items were excluded. We labeled factor 1 "Acceptance of loss." We reran the EFA. The factor structure was quite clear. All loadings were substantial. After these three rounds of EFA, we reached a three-factor nine-item structure with three items loaded on each factor. The item-factor structure was reported in Table 15.2. Next, we subjected this measurement model for confirmatory factor analysis (CFA) using the validation half of Sample A ($n = 279$).

Confirmatory Factor Analysis

To confirm the three-factor solution, CFA with Maximum Likelihood estimation was utilized. The model had a good fit: χ^2 [24] = 41.39, $p < 0.001$; χ^2/df = 1.72; root mean square error of approximation (RMSEA) = 0.05, and 90% confidence interval (CI) for RMSEA was (0.02, 0.08); comparative fit index (CFI) = 0.97; Tucker-Lewis index (TLI) = 0.95; standardized root mean square residual (SRMR) = 0.04; CD = 0.98. Only a few normalized residuals had an absolute value around 2. Standardized loadings were within the range of 0.49 and 0.86, which are reported in Table 15.1. The item-total correlations (ITC) were between 0.41 and 0.64. Comparing standardized loadings across factors, loadings on "Inner balance and calmness" and "Acceptance of loss" were quite strong, while loadings on "Transcending hedonism and materialism" were not as strong as those for the other two factors. When comparisons were made within the factors, the item "craving for things or pleasant feelings" was the strongest indicator for "Transcending hedonism and materialism." Similarly, feeling "a profound sense of peace" was the driving item for "Inner balance and calmness." All three items on "Acceptance of loss" had similar loadings. Turning

to associations among factors, "Acceptance of loss" was substantially correlated with the other two factors (0.53 with "Inner balance and calmness" and
0.46 with "Transcending hedonism and materialism" in the CFA model).
However, "Transcending hedonism and materialism" had a weak correlation (0.16) with "Inner balance and calmness," which was only marginally
significant ($p = 0.06$).

Multigroup CFA (MGCFA) was conducted to determine if the measurement model represented the data well in different groups (Bollen,
1989; Kline, 2016). Due to the small size of some groups, we used all 557
participants in Sample A. Assuming the same model form for different
groups, an unconstrained model with all parameters freely estimated for
different groups was first estimated (Acock, 2013; Bollen, 1989). We then
constrained all loadings to be the same across groups. An insignificant likelihood ratio test would suggest measurement invariance across groups.
Following this strategy, measurement invariance across gender groups was
first evaluated. The unconstrained model had adequate fit (χ^2 [78] = 154, p
< 0.001; χ^2/df = 1.9; RMSEA = 0.06; CFI = 0.93; TLI = 0.93; SRMR = 0.06).
The constrained model with all loadings set to be equal across gender groups
fitted data as well as the unconstrained model. The result indicated that the
three-factor nine-item model fitted both males and females equally well.
We extended the analysis to comparing factor means and factor variances.
The results indicated that females had lower means on all three factors, but
there was not enough evidence to suggest different factor variances across
gender groups. Measurement invariance across racial groups was also evaluated. Due to the relatively low number of racial minorities in the sample,
the comparisons were made between whites and non-whites. We found that
the measurement model fitted both whites and non-whites equally well with
only a few exceptions. While there was no sufficient evidence for unequal
loadings, white participants did have a lower mean on "Inner balance and
calmness," and the variances for "Acceptance of loss" and "Transcending
hedonism and materialism" were slightly greater among non-whites. The
model also fitted Christian and non-Christian groups equally well, a further
indication of measurement invariance.

To display group variations in a more straightforward way, three factor
scores were created, and group comparisons on the three factor scores are
reported in Table 15.3. Consistent with MGCFA, females scored lower on
"Acceptance of loss," "Transcending hedonism and materialism," and "Inner

Table 15.3 Bivariate correlation between equanimity factors (factor scores) and demographic and religious variables[a]

	Acceptance	Transcendence	Inner balance	IPS (summary score)
Female	−0.16***	−0.09*	−0.15***	−0.21***
White	−0.04	−0.01	−0.11*	−0.08
Christian	0.07	−0.06	0.11*	0.06
Nonreligious	−0.08	0.07	−0.10*	−0.05
Pray often	0.07	−0.03	0.18***	0.12**
Spirituality	0.09*	0.01	0.22***	0.16***
IPS (summary score)	0.81***	0.61***	0.70***	−

*** $p < 0.001$; ** $p < 0.01$; * $p < 0.05$.

[a] Nonreligious was coded as 1 for those who self-identified as atheist, were not sure if there is a God, or believed in nothing in particular. "Pray often" was measured by the question "How often do you pray or meditate" with five ordinal response choices: never (1), very little (2), some (3), frequently (4) and almost daily or more (5). Spirituality was measured by the question "How important is spirituality in your life" with five ordinal response choices ranging from 1 = Not at all important to 5 = Extremely important.

balance and calmness." Whites scored lower on "Inner balance and calmness," but Christians scored higher on this dimension. This was slightly different from the MGCFA results. The three factor scores were all strongly correlated with the summary score of the whole scale.

Conclusion

Using a sample of college students, this study proposed and initially evaluated the structure of a three-factor nine-item scale for measuring the concept of inner peace. The three-factor nine-item structure found from EFA using the calibration sample was confirmed in the CFA using the validation sample. Subsequent MGCFA affirmed measurement invariance across the gender groups, racial groups, and religious groups. Although the model fitted the data well, further evaluation of validity and reliability of the scale was needed.

Study 2: Reliability Assessment of the Inner Peace Scale

In this study we assessed test-retest reliability and internal consistency of the IPS.

Method

Participants and Procedures

In the fall semester of 2018, a total of 48 college students at a large, Midwestern US university participated in a randomized controlled trial on a mindfulness meditation intervention to improve concentration and well-being as a waiting-list control group for which they received cash rewards. The original study used the IPS in their two online surveys, which were 6 weeks apart. The 48 students in the control group were not contacted at all in the 6 weeks between the two online surveys. Of the 48 students, 46 completed both surveys. Data on the 46 students (Sample B) were used for test-retest reliability assessment. To assess the internal consistency, we relied on data collected from the 557 students of Sample A.

As reported in Table 15.1, Sample B (n = 46) was composed of 27 females (58.7%) and 19 males (41.3%), with a mean age of 21.8 (SD = 5.9). More than three=fourths of the sample were white (80.4%) and 91.3% were non-Hispanic. Eleven respondents self-identified as Christian (23.9%), eight participants self-identified as Catholic (17.3%), another eight participants as other religions, and 41.3% reported no specific religion or considered themselves as nonreligious.

Measure

In the two surveys involving the 46 students, only eight of the nine IPS items were included due to human error. The omitted item was "I maintain a balanced mind when bad things happen to me." As indicated in Table 15.1, it was the weakest indicator for the factor "Inner balance and calmness." As a result, we can only evaluate the test-retest reliability of the eight items. However, the internal consistency analysis was based on all the nine items identified in Study 1.

Results

Test-retest reliability. To quantify the test-retest reliability, we used the intra-class correlation coefficient (ICC) for absolute agreement derived from a two-way random-effects model (McGraw & Wong, 1996). The ICC for average measurements calculated for the summary IPS was 0.85 ($p < 0.0001$), indicating good test-retest reliability.

Internal consistency. Using data from the 557 students (Sample A), we calculated the Cronbach's α for the nine items, which was 0.73, indicating acceptable internal reliability. To take into consideration measurement error in assessing internal consistency, the scale reliability (SR) coefficient (Acock, 2013) was calculated for each latent factor. They are reported in Table 15.1. The internal consistency for "Inner balance and calmness" and "Acceptance of loss" were good (SR = 0.78 and SR = 0.73, respectively). The SR coefficient for "Transcending hedonism and materialism" (SR = 0.63) was a little lower than 0.7.

Discussion

The evaluation of the reliability of the IPS indicated that the scale had good test-retest reliability. The internal consistency was good for "Inner balance and calmness" and "Acceptance of loss" but was a bit weak for "Transcending hedonism and materialism." The results were consistent with the findings reported in Study 1. The loadings for indicators for "Transcending hedonism and materialism" were relatively lower than those for the other two factors. For example, the loading for the item "when I am in a very positive situation, I wish that it would last forever" was 0.49. This might due to the wording of the item. The question did not describe a specific situation, which might lead to more measurement errors. Frequency distribution indicated that a great majority of the sample reported that they either strongly agree or agree with the statement. The small standard deviation of the item also signaled homogeneity in responses to this item. The mean and the standard deviation on the other two items ("I am happiest when I get what I want" and "I find myself craving for things or pleasant feelings") were also lower than those of indicators for the other two factors. Taking all these together, the sample was relatively homogeneous on the factor of transcending hedonism and materialism in the direction of lower inner peace.

The dominant consumer culture in the US society might have contributed to the difficulties of measuring inner peace, which requires transcending superficial happy feelings and instant material gratification. Individuals in this culture are encouraged to pursue hedonistic happiness, and their personal achievements/successes are evaluated by wealth and material possession (Richins & Dawson, 1992). People in this culture would think it is legitimate to feel happiest when they get what they want, and they may not consider how desiring for things or pleasant feelings may inhibit their inner peace. As a result, respondents might interpret the two items without the term "craving" slightly differently from the item with the term "craving" which bears a negative connotation. A lower internal consistency might therefore result.

The lower internal consistency for this factor could also due to sample-specific characteristics. College students are young and may not be able to differentiate experiences associated with true happiness and those with instant gratification, which could be problematic for mental health in the long run. If this is the case, higher levels of measurement error could be a result. Future work should focus on improving the wording of the indicators for "Transcending hedonism and materialism" or using samples of community adults to evaluate the IPS.

Study 3: Validity Assessment of the Inner Peace Scale

In assessing the measurement validity of the IPS, we started with face and content validity (Carmines & Zeller, 1979). According to our conceptualization of inner peace, the scale covered all three theoretical dimensions of the concept, which suggested a certain level of content validity. After weeding out the extra items for the "Acceptance of loss," the final three-factor nine-item scale had obvious face validity. As indicated by the loadings reported in Table 15.1, all items were substantially loaded on the factor it measured. There were no significant cross-loadings suggested by the normalized residual matrix or the Lagrange multiplier tests. The correlations among the three factors (as reported in Study 1, the highest correlation is 0.53) were not high enough for us to suspect that they completely overlapped with each other. After this first step in validity evaluation, the focus of this study was on the construct validity of the IPS (Carmines & Zeller, 1979).

To establish construct validity, there should be evidence showing that the scale is sufficiently correlated with diverse, theoretically related variables

(Carmines & Zeller, 1979). We expected several theoretically relevant constructs to be substantially correlated with the sense of inner peace. First, a peaceful mind is a healthy mind. A person who lives in inner peace should suffer less from anxiety, depressive moods, rumination, and difficulties in emotion regulation. We expect strong negative correlations between IPS and symptoms of these mental health disorders. We believe that inner peace is an indicator for mental well-being. It should be positively associated with other indicators of well-being. For example, a person living in inner peace would have high levels of self-compassion and general psychological well-being. Research on mindfulness has found that the present-moment focus of mindfulness practices enhances the feeling of balance and equilibrium (Desbordes et al., 2015; Pagis, 2015). We also anticipated a positive correlation of IPS with mindfulness.

Method

Participants and Procedures
Sample A was used for construct validity assessment.

Measures
The following measures were used.

Center for Epidemiological Study–Depression (CESD; Radloff, 1977): Participants of Sample A completed the 20-item CESD scale, which assesses depressive symptoms (e.g., "I felt depressed"). Responses were scored on a 4-point Likert-type scale ranging from 0 (Not at all in the past 7 days) to 3 (Nearly every day in the past 7 days), with higher scores indicating more depressive symptoms.

Generalized Anxiety Disorder (GAD; Spitzer, Kroenke, Williams, & Lowe, 2006): The 7-item GAD scale was used to assess generalized anxiety disorder (e.g., "feeling nervous, anxious, or on edge"). Responses were scored on a 4-point Likert-type scale ranging from 0 (No days in the past 7 days) to 3 (5–7 days in the past 7 days), with higher scores indicating higher levels of GAD.

Rumination Scale (RS; Trapnell & Campbell, 1999): The Rumination subscale of the Rumination and Reflection Questionnaire was included in this study. The Rumination Scale assesses the tendency of ruminative negative thinking (e.g., "My attention is often focused on aspects of myself I wish

I'd stop thinking about"). Participants of Sample A completed the 8-item scale. Responses were scored on a 7-point Likert-type scale ranging from −3 (Strongly disagree) to 3 (Strongly agree), with higher scores indicating more ruminative thinking.

Psychological Well-Being Scale (PWB; Ryff, 1989): This 18-item scale has six subscales, including autonomy (e.g., "I have confidence in my own opinion, even if they are different from the way most people think"), self-acceptance (e.g., "I like most parts of my personality"), personal growth (e.g., "For me, life has been a continuous process of learning, changing, and growth"), environmental mastery ("The demands of everyday life get me down," reverse-coded), positive relations with others ("I have not experienced many warm and trusting relationships with others," reverse-coded), and purpose in life ("Some people wander aimlessly through life, I am not one of them"). Responses were scored on a 7-point Likert scale ranging from −3 (Strongly disagree) to 3 (Strongly agree) with higher scores indicating higher psychological well-being.

Mindful Attention Awareness Scale (MAAS; Brown & Ryan, 2003): Participants of Sample A completed the 15-item MAAS, which assesses mindfulness (e.g., "I rush through activities without being really attentive to them," reverse-coded). Responses were scored on a 5-point Likert-type scale ranging from 1 (Almost never) to 5 (Almost always), with higher scores indicating higher mindfulness.

Self-Compassion Scale (SCS; Raes, Pommier, Neff, & Van Gucht, 2011): This 12-item scale assesses six dimensions of self-compassion: self-kindness, common humanity, mindfulness, over-identification, isolation, and self-judgment (e.g., "I try to see my failings as part of the human condition"). Responses were scored on a 5-point Likert-type scale ranging from 1 (Almost never) to 5 (Almost always), with higher scores indicating higher self-compassion.

Difficulties in Eotion Regulation Scale (DERS; Gratz & Roemer, 2004): Several DERS subscales were used here: difficulties in fulfilling one's goals, impulsiveness, limited access to emotion regulation, lack of emotional awareness, and lack of emotional clarity ("I experience my emotions as overwhelming and out of control"). To shorten the length of the survey, we selected 9 items from the original 36 items. Responses were scored on a 5-point Likert-type scale ranging from 1 (Almost never) to 5 (Almost always). The responses were coded with higher scores indicating more difficulties in emotion regulation.

The validity and reliability of these scales were well-established in the literature. The Cronbach's α coefficients for these scales calculated with Sample A were within the range of 0.76 and 0.91.

Results and Discussion

The zero-order correlations of the summary score of the nine-item IPS with related scales are reported in Table 15.4. On one hand, IPS scores were strongly and negatively correlated with symptoms of mental disorders such as depressive symptoms ($r = -0.51$), anxiety ($r = -0.56$), rumination ($r = -0.58$), and difficulties in emotion regulation ($r = -0.55$). On the other hand, IPS scores were positively associated with psychological well-being ($r = 0.35$), self-compassion ($r = 0.056$), and mindfulness ($r = 0.32$).

Following the analytic-synthetic approach suggested by Mulaik and Millsap (2000), we utilized both EFA and CFA to further investigate the correlation of each dimension of IPS with dimensions of each of the above-mentioned mental health and well-being constructs, with factor-specific correlations reported in Table 15.5. In the analytic step, we started with EFA for each scale separately, which suggested the number of factors and factor-item structures emerged from our data. Although these mental health and well-being scales are well-established, we started with EFA because there is often no clear boundary between the confirmative and exploratory aspects of CFA when a new setting or a new sample is under consideration (Anderson

Table 15.4 Zero-order correlations among scale summary scores (Sample A)

	IPS	Cronbach's α
Inner Peace Scale (IPS)	—	0.73
Psychological well-being	0.35***	0.83
Mindfulness	0.32***	0.88
Self-compassion	0.56***	0.77
CES–D	−0.51***	0.91
Generalized anxiety disorder	−0.56***	0.91
Difficulties in emotion regulation	−0.55***	0.76
Rumination	−0.58***	0.86

*** $p < 0.001$.

Table 15.5 Correlations among latent factors of IPS and other related constructs[a] (Sample A, $n = 557$)

	Acceptance of loss	Transcending hedonism and materialism	Inner balance and calmness
Psychological Well-Being (PWB)			
WB1– Environmental mastery	0.27***	0.07	0.42***
WB2– Autonomy	0.20***	−0.05	0.28***
WB3– Positive relations	0.51***	0.22***	0.30***
WB4– Self-acceptance	0.57***	0.14*	0.52***
WB5– Personal growth	0.06	−0.17**	0.15**
WB6– Less sense of stagnation	0.42***	0.09	0.13*
Mindfulness (MAAS)			
Less autopiloting	0.35***	0.29***	0.16**
Awareness of the present	0.50***	0.23***	0.32***
Awareness of emotion	0.21***	0.03	0.02
Self-Compassion (SCS)			
Self-kindness, common humanity, and mindfulness	0.58***	0.33***	0.41***
Less overidentification, isolation, and self-judgment	0.29***	0.03	0.48***
Depressive Symptoms (CES–D)			
Depressive moods	−0.61***	−0.20***	−0.50***
Lack of well-being	−0.46***	−0.08	−0.42***
Negative relations	−0.53***	−0.13*	−0.35***
Generalized Anxiety Disorder (GADS)			
Generalized anxiety	−0.61***	−0.27***	−0.54***
Difficulties in Emotion Regulation (DERS)			
Lack of emotion awareness and clarity	−0.23***	−0.01	−0.34***
Limited access to emotion regulation	−0.68***	−0.24***	−0.48***
Rumination Scale (RS)			
Rumination	−0.65***	−0.34***	−0.49***

[a] Results from a set of standardized CFA conducted with sample A.

*** $p < 0.001$; ** $p < 0.01$; * $p < 0.05$.

& Gerbing, 1988). Results from EFA can inform us in model modification in CFA. In CFA, the theoretical latent structure of each of the instruments was first examined by evaluating how well the documented theoretical model fitted the data. Modifications were then made to improve fit based on information from EFA and the results from analyzing the standardized residual matrix and the Lagrange multiplier tests generated in CFA. Items with high uniqueness in EFA or with a standardized loading of less than 0.45 were deleted.

Theoretical factor structures of most scales were confirmed in these factor analyses. There were a few situations in which our factor analysis based on Sample A suggested modification. For example, the dimension of purpose of life of the PWB scale was not found in the student sample. Instead we found a factor that could be better labeled as a "sense of stagnation." The self-compassion scale displayed a two-factor structure in our analysis, with one factor manifested in all the positively termed items covering the self-kindness, common humanity, and mindfulness dimensions and the other manifested in all the reverse-coded items covering over-identification, isolation, and self-judgment dimensions.

After finalizing the CFA for each mental health and well-being scale, we took the synthetic step, in which the nine IPS items were added to each of the CFA models for correlations (standardized covariances) among latent factors. All models that generated these correlations had adequate fit. All CFI were greater than 0.94, and TLI was greater than 0.92. All RMSEA were smaller than 0.06 and the upper limit of their 90% CI were lower than 0.07. Although all χ^2 were significant, all χ^2/df were smaller than 3. Correlations estimated from these CFA were consistent with the theoretical expectations and most of them were statistically significant. Specifically, the "Acceptance of loss" had a correlation coefficient greater than 0.5 with the following constructs: positive relations (in PWB), self-acceptance (in PWB), awareness of the present (in Mindfulness), and self-kindness, common humanity, and mindfulness (in Self-Compassion). "Acceptance of loss" also had a strong negative correlation with depressive mood (in CES-D), negative relations (in CES-D), anxiety (GADS), rumination (RS), and limited access to emotion regulation (in DERS). Similarly, the correlations of "Inner balance and calmness" with the following constructs were quite strong: self-acceptance (in PWB), rumination (in RS), depressive moods (in CES-D), and anxiety (in GADS). The correlations of "Transcending hedonism and materialism" with these constructs were relatively small, but most of them were in the expected direction and statistically significant. Nevertheless, the two correlation analyses provided sufficient evidence for the construct validity of the IPS.

Study 4: Known Groups Analysis

A *known groups analysis* compares a measurement between a group of individuals known to have a certain characteristics or traits that are related to the measurement and a group without such traits. If the measurement can successfully discriminate between the two groups, the construct validity of the measurement is supported (Portney & Watkins, 2008). In this study, we extended the known groups analysis to the comparisons between groups with and without certain behaviors or experiences. As suggested by many sages in both Western and Eastern cultures, contemplative practices lead to inner peace. Prayer has been considered in different religions to be the most important practice for experiencing divine love and achieving inner peace (Lee, Poloma, et al., 2013). In many eastern traditions, such as Buddhism and Hinduism, meditation is central in the practice for liberating oneself from suffering and inner struggles (Cordaro et al., 2016; Hart, 1987). We expected that those who meditate or pray often would enjoy higher levels of inner peace. We also expect that groups that have gone through formal meditation training would report higher levels of inner peace compared to similar groups who have not received such training.

Methods

Participants and Procedures

Participants in Sample A were asked whether or not they meditate or pray and how often if they did. Of the 551 students who provided information on this question, 169 prayed/meditated frequently or almost daily or more; 245 students either never prayed/meditated or did very little. We compared these two groups on their IPS scores to evaluate the known-group validity of the scale.

In the fall semester of 2018, at a large, Midwestern US university, 98 college students (Sample C) participated in the same randomized trial as did the participants in Sample B. They were in the experimental group who received a 6-week mindfulness meditation training. All participants received cash rewards. The original study included the IPS in two online surveys: one took place before the intervention and one right after the 6-week intervention for both the experimental group (Sample C) and the control group (Sample B). Of the 98 students, 81 completed the training and participated in both surveys. As reported in Table 15.1, Sample C was composed of 57 females (70.4%) and 24 males (29.6%), with a mean age of 21 ($SD = 4.8$). More than two-thirds of the sample were white (69.2%), about 16.5% were black, and 97.5% were non-Hispanic. Thirty-seven percent of the respondents were self-identified as Christian, 17.3% self-identified as Catholic, 12.3% as other religions, and 39.5% considered themselves as without a specific religion or as nonreligious.

Measures. For sample A, all nine items of the IPS were included in the analysis. For Samples B and C, only eight of the nine IPS items were included in their two surveys. The omitted item was "I maintain a balanced mind when bad things happen to me."

Results and Discussion

In Sample A, comparing IPS scores between those who prayed or meditated regularly (mean = 24.72, $SD = 5.63$, $n = 159$) and those who never or seldom prayed/meditated (mean = 23.4, $SD = 5.77$, $n = 206$), the regular prayers/meditators reported a slightly higher mean score on IPS ($p = 0.02$; two-tailed t-test; Cohen's $d = 0.23$).

For participants who have gone through the 6-week meditation training (Sample C), the average IPS score elevated substantially (mean$_{before}$ = 20.05, SD_{before} = 4.75; mean$_{after}$ = 23.93, SD_{after} = 4.72; diff = 3.88, standard error [SE] = 0.46, $p < 0.000$; two-tailed t test). The effect size given by Cohen's d was 0.63, indicating the elevation in IPS was almost two-thirds of a standard deviation. Itemized analyses indicated that the greatest elevations were found among items for "Inner balance and calmness," with increases of about 1 standard deviation on both items. Elevations for the items for "Acceptance of loss" were also notable. However, the changes on items for "Transcending hedonism and materialism" were small and not statistically significant. For the control group (Sample B), comparing the IPS scores before and after the same 6-week interval, the average IPS score remained the same (mean$_{before}$ = 20.43, SD_{before} = 5.77; mean$_{after}$ = 20.39, SD_{after} = 5.31; diff = −0.04, $SE = 0.60$, $p = 0.90$ two-tailed t test). Item-specific analysis indicated that none of the items displayed noticeable changes after 6 weeks. The difference in difference (DID) of the summary IPS scores between the two groups was quite large (DID = 3.92, $p < 0.000$; Cohen's $d = 0.96$), with the change score for the group that had the 6-week meditation training being almost 1 standard deviation higher than that for the control group. The preceding results from known groups analyses rendered further support for the construct validity of the IPS.

Study 5: Cross-Culture Comparison

Although inner peace is considered a positive mental state in many cultures, not all cultures have inner peace as one of their "ideal affects," defined as how people want to feel or what the most desired feelings are (Lee, Lin, Huang, & Frederickson, 2013; Lu & Gilmour, 2004; Tsai et al., 2006). Researchers have argued that Western cultures generally prefer hedonic happiness, while Eastern cultures are more likely to pay attention to peace, contentment, and harmony (Lu, 2001). In a study involving Chinese and American undergraduate students, researchers found that Chinese students reported higher levels of peace of mind than did American students (Lee, Lin, et al., 2013). In contrast, members of American and European cultures emphasize more high-arousal emotions such as excited, elated, etc. (Tsai et al., 2006). In this study, we expect that individuals raised in the Chinese culture would score higher on the IPS due to the cultural preference for peace, contentment, and harmony (Cordaro et al., 2016; Lee, Lin, et al., 2013). Because the US culture prefers high-arousal emotions, we expect members of US culture to have lower levels of acceptance of loss and transcendence of hedonism and materialism.

Methods

Participants and Procedures
In March 2019, 106 Chinese undergraduate and graduate students from a major university located in Central China (Sample D) participated in a short online survey containing the Chinese version of the nine-item IPS on the Survey Monkey platform. We were allowed access to de-identified data for this sample. The mean age was 22.84 years ($SD = 2.35$) and 75.47% of the

sample was female. Due to the fact that religious beliefs and practices sometimes are politically sensitive in China, no information on faith background was collected. Sample A was also used in this study so that cross-culture comparison could be conducted. There were 31 students in Sample A who identified themselves as Asian without further differentiations in cultural origins. We deleted the 31 students from the analysis. Summary scores on IPS were created for both samples and compared against each other. Multigroup CFA was used to evaluate the measurement invariance of the IPS across two samples with different cultural backgrounds.

Results and Discussion

Difference in the average levels of the overall IPS for the Chinese and US samples was first evaluated. Because the Chinese sample had more females and was 2 years older on average, we controlled for gender and age in the comparison. After controlling for age and gender, the Chinese sample had an average IPS summary score about 1.68 points higher than that of the US sample ($p < 0.01$ Cohen's $d = 0.32$).

We followed the same strategy for MGCFA described in Study 1. The unconstrained model allowing all parameters for the two groups to vary fitted the data well (χ^2 [48] = 97.98, $p < 0.001$; $\chi^2/df = 2.04$; CFI = 0.96; TLI = 0.94; RSMEA = 0.06 with 90% CI [0.04, 0.07]; SRMR = 0.06). Further MGCFA indicated that there was not enough evidence to reject measurement invariance across the two samples. But the model allowing for different factor means across samples fitted the data significantly better than the one that didn't allow it. Closer examination indicated that the US sample had a lower mean on all three factors, but only the differences in the means for "Acceptance of loss" (effect size = −0.30; Acock, 2013) and "Transcending hedonism and materialism" (effect size = −0.45; Acock, 2013) were statistically significant. The effect size of the difference in "Transcending hedonism and materialism" signaled a substantial gap as the mean score on this factor for the US sample was almost half of a standard deviation lower than that of the Chinese sample. Further examinations on group difference in factor variances indicated that the variance of the factor "Transcending hedonism and materialism" for the US sample was more than double the size of that for the Chinese sample. The variance of the factor "Inner balance and calmness" for the US sample was also significantly higher. These results were consistent with our expectations and reflected cultural differences between the two groups; specifically, that US culture is more hedonistic and materialistic in general but also more diverse with respect to cultural values. Cross-culture comparison provided further support for construct validity of the IPS.

General Discussion and Conclusion

Although inner peace is frequently mentioned in philosophical and theological literature and in everyday life (a Google search produced more than 205 million results for "inner peace"), research on this multidimensional construct in the social sciences is lacking. Occasionally a single-item measure is used (Liu et al., 2015), or inner peace is integrated into a more general framework that incorporates material needs and group cohesion (Zucker et al., 2014). As a result, there are not many discussions on how we should conceptualize and measure this fundamental dimension of well-being of human life. Drawing on cross-cultural insights from philosophy, theology, and the social sciences, we developed a nine-item, three-dimensional instrument to measure inner peace, which we called the IPS. The dimensions included acceptance of loss, transcendence of hedonism and materialism, and inner balance and calmness. Our five empirical studies provided an initial psychometric evaluation of the new scale. The results from the five studies indicated good validity and reliability of IPS. The short length of the scale allows easy incorporation into standardized surveys.

To situate the IPS in the literature concerning positive human experiences and well-being, in Table 15.6, we juxtapose measures for closely related concepts documented in the literature so that the distinctive features of the IPS proposed in this study can be better seen.

The existing research literature regarding concepts related to peaceful mental states frequently conceive of them either as a subdomain of spirituality or an advanced spiritual experience. The measures listed in Table 15.6 generally reflect this conceptualization. An example for the former is the Serenity Scale developed as part of the measurement for spirituality (Kreitzer et al., 2009; Roberts & Aspy, 1993); the latter is exemplified by the "being at peace" portion of the Enlightenment Scale (Boyd-Wilson & Walkey, 2015). When it is not considered as part of the domain of spirituality, inner peace is often considered as an outcome of religious involvement (Ellison, Burdette, & Hill, 2009). This conceptualization and operationalization limit the application of these instruments when spirituality is not the major research consideration or with nonreligious groups. Boyd-Wilson and Walkey's measure mixed many other related concepts such as wholeness, being in the present moment, self-esteem, etc., due to the fact that the scale was developed to measure enlightenment. Wholeness, self-esteem, and well-being may be features of enlightenment. But there is room for debate whether or not many of the items are measuring peace per se.

Researchers in the field of positive psychology have recently started to study peaceful mental states such as tranquility and contentment as positive low-arousal affects (Berenbaum et al., 2018). Their definition for tranquility has a focus on acceptance, which is similar to one of the three dimensions in the IPS. Lee, Lin, et al.'s (2013) study treated peace of mind as a general mental state of peacefulness and harmony. Measures used in these studies tap mental states such as contentment, being at ease, and the feeling of harmony, which are related but still distinct from inner peace.

Comparing IPS and the five scales in Table 15.6 reveals some similarities. The feeling of peace found in all scales in Table 15.6 was included in IPS and labeled as "Inner balance and calmness." Similar to Boyd-Wilson and Walkey's and Kreitzer et al.'s scale, IPS also had a dimension of acceptance. Further examining the items on acceptance in Table 15.6, it was clear that the focus in these studies was on acceptance of undesirable and uncontrollable life events or situations. (e.g., "I accept things as they are rather than wish helplessly that they were better"; "I accept situations that I cannot change"). This was consistent with the "Acceptance of loss" factor in IPS. The major difference between IPS and the scales in Table 15.6 is found in the dimension of "Transcending hedonism and materialism," as well as excluding aspects that are not specifically related to inner peace (e.g., self-esteem).

Our conceptualization of inner peace focused on a balanced mind that is characterized by the absence of both self-imposed negative mental states triggered by undesirable life situations and heightened positive mental states due to hedonism and material gratification. The latter was discussed in some of the above-mentioned studies but they did not directly measure it (Boyd-Wilson & Walkey, 2015). A life pursuing hedonism by grasping external things such as possessions, positions, reputations, knowledge, etc. might make people happy in the short run, but they may not bring peace because of the transitory nature of life circumstances (Singer, 2007). Hedonistic lifestyles expressed through consumerism, which is spreading globally, are also not environmentally sustainable, suggesting a possible connection between inner peace and ecological well-being (Mayell, 2004). Hedonism, when it is associated with clinging to positive feelings, has been considered an aspect of complex defense mechanisms originating from lack of security, balance, and peace (Horney, 1950). The pursuit of positive thinking or feeling may involve inherent problems (Harris, 2008). According to this perspective, peace as a mental state necessitates the transcending of hedonism and materialism. A measurement for inner peace should intentionally measure this dimension. None of the scales in Table 15.6 tapped this dimension, which is therefore a *unique contribution* of the IPS. A global survey revealed that most people understand happiness in terms of inner harmony and peaceful relationships with others (Delle Fave et al., 2016), both of which are diminished by the selfish and unsustainable patterns of material acquisition fostered by a conceptualization of well-being that does not include peace as a core component.

The *transcending of hedonism and materialism* aspect of our conceptualization may be especially important for the development of *maturity* (moving beyond a state of being "dominated by impulses," especially hedonistic ones), which has been shown to change the "meaning and experience of happiness" (King, 2001, pp. 51, 56). Whereas an immature happiness rooted in positive affect might be the result of *avoiding* deep reflection on loss and regret, a strong foundation of inner peace may facilitate the successful *accommodation* of such losses into the development of a more mature personality (King, 2001) and a more contemplative way of living that fosters greater well-being for self and other (Baugher, 2019). This mature and thorough engagement with life on life's terms—including its negative aspects—is the way of complementarity (Bateson, 1971) and should be associated with a giving (meaningful) rather than taking (happy) orientation toward life (Baumeister et al., 2013), and with finding the true peace in the true good rather than the apparent peace in the apparent good (Aquinas, 1920).

The proposed IPS and its evaluation are not without limitations. First, samples used in the five studies were mainly college students. As suggested by the developmental view of human life, people grow from their life experiences. Therefore, older adults could have learned more about how to find and maintain inner balance from their richer life experiences and thus enjoy more inner peace than young adults. Although this is only a speculation, researchers have suggested that older people have more composure and more skills in dealing with life (Mirowsky & Ross, 1992). Future research should use samples, such as community adults, with a wider age distribution

Table 15.6 Measures for concepts similar to inner peace

Authors	Concept	Definition	Scale name	Scale features	Items
Boyd-Wilson &Walkey (2015)	Being at peace as part of enlightenment	No definition is given. The concept is considered as contained in the parent concept enlightenment, which is defined as "an ordinary way of being that once established means that an individual is authentic, compassionate, and at peace."	Being at Peace	15-item 5-point scale as a subscale of the Enlightenment Scale	1. In the "core" of me I'm content no matter what. 2. My life runs smoothly, even though challenges that arise. 3. Life isn't a big struggle anymore though it can be tough sometimes. 4. I have a sense of well-being. 5. Overall, things for me get better and better. 6. I trust my future. 7. I accept things as they are rather than wish helplessly that they were better. 8. Things for me have a basically peaceful feel to them. 9. My problems aren't problems now; they're just things I deal with in the normal flow of events. 10. I don't need to do or be or have anything more in order to feel whole. I feel whole now. 11. I don't get depressed and think I'm worthless. 12. I feel whole whether alone or with others. 13. I feel "centered in myself" even when interacting with others or doing something. 14. I understand who I am. 15. I don't feel that life has dished me out a bad deal.

Kreitzer et al. (2009)	Serenity	"A spiritual state that decreases stress and promotes optimal health, a sustained state of inner peace."	Brief Serenity Scale	22-item 5-point scale	Factor 1: Acceptance 1. I am forgiving of myself for past mistakes. 2. I take care of today and let yesterday and tomorrow take care of themselves. 3. In problem situations, I do what I am able to do and then accept whatever. 4. I accept situations that I can not change. 5. I try to place my problems in the proper perspective in any given situation. 6. I find ways to share my talents with others. 7. I attempt to deal with what is, rather than what was or what will be. 8. I feel that I have done the best I could in life. 9. I feel forgiving of those who have harmed me. 10. I feel serene. Factor 2: Inner Haven 11. I am aware of an inner source of comfort. 12. During troubled time, I experience an inner source of strength. 13. I experience peace of mind. 14. I am aware of inner peace. 15. I experience an inner quiet that does not depend on events. 16. When I get upset, I become peaceful by getting in touch with my inner self. 17. I experience an inner calm even when I am under pressure. 18. I can feel angry and observe my feeling of anger and separate myself from it and still feel an inner peace.

(continued)

Table 15.6 *Continued*

Authors	Concept	Definition	Scale name	Scale features	Items
					Factor 3: Trust 19. I trust that life events happen to fit a plan which is larger and more gentle than I can know. 20. I see the good in painful events that have happened to me. 21. Even though I do not understand, I trust in the ultimate goodness of the plan of things. 22. I trust that everything happens as it should.
Lee et al. (2013)	Peace of mind	"An internal state of peacefulness and harmony."	the Peace of Mind Scale	7-item 5-point Likert-type scale	1. My Mind is free and at ease. 2. I feel content and comfortable with myself in daily life. 3. My lifestyle gives me feelings of peace and stability. 4. I have peace and harmony in my mind. 5. it is difficult for me to feel settled. (Reverse). 6. The way I live brings me feelings of peace and comfort. 7. I feel anxious and uneasy in my mind (Reverse).
Berenbaum et al. (2018)	Tranquility	"One is at peace with one's current status, regardless of goal attainment."	Tranquility	3-item 5-point index	How much do you generally experience: (1) calm? (2) serene? (3) tranquil?
Ellison et al. (2009)	Tranquility	No definition is given in the study. The concept is used as a positive mental state as oppose to anxiety.	Tranquility	3-item 7-point index	How many of the last 7 days have you: (1) felt at ease? (2) felt content? (3) felt calm?

than college students. Second, we used convenience sampling, which limited the generalizability of the study's findings. For example, the cross-culture comparison would have been more informative if samples for both cultures were nationally representative.

We have already begun the process of developing better wording for our existing items or creating new items that better capture our three dimensions of inner peace. The multidisciplinary team at Harvard's Human Flourishing Program providing the following helpful suggestions, which demonstrate to us the value of engaging scholars from outside of our own discipline (sociology) to include such humanities as philosophy and theology. Some of our items focus on "mind" rather than "soul," or simply a sense of "I." Specific language will resonate with different groups: the notion of a "balanced mind" may not have a clear meaning with some populations. Others might prefer an item such as "I feel a profound sense of peace in my soul" or simply "I feel a profound sense of peace." Our items for transcending hedonism and materialism certainly need work, at least for Western audiences. A better wording suggested by colleagues is: "When things go wrong, I try to bury my sorrow in pleasure." The connection between this item and the domain seems quite direct, although social desirability may encourage a negative response. Another suggestion is about the term "positive situation" used in our items, which captures situations broader than hedonism and materialism because a positive situation could refer to any positive psychological states, such as a sense of being with God or even a state of inner peace. It would be better to make the item more specific. Such suggestions will have to undergo empirical validation, but, in the meantime, we affirm the value of multidisciplinary dialog.

The main purpose of this chapter was to introduce the IPS as a new measure for inner peace which contains "transcending hedonism and materialism"—an important dimension of the concept which is neglected in previous scales. Of course, this is just a start in our effort to conceptualize and measure inner peace for empirical research. The human experience of peace is rich and diverse. People have different levels of inner peace, experience it at different depths, move in or out of the state of inner peace, and transition from periodic states of inner peace to more constantly live in peace. Future studies should differentiate theoretically and empirically different levels and depths of inner peace, as well as different stages of dynamic processes of inner peace. Such research should also focus on mechanisms that contribute to or are detrimental to inner peace. For example, previous studies have found that a sensation-seeking tendency is linked to the de-sire for high-arousal emotions and experiences like happiness, excitement, and physical pleasure (Oishi, Schimmack, & Diener, 2001; Smith, Davison, Smith, Goldstein, & Perlstein, 1989; Zuckerman, 2015). How does this ten-dency relate to inner peace in general and its three dimensions in particular, especially the dimension of transcending of hedonism and materialism? Can the sensation-seeking tendency explain cross-cultural difference in the IPS? If inner peace, as we have defined it, is an engaged mental balance that can be learned and achieved, what are the strategies that one can take to cultivate this mental state?

In answering such questions, future research might find it helpful to con-nect inner and outer peace. In some Eastern traditions, for example, the notion of *karma* suggests that even if a person's mental state is currently peaceful, the harmful effects of their past deeds (and the deeds of others) may continue to cause disturbances that may unsettle their mental state long into the future. And although contemporary discussions sometimes portray inner peace as a form of escapism—retreating from the difficulties in the world into an experience of artificial bliss within a mental fortress—this is unlikely to contribute to healthy and sustainable forms of well-being for indi-viduals or communities. As the ancient Greeks put it, a peaceful "ordering of the soul" required that "such goods as friendship, pleasure, virtue, honor and wealth fit together as a whole" within an ideal "political order" (Kraut, 2018, n.p.). Similarly, in the fifth century AD Augustine's *City of God* devel-oped the ideal of the *Tranquillitas Ordinis* (the tranquility of order) to con-nect the inner experience of peace with an external harmony found in the right ordering of all things. One does not need to be a follower of Augustine to appreciate the ill effects on inner peace that flow from high levels of con-flict, injustice, and discord in the wider world. From this perspective, outer peace is a collective experience that arises from the right ordering of all things in the world, which would entail justice and healthy relationships. For Augustine, this would include right relationships of self to other people and to God, whereas the nonreligious might refer instead to right relationships to people and the natural environment.

Exploitative relationships are obviously contrary to both inner and outer peace. This is why we previously mentioned the peace-builder who seeks to create external conditions that foster peace. While working for peace, a peace-builder might hold peaceful beliefs and engage in practices that foster the state of inner peace. But this individual's state of inner peace will ultimately be incomplete unless there is a correspondingly high degree of right ordering in the world. For Augustine, complete inner peace in this world is not attainable. But it is always possible to cultivate the state of inner peace to some degree, just as it is possible to cultivate a trait of peacefulness.

Furthermore, we might imagine that a person who is *flourishing*, in the sense of having high levels of such well-being domains as happiness and life satisfaction, emotional and physical health, meaning and purpose, character and virtue, and satisfying social relationships (VanderWeele, 2017), would flourish even more if they also skillfully cultivated a state of inner peace *and* engaged in peace-building activities that more rightly ordered the world. If I am doing meaningful work in the world, but I am often agitated, or if I am happy but oblivious to injustice experienced by others, I am not fully flourishing. Inner peace and outer peace are both (at least partly) constitutive of full flourishing because my sense of wholeness requires a right ordering of both the self and the world. If I am out of balance in a psychological sense, I might produce great art for legions of adoring fans or engage in heroic actions as a first-responder in a manner that garners much public commendation, but my *complete* well-being will be limited. Likewise, if the world is out of balance—riven with injustice, polluted so that life-sustaining ecosystems are in decline—my own ability to thrive is necessarily compromised.

We recognize that "right ordering" is a highly contested term, and the point of our chapter is not primarily to explain the relationships between inner and outer peace. Nor have we attempted to advance a particularistic viewpoint of the meaning of peace. But we believe that it is necessary to begin to develop a framework that connects inner peace with engagement with the outer world (see also Delle Fave et al., 2016). In the final analysis, tradition-specific measures of inner peace may be needed in order to do justice to the distinct moral ecologies (Hunter & Olson, 2018) that give particularistic meaning to the term. We hope that our new measure of inner peace contributes to this broader project of linking inner and outer peace and situating the research within different moral ecologies. Although complete peace may remain elusive in a conflicted world, inner and outer peace surely make important contributions to the fullest possible experience of flourishing.

About the Authors

Juan Xi is Associate Professor in the Department of Sociology at the University of Akron and is author and co-author of more than 30 research articles and book chapters. Her recent research examines the impact of mindfulness meditation through a mindful approach to integrate qualitative and quantitative methods.

Matthew T. Lee is Director of Empirical Research at the Human Flourishing Program in the Institute for Quantitative Social Science at Harvard University and coauthor of *The Heart of Religion* (Oxford University Press, 2013). He is also a Distinguished Visiting Scholar of Health, Flourishing, and Positive Psychology at Stony Brook University's Center for Medical Humanities, Compassionate Care, and, and he previously served as Chair of the American Sociological Association's Section on Altruism, Morality, and Social Solidarity. His research explores pathways to human flourishing, benevolent service to others, and the integration of social science and the humanities.

Author Note

We thank Tyler VanderWeele, Laura Kubzansky, and Fr. Robert Gahl for their helpful suggestions on an earlier version of this chapter. The work was supported in part by a grant from the John Templeton Foundation. The views expressed in this chapter represent the perspective of the authors and do not reflect the opinions or endorsement of any organization. We have no known conflict of interest to disclose. Correspondence concerning this chapter should be directed to Juan Xi, Department of Sociology, University of Akron, Akron, OH, 44325-1905 (jx@uakron.edu).

References

Acock, A. C. (2013). *Discovering structural equation modeling using Stata* (Revised edition). College Station, TX: Stata Press.

Alcoholics Anonymous. (1953). *Twelve steps and twelve traditions*. New York: Alcoholics Anonymous World Services.

Alcoholics Anonymous. (2001). *Alcoholics Anonymous: The story of how thousands of men and women have recovered from alcoholism* (4th ed.). New York: Alcoholics Anonymous World Services.

Anderson, J. C., & Gerbing, D. W. (1988). Structural equation modeling in practice: A review and recommended two-step approach. *Psychological Bulletin, 103*(3) 411–423.

Aquinas, T. (1920). *Summa theologica.* http://www.newadvent.org/summa/3029.htm

Aurelias, M. (180/2006). *Meditations.* New York: Penguin.

Bateson, G. (1971). The cybernetics of "self": A theory of alcoholism. *Psychiatry, 34*, 1–18.

Baugher, J. (2019). *Contemplative caregiving: Finding healing, compassion & spiritual growth through end-of-life care.* Boulder, CO: Shambhala.

Baumeister, R. F., Vohs, K. D., Aaker J. L., & Garbinsky. E. N. (2013). Some key differences between a happy life and a meaningful life. *Journal of Positive Psychology, 8*, 505–516.

Belk, R. W. (1988). Third world consumer culture. In E. Kumcu & A. F. Firat (Eds.), *Research in marketing* (4th ed.) (pp. 113–127). Greenwich, CT: JAI.

Berenbaum, H., Huang, A. B., & Flores, L. E. (2018). Contentment and tranquility: Exploring their similarity and differences. *Journal of Positive Psychology, 14*, 252–259.

Bollen, K. A. (1989). *Structural equations with latent variables.* New York: Wiley.

Boyd-Wilson, B., & Walkey, F. H. (2015). The Enlightenment Scale: A measure of being at peace and open-hearted. *Pastoral Psychology, 64*, 311–325.

Brown, K. W., & Ryan, R. M. (2003). The benefits of being present: Mindfulness and its role in psychological well-being. *Journal of Personality and Social Psychology, 84*, 822–848.

Carmines, E. G., & Zeller, R. A. (1979). *Reliability and validity assessment.* Thousand Oaks, CA: SAGE Publications, Inc.

Cordaro, D. T., Glass, L., & Anderson, C. L. (2016). Contentment: Perceived completeness across cultures and traditions. *Review of General Psychology, 20*, 221–233.

Delle Fave, A., Brdar, I., Wissing, M. P., Araujo, U., Castro Solano, A., Freire, T., . . . Nakamura, J. (2016). Lay definitions of happiness across nations: The primacy of inner harmony and relational connectedness. *Frontiers in Psychology, 7*, 30, 1–23.

De Rivera, J., & Paez, D. (2007). Emotional climate, human security, and cultures of peace *Journal of Social Issues, 63*, 233–253.

Desbordes, G., Gard, T., Hoge, E. A., Holzel, B. K., Kerr, C., Lazar, S. W., . . . Vago, D. (2015). Moving beyond mindfulness: Defining equanimity as an outcome measure in meditation and contemplative research. *Mindfulness, 6*, 356–372.

Diener, E., Heintzelman, S. J., Kushlev, K., Tay, L., Wirtz, D., Lutes, L. D., & Oishi, S. (2017). Findings all psychologists should know from the new science on subjective well-being. *Canadian Psychology, 58*, 2, 87–104.

Diener, E., Lucas, R. E., & Scollon, C. N. (2006). Beyond the hedonic treadmill: Revising the adaptation theory of well-being. *American Psychologist, 61*, 305–314.

Ellison, C., Burdette, A. M., & Hill, T. D. (2009). Blessed assurance: Religion, anxiety, and tranquility among US adults. *Social Science Research, 38*, 656–667.

Ellsworth, P. C., & Smith, C. A. (1988). Shades of joy: Patterns of appraisal differentiating pleasant emotions. *Cognition and Emotion, 2*, 301–331.

Elster, J. (1983/2016). *Sour grapes: Studies in the subversion of rationality.* Cambridge: Cambridge University Press.

Fabrigar, L. R., Wegener, D. T., MacCallum, R. C., & Strahan, E. J. (1999). Evaluating the use of exploratory factor analysis in psychological research. *Psychological Methods, 4*, 272–299.

Farb, N. A. S., Segal, Z. V., Mayberg, H., Bean, J., McKeon, D., Fatima, Z., & Anderson, A. K. (2007). Attending to the present: Mindfulness meditation reveals distinctive neural models of self-reference. *Social Cognitive and Affective Neuroscience, 2*, 313–332.

Feng, Y. L. (1948). *A short history of Chinese philosophy.* New York: Macmillan.

Fleischman, P. R. (2004). *Cultivating inner peace: Exploring the psychology, wisdom and poetry of Gandhi, Thoreau, the Buddha, and others.* Onalaska, WA: Pariyatti.

Frankl, V. E. (1963). *Man's searching for meaning: An introduction to logotherapy* New York: Washington Square Press.

Fredrickson, B. L. (1998). What good are positive emotions? *Review of General Psychology, 2*, 300–319

Fox, J., Cashwell, C. S., & Picciotto, G. (2017). The opiate of the masses: Measuring spiritual bypass and its relationship to spirituality, religion, mindfulness, psychological distress, and personality. *Spirituality in Clinical Practice, 4*, 274–287.

Gratz, K. L., & Roemer, L. (2004). Multidimensional assessment of emotion regulation
and dysregulation: Development, factor structure, and initial validation of the difficulties in Emotion Regulation Scale. *Journal of Psychopathology and Behavioral
Assessment, 26*, 41–54.

Harris, R. (2008). *The happiness trap: How to stop struggling and start living*. Boston
MA: Trumpeter.

Hart, W. (1987). *The art of living: Vipassana meditation as taught by S. N. Goenka*
New York: HarperCollins.

Hayes, S. C. (2008). Foreword. In Harris, R. (Ed.), *The happiness trap: How to stop struggling and start living* (pp. ix–x). Boston MA: Trumpeter.

Hernandez, D. (2019). The noble abode of equanimity. *Tricycle,* Summer(57–59),
100–101.

Hone, L. C., Jarden, A., Schofield, G. M., & Duncan, S. (2014). Measuring flourishing: The
impact of operational definitions on the prevalence of high levels of wellbeing.
International Journal of Wellbeing, 4, 62–90.

Horney, K. (1950). *Neurosis and human growth: The struggle toward self-realization.*
New York: WW Norton.

Hunter, J. D., & Olson, R. S. (2018). *The content of their character: Inquiries into the varieties of moral formation.* New York: Finstock & Tew.

Kabat-Zinn, J. (2010). *Coming to our senses: Healing ourselves and the world through mindfulness.* London: Piatkus.

Kapstein, M. T. (2013). Stoics and bodhisattvas: Spiritual exercise and faith in two philosophical traditions. In M. Chase, S. R. L. Clark, & M. McGhee (Eds.), *Philosophy as
a way of life: Ancients and moderns—essays in honor of Pierre Hadot* (pp. 99–115).
New York: Wiley.

Kelly, T. M., Pransky, J., & Lambert, E. G. (2015). Realizing improved mental health
through understanding three spiritual principles. *Spirituality in Clinical Practice, 2*,
267–281.

Keyes, C. L. M. (2005). Mental illness and/or mental health? Investigating axioms of
the complete state model of health. *Journal of Counseling and Clinical Psychology, 73*,
539–548.

Keyes, C. L. M. (2011). Authentic purpose: The spiritual infrastructure of life. *Journal of
Management, Spirituality & Religion, 8*,–281–297.

King, L. A. (2001). The hard road to the good life: The happy, mature person. *Journal of
Humanistic Psychology, 41*(1), 51–72.

Kjell, O. N. E., Daukantaite, D., Hefferon, K., & Sikström, S. (2016). The harmony in life
scale complements the satisfaction with life scale: Expanding the conceptualization of
the cognitive component of subjective well-being. *Social Indicators Research, 126*, 2,
893–919.

Kline, R. B. (2016). *Principle and practice of structural equation modeling* (4th ed.).
New York: Guilford.

Kornfield, J. (2011). *Bring home the dharma: Awakening right where you are.* Boulder,
CO: Shambhala.

Kraut, R. (2018). Aristotle's ethics. *The Stanford Encyclopedia of Philosophy.* https://plato.
stanford.edu/archives/sum2018/entries/aristotle-ethics/

Kreitzer, M. J., Gross, C., Waleekhachonloet, O., Reilly-Spong, M., & Byrd, M. (2009). The Brief Serenity Scale: A psychometric analysis of a measure of spirituality and well-being. *Journal of Holistic Nursing, 27,* 7–16.

Lee, M. T. (2015). North central sociological association presidential address: The mindful society: Contemplative sociology, meta-mindfulness and human flourishing. *Sociological Focus, 48,* 271–299.

Lee, M. T., Pagano, M. E., Johnson, B. R. Post, S. G., Leibowitz, G. S., & Dudash, M. (2017). From defiance to reliance: Spiritual virtue as a pathway towards desistence, humility, and recovery among juvenile offenders. *Spirituality in Clinical Practice, 4,* 161–175.

Lee, M. T., Poloma, M. M., & Post, S. G. (2013). *The heart of religion: Spiritual empowerment, benevolence, and the experience of God's love.* New York: Oxford University Press.

Lee, Y. C., Lin, Y. C., Huang, C. L., & Fredrickson, B. (2013). The construct and measurement of Peace of Mind. *Journal of Happiness Studies, 14,* 571–590.

Liu, X., Xu, W., Wang, Y., Williams, J. M. G., Geng, Y., Zhang, Q., & Liu, X. (2015). Can inner peace be improved by mindfulness training: A randomized controlled trial. *Stress and Health, 31*(3), 245–254.

Lu, L. (2001). Understanding happiness: A look into the Chinese folk psychology. *Journal of Happiness Studies, 2,* 407–432.

Lu, L., & Gilmour, R. (2004). Culture, self and ways to achieve SWB: A cross-cultural analysis. *Journal of Psychology in Chinese Societies, 5,* 51–79.

Markides, K. (2001). *The mountain of silence: A search for orthodox spirituality.* New York: Doubleday.

Mayell, H. (2004). As consumerism spreads, Earth suffers, study says: About 1.7 billion people belong to the global "consumer class." National Geographic. https://www.nationalgeographic.com/environment/2004/01/consumerism-earth-suffers/

McDonald, M., & O'Callaghan, J. (2008). Positive psychology: A Foucauldian critique. *Humanistic Psychologist, 36,* 127–142.

McGraw, K., & Wong, S. P. (1996). Forming inferences about some Intraclass Correlation Coefficients. *Psychological Methods, 1,* 30–46.

Mirowsky, J., & Ross C. E. (1992). Age and depression. *Journal of Health and Social Behavior, 33,* 187–205.

Mulaik, S. A., & Millsap, R. E. (2000). Doing the four-step right. *Structural Equation Modeling, 7*(1), 36–73.

Myers, D. (1992). *The pursuit of happiness.* New York: Morrow.

Myers, D. G., & Diener, E. (1995). Who is happy? *Psychological Science, 6,* 10–19.

Nadler, S. (2016). Baruch Spinoza. *The Stanford Encyclopedia of Philosophy* (Summer 2016 Edition), Edward N. Zalta (Ed.), https://plato.stanford.edu/entries/spinoza/

Oishi, S., Schimmack, U., & Diener, E. (2001). Pleasures and subjective well-being. *European Journal of Personality, 12,* 153–167.

Pagis, M. (2015). Evoking equanimity: Silent interaction rituals in Vipassana meditation retreats. *Qualitative Sociology, 38,* 39–56.

Payton, A. R. (2009). Mental health, mental illness, and psychological distress: Same continuum or distinct phenomena? *Journal of Health and Social Behavior, 50,* 213–227.

Philippe, Fr. J. (2002). *Searching for and maintaining peace: A small treatise on peace of heart.* New York: Alba House.

Portney, L. G., & Watkins, M. (2008). *Foundations of clinical research: Applications to practice* (3rd ed.). Mahwah, NJ: Prentice Hall

Raes, F., Pommier, E., Neff, K. D., & Van Gucht, D. (2011). Construction and facto-rial validation of a short form of the Self-Compassion Scale. *Clinical Psychology & Psychotherapy, 18,* 250–255.

Radloff, L. S. (1977). The CES-D Scale: A self-report depression scale for research in the general population. *Applied Psychological Measurement, 1,* 385–401.

Richins, M. L., & Dawson, S. (1992). A consumer values orientation for materialism and its measurement: Scale development and validation. *Journal of Consumer Research, 19,* 303–316.

Roberts K., & Aspy C. (1993). Development of the serenity scale. *Journal of Nursing Measurement, 1,* 145–164.

Ryff, C. D. (1989). Happiness is everything, or is it? Explorations on the meaning of psy-chological well-being. *Journal of Personality and Social Psychology, 57,* 1069–1081.

Ryff, C. D. (2014). Psychological well-being revisited: Advances in the science and prac-tice of eudaimonia. *Psychotherapy and Psychosomatics, 83*(1),10–28.

Sachs, J. D. (2019). Addiction and unhappiness in America. In J. F. Helliwell, R. Layard, & J. D. Sachs (Eds.), *World happiness report 2019* (pp. 123–131). New York: Sustainable Development Solutions Network.

Safran, J. D., & Segal, Z. V. (1990). *Interpersonal process in cognitive therapy.* Lanham, MD: Rowman & Littlefield.

Schneider, K. (2011). Toward a humanistic positive psychology: Why can't we all just get along? *Existential Analysis, 22,* 32–38.

Seeley, R. B., & Burnside, W. (1838). *Twenty essays on the practical improvement of God's providential dispensations as a means of moral discipline to the Christian.* London: L&G Seeley.

Segal, Z. V., Williams, J. M. G., & Teasdale, J. D. (2013). *Mindfulness-based cognitive therapy for depression* (2nd ed.). New York: Guilford.

Singer M. A. (2007). *The untethered soul: The journey beyond yourself.* Oakland: New Harbinger.

Smith, B. D., Davison, R. A., Smith, D., Goldstein, H., & Perlstein., W. (1989). Senstation seeking and arousal: Effects of strong stimulation of electrodermal activation and memory task performance. *Personality and Individual Differences, 10,* 671–679.

Sointu, E. (2005). The rise of an ideal: Tracing changing discourses of wellbeing. *Sociological Review, 53,* 255–274.

Spinoza, B. (1677/1996). *Ethics.* New York: Penguin.

Spitzer, R., Kroenke, K., Williams, J. B. W., & Lowe, B. (2006). A brief measure for assessing generalized anxiety disorder: The GAD 7. *Archives of Internal Medicine, 166,* 1902–1907.

Sussman, S. (2010). A review of Alcoholics Anonymous/Narcotics Anonymous programs for teens. *Evaluation and the Health Professions, 33,* 26–55.

Sussman, S., Lisha, N., & Griffiths, M. (2011). Prevalence of the addictions: A problem of the majority or the minority? *Evaluation and the Health Professions, 34,* 1, 3–56.

Tsai, J. L., Knutson, B., & Fung, H. H. (2006). Cultural variation in affect valuation. *Journal of Personality and Social Psychology, 90,* 288–307.

Trapnell, P. D., & Campbell, J. D. (1999). Private self-consciousness and the five-factor model of personality: Distinguishing rumination from reflection. *Journal of Personality and Social Psychology, 76,* 284–304.

Vallerand, R. J. (2008). On the psychology of passion: In search of what makes people's lives most worth living. *Canadian Psychology, 49*(1), 1–13.

VanderWeele, T. J. (2017). On the promotion of human flourishing. *Proceedings of the National Academy of Sciences, 114,* 8148–8156.

Williams, M., & Penman, D. (2011). *Mindfulness: An eight-week plan for finding peace in a frantic world.* New York: Rodale.

Zucker, H., Ahn, R., Sindai, S. J., Blais, M., Nelson, B. D., & Burke, T. F. (2014). Development of a scale to measure individuals' ratings of peace. *Conflict and Health, 8*(17), 1–7.

Zuckerman, M. (2015). Sensation seeking: Behavior expressions and biosocial bases. In J. D. Wright (Ed.), *International Encyclopedia of the Social & Behavior Sciences* (2nd ed.) (pp. 607–614). Oxford: Elsevier Ltd.

16

Tradition-Specific Measures of Spiritual Well-Being

Tyler J. VanderWeele, Katelyn N. G. Long, and Michael J. Balboni

Abstract

Despite the fact that the vast majority of the world's population identifies with a religious tradition, spiritual well-being is an often-overlooked aspect of a person's overall well-being. Existing generic measures of spiritual well-being may be useful for some purposes, but are not sufficiently specific to capture the principal ends and concerns of most particular religious communities. Moreover, many of the generic spiritual well-being measures are often inapplicable to non-theistic or non-monotheistic religions. We thus propose that the study of well-being would be advanced by the development of tradition-specific measures of spiritual well-being across different religious traditions. To that end, we provide some conceptual background and develop a set of items for a measure of Christian spiritual well-being. Within the Christian religion, the measure is intended to be ecumenical in being broadly applicable across Catholic, Protestant, and Orthodox traditions. The items for the measure were developed in collaboration with Catholic, Protestant, and Orthodox theologians, pastors, priests, spiritual directors, and laity and covers the domains of beliefs, practices, service, communion with God, character, and relationships. We discuss a number of ways in which such a measure might be of use both for research purposes and for religious communities themselves to advance their own ends. We discuss the possible development of other tradition-specific measures of spiritual well-being in the context of a pluralistic society. These various measures of tradition-specific spiritual well-being may be of use in ensuring that empirical research on religion and well-being is not only of academic interest, but also serves the ends of religious communities themselves.

Tyler J. VanderWeele, Katelyn N. G. Long, and Michael J. Balboni, *Tradition-Specific Measures of Spiritual Well-Being*
In: *Measuring Well-Being*. Edited by: Matthew T. Lee, Laura D. Kubzansky, and Tyler J. VanderWeele, Oxford University
Press (2021). © Oxford University Press. DOI: 10.1093/oso/9780197512531.003.0017

Tradition-Specific Spiritual Well-Being

Efforts to assess well-being have increased considerably in the past decades, with growing acknowledgment that the subjective assessment of well-being provides an important complement to more objective measures (National Research Council, 2013; OECD, 2013). Efforts have been made to assess happiness and life satisfaction, meaning and purpose, personal growth, character, mastery, social relationships, and numerous other positive aspects of well-being (Ryff, 1989; Su, Tay, & Diener, 2014; VanderWeele, 2017a). Measures of well-being that assess a range of different domains of life that are important to people help to give a sense of what is and is not going well in a person's life.

One domain that is important to many people and that is often absent from these measures of well-being is *spiritual* well-being. A recent report from the Pew Foundation noted that 84% of the world's population identify with a particular religious tradition (Pew Religious Landscape Study, 2018); 68% of the world's population consider religion important in their daily life (Diener, Tay, & Myers, 2011); for many, it is the most important aspect of life. The neglect of spiritual well-being is thus an important omission in most assessments of well-being.

While certain generic measures of spiritual well-being have been put forward (Fisher, 2010; Paloutzian & Ellison, 1982), and may be useful for some purposes, they are arguably not sufficiently generic to apply to non-monotheistic or non-theistic religions, nor sufficiently specific to be of principal interest to most practicing religious communities. Other, even more generic measures of spiritual well-being have been criticized on the grounds of assessing principally psychological well-being rather than spiritual well-being (Koenig, 2008; Peterman, Fitchett, Brady, Hernandez, & Cella, 2002). The principal concerns and ends of most religious communities are more specific than the forms of well-being assessed by the generic measures. Notions of spiritual well-being will vary in important and dramatic ways across religious traditions. Thus, attempting to measure these goals and ends of religious practice will arguably require tradition-specific measures.

The development of new measures of tradition-specific spiritual well-being would facilitate an enhanced understanding and tracking of how various religious communities are faring and whether they perceive themselves as making progress toward those ends which they deem as of primary importance. Such tradition-specific measures of spiritual well-being could help supplement more generic measures of subjective well-being that are currently being used in the literature. The idea would not be so much the comparison of spiritual well-being across groups—indeed, with different tradition-specific measures this would not be possible—nor would the idea be to combine these spiritual well-being measures with those of more generic well-being. Rather, the hope of such measurement would be to acknowledge the importance of these ends of spiritual well-being to various religious communities and provide a way to assess progress toward these ends or lack thereof.

This chapter proposes such a measure of tradition-specific spiritual well-being for Christian religious communities. We provide conceptual background for the measure and describe the process of its development and refinement, along with a discussion of its potential limitations and directions for further development and use. If the approach of measuring spiritual well-being were to eventually be employed more broadly in a pluralistic context this would require the development of other tradition-specific measures (e.g., for Jewish, Muslim, Hindu, and other religious traditions). The development of such tradition-specific measures arguably requires researchers steeped in the religious tradition for which the measure is being proposed. Given this limitation, the present authors can thus, at best, present here a proposed measure of Christian spiritual well-being, describe its process of development, and hope that this might serve as a useful model for the development of other tradition-specific measures.

With regard to the Christian religion itself, while certain aspects of spiritual well-being have been assessed quantitatively in prior measures, such as the Measure of Christian Orthodoxy (Fullerton & Hunsberger, 1982), this measure is restricted only to beliefs and does not attempt to capture spiritual well-being more broadly. To the best of our knowledge, there is no prior quantitative measure of Christian spiritual well-being proposed in the academic literature that captures spiritual well-being across numerous domains. Part of the intent of this chapter is to fill this gap.

As we describe in more detail in the "Discussion" section, we believe that the development of these tradition-specific measures are of value not only for academic inquiry, but also for religious communities' capacity to track their own growth and evaluate their own efforts at enhancing spiritual well-being, as well as allowing religious leaders to identify areas of strength and weakness and enhance understanding around the determinants of spiritual well-being with the aim of improving it. Moreover, since it is indeed the case that so much of the world's population views religion and spiritual well-being as central, it would seem that any holistic assessment of well-being would arguably allow space for assessments of spiritual well-being as well. Thus, even in a pluralistic society, such tradition-specific measures of spiritual well-being might help supplement more generic well-being assessments.

Conceptual Background

In this section, we provide a brief description of the conceptual background underlying the measure; how, from a Christian perspective, the proposed measure of Christian spiritual well-being relates to other more general measures of well-being; and what the proposed measure does and does not capture. While some of the conceptual relations described here may be generalizable to other religious traditions, we recognize that the understanding of these relations will likely vary across traditions and thus recognize also the necessity of this conceptual work being carried out specifically for each tradition-specific measure. The comments here are intended only to pertain to the Christian tradition, and we recognize that even within that broad tradition there are likely to be various disagreements, a point to which we will return later.

We begin our description of conceptual background by examining the construct of Christian spiritual well-being in relation to more general notions of human flourishing or well-being. We have elsewhere provided in greater detail conceptualizations of human flourishing and spiritual well-being and their relations (VanderWeele, 2017a, 2020) and here give a more succinct summary to motivate the measure. We propose that *human flourishing* be understood as a state in which all aspects of a person's life are good (VanderWeele, 2017a). Within the Christian tradition, the final end of the human person is often described as some form of communion with God (Aquinas 1274/1948; Catholic Church, 2000; Westminster, 1647/2014). We might then define *eternal flourishing*, or *perfect well-being*, again understood within the Christian tradition, as final and complete communion with God. *Spiritual well-being*, in this life (which is the construct to be assessed by the proposed measure) might then be understood as a state in which one's life is, in all ways, oriented toward eternal flourishing or, arguably equivalently, as a state in which all aspects of a person's life are good with respect to his or her final end in God. *Temporal well-being* or *temporal flourishing* might then be understood as those aspects of human flourishing that pertain to the goods in this life, inclusive, for example, of happiness and life satisfaction, mental and physical health, meaning and purpose, character and virtue, and close social relationships (VanderWeele, 2017a). Thus understood, full human flourishing encompasses both spiritual and temporal well-being, with spiritual well-being, from a Christian perspective, being the component that is most central, that which brings a person to his or her final end in God.

It has long been understood in the Christian tradition that temporal flourishing and spiritual well-being, while often mutually supportive, can come into conflict. For example, a sense of calling to serve the poor by placing oneself in difficult or dangerous circumstances may be important for one's spiritual well-being but may compromise health or happiness. Acting on a calling to missions work in a different region or country, may likewise be constitutive of a person's spiritual well-being but may adversely affect social relations, especially, for example, if not understood or opposed by friends or family members. The potential conflict between temporal flourishing and spiritual well-being is also seen in Christian understandings of suffering. While suffering as an experience of the loss of some temporal good is to be understood as a deprivation, it can also be the source of transformation, of change and growth, of purification of desires, of reorientation to one's final end in God (John Paul II, 1984). When temporal goods and the spiritual life come into conflict, the latter is to be given priority as it constitutes the person's orientation to his or her final end in God.

However, spiritual well-being and temporal flourishing will often be consonant. Health of body and mind and a set of supportive relationships will often facilitate religious practices that promote spiritual well-being. Likewise, these religious practices can contribute to temporal flourishing by developing community, facilitating mental health, shaping character, and giving one a sense of understanding, meaning, purpose, and satisfaction (VanderWeele, 2017b). A person's temporal flourishing, including their health and happiness, is not irrelevant. Christian teaching is that the created order was shaped by God to be good. However, for a person in the fallen or broken order of the world to attain his or her final end in God, some giving up of aspects of temporal flourishing may be necessary for the sake of a greater spiritual well-being. Spiritual well-being does not eliminate, but rather relativizes and ultimately transforms, the importance of temporal flourishing.

The proposed measure is intended to assess the construct of Christian spiritual well-being, understood, as already described, as a state in which one's life is oriented toward eternal flourishing or as a state in which all aspects of a person's life are good with respect to his or her final end in God. As a measure, it can, at best, only assesses what is humanly assessable and, in the case of the present proposed measure, assessable by self-report. There are thus certainly aspects of spiritual well-being, understood as we have described, that are important but that cannot be included in the measure. The presence and operation of God's grace might be thought of as a central component of spiritual well-being in this life (Garrigou-Lagrange, 1999; Westminster, 1647/ 2014), but it is not one that can be readily assessed by human capacities. The measure will thus, of necessity, have important omissions. As any assessment of an abstract concept, it will not be wholly adequate. It will not capture the fullness or complexity of the underlying construct. For reasons alluded to in the introduction and revisited in our concluding discussion, we believe that some measure will be preferable to no attempt at quantification at all, but the limitations of the approach and the acknowledgment of what cannot be measured is, of course, important as well.

Process of Measure Development

In this section we provide a brief description of the process of development and refinement of the proposed Christian spiritual well-being measure. The authors initially proposed six domains of Christian spiritual well-being in light of the preceding conceptual considerations. These six domains were beliefs, practices, service, communion with God, Christian character, and relationships. The domains thus include (i) cognitive components (beliefs) with the items principally following historic Christian creeds, supplemented by a statement on the Scriptures; (ii) practices to sustain Christian faith and commitment including prayer, learning, service attendance, sacraments, reflection, and confession; (iii) service, including helping those in need, supporting the Christian community, the sharing of one's faith, and financial or material giving; (iv) communion with God including various relational, experiential, and cognitive aspects; (v) character with reference to the theological virtues of faith, hope, and love (Aquinas 1274/1948; Pieper, 1966), but also reference to a sense of calling and to growth in holiness; and (vi) relationships including love of others, forgiveness, and spiritual social support. Within various spiritual theologies (Garrigou-Lagrange, 1999; McGinn, Meyendorf, & Leclercq, 1986) each of these is seen as contributing to a person's movement toward his or her final end in God. The domain constituted by communion with God is arguably that which comes closest to approximating the final end itself. However, with spiritual well-being understood, as we have described, as a state in which one's life is oriented toward eternal flourishing or as a state in which all aspects of a person's life are good with respect to his or her final end in God, each of the other domains is important in that orientation and movement toward that end.

After discussion among authors, an initial set of items was proposed within each of the domains. The domains and sets of items were sent out for feedback from various Catholic, Protestant, and Orthodox theologians, spiritual directors, priests, pastors, and scholars. Feedback was solicited with respect to the overall conception of the measure, including the domains, the specific item wording, and any important potentially assessable aspects of Christian spiritual well-being that were absent from the proposed set of items. Item wording was refined in response to feedback, and new items were added in response to suggestions pertaining to what was missing and how the item set might be supplemented. The authors undertook several rounds of such feedback from a diverse range of sources. An interdisciplinary group of scholars likewise provided similar feedback. Finally, feedback was obtained through a series of focus groups in both Catholic and Protestant settings. Focus group members likewise provided suggestions on specific item wording, on the overall conceptualization, and on what might be absent. The authors finalized the proposed set of items following three such focus groups.

A decision was made to keep the proposed measure ecumenical, with the hope of being applicable to the Christian faith across Catholic, Protestant, and Orthodox traditions. In each of these different Christian traditions, a slightly modified set of items and wordings might be preferable. Nevertheless, it was thought that it would be more desirable to develop a measure that could be employed across multiple contexts than to provide numerous slight adaptations. Moreover, within the Protestant tradition, the pursuit of more specific denominationally tailored measures might then result in a proliferation of such measures across Lutheran, Presbyterian, Methodist, Baptist, and Pentecostal denominations, and perhaps even subdivisions within each of these denominations. There is of course tension between a measure ideally shaped for a specific religious community versus one that is broadly applicable. We recognize that the very decision to pursue a tradition-specific measure of spiritual well-being for the Christian faith itself constitutes a move toward specificity from more generic spiritual well-being measures

(Paloutzian & Ellison, 1982; Peterman et al., 2002). We do not think there is a right, a wrong, or an ideal, level of specificity. A particular decision entails a set of tradeoffs. The decision here to pursue a measure of Christian tradition-specific measure of spiritual well-being while still attempting to encompass the major traditions within the Christian faith was shaped by the perceived need for a measure that had Christian ends in view, but with the hope of broad adoption.

However, the attempt to develop a measure applicable across Catholic, Protestant, and Orthodox traditions thus entailed certain challenges. Various potential items concerning devotional practices with respect to the saints, for example, were excluded because this is not a part of most Protestant practices, even though these items were suggested by Catholic and Orthodox reviewers and focus group participants. Reference to explicit frequency with regard to Scripture reading, emphasized by some evangelical focus group participants, was left more ambiguously worded and included in the more general statements about efforts to "learn more about my faith" since the manner in which the Scriptures are read, received, and taught vary across these traditions. Reference to frequency was likewise absent from the statement about participation in the sacraments and the Eucharist since these practices vary considerably across different Christian traditions. Instead emphasis was placed on the sacraments or the Eucharist being "an important part of my Christian faith" as this would constitute a relatively shared understanding. More generally, there was some tension throughout with regard to preferred item wording across members of Catholic versus Protestant focus groups. While such preferences were manifest as well with feedback from priests, pastors, theologians, and spiritual directors, the preferences emerged even more strongly with lay community members and parishioners. The authors tried to achieve a compromise in navigating these item wording preferences and to avoid any wording which elicited persistent confusion or puzzlement. Such compromises were again necessary in the attempt to keep the measure of Christian spiritual well-being ecumenical across major Christian traditions.

In spite of these efforts toward inclusiveness, we recognize also that some of the proposed items may not be viewed as appropriate in certain liberal mainline Protestant denominations. Christian communities that do not emphasize historic creeds may not see the belief items, for example, as appropriate. We acknowledge that not every item would be seen as constituting *spiritual well-being* to every group that self-identifies as Christian. However, through

490 ADVANCING THE CONVERSATION ABOUT MEASUREMENT

the process of development and refinement just described we believe that there are very substantial portions of those who identify with the Christian faith for which the items would constitute a reasonable spiritual well-being assessment. In light of the extraordinary diversity within Christianity, a truly universally acceptable measure does not seem possible. In settings in which some of the items presented here are not viewed as appropriate, they could be modified or set aside. For many, however, we believe the full set of items may be viewed as useful and suitable.

Proposed Measure of Christian Spiritual Well-Being

Following the process of development just described, the proposed items for the spiritual well-being measure across the six domains of beliefs, practices, service, communion with God, Christian character, and relationships are given here. There are 30 items total; each of the six domains has between four and six items. The items themselves might be scored from 1 to 7, with specific anchors corresponding to 1 = Strongly Disagree, 2 = Disagree, 3 = Slightly Disagree, 4 = Neither Agree or Disagree, 5 = Slightly Agree, 6 = Agree, 7 = Strongly Agree. Alternatively, if space is limited with regard to including various anchors, the items might be scored from 0 to 10 with 0 = Strongly Disagree to 10 = Strongly Agree. Further research following data collection efforts will consider the advantages and disadvantages of these different scoring strategies. Depending on the intended purpose or use of the measure, the individual item responses may be of interest, item scores might be averaged within domains, or the domain means or item responses themselves might be averaged to form an overall summary measure. The 30 items are as follows:

Beliefs:
  I believe in one God as three persons: Father, Son, and Holy Spirit
  I believe that through Jesus Christ's life, death, and resurrection, God
    brought salvation
  I believe that God brings grace through the Holy Spirit and the Church
  I believe Jesus will return to fully bring life everlasting
  I believe that the Scriptures of the Old and New Testament guide us to
    salvation

Practices:

I intentionally take time each day to practice prayer.

I regularly devote time to learn more about my faith.

I regularly attend church services.

I participate in the sacraments such as Eucharist or Holy Communion as an important part of my Christian faith.

I regularly reflect on my life to understand what I have done wrong and how to improve.

Confessing my sins is an important part of my spiritual life.

Service:

I help those in need as a way of living out my Christian faith.

I use the gifts God has given me to support the Christian community.

I tell others who are not Christian about my faith.

I give financially what I should and use my resources in ways that advance the kingdom of God.

Communion with God:

I have come closer to God through my prayer and spiritual practices.

I intentionally seek God's presence in my daily life.

I am growing in my understanding of who God is.

I have a meaningful relationship with God.

God loves me and cares about me.

Christian Character:

I always have complete faith in God's plan of salvation.

My hope in God directs all of my desires and actions.

I love God above all else.

My calling to be a Christian guides my life's work.

I try to actively improve good habits and combat sinful ones.

I allow the Holy Spirit to guide me in growing holiness in life.

Relationships:

I love my neighbor as myself.

I have forgiven those who have hurt me.

There are people in my life with whom I talk to about deep spiritual matters.

There are people in my community who regularly support me in my faith.

Short Form of the Measure

Alternatively, as a very brief short form of the Christian spiritual well-being measure, one item might be selected in each of the six domains as follows, with scoring as described previously. Future research following data collection efforts will assess whether other choices of the single item for each domain might be preferable from an empirical standpoint. The current proposed six items for the short form of the Christian spiritual well-being assessment are as follows:

Beliefs: I believe that through Jesus Christ's life, death, and resurrection, God brought salvation.
Practice: I intentionally take time each day to practice prayer.
Service: I use the gifts God has given me to support the Christian community.
Communion: I have a meaningful relationship with God.
Character: My calling to be a Christian guides my life's work.
Relationships: I love my neighbor as myself.

Discussion

In this chapter, we have proposed a preliminary measure of tradition-specific spiritual well-being applicable to the Christian faith. The measure is intended to be broadly ecumenical across Catholic, Protestant, and Orthodox traditions and across the domains of beliefs, practices, service, communion with God, character, and relationships. It is intended to capture, albeit relatively crudely, a person's orientation to, as understood by the Christian faith, one's final end in God.

Further research will focus on collecting data on this measure in different Christian and church contexts. The distribution of responses will be assessed, the psychometric properties of the measure will be evaluated, work will be done on assessing the advantages and disadvantages of different scoring strategies, and the measure will eventually be used for the purposes of tracking, assessment, and evaluation in some of the ways described here.

Specifically, we believe the measure may be of use and interest to Christian communities in different ways. One straightforward way in which the measure may be of interest to religious communities is as an assessment tool: as a means by which a pastor or priest or other religious leader could assess the perceived spiritual well-being strengths, as well as areas in need of attention or care, within a community, congregation, or parish. For example, this may be useful in determining what aspects of spiritual life to focus on in teaching or in the development of new programs. A second potential use may be the assessment and evaluation of the effectiveness of various programs or new efforts that are put in place to foster spiritual growth. This could be done within the context of a before-and-after study or, more ambitiously, a randomized trial. While the general form of a randomized trial with a tradi-tional "treatment" and "control" group may be unacceptable in the context of many religious community settings, randomization of, for example, two different types of spiritual retreats or a wait-list randomization (e.g., ran-domization to participate in the program either now or later) may, in some contexts, be considered acceptable. In any case, such designs may help eval-uate the efficacy of the proposed program and activities and do so using a set of outcomes, captured by the Christian spiritual well-being measure, that are closely aligned to the goals and ends of the community itself. A third poten-tial use may simply be as a tool for individual self-reflection. The process of providing responses to the proposed measure's various items may provide opportunity for self-reflection and self-evaluation, and the measure may be used as a guide for decisions on further efforts or changes in life or on seeking support. The measure could be used for this purpose on a single occasion and might also be useful for identifying and exploring changes in spiritual well-being over time.

The measure is based on self-report and, as such, is subject to the usual limitations of self-report. The items themselves may be interpreted differ-ently by different individuals, and the scoring (e.g., what constitutes a "6" versus a "7") might likewise be interpreted differently across persons. This makes comparisons across individuals or across communities potentially problematic. Nevertheless, for the uses just described the self-report na-ture is not necessarily problematic. Despite the measure employing self-reporting, it may still be useful for a religious leader to get a sense of the perceived strengths and weaknesses of a community. In the context of a ran-domized program or intervention evaluation, self-report biases will be bal-anced across groups by randomization itself. For the purposes of reflection or the tracking of an individual over time, likewise the self-report nature of the measure is not necessarily problematic. The appropriateness of a measure depends on its use, and, for these various uses, the measure might often be appropriate. However, even in these aforementioned contexts, due caution is needed. Programs or activities that make participants more aware of the possibilities of growth, high standards or aspirations, the spiritual lives of the saints, or the need for humility may end up altering an individual's interpretation of the scores themselves (e.g., individuals might rate themselves lower on a variety of items after studying the life of an important faithful historical figure). In contexts in which this may be an important component of the program to be evaluated, further caution in interpretation is certainly warranted. Relatedly, a person might, for a period of time, not feel particularly close to God and yet through this process be experiencing a deepening of their spirituality, an experience which, in its more extreme forms, is sometimes referred to as a "dark night of the soul" (Saint John of the Cross, 1585). For all of these reasons, interpretation of results must be handled carefully. However, the hope and intent of the measure is that it be used by religious communities in many of these aforementioned ways while maintaining awareness of the caveats and limitations.

It may be desirable also to supplement the subjective self-report evaluations that constitute the measure with additional more objectively reported questions concerning the actual frequency of service attendance, the time spent in prayer, the amount of money given, the number of people with whom one has discussed the Christian faith, the number of hours spent volunteering, etc. However, as with subjective assessments, more objective measures also need to be interpreted carefully since life circumstances can vary considerably. A larger absolute amount given to charity may not indicate greater generosity depending on, for example, the extent of one's income, the size of the family one is supporting, etc. However, the subjective measures and the more objective measures, taken together, may provide a fuller picture of spiritual well-being.

The measure proposed here was for spiritual well-being as it pertains to the Christian faith. In the introduction, we suggested the possibility of supplementing general measures of well-being with tradition-specific measure of spiritual well-being. For such a proposal to be reasonable within the context of a pluralistic society, other tradition-specific measures of spiritual well-being would need to be developed as well. We recognize that the challenges in producing a Jewish, Muslim, Hindu, or Buddhist measure will likely be distinct from the challenges encountered in the development and refinement of this measure of Christian spiritual well-being. No measure will be wholly adequate. Some of the challenges are likely to be similar, including dealing with multiple traditions present within what is often referred to as the same religion, deciding on specific items and appropriate item wording, and appropriately acknowledging what cannot be assessed. It is possible that some of the lessons and challenges documented here might be useful in the development of other tradition-specific measures, but we acknowledge that many, and additional, challenges might well be quite different. The development of other tradition-specific measures may also be useful in facilitating dialogue and in clarifying differences and commonalities in the understanding of spiritual well-being and in the beliefs and truth claims of different religious traditions.

We do, however, believe that supplementing general measures of well-being with tradition-specific measures of spiritual well-being is important in evaluating human progress. As noted earlier, the vast majority of the world's population identifies with a religious tradition, and, for most, this is an important part of their daily life (Diener et al., 2011; Pew Religious Landscape Study, 2018); for many, it is the most important part. The use of measures of tradition-specific spiritual well-being would facilitate an understanding and tracking of how various religious communities are faring and whether they perceive themselves as making progress toward attaining those ends which they deem most important. Such measurement would acknowledge the importance of these ends of spiritual well-being to various religious communities. It would furthermore provide a way to assess progress toward these ends or lack thereof, and to facilitate the capacity of bringing an empirically informed case for promoting these ends into policy discussions. Such advocacy would need to likewise acknowledge the competing interests and ends of other communities and carry out these discussions in the context of a country's full political life. However, the use of such measures may help religious communities themselves in the discernment of how various government policies do, or do not, affect these communities' principal priorities. If these are the matters that many people care most about, it seems this should at least be acknowledged and taken into account in policy decisions and considerations of societal progress.

Social science research on religion has sometimes been criticized from theological perspectives for simplifying and instrumentalizing religion (Bishop, 2009; Shuman & Meador, 2002). The conception of religion and spirituality is sometimes criticized as being very thin, reductionistic, and not engaged with religion's chief concerns about God, salvation, life after death, or with specific beliefs. It is moreover argued that much social-scientific research promotes using religion to advance health or various temporal or secular ends while in fact neglecting religion's own goals and internal goods. The research may sometimes promote the replacing of the true meaning of faith with a self-interested individualism which enlists religious faith to simply get what one wants (Shuman & Meador, 2002). From the perspective of communities of faith, these concerns are important. However, we would argue that rather than abandoning social-scientific methods in light of these concerns, a preferable approach would be to broaden the conceptualizations of religion along with the set of outcomes examined when employing such empirical quantitative methodology. The measure of Christian spiritual well-being that we have proposed here provides an outcome measure shaped by the principal aims of many Christian religious communities and may help better align quantitative research efforts with the primary ends of Christian communities themselves. The use of these outcome measures, shaped by the ends of religious communities, may allow for research that is not only of academic interest, but also of use and benefit to the religious communities themselves. The possibility of this being so would likely be enhanced further by additional and ongoing dialogue between researchers and religious communities (Balboni & Balboni, 2018; Long, Gregg, VanderWeele, Oman, & Laird, 2019; VanderWeele, 2017c). We hope that this proposed measure of Christian spiritual well-being, focused on the tradition-specific ends of Christianity itself, will help make that possibility a reality.

About the Authors

Tyler J. VanderWeele is the John L. Loeb and Frances Lehman Loeb Professor of Epidemiology in the Departments of Epidemiology and Biostatistics at the Harvard T. H. Chan School of Public Health, Director of the Human Flourishing Program, and Co-Director of the Initiative on Health, Religion, and Spirituality at Harvard University. His research concerns methodology for distinguishing between association and causation in observational studies, and his empirical research spans psychiatric, perinatal, and social epidemiology; the science of happiness and flourishing; and the study of religion and health, including both religion and population health and the role of religion and spirituality in end-of-life care. He has published more than 300 papers in peer-reviewed journals and is author of the book *Explanation in Causal Inference* (Oxford University Press, 2015).

Katelyn N. G. Long is John and Daria Barry Postdoctoral Fellow at the Human Flourishing Program at Harvard University and a postdoctoral fellow at the Harvard T. H. Chan School of Public Health. Her current work focuses on determinants of well-being, group dynamics of religion on human flourishing, and the development of tradition-specific spiritual well-being measures. She completed her doctoral studies at Boston University School of Public Health, where her dissertation focused on the role of faith-based and charitable health providers in health systems. Her other public health work has been in the areas of chronic disease prevention, adolescent health, mental health, and positive deviance in vulnerable communities.

Michael J. Balboni is an instructor at Harvard Medical School in the department of psychiatry at Brigham & Women's Hospital. As a theologian, his focus has included the development of a theology of medicine and a concentration in the theological underpinnings related to spiritual care in a pluralistic, secular medical context. As a researcher, his empirical projects have focused on spirituality and religion and their associations with end-of-life medical utilization and patient outcomes. He is co-editor of *Spirituality and Religion Within the Culture of Medicine: From Evidence to Practice* (Oxford University Press, 2017), and the co-author (together with Tracy Balboni) of *Hostility to Hospitality: Spirituality and Professional Socialization Within Medicine* (Oxford University Press, 2018). He is a Congregational minister in Boston.

Author Note

We thank the John Templeton Foundation for Grant 61075 "Religious Communities and Human Flourishing" in support of this work. Additional support was provided by the Lee Kum Sheung Center for Health and Happiness. We thank Daniel Hall, John Grieco, Susan Holman, Matthew Lee, Jeffrey Hanson, Matthew Wilson, Andrew Fassett, Jason Harris, Tracy Balboni, Harold Koenig, Gloria White-Hammond, Robert Gahl, Ryan Gregg, and focus group participants at the Bay Church, Concord, California, and at Boston College Catholic Student Center for helpful discussions and for comments on the proposed measure and items. The views expressed in this chapter represent the perspectives of the authors and do not reflect the opinions or endorsement of any organization. We have no known conflict of interest to disclose. Correspondence concerning this chapter should be directed to Tyler J. VanderWeele, Harvard T. H. Chan School of Public Health, Departments of Epidemiology and Biostatistics, 677 Huntington Avenue, Boston, MA 02115 (tvanderw@hsph.harvard.edu).

References

Aquinas, T. (1274/1948). *Summa theologica. Complete English translation in five volumes.* Notre Dame, IN: Ave Maria Press.

Balboni, M. J., & Balboni, T. A. (2018). *Hostility to hospitality: Spirituality and professional socialization within medicine.* New York: Oxford University Press.

Bishop, J. P. (2009). Biopsychosociospiritual medicine and other political schemes. *Christian Bioethics, 15,* 254–276.

Catholic Church. (2000). *Catechism of the Catholic church* (2nd ed.). Vatican City: Libreria Editrice Vaticana.

Diener, E., Tay, L., & Myers, D. G. (2011). The religion paradox: If religion makes people happy, why are so many dropping out? *Journal of Personality and Social Psychology, 101,* 1278–1290.

Fisher, J. (2010). Development and application of a spiritual well-being questionnaire called SHALOM. *Religions, 1*(1), 105–121.

Fullerton, J. T., & Hunsberger, B. (1982). A unidimensional measure of Christian orthodoxy. *Journal for the Scientific Study of Religion, 21,* 317–326.

Garrigou-Lagrange, R. (1999). *Three ages of the interior life.* Charlotte, NC: TAN.

John Paul II (1984). Salvifici Doloris. *Apostolic Letter* (Freurary 11). Rome, Italy.

Koenig, H. G. (2008). Concerns about measuring "Spirituality" in research. *Journal of Nervous and Mental Disease, 196,* 349–355.

Long, K. N. G., Gregg, R. J., VanderWeele, T. J., Oman, D., & Laird, L. D. (2019). Boundary Crossing: Meaningfully engaging religious traditions and religious institutions in public health. *Religions, 10*(7), 412.

McGinn, B., Meyendorf, J., & Leclercq, J. (1986). *Christian spirituality. Volumes I–III.* Abingdon, UK: Routledge.

National Research Council. (2013). *Subjective well-being.* Washington, DC: National Academies Press.

OECD. (2013). *Guidelines on measuring subjective well-being.* Paris: OECD.

Paloutzian, R. F., & Ellison, C. W. (1982). Loneliness, spiritual well-being, and the quality of life. In L. A. Peplau & D. Perlman (Eds.), *Loneliness: A sourcebook of current theory, research and therapy* (pp. 224–237). New York: John Wiley & Sons.

Peterman A. H., Fitchett, G., Brady, M. J., Hernandez, L., & Cella, D. (2002). Measuring spiritual well-being in people with cancer: The Functional Assessment of Chronic Illness Therapy–Spiritual Well-Being Scale (FACIT-Sp). *Annals of Behavioral Medicine, 24,* 49–58.

Pew Religious Landscape Study. (2018). www.pewforum.org/religious-landscape-study/

Pieper, J. (2011). *Faith, hope, love.* San Francisco: Ignatius Press.

Ryff, C. D. (1989). Happiness is everything, or is it? Explorations on the meaning of psychological well-being. *Journal of Personality and Social Psychology, 57,* 1069–1081.

Saint John of the Cross. (1585/2003). *The dark night of the soul.* Mineola, NY: Dover Publications.

Shuman J. J., & Meador K. G. (2002). *Heal thyself: Spirituality, medicine, and the distortion of Christianity.* New York: Oxford University Press.

Su, R., Tay, L., & Diener, E. (2014). The development and validation of the comprehensive inventory of thriving (CIT) and the brief inventory of thriving (BIT). *Applied Psychology: Health and Well-Being, 6,* 251–279.

VanderWeele, T. J. (2017a). On the promotion of human flourishing. *Proceedings of the National Academy of Sciences of the United States of America, 31,* 8148–8156.

VanderWeele, T. J. (2017b). Religious communities and human flourishing. *Current Directions in Psychological Science, 26,* 476–481.

VanderWeele, T. J. (2017c). Religion and health: A synthesis. In J. R. Peteet & M. J. Balboni (Eds.), *Spirituality and religion within the culture of medicine: From evidence to practice* (pp. 357–401). New York: Oxford University Press.

VanderWeele, T. J. (2020). Spiritual well-being and human flourishing: Conceptual, causal, and policy relations. In A. Cohen (Ed.), *Religion and human flourishing.* Waco, TX: Baylor University Press.

Westminster. (1647/2014). *Westminster shorter catechism.* Radford, VA: SMK Books.

PART 4

SCHOLARLY DIALOGUE ON THE SCIENCE OF WELL-BEING

17

Current Recommendations on the Selection of Measures for Well-Being

*Tyler J. VanderWeele, Claudia Trudel-Fitzgerald, Paul V. Allin,
Colin Farrelly, Guy Fletcher, Donald E. Frederick, Jon Hall,
John F. Helliwell, Eric S. Kim, William A. Lauinger, Matthew T. Lee,
Sonja Lyubomirsky, Seth Margolis, Eileen McNeely, Neil G. Messer,
Louis Tay, K. Vish Viswanath, Dorota Węziak-Białowolska,
and Laura D. Kubzansky*

Abstract

Measures of well-being have proliferated over the past decades. Very little guidance has been available about which measures to use in particular contexts. This chapter provides a series of recommendations, based on the present state of knowledge and the existing measures available, of which measures might be preferred in which contexts. The recommendations came out of an interdisciplinary workshop on the measurement of well-being and are shaped around the number of items that can be included in a survey and also based on the differing potential contexts and purposes of data collection such as, for example, government surveys, multiuse cohort studies, or studies specifically about psychological well-being. The recommendations are not intended to be definitive but instead to stimulate discussion and refinement and provide guidance to those relatively new to the study of well-being.

Over the past several years, interest in the measurement and promotion of well-being has increased exponentially with calls for societal transformation and a new vision for health that places well-being at the center

Tyler J. VanderWeele, Claudia Trudel-Fitzgerald, Paul V. Allin, Colin Farrelly, Guy Fletcher, Donald E. Frederick, Jon Hall, John F. Helliwell, Eric S. Kim, William A. Lauinger, Matthew T. Lee, Sonja Lyubomirsky, Seth Margolis, Eileen McNeely, Neil G. Messer, Louis Tay, K. Vish Viswanath, Dorota Węziak-Białowolska, and Laura D. Kubzansky, *Current Recommendations on the Selection of Measures for Well-Being* In: *Measuring Well-Being*. Edited by: Matthew T. Lee, Laura D. Kubzansky, and Tyler J. VanderWeele, Oxford University Press (2021). © Oxford University Press. DOI: 10.1093/oso/9780197512531.003.0018

(Plough, 2015). As research on well-being as both an outcome (or a target for monitoring) and as a predictor of other health-related outcomes has expanded dramatically, conceptions and measures of well-being have likewise proliferated. Consequently, it can be challenging to compare ideas and findings across different measures and conceptions. For example, well-being can be characterized by objective measures, also referred to as measures related to "standard of living," and by subjective measures based on the cognitive and affective judgments a person makes about their life (Stiglitz, Sen, & Fitoussi, 2010). Objective aspects of well-being will, of course, also influence subjective well-being levels (Patel et al., 2018). Many countries routinely collect data on various factors that are considered indicators of objective well-being, including measures of educational attainment, safety, income, life expectancy, and so forth. Only a few countries have begun to collect data on subjective well-being measures, notably life satisfaction and happiness, on a regular basis. However, subjective well-being has been an important area of research in psychology for decades (Myers & Diener, 2018), and increasingly in other academic disciplines as well (Ngamaba, 2018). Subjective well-being is moreover not merely the absence of mental illness; indeed, measures of subjective well-being predict strongly and independently subsequent mental illness above and beyond baseline measures of mental illness (Wood & Joseph, 2010). The focus of this chapter is to provide a set of recommendations concerning measuring subjective well-being.

At least three conceptual approaches to evaluating subjective well-being are commonly used, including hedonic, evaluative, and eudaimonic conceptions of well-being (Kahneman, Diener, & Schwarz, 2003; National Research Council, 2013; OECD, 2013; Ryff, 1989). A hedonic perspective focuses on well-being understood as whether one feels happy or experiences pleasure and lacks pain; an evaluative perspective focuses on well-being defined by one's view of, or overall satisfaction with, life or different domains of life. Closely related desire fulfillment theories, while receiving considerable attention in philosophy (Fletcher, 2016) have only recently been empirically operationalized (Chapter 13, in this volume). A eudaimonic perspective focuses on whether individuals feel they have attained self-realization or if they are fully functioning or fulfilling a sense of purpose. There is general agreement that well-being itself is a broadly multidimensional construct that extends beyond simply feeling happy or being satisfied with life (OECD, 2019; Stiglitz, Sen, & Fitoussi, 2016).

A distinction might also be drawn between "psychological well-being," which concerns assessment of an individual's various psychological states, versus "subjective well-being," which includes an individual's subjective assessment of any aspect of their life (e.g., finances, physical health). While these two terms are often used interchangeably, neither of these categories encompasses the other. Psychological states can be assessed by direct observation (e.g., of textual communication) rather than subjective self-report; conversely, one can report subjectively on states that are not psychological, like one's physical health. In this chapter, we use "psychological well-being" or "subjective well-being" in their more general descriptive senses rather than to refer to any specific measures.

Despite measurement and conceptual challenges, the recent proliferation of studies on well-being has provided an exciting array of results and novel insights. However, there is, as yet, little guidance about what to measure or which scale to use for any particular investigation. Answers to these kinds of questions inevitably depend on the context, the resources available, and the goals of measurement. Different measures may be better suited to studying the determinants of well-being versus understanding the effects of aspects of well-being on other outcomes. Although a number of good overviews of different subjective well-being measures are available (Hone, Jarden, Schofield, & Duncan, 2014; National Research Council, 2013; OECD, 2013; Su, Tay, & Diener, 2014; Tay, Chan, & Diener, 2014), these generally provide a compendium of existing measures (or information on where to find the measures) rather than specific guidance regarding which measures to use in what contexts. In this chapter, we put forward a series of recommendations for selecting measures of subjective well-being across different contexts, focusing on the use of subjective rather than objective measures.

Methods

These recommendations arose out of an interdisciplinary workshop on the measurement of well-being hosted at Harvard University in April 2018, and drawing upon a multidisciplinary group of well-being experts from around the world. Discussions of well-being measures are often confined to experts within a single discipline. However, greater understanding of both the science of well-being and its measurement issues may be gained from considering research on well-being in studies across multiple disciplines. Thus, the workshop conveners, directors of the Lee Kum Sheung Center for Health and Happiness and of the Human Flourishing Program (both at Harvard University), identified workshop participants by seeking scholars who have actively contributed to the study of well-being and who also, together, could broadly represent numerous disciplines including psychology, sociology, economics, political science, public health, medicine, statistics, philosophy, and theology. In addition to individual workshop presentations and discussions about the study of well-being from a range of disciplinary perspectives, several sessions were devoted to questions of measurement recommendations. Building on these discussions, an initial set of recommendations was drafted and all workshop participants were invited to comment and contribute. Final recommendations, further refined in subsequent discussion and written exchange, are presented here.

A key component driving the discussion and ensuing recommendations was recognition that there will not be a one-size-fits-all recommendation for measuring well-being. Recommendations must be informed by careful consideration of each type of research or reporting endeavor and the likely constraints on the number of items that can be used to measure well-being in specific contexts (e.g., government surveys, multiuse cohort studies, studies specifically about well-being). Thus, different recommendations are made depending on the purpose for which a well-being measure is sought, with rationale provided for the choice of measures. These recommendations are not intended to be definitive, but rather constitute the consensus of our interdisciplinary panel of experts given the present state of knowledge and the measures currently available. Our goals are to provide practical guidance for the present moment and stimulate debate and discussion, which we expect will refine well-being measurement further as new research in this area emerges. Recommendations are organized according to their intended use and, within each section, giving consideration to the options available depending on the number of items a given project might be able to accommodate.

Results

Psychological Well-Being in Government Surveys

Government surveys are frequently designed for the purposes of monitoring and surveillance. Our recommendations for assessing psychological well-being in government surveys with a very limited number of items follows that of the UK's Measuring National Well-Being Programme. In 2010, the UK government committed to assessing national levels of well-being (Allin & Hand, 2017). To accomplish this, the UK's Office for National Statistics established a Measuring National Well-Being Programme to identify key areas that mattered most to people and to make an initial proposal for domains and specific measures. This Programme drew on existing frameworks in the well-being literature, including prior work by the Organisation for Economic Cooperation and Development (OECD) (Hall, Giovannini, Morrone, & Ranuzzi, 2010), and aimed to incorporate items for subjective well-being already used in the international well-being literature. They included items related to hedonic, evaluative, and eudaimonic well-being, but also tried to keep the number of questions limited to avoid excessive costs and enable widespread use. The questions were tested in the Annual Population Survey of households, and a final set of four questions has now been included on the annual UK National Survey since 2011 (Allin & Hand, 2017). Based on the thoughtful engagement of the UK's Measuring National Well-Being Programme, the choice of questions already widely used in well-being research, the range of questions administered, and the successful record of data collection on these questions, we recommend using this same four-question set for obtaining a brief assessment of psychological well-being via government surveys or other large-scale population-wide monitoring instrument. Although other countries and organizations have also included additional well-being questions, such as those included in the European Social Survey, these constitute a much longer list of questions and may be less suitable for very brief well-being assessments. The four questions from the UK National Survey are:

1. Overall, how satisfied are you with life as a whole these days?
2. Overall, to what extent do you feel the things you do in your life are worthwhile?
3. Overall, how happy did you feel yesterday?
4. Overall, how anxious did you feel yesterday?

Questions are asked using a 0–10 response scale, where 0 is "Not at all" and 10 is "Completely." This limited set is easily incorporated into existing surveys and relatively quick to administer. Moreover, any monitoring body using these items could immediately compare their findings with UK statistics. The four questions draw from each of the broad conceptual approaches to psychological well-being: evaluative well-being (item 1 [life satisfaction]), eudaimonic well-being (item 2 [purpose/meaning in life]), and hedonic well-being and ill-being, respectively (items 3 [positive affect] and 4 [negative affect]). Gallup, OECD, and other large-scale organizations engaged in monitoring subjective well-being also use these items in assessing evaluative and eudaimonic well-being (i.e., life satisfaction and worthwhile activities, respectively; OECD, 2013). The items evaluating hedonic well-being and ill-being query positive and negative affect, respectively, and sample from the person's experience of the prior day. While enquiring only about a single day may not be representative of life more broadly and is perhaps less suitable for etiologic research purposes, it does provide an assessment of positive and negative affect for the country or region as a whole when responses are averaged over numerous persons on different days (Allin & Hand, 2017). Thus, they may be useful for monitoring and tracking. While some have aggregated the four questions by taking a sum score across the items (Benson, Sladen, Liles, & Potts, 2019), items represent distinct conceptual domains and are generally reported separately.

When even four items are too many to include on a given survey, for an even briefer *two-item survey*, we recommend assessing evaluative and eudaimonic well-being using the life satisfaction (item 1) and worthwhile activity (item 2) questions. These two items have been used extensively, have broad conceptual coverage, and, across numerous individual items, show some of the highest and most consistent correlations with much broader well-being measures (Cheung & Lucas, 2014; Helliwell, Layard, & Sachs, 2016; OECD, 2013). When it is possible to include only a *single item*, we recommend assessing evaluative well-being (item 1). Although measuring life satisfaction alone is subject to numerous limitations (Allin & Hand, 2017; Kahneman et al., 2003; Ryff, 1989; VanderWeele, 2017), if only one question can be included, life satisfaction does provide a relatively broad assessment and has been found to perform similarly compared to multiple-item life satisfaction scales in prior work (Cheung & Lucas, 2014). Moreover, this item has been used in surveys around the world (Helliwell et al., 2016), which allows comparisons across countries. For more substantial assessments, perhaps targeted not only for monitoring but also for research, see also the following sections.

Psychological Well-Being in Multiuse Cohort Studies

Increasingly, multipurpose cohort studies have been seeking well-being items to include in data collection instruments for use with explanatory research (rather than monitoring and surveillance) that may examine well-being either as an outcome (i.e., dependent variable) or as a predictor (i.e., independent variable/exposure) of other outcomes. When considering well-being as an outcome, a broader conceptualization can be appropriate, but specific aspects of well-being can also be examined. When considering well-being as a predictor of other health-related outcomes, more specific conceptualizations are likely to be useful, with a particular focus on items that predict future changes in health and behavior. For many multiuse cohort studies, space constraints often make it possible to include only a handful of items. In these circumstances, we recommend the following six questions drawn from the evaluative, eudaimonic, hedonic, and other domains. The items could be used as predictors or as outcomes in etiologic research.

1. Overall, how satisfied are you with life as a whole these days?
2. Overall, to what extent do you feel the things you do in your life are worthwhile?
3. In general, how happy or unhappy do you usually feel?
4. I have a sense of direction and purpose in life.
5. Overall, I expect more good things to happen to me than bad.
6. If something can go wrong for me, it will (reverse-coded).

The first two items are scored from 0 = Not at all to 10 = Completely. The third item is scored from 0 (Extremely Unhappy) to 10 (Extremely Happy) and the fourth item from 0 (Strongly Disagree) to 10 (Strongly Agree). The fifth and sixth items have traditionally been scored from 1 (Strongly Disagree) to 5 (Strongly Agree), but could also be scored from 0 to 10 for consistency with the others.

Including the first two questions has the advantages discussed earlier. For item 3, unlike the question used in the UK survey, which asks about happiness level on the previous day, the question here is phrased according to general levels of happiness (Fordyce, 1988). This may be more suitable for individual-level etiologic research purposes because it captures a more stable, enduring experience in contexts where well-being is inquired only sporadically (Hudson, Lucas, & Donnellan, 2017). Among the various dimensions of psychological well-being, purpose and optimism are among those that are most consistently and strongly related to physical health outcomes, including all-cause mortality in prospective studies (Trudel-Fitzgerald et al., 2019); thus, we suggest two questions to capture each of these domains. The optimism items (5 and 6) are drawn from the Life Orientation Test-Revised (LOT-R; Scheier, Carver, & Bridges, 1994) using the items most predictive of mortality. For purpose, the worthwhile activities item (2) is supplemented by an item (4) from the purpose subscale of the Psychological Well-Being Scale (Ryff, 1989).

Studies of Psychological Well-Being

The greatest progress in the science of well-being will likely come from large studies designed specifically to measure and study well-being itself. For this purpose, we recommend scales and inventories that include assessment of multiple aspects of psychological well-being, including life satisfaction, positive affect, meaning, purpose, and personal growth, among others. Some have argued that composite measures of well-being that aggregate across these various dimensions can be useful in gaining a broad perspective on potential determinants of overall well-being and might be valuable as a focus for policy (e.g., Su et al., 2014). Evidence suggests that the overall aggregates of various different multidimensional well-being scales are themselves often strongly correlated (Goodman, Disabato, Kashdan, & Kaufman, 2018) and thus contain very similar information, though, if dichotomized, differing dichotomization schemes can of course lead to different conclusions concerning, for example, prevalence (Hone et al., 2014). From a scientific perspective, however, when seeking to understand the causes and consequences of distinct aspects of psychological well-being, the use of more specific measures is necessary. In fact, different dimensions of psychological well-being very likely have different causes and different effects (Baumeister, Vohs, Aaker, & Garbinsky, 2013; Trudel-Fitzgerald et al., 2019). It is thus the specific dimensions included within a scale or inventory that will likely be most relevant for the scientific study of well-being since aggregate measures are often similar. This perspective shapes the remainder of the recommendations in this chapter. Various validated scales that measure specific dimensions of psychological well-being, such as those developed by Diener, Emmons, Larsen, and Griffin

(1985); Ryff (1989); Lyubomirsky and Lepper (1999); Keyes (2002); Su et al. (2014); Warwick Medical School (2018), and others, might be used for this purpose.

When seeking to study specific dimensions of psychological well-being, we recommend, when possible, the use of at least two different scales designed to assess the same construct as a sensitivity analysis for the robustness of the conclusions being drawn. For example, for meaning and purpose, one might use both the purpose subscale from the Psychological Well-Being Scale (Ryff, 1989) and Meaning in Life questionnaire (Steger, Frazier, Oishi, & Kahler, 2006) in the same study. Such practice may also help address aspects of measurement that have not yet, or only recently, been adequately conceptualized. For instance, while meaning and purpose in life are often combined in measures designed to capture a single construct, recent empirical and conceptual work has suggested three distinct facets (Martela & Steger, 2016). The use of more than one scale to assess the same construct may help facilitate such insights.

If a study seeks to examine numerous domains of psychological well-being, either as a predictor or as an outcome, then a broad multidimensional inventory will most likely be desirable because such a measure can be considered either as a single composite or by specific subdomains. Among the existing available measures that include multiple items for many different dimensions, we recommend the 54-item Comprehensive Inventory of Thriving (CIT; Su et al., 2014). This inventory was created based on a prior survey of other multidimensional approaches to and measures of psychological well-being (e.g., Diener et al., 1985, 2009; Ryff, 1989; Scheier et al., 1994; Seligman, 2011) and includes multiple items per dimension. The CIT includes three items each for 18 facets that are grouped within the following seven dimensions: relationships (support, community, trust, respect, loneliness, belonging), engagement, mastery (skills, learning, accomplishment, self-efficacy, self-worth), autonomy, meaning, optimism, and subjective well-being (life satisfaction, positive feelings, absence of negative feelings) ($\alpha = 0.71$–0.96 across varied populations; Su et al., 2014). Its psychometric properties and measurement invariance have also been examined in cross-cultural settings (Wiese, Tay, Su, & Diener, 2018). Once again, we recommend that, if possible, the study of each CIT construct be supplemented by the use of other scales (e.g., Diener et al., 1985; Keyes, 2002; Lyubomirsky & Lepper, 1999; Martela & Steger, 2016; Ryff, 1989; Scheier et al., 1994; Steger et al., 2006) purportedly assessing the same construct.

Human Flourishing

Human flourishing or complete human well-being is the broadest possible construct under the study of well-being. Notably, it has been conceptualized as "the achievement of all goods, purposes and ends of human existence" (Messer, 2013) or as "a state in which all aspects of a person's life are good" (VanderWeele, 2017). Such ends and goods include not only psychological well-being but also physical health, a domain that is absent from many of the scales discussed earlier, and character, and it could also include both objective and subjective assessments. As before, we will focus here on the subjective aspects. Important to note is that, because it is so broad, the construct of flourishing should ideally capture, among other things, multiple facets of psychological well-being (e.g., hedonic, evaluative, and eudaimonic) as relevant subcomponents of the larger experience. As such, in many research contexts, "flourishing" makes sense principally as an outcome rather than as a predictor. It would make little sense to examine the effects of flourishing on subsequent physical health if the flourishing construct itself includes physical health. However, assessing flourishing is useful in other contexts (e.g., examining the effect of individual employee flourishing on various objective outcomes including productivity or turnover).

Developing valid measures is a complex process, especially when the construct is as broad as flourishing. There may be tension between capturing as many domains as possible versus the danger of including domains that are relatively less important or trivial. A focus on those dimensions of human well-being that are ends in themselves and nearly universally desired may help shape consensus on what to measure (VanderWeele, 2017). A number of conceptualizations and measures of flourishing have been developed (Diener et al., 2009; Hone et al., 2014; Huppert & So, 2013; Keyes, 2002; Seligman, 2011; VanderWeele, 2017), though many of these do not include physical health. To enhance reliability and make it possible to consider various dimensions separately, we believe at least two or three items per domain assessed would be desirable. Several existing approaches make use of only one item per domain (Diener et al., 2009; Huppert & So, 2013). For a longer multi-item comprehensive assessment of subjective flourishing, because of its breadth, as noted earlier, we recommend supplementing Su et al.'s (2014) CIT described earlier, which covers multiple dimensions of psychological well-being, with a multi-item assessment of physical health such as the 12-Item Short-Form Health Survey (SF-12; Ware, Kosinski, & Keller, 1996).

The SF-12 is widely used, has demonstrated good psychometric properties (e.g., 2-week test-retest reliability, $r = 0.86$ in UK adults and 0.89 in US adults, [Ware et al.,1996]; $\alpha = 0.70$ to 0.89 across samples of older adults [Resnick & Nahm, 2001]), and it captures the dimension of physical health that is absent from the CIT. For a brief 10-item flourishing measure that may also permit separate consideration of domains, we recommend VanderWeele's (2017) Flourishing Index, which comprises two items for each of the following domains: happiness and life satisfaction, mental and physical health, meaning and purpose, character and virtue, and close social relationships. These items were chosen from among those most commonly used and previously validated prior well-being scales. The scale has had some degree of empirical validation ($\alpha = 0.89$, Węziak-Białowolska, McNeely, & VanderWeele, 2019a), and its psychometric properties and measurement invariance have also been recently examined in cross-cultural settings (Węziak-Białowolska, McNeely, & VanderWeele, 2019b).

Discussion

As noted earlier, our recommendations are provisional, drawing on the current state of knowledge and the existing validated measures available. Although recommending a set of validated items, as in many cases described earlier, is not comparable to the process of validating a set of items when combined into a new measure, we hope these recommendations will help facilitate subsequent research on well-being and on its measurement. Here, we consider a number of other future developments that may further improve our ability to measure, study, and track well-being.

In the preceding discussion, for settings in which only a single well-being item will be used, we recommended the question, "Overall, how satisfied are you with life as a whole these days?" While investigators have generally referred to this item as a "cognitive" or "evaluative" measure of psychological well-being, it does place strong emphasis on satisfaction rather than on whether all facets of life are in fact good. This could be problematic. A person can be satisfied and addicted to narcotics, or satisfied and completely socially isolated. It is not clear that it is reasonable in such cases to say that human well-being is high. Although unusual examples, they demonstrate the potential that assessing life satisfaction alone which, out of context, may not represent an accurate portrait of well-being or flourishing in life as a whole. This critique may be less relevant to other forms of life evaluation that do not make explicit reference to "satisfaction," including the Cantril Ladder (Helliwell et al., 2016). However, the latter requires considerably more space than the simple life satisfaction question, but it may be preferable if there are not strict constraints on space. Other single-item measures that might more holistically consider self-report evaluations of well-being across the whole of life and that are less focused only on the satisfaction of desires might deserve further study, such as "All aspects of my life at present are good," or "All is well with my life." Whether they perform better than the widely studied life satisfaction item just mentioned requires further research and assessment. Until better studied, it may be desirable, when possible, to include at least two single-item overall evaluative measures.

While existing measures capture a number of important dimensions, other aspects of well-being are absent, as pointed out by philosophers and others (e.g., Fletcher, 2016). First, few well-being scales make any attempt to capture the value of existing knowledge or processes necessary for acquiring it. Second, most scales focus almost exclusively on individual well-being. Although some measures include items assessing the quality of an individual's social relationships, broader community well-being is often overlooked. Examining community well-being (e.g., within a family, city, or nation) may also be important for a broader understanding of the determinants and consequences of individual well-being (Allin & Hand, 2017; Phillips & Wong, 2017). It may thus be useful to supplement measures of individual well-being, and their aggregates, with measures of community well-being (Allin & Hand, 2017; Phillips & Wong, 2017; VanderWeele, 2019; VanderWeele, McNeely, & Koh, 2019).

Third, although some measures of *spiritual* well-being are available (Paloutzian & Ellison, 1982; Peterman, Fitchett, Brady, Hernandez, & Cella, 2002), the most widely used *general* well-being scales do not capture spiritual well-being. This is potentially problematic. For much of the world's population, some notion of spirituality or religion is highly important (Diener, Tay, & Myers, 2011; Pew Religious Landscape Study, 2018), and many consider it the most important aspect of well-being. Including spiritual well-being items within general well-being scales is challenging because, to a greater extent than with other aspects of well-being, the way in which this construct is understood likely varies across religious and spiritual traditions. Thus, tradition-specific measures of spiritual well-being may be an important and necessary step forward (Chapter 16, in this volume). Such measures could potentially supplement more generic and universal well-being measures.

Fourth, although many psychological well-being scales include some notion of autonomy, they are often framed negatively and principally assess whether individuals feel they can make decisions free from influence of others. While useful in many contexts, in some cultures, this formulation may be considered relatively less essential to well-being. The existing measures, moreover, often do not capture positive notions of having freedom to pursue what is important in life. Existing negatively framed autonomy scales might thus be supplemented with an item like "I am free to pursue what is most important" or, like Gallup's question, "Are you satisfied or dissatisfied with your freedom to choose what you do with your life?" Such items may also help to capture aspects of well-being that are important to some individuals but not to others. For example, artists who cannot pursue artistic expression, creation, and aesthetic experience may feel their well-being is severely compromised. However, for others, the absence of art for a time, even if they enjoy it, may not similarly substantially compromise well-being. An item such as "I am free to pursue what is most important" may help address these nuances. Such ideas arguably bear some correspondence to Sen's capabilities approach to well-being (Sen, 1999), although its empirical operationalizations have tended to focus on more objective measures (Alkire, 2002; Alkire & Santos, 2010).

Fifth, more work could be done examining important cross-cultural variations in which aspects of well-being are considered most important in different contexts and whether current measures of well-being, mostly developed in Western and high-income countries, may be missing other elements important in other cultures. Future well-being measure development and refinement might consider these potential omissions.

Conclusion

The recommendations in this chapter are not intended to be definitive but rather to (1) provide guidance for those needing to make practical decisions about well-being measurement today and (2) prompt further discussion and debate that will eventually lead to further refinement. That well-being is measured—and how it is measured—is critical. What investigators, practitioners, and policy-makers measure shapes what they discuss, what priorities they set, and what they aim for. Studies to advance our understanding of the distribution, determinants, and consequences of well-being are essential in efforts to try to improve well-being. However, such studies cannot take place without proper measurement, which in turn is shaped by the purposes and constraints (e.g., regarding number of items) of any particular study. If the well-being of individuals and nations does not get measured, then the focus will likely shift to other indicators, such as only income or physical health. We hope that the recommendations offered here might facilitate more frequent, effective, and impactful measurement of well-being.

About the Authors

Tyler J. VanderWeele is the John L. Loeb and Frances Lehman Loeb Professor of Epidemiology in the Departments of Epidemiology and Biostatistics at the Harvard T. H. Chan School of Public Health, Director of the Human Flourishing Program, and Co-Director of the Initiative on Health, Religion, and Spirituality at Harvard University. His research concerns methodology for distinguishing between association and causation in observational studies, and his empirical research spans psychiatric, perinatal, and social epidemiology; the science of happiness and flourishing; and the study of religion and health, including both religion and population health and the role of religion and spirituality in end-of-life care. He has published more than 300 papers in peer-reviewed journals, and is author of the book *Explanation in Causal Inference* (Oxford University Press, 2015).

Claudia Trudel-Fitzgerald is Research Scientist at the Lee Kum Sheung Center for Health and Happiness and the Department of Social and Behavioral Sciences at the Harvard T. H. Chan School of Public Health. She is also a licensed clinical psychologist specializing in cognitive behavioral-therapy. Her research projects target the role of positive and negative emotions in the maintenance and decline of physical health as well as longevity.

Paul V. Allin is Visiting Professor in statistics at the Department of Mathematics, Imperial College London, and coauthor of *The Wellbeing of Nations: Meaning, Motive and Measurement* (Wiley, 2014). He also chairs the UK Statistics User Forum and the Advisory Panel of the What Works Centre for Wellbeing, following a career as a professional statistician, researcher, and policy analyst in various UK government departments and agencies, latterly as the first director of the Measuring National Wellbeing Programme. His current research interests are the measurement of national well-being and progress, and the use of these measures in politics, policy, business, and everyday life.

Colin Farrelly is Professor and Queen's National Scholar in the Department of Political Studies at Queen's University, in Kingston, Ontario. He is the author of *Genetic Ethics: An Introduction* (Polity Books, 2018) and *Biologically Modified Justice* (Cambridge University Press, 2016). The themes of reason, science, progress, and optimism inform his curiosity-driven research interests and interdisciplinary focus.

Guy Fletcher is Senior Lecturer in Philosophy at the University of Edinburgh, UK. His work examines the nature of moral discourse, philosophical theories of well-being, and theories of prudential discourse. He edited the *Routledge Handbook of Philosophy of Well-Being* (Routledge, 2015) and co-edited *Having It Both Ways: Hybrid Theories in Meta-Normative Theory* (Oxford University Press, 2014). He is author of *An Introduction to the Philosophy of Well-Being* (Routledge, 2016) and has another book, *Dear Prudence: The Nature and Normativity of Prudential Discourse* (Oxford University Press, 2021).

Donald E. Frederick is an Associate—and former Postdoctoral Fellow—at the Human Flourishing Program in the Institute for Quantitative Social Science at Harvard University. He currently works on understanding the intersection of technology and flourishing as well as developing technology to promote flourishing based on social science research. His past research focused on the psychology of work and its relationship(s) to flourishing.

Jon Hall works at the United Nations Development Programme. He has spent 20 years thinking about how metrics for progress influence the direction of nations and led the Global Project on Measuring the Progress of Societies at the Organisation for Economic Co-Operation and Development for 5 years.

John F. Helliwell is a Distinguished Fellow of the Canadian Institute for Advanced Research. He is also Professor Emeritus of Economics at the University of British Columbia and a Research Associate of the National Bureau of Economic Research. He was previously a member of the National Statistics Council (2001–2015). His books include *Globalization and Well-Being* (University of British Columbia Press, 2002), *Well-Being for Public Policy* (Oxford University Press, 2009), *International Differences in Well-Being* (Oxford University Press, 2010), and the *World Happiness Report* (Sustainable Development Solutions Network). His current research is mainly on the sources and consequences of subjective well-being, with a special focus on the social determinants of well-being and the policy applications of well-being research.

Eric S. Kim is Assistant Professor in the Department of Psychology at the University of British Columbia. His program of research aims to identify, understand, and intervene in the individual and environmental dimensions of psychological well-being that enhance healthy lifestyle behaviors and reduce the risk of age-related chronic conditions. He enjoys spending time at the intersection of several disciplines and in his work integrates perspectives from psychology, biostatistics, social epidemiology, cardiology, and translational science.

William A. Lauinger is Associate Professor of Philosophy and Coordinator of the Ethics Program at Chestnut Hill College in Philadelphia, Pennsylvania. He is the author of *Well-Being and Theism: Linking Ethics to God* (Continuum, 2012) and various articles in ethics and the philosophy of religion. Most of his research focuses on human well-being: on what it is, how to attain it, and how it connects to other important phenomena, such as morality and religion.

Matthew T. Lee is Director of Empirical Research at the Human Flourishing Program in the Institute for Quantitative Social Science at Harvard University and coauthor of *The Heart of Religion* (Oxford University Press, 2013). He is also a Distinguished Visiting Scholar of Health, Flourishing, and Positive Psychology at Stony Brook University's Center for Medical Humanities, Compassionate Care, and Bioethics, and he previously served as Chair of the American Sociological Association's Section on Altruism, Morality, and Social Solidarity. His research explores pathways to human flourishing, benevolent service to others, and the integration of social science and the humanities.

Sonja Lyubomirsky is Distinguished Professor and Vice Chair in the Department of Psychology at the University of California, Riverside, where she has been recognized with the Faculty of the Year (twice) and Faculty Mentor of the Year Awards. Dr. Lyubomirsky's research focuses on how to increase happiness and positive emotions, with a focus on expressing gratitude, practicing kindness, and boosting connection as interventions. She is the author of *The How of Happiness* (Penguin, 2007) and *The Myths of Happiness* (Penguin, 2013), translated in 36 countries. She has received many honors, including the Diener Award for Outstanding Midcareer Contributions in Personality Psychology, the Christopher J. Peterson Gold Medal, the Distinguished Research Lecturer Award, and a Positive Psychology Prize.

Seth Margolis is a fifth-year graduate student in the Department of Psychology at the University of California, Riverside. He works with Dr. Sonja Lyubomirsky in her Positive Activities and Well-Being Laboratory. His research focuses on well-being measurement, quantitative methodology, and personality interventions that boost well-being.

Eileen McNeely is the founder and Director of SHINE, the initiative for the sustainability of health and human capital in the workplace, at the Harvard T. H. Chan School of Public Health. She conducts research and teaches in the Environmental Occupational Medicine and Epidemiology Program. She has worked as a consultant, researcher, clinician, and educator in the field for more than 20 years.

Neil G. Messer is Professor of Theology at the University of Winchester, UK, and the author of several books including *Theological Neuroethics: Christian Ethics Meets the Science of the Human Brain* (Bloomsbury, 2017) and *Science in Theology: Encounters Between Science and the Christian Tradition* (Bloomsbury, 2020). He has been a Guest Professor in the Center for Theology, Science, and Human Flourishing at the University of Notre Dame, and is Co-convener of the joint Theology and Neuroethics Interest Group of the Society of Christian Ethics, Society of Jewish Ethics, and Society for the Study of Muslim Ethics. His research is concerned with the intersections of Christian theology, ethics, healthcare, and the biosciences.

Louis Tay is Associate Professor of Industrial-Organizational Psychology at Purdue University. His research interests are in well-being, methodology, and measurement. He is the co-editor of the books *Handbook of Well-Being* (DEF Publishers, 2018) and *Big Data in Psychological Research* (APA Books, 2020). He serves as an associate editor at *Organizational Research Methods*.

K. "Vish" Viswanath is Lee Kum Kee Professor of Health Communication in the Department of Social and Behavioral Sciences at the Harvard T. H. Chan School of Public Health and in the McGraw-Patterson Center for Population Sciences at the Dana-Farber Cancer Institute. He is the co-editor of four books and monographs: *Mass Media, Social Control and Social Change* (Iowa State University Press, 1999), *Health Behavior and Health Education: Theory, Research & Practice, 5th Ed.* (Jossey Bass, 2015), *The Role of Media in Promoting and Reducing Tobacco Use* (National Cancer Institute, 2008), and *A Socioecological Approach to Addressing Tobacco-Related Health Disparities* (National

Cancer Institute, 2017) and has written more than 250 papers and book chapters. His work, drawing from literature in communication science, social epidemiology, and social and health behavior sciences, focuses on translational communication science to influence public health policy and practice with a particular focus on communication inequalities and health disparities.

Dorota Węziak-Białowolska is Research Scientist at the Sustainability and Health Initiative for NetPositive Enterprise at Harvard T. H. Chan School of Public Health. She previously worked for the European Commission Joint Research Centre where she coordinated projects on measuring poverty, well-being, and quality of life in the regional setting. Her research interests are in methodology, including psychometrics, composite indicators, impact assessment, and evaluation; and her recent projects focus on applied well-being and health in the workplace setting.

Laura D. Kubzansky is Lee Kum Kee Professor of Social and Behavioral Sciences and co-Director of the Lee Kum Sheung Center for Health and Happiness at the Harvard T.H. Chan School of Public Health. Dr. Kubzansky has published extensively on the role of psychological and social factors in health. Ongoing research includes studying biobehavioral mechanisms linking emotions, social relationships, and health; defining, measuring, and modifying aspects of well-being; and workplace conditions in relation to well-being. She has served on the leadership team for multiple training programs for junior scholars and is principal investigator or co-investigator on numerous grants.

Author Note

The research was supported by the John Templeton Foundation (Grant 61075) to Dr. Tyler J. VanderWeele and by funding from the Lee Kum Sheung Center for Health and Happiness at the Harvard T. H. Chan School of Public Health and the Human Flourishing Program at Harvard University. This set of recommendations came about as a result of an interdisciplinary workshop on the measurement of well-being of which the authors were a part. The critical intellectual content of the chapter was shaped by all authors and would not have been possible without their participation. The chapter represents the collective thought of the author list. The chapter was drafted by Tyler J. VanderWeele, Claudia Trudel-Fitzgerald, and Laura D. Kubzansky. All authors provided critical review, feedback, additions, further references, and guidance. The views expressed in this chapter represent the perspectives of the authors and do not reflect the opinions or endorsement of any organization. We have no known conflict of interest to disclose. Correspondence concerning this chapter should be directed to Tyler J. VanderWeele, Harvard T. H. Chan School of Public Health, Departments of Epidemiology and Biostatistics, 677 Huntington Avenue, Boston, MA 02115 (tvanderw@hsph.harvard.edu). The present chapter is a slightly edited reprint of: VanderWeele, Trudel-Fitzgerald, Allin, et al. (2020). Current recommendations on the selection of measures for well-being. *Preventive Medicine, 133*.https://doi.org/10.1016/j.ypmed.2020.106004

References

Alkire, S. (2002). *Valuing freedoms: Sen's capability approach and poverty reduction.* Oxford: Oxford University Press.

Alkire, S., & Santos, M. E. (2010). *Acute multidimensional poverty: A new index for developing countries.* United Nations Development Programme Human Development Report Office Background Paper. New York: UN Development Programme.

Allin, P., & Hand, D. J. (2017). New statistics for old?—Measuring the wellbeing of the UK. *Journal of the Royal Statistical Society, Series A, 180,* 1–22.

Baumeister, R. F, Vohs, K. D., Aaker, J. L., & Garbinsky, E. N. (2013). Some key differences between a happy life and a meaningful life. *Journal of Positive Psychology, 8*(6), 505–516.

Benson, T., Sladen, J., Liles, A., & Potts, H. W. W. (2019). Personal Wellbeing Score (PWS)—a short version of ONS4: Development and validation in social prescribing. *BMJ Open Quality, 8,* e000394. doi:10.1136/bmjoq-2018-000394

Cheung, F., & Lucas, R. E. (2014). Assessing the validity of single-item life satisfaction measures: Results from three large samples. *Quality of Life Research, 23*(10), 2809–2818.

Diener, E., Tay, L., Myers, D. G. (2011). The religion paradox: If religion makes people happy, why are so many dropping out? *Journal of Personality and Social Psychology 101,* 1278–1290.

Diener, E., Wirtz, D., Tov, W., Kim-Prieto, C., Choi, D., Oishi, S., & Biswas-Diener, R. (2009). New measures of well-being: Flourishing and positive and negative feelings. *Social Indicators Research, 39,* 247–266.

Diener, E., Emmons, R. A., Larsen, R. J., & Griffin, S. (1985). The satisfaction with life scale. *Journal of Personality Assessment, 49,* 71–75.

Fletcher, G. (2016). *The Routledge handbook of philosophy of well-being.* Abingdon, UK: Routledge.

Fordyce, M. W. (1988). A review of research on the happiness measures: A sixty second index of happiness and mental health. *Social Indicators Research, 20,* 355–381.

Goodman, F. R., Disabato, D. J., Kashdan, T. B., & Kauffman, S. B. (2018). Measuring well-being: A comparison of subjective well-being and PERMA. *Journal of Positive Psychology, 13*(4), 321–32.

Hall, J., Giovannini, E., Morrone, A., Ranuzzi, G. (2010). A framework to measure the progress of societies. *Working Paper 34, STD/DOC(2010)5.* Paris: Statistics Directorate, Organisation for Economic Co-operation and Development. http://kniknowledgebase.org/wp-content/uploads/2015/08/A_Framework_to_Measure_   the_Progress_of_Societies.pdf

Helliwell, J., Layard, R., & Sachs, J. (2016). *World happiness report 2016, Update (Vol. I).* New York: Sustainable Development Solutions Network.

Hone, L. C., Jarden, A., Schofield, G. M., & Duncan, S. (2014). Measuring flourishing: The impact of operational definitions on the prevalence of high levels of wellbeing. *International Journal of Wellbeing, 4*(1), 62–90.

Hudson, N. W., Lucas, R. E., & Donnellan, M. B. (2017). Day-to-day affect is surprisingly stable: A two-year longitudinal study of well-being. *Social Psychological and Personality Science, 8*(1), 45–54.

Huppert, F. A., & So, T. T. (2013). Flourishing across Europe: Application of a new conceptual framework for defining well-being. *Social Indicators Research, 110*(3), 837–61.

Kahneman, D., Diener, E., & Schwarz, N. (2003). *Well-being: The foundations of hedonic psychology.* New York: Russell Sage Foundation.

Keyes, C. L. (2002). The mental health continuum: From languishing to flourishing in life. *Journal of Health and Social Behavior, 43*(2), 207–222.

Lyubomirsky, S., & Lepper, H. (1999). A measure of subjective happiness: Preliminary reliability and construct validation. *Social Indicators Research, 46*, 137–155.

Martela, F., & Steger, M. F. (2016). The three meanings of meaning in life: Distinguishing coherence, purpose, and significance. *Journal of Positive Psychology, 11*(5), 531–545.

Messer, N. (2013). *Flourishing: Health, disease and bioethics in theological perspective.* Grand Rapids, MI: Eerdmans Publishing.

Myers, D. G., & Diener, E. (2018). The scientific pursuit of happiness. *Perspectives on Psychological Science, 13*(2), 218–225.

National Research Council. (2013). *Subjective well-being.* Washington, DC: National Academies Press.

Ngamaba, K. H. (2018). Income inequality and subjective well-being: A systematic review and meta-analysis. *Quality of Life Research, 27*(3), 577–596.

OECD. (2013). *Guidelines on measuring subjective well-being.* Paris: OECD.

OECD. (2019). *How's life?* Paris: OECD.

Paloutzian, R. F., & Ellison, C. W. (1982). Loneliness, spiritual well-being, and the quality of life. In L. A. Peplau & D. Perlman (Eds.), *Loneliness: A sourcebook of current theory, research and therapy* (pp. 224–237). New York: John Wiley & Sons.

Patel, V., Saxena, S., Lund, C., Thornicroft, G., Baingana, F., Bolton, P., . . . Herrman, H. (2018). The Lancet Commission on global mental health and sustainable development. *Lancet, 392*(10157), 1553–1598.

Peterman, A. H., Fitchett, G., Brady, M. J., Hernandez, L., & Cella, D. (2002). Measuring spiritual well-being in people with cancer: The Functional Assessment of Chronic Illness Therapy–Spiritual Well-Being Scale (FACIT-Sp). *Annals of Behavioral Medicine, 24*, 49–58.

Pew Religious Landscape Study. (2018). http://www.pewforum.org/religious-landscape-study/, Accessed date: 24 July 2020.

Phillips, R., & Wong, C. (2017). *Handbook of community well-being research.* Dordrecht: Springer.

Plough, A. L. (2015). Building a culture of health: A critical role for public health services and systems research. *American Journal of Public Health, 105*(Suppl 2), S150–2.

Resnick, B., & Nahm, E. S. (2001). Reliability and validity testing of the revised 12-item Short-Form Health Survey in older adults. *Journal of Nursing Measurement, 9*(2), 151–161.

Ryff, C. D. (1989). Happiness is everything, or is it? Explorations on the meaning of psychological well-being. *Journal of Personality and Social Psychology, 57*, 1069–1081.

Scheier, M. F., Carver, C. S., & Bridges, M. W. (1994). Distinguishing optimism from neuroticism (and trait anxiety, self-mastery, and self-esteem): A reevaluation of the Life Orientation Test. *Journal of Personality and Social Psychology, 67*(6), 1063–1078.

Seligman, M. E. P. (2011). *Flourish: A visionary new understanding of happiness and well-being.* New York: Free Press.

Sen, A. (1999). *Development as freedom.* New York: Knopf.

Steger, M. F., Frazier, P., Oishi, S., & Kaler, M. (2006). The meaning in life questionnaire: Assessing the presence of and search for meaning in life. *Journal of Counseling Psychology, 53*(1), 80–93.

Stiglitz, J. E., Sen, A., & Fitoussi, J. P. (2010). *Mismeasuring our lives.* New York: New Press.

Stiglitz, J., Sen, A., & Fitoussi. (2016). *Report by the Commission on the Measurement of Economic Performance and Social Progress*. Paris: Commission on the Measurement of Economic Performance and Social Progress.

Su, R., Tay, L., & Diener, E. (2014). The development and validation of the Comprehensive Inventory of Thriving (CIT) and the Brief Inventory of Thriving (BIT). *Applied Psychology: Health and Well-Being, 6*, 251–279.

Tay, L., Chan, D., & Diener, E. (2014). The metrics of societal happiness. *Social Indicators Research, 117*, 577–600.

Trudel-Fitzgerald, C., Millstein, R. A., von Hippel, C., Howe, C. J., Tomasso, L. P., Wagner, G. R., & VanderWeele, T. J. (2019). Psychological well-being as part of the public health debate? Insight into dimensions, interventions, and policy. *BMC Public Health, 19*(1), 1–11.

VanderWeele, T. J. (2017). On the promotion of human flourishing. *Proceedings of the National Academy of Sciences of the United States of America, 31*, 8148–8156.

VanderWeele, T. J. (2019). Measures of community well-being: A template. *International Journal of Community Well-Being, 2*, 253–275, https://doi.org/10.1007/s42413-019-00036-8

VanderWeele, T. J., McNeely, E., & Koh, H. K. (2019). Reimagining health—flourishing. *Journal of the American Medical Association, 321*(17), 1667–1668.

Ware, J. E, Kosinski, M., & Keller, S. D. (1996). 12-Item Short-Form Health Survey: Construction of scales and preliminary tests of reliability and validity. *Medical Care, 34*, 220–233.

Warwick Medical School. (2018). Warwick-Edinburgh Mental Wellbeing Scale (2018 version). https://warwick.ac.uk/fac/sci/med/research/platform/wemwbs

Węziak-Białowolska, D., McNeely, E., & VanderWeele, T. J. (2019a). Flourish index and secure flourish index—validation in workplace settings. *Cogent Psychology, 6*, 1598926.

Węziak-Białowolska, D., McNeely, E., & VanderWeele, T. J. (2019b). Human flourishing in cross cultural settings: Evidence from the US, China, Sri Lanka, Cambodia and Mexico. *Frontiers in Psychology, 10*, 1269, https://doi.org/10.3389/fpsyg.2019.01269.

Wiese, C. W, Tay, L., Su, R., & Diener, E. (2018). Measuring thriving across nations: Examining the measurement equivalence of the Comprehensive Inventory of Thriving (CIT) and the Brief Inventory of Thriving (BIT). *Applied Psychology: Health and Well-Being, 10*(1), 127–148.

Wood, A. M., & Joseph, S. (2010). The absence of positive psychological (eudemonic) well-being as a risk factor for depression: A ten year cohort study. *Journal of Affective Disorders, 122*(3), 213–217.

18

Advancing the Science of Well-Being

A Dissenting View on Measurement Recommendations

Carol D. Ryff, Jennifer Morozink Boylan, and Julie A. Kirsch

Abstract

We question use of the term "well-being" to encompass notably distinct phenomena (objective indicators of socioeconomic status and health, subjective indicators of psychological experience) and dispute characterization of the field of well-being as relatively new. We also call for greater interplay between government surveys and multi-use cohort studies, both of which increasingly focus on well-being. The Midlife in the United States (MIDUS) study is presented as an example of how to negotiate distinct disciplinary priorities in broad-based studies of well-being and health, including those that take context seriously. We conclude with explanations for why we do not endorse any of the measurement recommendations (single-item measures, 4-6 item measures, multi-item assessments) put forth in the preceding chapter, arguing that the ultra-short assessments ignore extensive prior science documenting the complex, multi-faceted nature of well-being, while the proposed longer assessment (Comprehensive Inventory of Thriving, CTI) suffers from multiple problems including a questionable conceptual foundation, inadequate evidence of validity and reliability, and highly redundant items.

We appreciate the opportunity to respond to the "Current Recommendations on the Selection of Measures for Well-Being" (Chapter 17) endorsed by many contributors to this volume. It is worthwhile to engage in scholarly debate and discussion about how to best advance growing interest in assessing human well-being. We have multiple concerns with the current recommendations and have organized our thoughts around four overarching issues. Building

Carol D. Ryff, Jennifer Morozink Boylan, and Julie A. Kirsch, *Advancing the Science of Well-Being* In: *Measuring Well-Being*. Edited by: Matthew T. Lee, Laura D. Kubzansky, and Tyler J. VanderWeele, Oxford University Press (2021).
© Oxford University Press. DOI: 10.1093/oso/9780197512531.003.0019

from these, a final section distils our specific responses to each of the targeted recommendations, none of which we endorse. We offer these objections not to be contentious or unappreciative of the work of others, but rather to provide honest assessments of why they seem seriously problematic. Ultimately, the arbiters of such matters will not be the authors of the current volume, including ourselves, but rather members of the scientific community and government officials who must make difficult decisions in how to assess well-being. We hope this exchange will inform their decisions.

The Downside of Calling Everything Well-Being

Nomenclature matters. It defines what we are interested in, specifies what it should be named, and, importantly for science, encompasses the operational procedures involved in obtaining its measurement. In our view, using "well-being" as an umbrella term that applies to notably distinct phenomena (e.g., Messer, 2013; VanderWeele, 2017) is problematic. That is, we question whether science is usefully advanced by calling a host of distinct phenomena, such as objective indicators of socioeconomic status (educational attainment, income, standard of living), diverse indicators of health (health conditions, functional capacities, life expectancy), and multiple subjective indicators (happiness, life satisfaction, purpose, self-realization) *all* "well-being." Such inclusiveness, in our view, muddles important scientific agendas regarding what it means to be well, for whom opportunities of wellness are or are not available, and what health consequences well-being may have.

We propose that a better approach distinguishes among these different factors to focus on critical questions, such as what key sociodemographic, experiential, and contextual factors influence *people's inner sense of how their lives are going* (i.e., *subjective well-being*). Thus, we favor calling objective measures what they are: indicators of position in the surrounding social structure (e.g., education, economic status), indicators of chronic and acute stress exposures (e.g., caregiving responsibilities, job change), and indicators of physical health (e.g., chronic conditions, health symptoms, functional capacities, biomarkers). So doing draws attention to important measurement issues in all of these domains but, more importantly, provides clear conceptual and empirical foundations for scientific investigation of *how, and for whom, these objective factors shape inner experiences of subjective well-being.*

We also challenge the characterization of the field of well-being as something relatively new that has emerged in recent decades. In fact, subjective well-being as a domain of scientific inquiry has been present in social scientific studies, including population-based endeavors, since the middle of the past century (Andrews, 1974; Bradburn & Noll, 1969; Gurin, Veroff, & Feld, 1960). Beyond that, scholarly interest in well-being has been part of the human journey since the ancient Greeks. Our Chapter 4 in this volume revisits parts of that distant literature to show how it has shaped numerous conceptual and empirical approaches to well-being in our era. Without attending to this past, science fails to be cumulative. This matters not only for conceptual reasons regarding how well-being should be formulated but, more importantly, for what decades of empirical science has revealed regarding the antecedents and consequents of diverse aspects of well-being. Too many of the key sources cited in the recommendations chapter, most of which are relatively recent, neglect this larger literature.

Ships Passing in the Night: Government Surveys and Multiuse Cohort Studies

A strength behind the proposed recommendations is that they jointly consider assessments of well-being in government surveys *and* in multiuse cohort studies. These two worlds, both typically supported by taxpayer resources, seem to rarely intersect. A compelling case can be made, however, that these large realms—one oriented toward informing government policies and practices and the other toward generating new findings on the science of health—need to more frequently engage one another. In our view, scientific evidence about well-being and health from multiuse cohort studies can and should inform what aspects of well-being are important to include in big government surveys such as the UK National Wellbeing Programme or the Organization for Economic Cooperation and Development (OECD).

We highlight evidence from the Midlife in the United States (MIDUS) Survey, the Health and Retirement Study (HRS), and the English Longitudinal Study of Ageing (ELSA) to underscore these points. A proliferation of recent findings have documented the protective influence of eudaimonic aspects of well-being, particularly purpose in life, in reducing risk for major depression (Keyes, 2002; Rottenberg, Devendorf, Panaite, Disabato, & Kashdan, 2019), multiple disease outcomes (Boyle, Buchman, & Bennett, 2010; Kim,

Sun, Park, Kubzansky, & Peterson, 2013; Kim, Sun, Park, & Peterson, 2013), and extending length of life (Hill & Turiano, 2014; Steptoe, Deaton, & Stone, 2015). Intervening biological and brain-based mechanisms have also been explicated (Hafez et al., 2018; Heller et al., 2013; Morozink, Friedman, Coe, & Ryff, 2010; Schaefer et al., 2013; Zilioli, Slatcher, Ong, & Gruenewald, 2015).

Such evidence from cohort studies suggests that those making choices about what to include in government surveys would be wise to include quality assessments of eudaimonic well-being. Unfortunately, the proposed items put forth in the recommendations bear little likeness to the actual assessment of diverse aspects of well-being in cohort studies that have generated scientific findings linking these aspects of well-being to health. What is thus perpetuated is a problematic disconnect between the emerging scientific findings and policy-oriented government surveys.

Relatedly, and in recognition that survey costs and efficiencies are paramount in adjudicating what to assess, it is important to consider whether good societies are well served by focusing on extremely limited questions, mostly about happiness and life satisfaction, at the expense of other critical aspects of well-being, such as citizens' perceptions of whether they are able to pursue meaningful and purposeful lives, whether they see themselves as able to make the most of their personal talents and capacities, or whether they have positive self-regard. Government surveys and cohort studies that neglect this wider scope of what well-being is, as distilled from decades of science and distant philosophy, are ultimately short-sighted. They are pursuits that effectively ensure that what is learned or gets translated to public practice will fall short of the subject matter they seek to advance.

In reflecting about these issues, we also note growing evidence that eudaimonic well-being is modifiable. Diverse interventions to improve well-being now demonstrate reduced rates of depression and anxiety as well as improved subjective health (Cantarella, Borella, Marigo, & De Beni, 2017; Fava, 2016; Friedman et al., 2019; Ruini, 2017). These psychotherapeutic and psychosocial practices have been carried out with healthy populations as well as among patients with mental illness (Weiss, Westerhof, & Bohlmeijer, 2016). Such interventions build on the multifaceted nature of eudaimonia, which likely contributes to why they are efficacious: that is, these initiatives address, at the individual level, unique strengths and weaknesses across multiple aspects of well-being.

Taken together, we view the highly streamlined measurement recommendations as conveying a comparative devaluing of the richness of subjective well-being relevant to the space allotted in government and co-hort surveys to other topics, such as socioeconomic status (education, in-come, wealth, financial stress, insurance), health behaviors and practices (diet, alcohol use, exercise, sleep), and healthcare utilization and diverse health outcomes (chronic conditions, symptoms, functional capacities, biomarkers). The implicit message is that how people think and feel about their well-being is simple, not complicated, and can be easily captured with a handful of items. This stance guarantees impoverished knowledge and thereby limits scientific and translational impact. Put succinctly, the pro-posed recommendations reveal a capitulation to the view that well-being is inherently less important, less multifaceted, and less consequential than ex-tant science shows it to be.

Negotiating Distinct and Often Competing Disciplinary Priorities

Sitting in the background of the proposed measurement recommendations and our responses to them are differing disciplinary priorities. In our view, these point to contrasting strengths and weaknesses across scientific fields that need to be recognized and negotiated. Population sciences (de-mography, epidemiology, sociology) have the great strength of capturing sociodemographic diversity and sampling representativeness. Historically, however, these disciplines have fallen short when it comes to the comprehen-sive assessment of complex psychological and social constructs. Alternatively, small-sample disciplines, exemplified by numerous subfields of psychology (cognition, emotion, motivation, personality, well-being) have the strength of attending carefully to the conceptualization and operationalization of their key constructs, including a commitment to rigorous psychometric evaluations. However, they have traditionally shown little, if any, concern for sociodemographic diversity among those they study and even less commit-ment to sampling representativeness.

These contrasting strengths and weaknesses are insufficiently recog-nized in the proposed recommendations. Indeed, the "voice" behind the recommendations is population science and practice, exemplified by cohort studies and government surveys, but the subject matter under consideration comes from psychological science and human development. We see it as in-formative to note the history of the MIDUS Survey, which was an explicit endeavor seeking to negotiate constructively these different disciplinary priorities (see Ryff & Krueger, 2018). Conceived by a multidisciplinary team of scientists representing most of the aforementioned fields (e.g., epidemiology, demography, economics, multiple subfields of psychology, sociology, human development), there was considerable tension at the outset regarding how limited resources should be best allocated. Two equally important objectives were center stage: (1) achieving high-quality samples defined in terms of population coverage and representativeness and (2) achieving high-quality assessment of key constructs, including psychosocial factors (personality, emotion, well-being, social relationships, diverse stress exposures) as well as numerous aspects of health. A key achievement of the MIDUS Survey was to demonstrate that the usual commitment to ultra-short-form assessments of these domains in a large cohort study was neither necessary nor wise.

Focusing only on assessments of well-being, MIDUS included comprehensive measures that covered multiple indicators of hedonic well-being (e.g., overall life satisfaction, domain-specific life satisfaction, positive and negative affect measured with multiple established scales) and eudaimonic well-being (autonomy, environmental mastery, personal growth, positive relations with others, purpose in life, self-acceptance), along with scales of optimism, sense of control, and a host of social relational measures (social support given and received, quality of ties to spouse/partner, children, friends). Importantly, response rates for these lengthy assessments and many other measures across multiple waves of data collection, have been high (81–89%). Building on the MIDUS experience, we note that other large national studies, such as the Health and Retirement Study, have adopted many MIDUS measures. These developments challenge the view that big population studies or government surveys are inherently unsuited for using the well-validated, multi-item scales needed to adequately operationalize core psychosocial constructs.

What has been learned over the past three decades is that this commitment to quality measurement of key constructs has been greatly endorsed by the scientific community: MIDUS has more than 20,000 unique data users who have contributed more than 1,400 publications, many appearing in top-tier journals in diverse fields. Pertinent to the present focus, many of these publications concern assessments of psychological well-being, affect, and emotion—the findings from which have advanced knowledge of numerous sociodemographic factors that predict these outcomes (age, gender, socioeconomic status, race) and many more that link such outcomes to diverse aspects of health, including biological risk factors and brain-based assessments. The key point here is to use the MIDUS study as a critical illustration that the push toward ultra-short-form assessments is not required in top-tier population studies. Beyond that, and of far greater importance, is that the scientific advances that follow from such a commitment to high-quality assessment of complex psychosocial constructs are deep and wide.

Taking Context Seriously

Emphasized in the abstract of the proposed recommendations was the need to carefully consider "what measures might be preferred in *which contexts.*" We agree that context should be taken seriously but observe that so doing is at odds with recommendations for highly streamlined assessments of well-being. In our view, the evidence documenting the highly contextualized nature of well-being is too extensive to support advocacy for extremely limited measures. For example, a prior review of more than 200 studies of well-being (Ryff, 2014) revealed richly distinct patterns of findings depending on whether the context was examining the challenges of aging, experiences in family life (e.g., death of child, caregiving, non-normative parenting), work contexts (e.g., paid/unpaid work; career pursuits; work–family conflict; volunteering), or specific health conditions (e.g., fibromyalgia, cancer survivors, frailty).

More recently, socioeconomic equality has emerged as one of the most pressing issues of our time (Kirsch, Love, Radler, & Ryff, 2019), with extensive findings showing the lingering effects of the Great Recession (Burgard & Kalousova, 2015), particularly among those who were already disadvantaged. Such work includes evidence of compromised well-being and increased psychological distress, assessed comprehensively (Goldman, Glei, & Weinstein, 2018). Moreover, certain aspects of well-being previously found to be protective in the face of inequality (Morozink et al., 2010) have been shown to be disabled among those exposed to high Recession hardships (Kirsch & Ryff, 2016).

Racial disparities in well-being also call for wide-ranging, comprehensive assessments, particularly in light of prior findings documenting that blacks scored higher than whites on multiple aspects of flourishing (Keyes, 2009). These outcomes are evident despite sobering racial disparities in morbidity and mortality (Williams, 2012). Such paradoxes require thoughtful and nuanced approaches that build from comprehensive and diverse measures of well-being.

Finally, at the level of broad comparisons across cultural contexts, the need for wide-ranging assessments of well-being is clearly evident. Cultural theories of individualism versus collectivism lead to distinct predictions, some of which have been examined in findings based on probability samples from Japan and the United States. Findings have underscored cultural differences in how well-being is linked with biological health: overall patterns underscore the reduced importance of hedonic well-being for Japanese compared to US adults (Kitayama & Park, 2017; Miyamoto et al., 2013; Yoo, Miyamoto, Rigotti, & Ryff, 2017). Happiness, inscribed in the US Declaration of Independence, in fact, emerges as more significant for the health (measured objectively) of adults in this country, and concomitantly, negative affect is not found to be linked with poor health in Japan. Without careful attention to guiding theoretical frameworks and quality assessment of multiple aspects of well-being, these differences could not have become known.

In short, we strongly endorse the need to study well-being in diverse life contexts defined by sociodemographic and cultural factors as well as by work and family life. Critically needed in such inquiries are high quality, comprehensive assessments of well-being because extant research has made clear that distinctions among varieties of well-being matter uniquely depending on the context. These diverse patterns of outcomes offer their own version of sensitivity analyses by clarifying which aspects of well-being are, and are not, tied to distinct life contexts and challenges.

How Science Best Proceeds

Drawing on preceding points, we close with targeted responses to the specific measurement recommendations put forth by VanderWeele et al. in Chapter 17. In brief, we do not endorse any of them.

The most extreme recommendation pertains to what should be used for a single-item assessment of well-being. Here they propose using a single question about life satisfaction. They also recommend including an additional item on worthwhile activities when two-item measures are used. These suggestions fail to recognize major advances in the scientific study of well-being over the past 30 years: the central message of such work is that well-being is complex and multidimensional in structure. Advocating for a single item is the equivalent of recommending a single item to assess socio-economic status, depression, anxiety, or intelligence, which no one would do. Through extensive scientific research, each of those domains is now recognized to be complex and multifaceted. Measures for them must therefore be commensurate with what they are known to encompass. The same perspective now applies to the domain of psychological well-being.

The next-level recommendation is that four questions from the UK National Survey, conducted annually since 2011, are proposed for obtaining brief assessment of psychological well-being via government surveys. Despite their repeated usage and contributions to useful knowledge, these questions are unacceptable standard bearers or exemplars for how to assess well-being in other endeavors. That is to say, we are not advocating that such items be abolished, but rather than we oppose their adoption in future studies. Why?

The answer has to do with item content. Two of the four items cover hedonic well-being: "Overall, how satisfied are you with life as a whole these days?" and "Overall, how happy did you feel yesterday?" A third item covers eudaimonic well-being: "Overall, to what extent do you feel that the things you do in your life are worthwhile?" The fourth item is the following: "Overall, how anxious did you feel yesterday?" That two items pertain to how one felt *yesterday* is notably problematic, given growing evidence documenting within-person variability in affect across days (Brose, Schmiedek, Gerstorf, & Voelkle, 2019). The most flawed item pertains to anxiety. Negative affect has been extensively measured in studies of well-being (see later comments on the Comprehensive Inventory of Thriving), but none of this prior work has included assessment of anxiety. Like depression, anxiety is known to be psychologically complex and requires multiple items to be credibly assessed.

The next recommendation is for six items that should be used in multicohort studies that have space constraints. The proposed items are described as covering evaluative, eudaimonic, hedonic well-being, and other domains. Justification is not provided for why optimism is privileged with two of the six items, whereas all other domains are represented with a single item. For all items, no sound conceptual or empirical rationales are offered as to why they represent the putative domains of interest. Most concerning is that all of the recommendations for short-form assessments constitute a capitulation to the view that well-being is simple and can be credibly assessed with a handful of items. Extensive science assembled over the past 30 years challenges this view and, along the way, points to many better measurement alternatives.

Our primary objection pertains to what is put forth for a longer multi-item comprehensive assessment of subjective flourishing, namely, the Comprehensive Inventory of Thriving (CIT; Su, Tay, & Diener, 2014). For multiple theoretical and empirical reasons, we do not believe the CIT warrants this endorsement. First, although the measure claims to be theory-driven, no theory supports the opening announcement that psychological well-being consists of seven core dimensions, none of which is defined. The core dimensions are arrayed in a table that cross-classifies them with the key instruments from which they were derived. Some are misclassified. For example, Judge's self-esteem scale is listed as a dimension of mastery, which it is not; Ryff's self-acceptance scale is listed as a dimension of subjective well-being, which it is not; Ryff's personal growth scale, key in operationalizing Aristotle's eudaimonia, is missing.

Second, without explanation, some of the proposed seven dimensions are then elaborated with underlying facets. For example, the relationship dimension is broadened to include six facets (support, community, trust, respect, loneliness, belonging), mastery is broadened to include five facets (skills, learning, accomplishment, self-efficacy, self-worth), and subjective well-being is broadened to include three facets (life satisfaction, positive feeling, negative feeling). The remaining dimensions (engagement, autonomy, meaning, optimism) have only one facet.

The resulting 18 facets, around which subsequent measurement work proceeds, thus come with no conceptual formulation. Instead, a series of seemingly arbitrary decisions determine what falls under the broad umbrella of thriving (e.g., if loneliness is part of the relationship domain, why is boredom not included in the engagement domain?). Given the lack of a sound conceptual foundation, a major concern regarding the CIT is that many of its proposed dimensions are already operationalized with widely used short scales (e.g., LOT for optimism, UCLA loneliness scale, Ryff scales for multiple dimensions of eudaimonic well-being).

Methodological concerns abound with the validity and reliability of the CIT. Regarding the samples utilized, none of the five samples was a probability sample, nor was any information provided on the recruitment approach or response rates. The first sample, which was crucial in testing and selecting three items for each of the 18 facets of well-being, was based exclusively on college undergraduates despite extensive evidence that well-being varies systematically by age and socioeconomic status (as reviewed in our Chapter 4). The second sample consisted of adults over the age of 60, and the third sample consisted of individuals with annual incomes of less than $20,000. No rationale was provided for either recruitment strategy. The remaining two samples included "adults representing different age groups, diverse occupations, and a wide range of income and education levels" (p. 257). No detailed information on participant recruitment than what was just quoted was provided. Collectively, these samples do not constitute a sound basis from which to assess merits of the instrument for population-based samples.

Items included in the CIT are highly redundant. Positive feelings, a facet of subjective well-being, are assessed with these items: "I feel positive most of the time," "I feel happy most of the time," "I feel good most of the time." This content is at odds with emotions included in prominent, widely used measures of positive affect, such as the Positive and Negative Affect Schedule (PANAS; e.g., cheerful, in good spirits, happy, peaceful, satisfied, full of life; Watson, Clark, & Tellegen, 1988). Similarly, negative feelings, another facet of subjective well-being, are assessed with these items: "I feel negative most of the time," "I experience unhappy feelings most of the time," "I feel bad most of the time." Not only are these items mirror opposites of the positive items, they neglect the negative emotions included in well-used measures (e.g., sad, nervous, restless, hopeless, worthless, afraid, irritable, ashamed, upset). Redundancy in item content translates to problems in α coefficients, which are extremely high: all are greater than 0.71, with the majority (70%) ranging from 0.85 to 0.96. These coefficients document that the items within the 18 facets are fundamentally equivalent.

Critically missing are item-to-scale correlations, the starting point for discerning the putative distinctness of the 18 facets/7dimensions of thriving. Indices of model fit are provided, but factor loadings from the multigroup confirmatory factor analyses are only available on the website of the first author. These factor loadings demonstrate considerable variability across samples (range from 0.43–1.0), undermining the conclusion that the validation analysis replicated in unique samples.

Intercorrelations among the 18 facets are likewise very high (>0.60, with some >0.80), suggesting notable blurring among the 18 subscales. Tests of convergent validity with established measures are compromised by the fact that the items used to generate the CIT were taken from these instruments (Flourishing Scale [FS], Satisfaction with Life Scale [SWLS], Self-Mastery Scale [SMS], Life Orientation Test-Revised [LOT-R], Core Self-Evaluations Scale [CSES]) used to validate the new inventory. The obtained correlations are thus inflated by overlapping content. Tests of predictive validity, using assessed self-reported health measured at the same time, are likewise of limited value, given known positivity/negativity biases that come from using the same source to measure both well-being and health (i.e., those who rate their well-being favorably tend to rate their health favorably [or the alternative]). Finally, evidence of incremental validity over prior measures is unsurprising given that the prior measures assessed only single or limited dimensions of thriving.

For the all of preceding reasons, we do not endorse the use of the CIT (or the shorter-form BIT) in future scientific research or government studies. Efforts to validate the instrument reveal multiple problems that are compounded by limited samples and the starting selection of highly redundant items. This overall profile does not add up to a compelling case for adopting the CIT. However, as stated at the beginning of this dissenting view, we acknowledge that those orchestrating the government surveys or the multiuse cohort studies will make the ultimate decisions about what instruments should be used in what contexts. What we have tried to do in this essay is articulate the reasoning behind our opposition to all of the proposed recommendations put forth by VanderWeele et al. (Chapter 17) in hopes of advancing scholarly exchange about how to best assess well-being going forward.

About the Authors

Carol D. Ryff is Director of the Institute on Aging and Hilldale Professor of Psychology at the University of Wisconsin-Madison. She studies psychological well-being: how it varies by sociodemographic factors and how it matters for health, including diverse disease outcomes, length of life, physiological regulation, and neural circuitry. She is Principal Investigator of the Midlife in the United States (MIDUS) longitudinal study and its sister study, Midlife in Japan (MIDJA). An integrative theme across these studies is resilience—the capacity to maintain or regain well-being and health in the face of adversity.

Jennifer Morozink Boylan is Assistant Professor of Health and Behavioral Sciences at the University of Colorado Denver. She received her PhD in biological psychology from the University of Wisconsin-Madison and completed postdoctoral fellowships in the Health Disparities Research Scholars Program at the University Wisconsin-Madison School of Medicine and Public Health and in the Cardiovascular Behavioral Medicine Program at the University of Pittsburgh. Her program of research centers on conceptualizing positive psychological characteristics and their potential influence on physical health, situating psychological risk and protective factors within broader social contexts (e.g., socioeconomic status, race, and culture), and examining biological mechanisms underlying how the social environment affects disease pathophysiology.

Julie A. Kirsch, is a postdoctoral fellow at the University of Wisconsin-Madison Center for Tobacco Research and Intervention. She studies the intersections between inequality, health, and well-being and psychosocial pathways to mitigating the consequences of socioeconomic adversity. Her research reflects integrative work that spans psychological and health sciences.

Author Note

This work was supported by the John D. and Catherine T. MacArthur Foundation Research Network and National Institute on Aging (P01-AG020166, U19-AG051426), with additional support provided by the John Templeton Foundation and the Lee Kum Sheung Center for Health and Happiness. The views expressed in this chapter represent the perspectives of the authors and do not reflect the opinions or endorsement of any organization. We have no known conflict of interest to disclose. Correspondence concerning this chapter should be directed to Carol D. Ryff, Institute on Aging, 2245 Medical Science Center, University of Madison, WI 53706 (cryff@wisc.edu).

References

Andrews, F. M. (1974). Social indicators of perceived life quality. *Social Indicators Research, 1*(3), 279–299.

Boyle, P. A., Buchman, A. S., & Bennett, D. A. (2010). Purpose in life is associated with a reduced risk of incident disability among community-dwelling older persons. *American Journal of Geriatric Psychiatry, 18*(12), 1093–1102.

Bradburn, N. M., & Noll, C. E. (1969). *The structure of psychological well-being: By Norman M. Bradburn with the assistance of C. Edward Noll.* Aldine. http://books.google.com/books?id=La2lNAEACAAJ&pgis=1

Brose, A., Schmiedek, F., Gerstorf, D., & Voelkle, M. C. (2019). The measurement of within-person affect variation. *Emotion.* https://doi.org/10.1037/emo0000583

Burgard, S. A., & Kalousova, L. (2015). Effects of the Great Recession: Health and well-being. *Annual Review of Sociology, 41*(1), 181–201.

Cantarella, A., Borella, E., Marigo, C., & De Beni, R. (2017). Benefits of well-being training in healthy older adults. *Applied Psychology: Health and Well-Being, 9*(3), 261–284.

Fava, G. A. (2016). Well-being therapy: Current indications and emerging perspectives. *Psychotherapy and Psychosomatics, 85*(3), 136–145.

Friedman, E. M., Ruini, C., Foy, C. R., Jaros, L., Love, G., & Ryff, C. D. (2019). Lighten UP! A community-based group intervention to promote eudaimonic well-being in older adults: A multi-site replication with 6 month follow-up. *Clinical Gerontologist, 42*(4), 387–397.

Goldman, N., Glei, D. A., & Weinstein, M. (2018). Declining mental health among disadvantaged Americans. *Proceedings of the National Academy of Sciences of the United States of America, 115*(28), 7290–7295.

Gurin, G., Veroff, J., & Feld, S. (1960). *Americans view their mental health: A nationwide interview survey.* Oxford: Basic.

Hafez, D., Heisler, M., Choi, H. J., Ankuda, C. K., Winkelman, T., & Kullgren, J. T. (2018). Association between purpose in life and glucose control among older adults. *Annals of Behavioral Medicine, 52*(4), 309–318.

Heller, A. S., van Reekum, C. M., Schaefer, S. M., Lapate, R. C., Radler, B. T., Ryff, C. D., & Davidson, R. J. (2013). Sustained striatal activity predicts eudaimonic well-being and cortisol output. *Psychological Science, 24*(11), 2191–2200.

Hill, P. L., & Turiano, N. A. (2014). Purpose in life as a predictor of mortality across adulthood. *Psychological Science, 25*(7), 1482–1486.

Keyes, C. L. M. (2002). The mental health continuum: From languishing to flourishing in life. *Journal of Health and Social Behavior, 43*(2), 207–222.

Keyes, C. L. M. (2009). The black-white paradox in health: Flourishing in the face of social inequality and discrimination. *Journal of Personality, 77*(6), 1677–1706.

Kim, E. S., Sun, J. K., Park, N., & Peterson, C. (2013). Purpose in life and reduced incidence of stroke in older adults: The Health and Retirement Study. *Journal of Psychosomatic Research, 74*(5), 427–432.

Kim, E. S., Sun, J. K., Park, N., Kubzansky, L. D., & Peterson, C. (2013). Purpose in life and reduced risk of myocardial infarction among older US adults with coronary heart disease: A two-year follow-up. *Journal of Behavioral Medicine, 36*(2), 124–133.

Kirsch, J. A., & Ryff, C. D. (2016). Hardships of the great recession and health: Understanding varieties of vulnerability. *Health Psychology Open, 3*(1).

Kirsch, J. A., Love, G. D., Radler, B. T., & Ryff, C. D. (2019). Scientific imperatives vis-à-vis growing inequality in America. *American Psychologist, 74*(7), 764–777.

Kitayama, S., & Park, J. (2017). Emotion and biological health: The socio-cultural moderation. *Current Opinion in Psychology, 17*, 99–105.

Miyamoto, Y., Boylan, J. M., Coe, C. L., Curhan, K. B., Levine, C. S., Markus, H. R., . . . Ryff, C. D. (2013). Negative emotions predict elevated interleukin-6 in the United States but not in Japan. *Brain, Behavior, and Immunity, 34*, 79–85.

Morozink, J. A., Friedman, E. M., Coe, C. L., & Ryff, C. D. (2010). Socioeconomic and psychosocial predictors of interleukin-6 in the MIDUS national sample. *Health Psychology, 29*(6), 626–635.

Park, J., Kitayama, S., Miyamoto, Y., & Coe, C. L. (2019). Feeling bad is not always unhealthy: Culture moderates the link between negative affect and diurnal cortisol profiles. *Emotion*. https://doi.org/10.1037/emo0000605

Rottenberg, J., Devendorf, A. R., Panaite, V., Disabato, D. J., & Kashdan, T. B. (2019). Optimal well-being after major depression. *Clinical Psychological Science, 7*(3), 621–627.

Ruini, C. (2017). *Positive psychology in the clinical domains: Research and practice.* Basel, Switzerland: Springer International. https://doi.org/10.1007/978-3-319-52112-1

Ryff, C. D. (2014). Psychological well-being revisited: Advances in the science and practice of eudaimonia. *Psychotherapy and Psychosomatics, 83*(1), 10–28.

Ryff, C. D., & Krueger, R. F. (2018). *The Oxford handbook of integrative health science.* New York: Oxford University Press.

Schaefer, S. M., Morozink Boylan, J., van Reekum, C. M., Lapate, R. C., Norris, C. J., Ryff, C. D., & Davidson, R. J. (2013). Purpose in life predicts better emotional recovery from negative stimuli. *PLoS ONE, 8*(11), e80329. https://doi.org/10.1371/journal.pone.0080329

Steptoe, A., Deaton, A., & Stone, A. A. (2015). Subjective wellbeing, health, and ageing. *Lancet, 385*(9968), 640–648.

Su, R., Tay, L., & Diener, E. (2014). The development and validation of the Comprehensive Inventory of Thriving (CIT) and the Brief Inventory of Thriving (BIT). *Applied Psychology: Health and Well-Being, 6*(3), 251–279.

VanderWeele, T. J. (2017). On the promotion of human flourishing. *Proceedings of the National Academy of Sciences of the United States of America, 31*, 8148–8156.

Watson, D., Clark, L. A., & Tellegen, A. (1988). Development and validation of brief measures of positive and negative affect: The PANAS scales. *Journal of Personality and Social Psychology, 54*(6), 1063–1070.

Weiss, L. A., Westerhof, G. J., & Bohlmeijer, E. T. (2016). Can we increase psychological well-being? The effects of interventions on psychological well-being: A meta-analysis of randomized controlled trials. *PLoS ONE, 11*(6), 1–16.

Williams, D. R. (2012). Miles to go before we sleep: Racial inequities in health. *Journal of Health and Social Behavior, 53*(3), 279–295.

Yoo, J., Miyamoto, Y., Rigotti, A., & Ryff, C. D. (2017). Linking positive affect to blood lipids: A cultural perspective. *Psychological Science, 28*(10), 1468–1477.

Zilioli, S., Slatcher, R. B., Ong, A. D., & Gruenewald, T. L. (2015). Purpose in life predicts allostatic load ten years later. *Journal of Psychosomatic Research, 79*(5), 451–457.

19

Response to "Advancing the Science of Well-Being: A Dissenting View on Measurement Recommendations"

Tyler J. VanderWeele, Claudia Trudel-Fitzgerald,
and Laura D. Kubzansky

Abstract

This chapter responds to the criticisms offered in Chapter 18 of the recommendations made in Chapter 17. We respond to concerns about the use of the term "well-being" and the use of single-item measures, as well as about the Comprehensive Inventory of Thriving, while offering further justification of the original recommendations. Our view is that it is better to include one, or a small number, of well-being items, rather than none at all, and that it is likewise preferable to offer some guidance, rather than none, for those new to research on well-being.

We appreciate the comments offered by Ryff et al. (Chapter 18, in this volume) on the importance of nomenclature and the related history of disciplines, the multidimensional nature of subjective well-being, and the context in which measurement occurs. These are indeed critical aspects of the complexity inherent to the topic of well-being measurement. Much of the discussion of Ryff et al. (Chapter 18) we agree with, and much of it is not at odds with what was recommended in our chapter (Chapter 17, in this volume).

In particular, Ryff et al. recommended that investigators avoid using "well-being" as an umbrella term when referring to distinct constructs. We appreciate the more detailed discussion of this issue and, in fact, entirely agree that the indicators like socioeconomic status and educational attainment

Tyler J. VanderWeele, Claudia Trudel-Fitzgerald, and Laura D. Kubzansky, *Response to "Advancing the Science of Well-Being: A Dissenting View on Measurement Recommendations"* In: *Measuring Well-Being*. Edited by: Matthew T. Lee, Laura D. Kubzansky, and Tyler J. VanderWeele, Oxford University Press (2021). © Oxford University Press. DOI: 10.1093/oso/9780197512531.003.0020 (often used to characterize "objective well-being") are different from those capturing physical health, which are also different from those representing subjective psychological well-being (e.g., happiness, life satisfaction, purpose in life). Objective well-being indicators are not only distinct from subjective well-being indicators, but the former are often drivers of the latter (Kubzansky et al., 2018; Patel et al., 2018). Confusion can indeed arise when having these multiple referents for "well-being." However, a number of overall well-being indices created for the purposes of tracking country-level (or other administrative units) performance concerning growth and development (e.g., Stiglitz, 2016) actually include both subjective and objective indicators. It is difficult to insist on terminology when it is used by others in a variety of ways. Nevertheless, distinguishing these constructs and terms will foster careful consideration about the various contexts in which measures of subjective well-being are needed, as well as facilitate further research about relationships between the social context, social inequality, and subjective well-being—as discussed further later.

We also completely agree that interest in, and the study, of well-being is not in its infancy. Ryff et al. referred to interest in the topic since the ancient Greeks. While reflection upon human well-being is indeed millennia old, the measurement and empirical study of subjective well-being is comparatively recent. Although the empirical study of subjective well-being has been ongoing in important ways for decades, there can be no doubt that interest in and attention to this area of research has expanded dramatically in recent years, along with accompanying knowledge.

We endorse Ryff et al.'s insistence that well-being is multidimensional and complex. We also understand their concern about reducing well-being measurement to a single item, which was central in their objection to the recommendations for government surveys and multiuse cohort studies. We agree that, whenever it is possible to advocate for longer well-being assessments, it would be beneficial for the field to do so. However, we have been in situations in which investigators are willing to include one, and only one, subjective well-being item in their survey. Our view is that it is better to include one than none at all. Moreover, it is worth noting that other researchers have previously demonstrated that single life satisfaction measures can in some contexts perform similarly to multi-item ones (Cheung & Lucas, 2014). In our own work, when developing a 40-item well-being index covering numerous domains of flourishing (Lee et al., 2020; VanderWeele,

2017), we found correlations of the single life satisfaction item "Overall, how satisfied are you with life as a whole these days?" of magnitude 0.70 to 0.75 with the entire 40-item index. Similarly strong correlations with the full index held for "Overall, to what extent do you feel the things you do in your life are worthwhile?" and with "All is well with my life." In parallel, a recent narrative review found that both single- and multi-item measures of life satisfaction are reliably associated with mortality risk (Trudel-Fitzgerald et al., 2019a). Although the review found happiness captured by a single item was not as reliably associated with mortality across a handful of studies (Trudel-Fitzgerald et al., 2019a), one-item measures of happiness have been associated with other health-related outcomes, such as lifestyle behaviors over time (e.g., smoking, physical activity, diet quality; Trudel-Fitzgerald et al., 2019b). The Japanese term *Ikigai* is another construct that has mostly been assessed using a single item, which has shown fairly consistent associations with subsequent health outcomes and mortality risk (Boehm & Kubzansky, 2012; Trudel-Fitzgerald et al., 2019a). Thus, while we completely agree that most constructs are more accurately captured with multiple items (e.g., personal growth, positive affect, meaning in life), we also believe there is sometimes valuable insight to be gained even with a single item, when it is a good one. Moreover, for researchers who are skeptical about the empirical assessment of well-being and may not want to attempt its assessment or devote a great deal of time or questionnaire "real estate" to the endeavor, it is arguably best to start somewhere using either a single or just a few items, rather than to abandon the undertaking altogether. As was noted in our chapter, if, in government or multipurpose cohort studies, it is possible to have longer assessments, we would absolutely be in favor of using more comprehensive, multi-item measures, and we would not then recommend these very brief assessments.

With regard to our measurement recommendations for specific items, we suggested the life satisfaction question because it has already been used so widely, both in scientific research and government surveys, and is recommended by the Organisation for Economic Co-operation and Development (OECD, 2013). The question on worthwhile activities (which we suggested as a complement to the life satisfaction item, if it is possible to include only two items) is likewise widely employed, including in the UK national program of personal well-being since 2011 (Office for National Statistics, 2018); a similar item is also recommended in the OECD guidelines (2013). Worthwhile activities tap into eudaimonic well-being which, as underscored by Ryff et al., is an important aspect of well-being that has been related to a wide variety of outcomes, including physical health (Boehm & Kubzansky, 2012; Chapter 5, in this volume). To maximize comparability with past research we suggested the life satisfaction question if only one item is possible; however, it is indeed plausible that it would be of greater benefit to society to replace that life satisfaction question with one on worthwhile activities or with some other item. Indeed, this was explicitly raised in the discussion section of our chapter as an important area for future research. While Ryff et al. expressed concerns about empirical evidence to support the value of the worthwhile activities question, this eudaimonic well-being item has been used in etiologic long-term research and predicts numerous health and other outcomes over time (Steptoe & Fancourt, 2019). This work is relatively recent, but, as noted earlier, the field is developing rapidly. The happiness and anxiety items were the third and fourth items we recommended for use in government surveys if space allowed. Ryff et al. criticized these items with respect to their reference to "yesterday" given the intraperson variability. We are sympathetic to this issue. However, as we noted, while we agree that these items would be less suitable in etiologic longitudinal research on a cohort of individuals, when they are sampled over many persons on different days, they provide a representative aggregate of individuals' self-assessed happiness and anxiety, respectively, over time for a nation. In the section on multiuse cohort studies, when the same group of individuals is followed over time, one would desire a measure with less day-to-day variability and thus we modified our recommendations accordingly (i.e., by selecting items that do not refer to "yesterday" as the time frame). In most government surveys, it is not possible to use the data for individual-level longitudinal panel research.

Regarding items recommended for multiuse cohort studies, counter to Ryff et al.'s claim, we did provide a rationale for our choices. For example, we suggested the use of items related to purpose and optimism based in part on their predictive validity for outcomes most people care about; for instance, numerous studies have demonstrated that these represent key psychological constructs that predict mortality (Cohen, Bavishi, & Rozanski, 2016; Rozanski, Bavishi, Kubzansky, & Cohen, 2019; Trudel-Fitzgerald et al., 2019a) as well as health-related behaviors and biomarkers (e.g., allostatic load, antioxidants; Chapter 5, in this volume). Furthermore, we did not recommend optimism as the only facet of well-being to receive two items in multiuse cohort studies, but also suggested that investigators measure purpose with two items. Many existing multiuse cohort studies arise out of biomedical research contexts and have the study of health as one of their central motivations. Focusing on health in cohort studies is, of course, not a necessity, and interest seems to be increasing in the social sciences for collaborating on the development of very large multiuse cohort studies for a range of purposes. However, many cohort studies in biomedicine have not included measures of well-being as it has not been a central focus of their investigations. For investigators interested in evaluating relationships between subjective well-being and a range of other health outcomes by using these cohort studies, capacity to predict physical health and mortality can be used as a persuasive argument for convincing skeptics about the utility of including items on well-being. Moreover, such arguments may be more effective if it is possible to recommend a limited set of items rather than taking an all-or-nothing stance. Thus, rather than implying that measurement of well-being is "less important, less multifaceted, and less consequential," as suggested by Ryff et al., we hope that our recommendations of both shorter and longer measures of well-being will result in a wider and more comprehensive use and study of these constructs.

In addition, we respectfully disagree with Ryff et al.'s claim that our entire recommendations document was shaped solely around a population or demographic perspective. That perspective was certainly dominant in the recommendations for government surveys and multiuse cohorts because a population perspective is often the motivation for such studies. However, after reviewing issues related to those types of studies, we went on to discuss recommendations for studies focused principally on well-being, wherein theoretically rich perspectives, such as from the psychological sciences and human development, are more dominant. Regarding the recommendations given in that section, Ryff et al. expressed skepticism regarding the use of the Comprehensive Inventory of Thriving (CIT; Su, Tay, & Diener, 2014) because of concerns about the psychometric quality of the measure. We would like to point out that in our recommendations the CIT was suggested not for use principally as an aggregate measure of well-being, but rather as a way to obtain an inventory of numerous different facets of well-being. One may use each of the facets without aggregating or without endorsing the conceptual grouping in domains of the different facets. As noted in our chapter, this scale was recommended on the grounds of its breadth of coverage. Moreover, the original authors reported that the CIT subscales are correlated but distinguishable from each other, a factor structure that was found in all five of their original validation samples (Su et al., 2014). There has also been further cross-cultural psychometric evaluation (Wiese, Tay, Su, & Diener, 2018). Following predictions one would make based on prior work (Boehm & Kubzansky, 2012; Pressman, Jenkins, & Moskowitz, 2019; Chapter 5, in this volume), validation studies demonstrated that higher scores on several CIT subdomains—particularly Life Satisfaction, Positive Emotions, Optimism, and Accomplishment—separately correlated with fewer medical problems, higher levels of physical functioning, and more frequent engagement in healthy behaviors (Su et al., 2014).

Ryff et al. also criticized the fact that many of the CIT items were overlapping or very closely related to prior scales on the basis that this compromised "tests of convergent validity with established measures." However, in our view, the overlap with prior well-validated items is in fact a strength. Again, our recommendations regarding this measure did not pertain to its conceptual underpinnings per se, but rather to the inventory of different aspects of well-being, as providing a number of well-studied items derived from prior work that covers very many facets of subjective well-being. Moreover, we did recommend that, whenever possible, each construct should be measured by more than one scale to help facilitate new insights and possible conceptual distinctions that may be obscured by a single scale and set of items. Notably, we suggested drawing on Ryff's Psychological Well-Being scales (Ryff, 1989) for this, among others. This would arguably help facilitate the rich theorization that Ryff et al. desire and have contributed to. Unfortunately, Ryff et al. did not seem to acknowledge this important aspect of the recommendations.

In their section about the importance of context, Ryff et al. also pointed to the need for acknowledging factors related to subjective well-being, including life events, socioeconomic inequalities, cultural differences, and racial disparities. We concur that these are key social determinants of subjective well-being that should be considered in both scientific research and government surveys. To date, most scientific research on subjective well-being has relied on samples from high-income countries, circumscribed to certain races and cultures, which may not be generalizable to other populations. Yet, as underlined by Ryff et al. and elsewhere in this book (Chapter 5), it remains unclear as of now whether constructs of subjective well-being are conceived similarly across race, cultures, and countries worldwide given documented differences in the experience, value, and understanding of well-being (Choi & Chentsova-Dutton, 2017; Diener, Lucas, & Oishi, 2018; Ma, Tamir, & Miyamoto, 2018; Ryff, 2017). Thus, we fully endorse the perspective that careful assessment of subjective well-being in different populations is critically warranted.

Any set of concrete recommendations will have limitations. However, for those relatively new to the field who may be interested in measuring subjective well-being, we do believe that some guidance is of help. Very little has been offered beyond a description of the array of options (e.g., Lindert, Bain, Kubzansky, & Stein, 2015; Linton, Dieppe, & Medina-Lara, 2016; Salsman et al., 2014), perhaps except from the OECD Guidelines on measuring subjective well-being (OECD, 2013), which are intended for national statistical offices primarily. Ryff et al. proposed a number of criticisms with respect to the concrete recommendations that we put forward. We believe some of these are inaccurate and have tried to address the inaccuracies in our discussion here, some criticisms are reasonable but arguably inescapable, some dismissed a context we think is important (i.e., single-item measures), and some do indeed point to limitations in current recommendations and in our current knowledge. As stated explicitly in our chapter, the recommendations are meant to be provisional and to prompt debate and, hopefully, over time, refinement. For example, we believe the question as to which single-item measure should be used to assess subjective well-being if only one is possible is an important and open topic for further research. Unfortunately, Ryff et al. did not explicitly offer their own alternative recommendations. We again believe some guidance is better than none for those new to work on well-being. An alternative possibility might be to suggest that the first author of the dissent's own Psychological Well-Being Scale (Ryff, 1989) be put forward. Indeed, in our section on using at least two scales, when possible, for each well-being construct, we suggested drawing on Ryff's Psychological Well-Being scales, among others. However, whether it would be possible to get governments around the world to administer a multiple-item multidomain well-being assessment is open to question. If this were to occur, we would be delighted, as it would enrich our knowledge of global subjective well-being considerably. However, we suspect that, at least initially, encouraging the use of a handful of items may well be a more successful approach in broadening the assessment and the study of well-being.

About the Authors

Tyler J. VanderWeele is the John L. Loeb and Frances Lehman Loeb Professor of Epidemiology in the Departments of Epidemiology and Biostatistics at the Harvard T. H. Chan School of Public Health, Director of the Human Flourishing Program, and Co-Director of the Initiative on Health, Religion, and Spirituality at Harvard University. His research concerns methodology for distinguishing between association and causation in observational studies, and his empirical research spans psychiatric, perinatal, and social epidemiology; the science of happiness and flourishing; and the study of religion and health, including both religion and population health and the role of religion and spirituality in end-of-life care. He has published more than 300 papers in peer-reviewed journals and is author of the book *Explanation in Causal Inference* (Oxford University Press, 2015).

Claudia Trudel-Fitzgerald is Research Scientist at the Lee Kum Sheung Center for Health and Happiness and the Department of Social and Behavioral Sciences at the Harvard T. H. Chan School of Public Health. She is also a licensed clinical psychologist specializing in cognitive behavioral-therapy. Her research projects target the role of positive and negative emotions in the maintenance and decline of physical health as well as longevity.

Laura D. Kubzansky is Lee Kum Kee Professor of Social and Behavioral Sciences and Co-Director of the Lee Kum Sheung Center for Health and Happiness at the Harvard T. H. Chan School of Public Health. Dr. Kubzansky has published extensively on the role of psychological and social factors in health. Ongoing research includes studying biobehavioral mechanisms linking emotions, social relationships, and health; defining, measuring, and modifying aspects of well-being; and workplace conditions in relation to well-being. She has served on the leadership team for multiple training programs for junior scholars and is principal investigator or co-investigator on numerous grants.

Author Note

This work was supported in part by a grant from the John Templeton Foundation and by the Lee Kum Sheung Center for Health and Happiness. The views expressed in this chapter represent the perspectives of the authors and do not reflect the opinions or endorsement of any organization. We have no known conflict of interest to disclose. Correspondence concerning this chapter should be directed to Tyler J. VanderWeele, Harvard T. H. Chan School of Public Health, Departments of Epidemiology and Biostatistics, 677 Huntington Avenue, Boston, MA 02115 (tvanderw@hsph.harvard.edu).

References

Boehm, J. K., & Kubzansky, L. D. (2012). The heart's content: The association between positive psychological well-being and cardiovascular health. *Psychological Bulletin, 138*(4), 655–691.

Cheung, F., & Lucas, R. E. (2014). Assessing the validity of single-item life satisfaction measures: Results from three large samples. *Quality of Life Research, 23*(10), 2809–2818.

Choi, E., & Chentsova-Dutton, Y. E. (2017). The relationship between momentary emotions and well-being across European Americans, Hispanic Americans, and Asian Americans. *Cognition & Emotion, 31*(6), 1277–1285.

Cohen, R., Bavishi, C., & Rozanski, A. (2016). Purpose in life and its relationship to all-cause mortality and cardiovascular events: A meta-analysis. *Psychosomatic Medicine, 78*(2), 122–133.

Diener, E., Lucas, R. E., & Oishi, S. (2018). Advances and open questions in the science of subjective well-being. *Collabra: Psychology, 4*(1), 15.

Kubzansky, L. D., Huffman, J. C., Boehm, J. K., Hernandez, R., Kim, E. S., Koga, H. K., . . . Labarthe, D. R. (2018). Positive psychological well-being and cardiovascular disease: JACC Health Promotion Series. *Journal of the American College of Cardiology, 72*(12), 1382–1396.

Lee, M. T., Weziak-Bialowolska, D., Mooney, K. D., Lerner, P. J., McNeely, E., & VanderWeele, T. J. (2020). Self-assessed importance of domains of flourishing: Demographics and correlations with well-being. *Journal of Positive Psychology*, https://doi.org/10.1080/17439760.2020.1716050.

Lindert, J., Bain, P. A., Kubzansky, L. D., & Stein, C. (2015). Well-being measurement and the WHO health policy Health 2010: Systematic review of measurement scales. *European Journal of Public Health, 25*(4), 731–740.

Linton, M. J., Dieppe, P., & Medina-Lara, A. (2016). Review of 99 self-report measures for assessing well-being in adults: Exploring dimensions of well-being and developments over time. *BMJ Open, 6*(7), e010641.

Ma, X., Tamir, M., & Miyamoto, Y. (2018). A socio-cultural instrumental approach to emotion regulation: Culture and the regulation of positive emotions. *Emotion, 18*(1), 138–152.

OECD. (2013). *Guidelines on measuring subjective well-being*. Paris: OECD.

Office for National Statistics. (2018). Well-being. https://www.ons.gov.uk/peoplepopulationandcommunity/wellbeing.

Patel, V., Saxena, S., Lund, C., Thornicroft, G., Baingana, F., Bolton, P., . . . Herrman, H. (2018). The Lancet Commission on global mental health and sustainable development. *Lancet, 392*(10157), 1553–1598.

Pressman, S. D., Jenkins, B. N., & Moskowitz, J. T. (2019). Positive affect and health: What do we know and where next should we go? *Annual Review of Psychology*. DOI:10.1146/annurev-psych-010418-102955

Rozanski, A., Bavishi, C., Kubzansky, L. D., & Cohen, R. (2019). Association of optimism with cardiovascular events and all-cause mortality: A systematic review and meta-analysis. *JAMA Network Open, 2*(9), e1912200.

Ryff, C. D. (1989). Happiness is everything, or is it? Explorations on the meaning of psychological well-being. *Journal of Personality and Social Psychology, 57*, 1069–1081.

Ryff, C. D. (2017). Eudaimonic well-being, inequality, and health: Recent findings and future directions. *International Review of Economics, 64*(2), 159–178.

Salsman, J. M., Lai, J. S., Hendrie, H. C., Butt, Z., Zill, N., Pilkonis, P. A., . . . Cella, D. (2014). Assessing psychological well-being: Self-report instruments for the NIH Toolbox. *Quality of Life Research, 23*(1), 205–215.

Steptoe, A., & Fancourt, D. (2019). Leading a meaningful life at older ages and its relationship with social engagement, prosperity, health, biology, and time use. *Proceedings of the National Academy of Sciences of the United States of America, 116*(4), 1207–1212.

Stiglitz, J., Sen, A., & Fitoussi. (2016). *Report by the Commission on the Measurement of Economic Performance and Social Progress*. Paris: Commission on the Measurement of Economic Performance and Social Progress.

Su, R., Tay, L., Diener, E. (2014). The development and validation of the Comprehensive Inventory of Thriving (CIT) and the Brief Inventory of Thriving (BIT). *Applied Psychology: Health and Well-Being, 6*, 251–279.

Trudel-Fitzgerald, C., Millstein, R. A., von Hippel, C., Howe, C. J., Tomasso, L. P., Wagner, G. R., & VanderWeele, T. J. (2019a). Psychological well-being as part of the public health debate? Insight into dimensions, interventions, and policy. *BMC Public Health, 19*(1), 1–11.

Trudel-Fitzgerald, C., James, P., Kim, E. S., Zevon, E. S., Grodstein, F., & Kubzansky, L. D. (2019b). Prospective associations of happiness and optimism with lifestyle over up to two decades. *Preventive Medicine, 126*, 105754.

VanderWeele, T. J. (2017). On the promotion of human flourishing. *Proceedings of the National Academy of Sciences of the United States of America, 31*, 8148–8156.

Wiese, C. W, Tay, L., Su, R., & Diener, E. (2018). Measuring thriving across nations: Examining the measurement equivalence of the Comprehensive Inventory of Thriving (CIT) and the Brief Inventory of Thriving (BIT). *Applied Psychology: Health and Well-Being, 10*(1), 127–148.

20

Response to Response

Growing the Field of Well-Being

Carol D. Ryff, Jennifer Morozink Boylan, and Julie A. Kirsch

Abstract

We challenge the view that "one is better than none" on grounds that single-item assessments perpetuate a simplistic view of well-being, which is out of touch with how the field has progressed over recent decades. We also question blanket advocacy for measures in the absence of substantive scientific questions that require thoughtful engagement with the prior literature to make sound measurement choices. Substantive illustrations, invoking research on well-being and health in different cultural and socioeconomic contexts, are provided. Quality control is also essential in making sound measurement choices. Numerous contenders fail at this juncture because they have no conceptual foundation and also lack rigorous psychometric analyses documenting their empirical credibility. Another critical element in adjudicating measurement quality is extent of prior usage: that is, evidence that the measures have taken hold in the scientific community, indicated by citation counts and number of published studies. We conclude that all such quality control criteria were inadequately addressed or missing in the measurement recommendations put forth in Chapter 17.

We appreciate clarifications from VanderWeele et al. about areas of agreement that exist in this exchange (Chapter 19): why it is not useful to call everything "well-being," that the science of well-being is not in its infancy, and that well-being is complex and multifaceted. However, other parts of their response to our dissenting view bring into high relief areas of notable

Carol D. Ryff, Jennifer Morozink Boylan, and Julie A. Kirsch, *Response to Response* In: *Measuring Well-Being*. Edited by: Matthew T. Lee, Laura D. Kubzansky, and Tyler J. VanderWeele, Oxford University Press (2021). © Oxford University Press. DOI: 10.1093/oso/9780197512531.003.0021 disagreement that we distill here. Our intent is to sharpen scholarly discussion about how the field of well-being best moves forward.

"One Is Better Than None" Is Mistaken

The view that a single-item assessment of well-being is better than no assessment is, in our view, without merit and should be relegated to the past. Such a stance perpetuates a simplistic view of well-being that fails to embrace how the field has progressed. Few would endorse a recommendation for a single-item assessment of depression, anxiety, personality, cardiovascular risk, or socioeconomic status because guiding conceptualizations and operational definitions in each of these areas are, after decades of inquiry, recognized to be complex and multidimensional—not just a single thing. Given the past 50 years of research on subjective well-being, we believe the time has arrived for scientists and practitioners to similarly acknowledge that there is no single question, or even handful of questions, that do justice to this fundamentally important realm of human experience, which is increasingly known to matter for many aspects of health. The crux of the matter is this: simplistic measures of well-being effectively guarantee simplistic findings. Such a practice undermines progress in the field, including development of policies and interventions to promote well-being in its various forms.

Blanket Advocacy Is at Odds with Good Science

We are wary of advocacy for specific measures proffered in the absence of substantive scientific questions. What makes such blanket recommendations imprudent is that the relevance of any particular indicator of well-being likely varies depending on the specific objectives of the study and relevant contextual factors. Stated otherwise, scientists and policy-makers are far more likely to make good choices among the diverse well-being scales available by thinking through the options vis-à-vis the core aims of their planned studies. So doing requires serious engagement with the prior literature in targeted research areas. In writing winning grant proposals or compelling journal articles, it would be folly to defend measurement choices by citing recommendations that are disconnected from substantive scientific questions. More persuasive and likely critical in peer review is the presentation of measurement rationales based on goals of the project, guiding theoretical models, related prior findings, contextual considerations, and feasibility issues. We offer two substantive illustrations to underscore these points. The first invokes differing cultural contexts and the second differing socioeconomic contexts.

Prior work in cultural psychology revealed that well-being is conceptualized and experienced differently across sociocultural contexts related to distinctions between collectivism and individualism, also framed in terms of interdependent and independent cultures. Drawing on these ideas, recent findings show that how well-being matters for health varies by cultural context. For example, within *independent* cultural contexts, like the United States, well-being is personal and individual in scope, and higher levels of nearly all dimensions of well-being (hedonic and eudaimonic) predict better mental and physical health (see findings reviewed in our Chapter 18). In contrast, within *interdependent* cultural contexts, like Japan, well-being is relational and collective in scope, which calls for greater emphasis on social connectedness as a key aspect of well-being (Yoo, Miyamoto, & Ryff, 2016). How positive and negative emotions are experienced and matter for health also varies by cultural context. In Japan, positive and negative emotions are more likely to co-occur—hence, the idea of dialectical emotions (Miyamoto & Ryff, 2010), which in turn are tied with fewer health symptoms in Japan compared to the United States. Furthermore, positive affect often does not predict better health outcomes, including biological measures, in Japanese adults (Boylan, Tsenkova, Miyamoto, & Ryff, 2017; Kitayama & Park, 2017; Yoo, Miyamoto, Rigotti, & Ryff, 2017). Negative affect, which is known to predict poorer health in the United States (e.g., interleukin-6, diurnal cortisol) likewise does not predict poor health in Japan (Miyamoto et al., 2013; Park, Kitayama, Miyamoto, & Coe, 2019). Alternatively, eudaimonic well-being, especially purpose in life and what makes life worth living (known as *ikigai* in Japan) appear to be valued and health-relevant in both cultural contexts (Ryff et al., 2014). Comparative studies have also made clear the need to distinguish between low- and high-arousal emotions, given emphasis on high arousal in the United States and low arousal in Japan (Clobert et al., 2019). In sum, research on culture, well-being, and health underscores that judicious measurement choices require attending to prior scientific findings infused with attentiveness to distinct sociocultural meaning systems and differing philosophical, religious, and political traditions. Indiscriminate measurement recommendations in such inquiries are deeply problematic.

Differing socioeconomic contexts call for attending to prior research and theory as well. Here, we question the observation by VanderWeele et al. that most prior research on subjective well-being has relied on "samples from high-income countries, circumscribed to certain races and cultures, which may not be generalizable to other populations." This claim overlooks the high volume of health inequalities research within the United States that documents notable variation in well-being and health as a function of socioeconomic status and ethnic minority status. Thus, although the United States is, relatively speaking, a high-income country, extensive science documents widespread and increasing disparities in wealth and their health concomitants. What do such disparities mean for judicious choices of measures of well-being? According to the reserve capacity model, a conceptual framework of social inequality and health, individuals who are socioeconomically disadvantaged are posited to have a smaller reserve of psychosocial resources, including lower levels of psychological well-being (Matthews & Gallo, 2011). Previous work has shown that indicators of lower socioeconomic status are associated with lower levels of well-being, including optimism and life satisfaction (Boehm, Chen, Williams, Ryff, & Kubzansky, 2015) and purpose in life (Ryff & Singer, 2008). Nonetheless, there is notable variability within socioeconomic strata, and some individuals who are lower in socioeconomic status maintain high levels of well-being (Ryff, Magee, Kling, & Wing, 1999; Markus, Ryff, Barnett, & Palmersheim, 2004). Furthermore, most dimensions of eudaimonic well-being and positive affect were found to attenuate the relationship between lower educational attainment and higher levels of inflammation (Morozink, Friedman, Coe, & Ryff, 2010)—that is, they emerge as protective resources even among the less educated. A summary of related findings on health inequalities from the Midlife in the United States (MIDUS) survey implicates other psychological resources as well, such as sense of control and conscientiousness, along with an array of vulnerability factors (negative affect, neuroticism, anger, anxiety; Kirsch, Love, Radler, & Ryff, 2019). Thus, the scope of psychological factors to consider in research on socioeconomic disparities, which are worsening over time—and their implications for health—is deep and wide. Theoretical considerations matter, such as the idea that some psychological protective factors may be undermined by pervasive socioeconomic disadvantage and even transformed into sources of vulnerability (Shanahan, Hill, Roberts,

Eccles, & Friedman, 2014). Purpose in life, for example, typically conceived as a protective resource, emerged as a vulnerability factor for poorer health among those with low educational status who also experienced greater hardship from the Great Recession (Kirsch & Ryff, 2016). Thus, future research needs to attend to which psychosocial resources, including aspects of wellbeing, are at risk for being undermined, and which may be more resilient to the forces of inequality. This perspective calls for psychological measurement that is broad in scope, as just illustrated.

The larger message from the preceding two examples is that contextual influences on well-being and health, which are critically needed in future science, demand comprehensive measurement choices built on prior scientific findings in targeted areas. Such endeavors are not usefully orchestrated by adopting thin (few items), context-free measurement recommendations.

Quality Control in Choosing Among Measures of Well-Being

We appreciate the challenges faced by newcomers to the field of well-being, with its long history of empirical work guided by different approaches (as distilled in our Chapter 4) and the accompanying proliferation of new measures in recent years. At the core of this panorama of possibilities is a key issue: What constitutes quality measurement of well-being? Numerous contenders fail at this juncture and are not worthy of serious consideration.

A first critical element in adjudicating quality is whether the formulation is clearly and coherently defined, ideally by drawing on relevant theory and/ or philosophy. No such conceptual foundation undergirds the measurement recommendations of VanderWeele et al. in Chapter 17. Indeed, many terms invoked (flourishing, hedonic, eudaimonic) are themselves not clearly defined or linked with prior conceptualizations. Instead, the focus is exclusively on specific items, most of which did not come from coherent, well-validated models of well-being.

The second critical element of quality is that measures of well-being must emerge from rigorous psychometric analyses, starting with explication of how the items were generated: Based on what procedures and what guiding constructs? Next are multiple steps in refining item pools (via examination of item-to-scale correlations as well as assessments of face and content validity). Whether the multidimensionality of the model is empirically supported (confirmatory factor analysis) must be assessed, along with how well the scales align with other purportedly similar as well as different constructs (convergent and discriminant validity). Unfortunately, few measures recommended by VanderWeele et al. in Chapter 17 come with compelling psychometric evidence that they are, in fact, valid and reliable indicators of the constructs they purport to assess. Here we note that α coefficients (indices of internal consistency) are not a substitute for painstaking psychometric validation. Regarding VanderWeele et al.'s, recommendation of the Comprehensive Inventory of Thriving (CIT) for comprehensive assessment of well-being, we will not repeat our previous points about its lack of theory and its problematic psychometric features. Instead, we note a further marked deficiency relative to other measurement options: namely, minimal scientific usage.

Thus, the third critical element in adjudicating quality is whether the proposed new measures have taken hold in the scientific community, as indicated by citation counts and number of published studies. These are useful components of measurement quality because they reflect individual decisions made by wide-ranging investigators about what measures to use in their own studies. Presumably such choices are based on evaluation of prior usage as well as consideration of the two previously mentioned criteria: namely, the merits of the guiding conceptual model and the psychometric rigor with which the scales were generated.

We conclude this section by noting that the Ryff (1989) model of well-being fares well according to the preceding three quality control criteria. That is, it emerged from a rich integration of multiple theoretical perspectives, and the process of translating the conceptual model to assessment tools was comprehensive and psychometrically rigorous. The model also took hold in the scientific community, with more than 1,200 publications generated and the scales translated to 40 different languages. Here we respond to VanderWeele et al.'s probe in Chapter 19 as to why we do not offer our own recommendations, including advocating for use of the Ryff (1989) scales. The reason, as articulated earlier, is that we believe measurement choices are best made via careful consideration of guiding scientific questions, relevant prior findings, and contextual considerations. In short, we do not favor blanket recommendations for *any* extant measures of well-being, including the Ryff scales. It is worth noting that Ryff has never explicitly advocated for use of her model; rather she has marveled at its widespread usage (Ryff, 2018).

Summary: Advancing Well-Being Research Via Quality Science on Compelling Questions

The gist of our thoughts about advancing well-being research are distilled as follows. First, researchers, policy-makers, and practitioners need to recognize that well-being is multiple things—the time has passed since it can be captured with a single question about life satisfaction, happiness, or meaning. Second, in deciding which among many possible measures to use, choices will inevitably vary depending on the guiding questions of the research along with theoretical and contextual considerations. In situations where limited prior findings offer guidance, it is wise to include multiple measures from different conceptual approaches to maximize the prospect of learning which measures matter under which conditions and for whom. Third, quality control concerns must be invoked. This requires careful evaluation of the conceptual background for differing approaches and the rigor with which related measures have been generated and evaluated. An undeniable marker of quality is scope of prior usage—the array of important scientific findings that have grown up around the measures.

About the Authors

Carol D. Ryff is Director of the Institute on Aging and Hilldale Professor of Psychology at the University of Wisconsin-Madison. She studies psychological well-being—how it varies by sociodemographic factors and how it matters for health, including diverse disease outcomes, length of life, physiological regulation, and neural circuitry. She is Principal Investigator of the Midlife in the United States (MIDUS) longitudinal study and its sister study, Midlife in Japan (MIDJA). An integrative theme across these studies is resilience—the capacity to maintain or regain well-being and health in the face of adversity.

Jennifer Morozink Boylan is Assistant Professor of Health and Behavioral Sciences at the University of Colorado Denver. She received her PhD in biological psychology from the University of Wisconsin-Madison and completed postdoctoral fellowships in the Health Disparities Research Scholars Program at the University Wisconsin-Madison School of Medicine and Public Health and in the Cardiovascular Behavioral Medicine Program at the University of Pittsburgh. Her program of research centers on conceptualizing positive psychological characteristics and their potential influence on physical health, situating psychological risk and protective factors within broader social contexts (e.g., socioeconomic status, race, and culture), and examining biological mechanisms underlying how the social environment affects disease pathophysiology.

Julie A. Kirsch, MS, is a postdoctoral fellow at the University of Wisconsin-Madison Center for Tobacco Research and Intervention. She studies the intersections between inequality, health, and well-being and psychosocial pathways to mitigating the consequences of socioeconomic adversity. Her research reflects integrative work that spans psychological and health sciences.

Author Note

This work was supported by the John D. and Catherine T. MacArthur Foundation Research Network and National Institute on Aging (P01-AG020166, U19-AG051426), with additional support provided by the John Templeton Foundation and the Lee Kum Sheung Center for Health and Happiness. The views expressed in this chapter represent the perspectives of the authors and do not reflect the opinions or endorsement of any organization. We have no known conflict of interest to disclose. Correspondence concerning this chapter should be directed to Carol D. Ryff, Institute on Aging, 2245 Medical Science Center, University of Madison, WI 53706 (cryff@wisc.edu).

References

Boehm, J. K., Chen, Y., Williams, D. R., Ryff, C., & Kubzansky, L. D. (2015). Unequally distributed psychological assets: Are there social disparities in optimism, life satisfaction, and positive affect? *PLoS ONE, 10*(2), 1–16.

Boylan, J. M., Tsenkova, V. K., Miyamoto, Y., & Ryff, C. D. (2017). Psychological resources and glucoregulation in Japanese adults: Findings from MIDJA. *Health Psychology, 36*(5), 449–457.

Clobert, M., Sims, T. L., Yoo, J., Miyamoto, Y., Markus, H. R., Karasawa, M., & Levine, C. S. (2019). Feeling excited or taking a bath: Do distinct pathways underlie the positive affect-health link in the US and Japan? *Emotion*. Advance online publication. doi:10.1037/emo0000531

Kirsch, J., & Ryff, C. D. (2016). Hardships of the Great Recession and health: Understanding varieties of vulnerability. *Health Psychology Open, 3*(1), doi:10.1177/2055102916652390

Kirsch, J. A., Love, G. D., Radler, B. T., & Ryff, C. D. (2019). Scientific imperatives vis-à-vis growing inequality in America. *American Psychologist, 74*(7), 764–777.

Kitayama, S., & Park, J. (2017). Emotion and biological health: The socio-cultural moderation. *Current Opinion in Psychology, 17*, 99–105.

Markus, H. R., Ryff, C. D., Barnett, K. L., & Palmersheim, K. A. (2004). In their own words: Well-being at midlife among high school and college educated adults. In O. G. Brim, C. D. Ryff, & R. C. Kessler (Eds.), *How healthy are we?: A national study of well-being at midlife* (pp. 273–319). Chicago, IL: University of Chicago.

Matthews, K. A., & Gallo, L. C. (2011). Psychological perspectives on pathways linking socioeconomic status and physical health. *Annual Review of Psychology, 62*, 501–530.

Miyamoto, Y., Boylan, J. M., Coe, C. L., Curhan, K. B., Levine, C. S., Markus, H. R., . . . Ryff, C. D. (2013). Negative emotions predict elevated interleukin-6 in the United States but not in Japan. *Brain, Behavior, and Immunity, 34*, 79–85.

Miyamoto, Y., & Ryff, C. D. (2010). Cultural differences in the dialectical and non-dialectical emotional styles and their implications for health. *Cognition & Emotion, 25*(1), 22–39.

Morozink, J. A., Friedman, E. M., Coe, C. L., & Ryff, C. D. (2010). Socioeconomic and psychosocial predictors of interleukin-6 in the MIDUS national sample. *Health Psychology, 29*(6), 626 635.

Park, J., Kitayama, S., Miyamoto, Y., & Coe, C. L. (2019). Feeling bad is not always unhealthy: Culture moderates the link between negative affect and diurnal cortisol profiles. *Emotion.* Advance online publication. https://doi.org/10.1037/emo0000605

Ryff, C. D. (1989). Happiness is everything, or is it?: Explorations on the meaning of psychological well-being. *Journal of Personality and Social Psychology, 57,* 1069–1081.

Ryff, C. D. (2018). Well-being with soul: Science in pursuit of human potential. Perspectives on *Psychological Science, 13*(2), 242–248.

Ryff, C. D., Love, G. D., Miyamoto, Y., Markus, H. R., Curhan, K. B., Kitayama, S., Park, J., Kawakami, N., Kan, C., & Karasawa, M. (2014). Culture and the promotion of well-being in East and West: Understanding varieties of attunement to the surrounding context. In G. A. Fava & C. Ruini (Eds.), *Increasing psychological well-being in clinical and education settings: Interventions and cultural contexts* (pp. 666–679). New York, NY, Springer.

Ryff, C. D., Magee, W. J., Kling, K. C., & Wing, E. H. (1999). Forging macro-micro linkages in the study of psychological well-being. In C. D. Ryff & V. W. Marshall (Eds.), *The self and society in aging processes* (pp. 247–278). New York: Springer.

Ryff, C. D., & Singer, B. H. (2008). Know thyself and become what you are: A eudaimonic approach to psychological well-being. *Journal of Happiness Studies, 9,* 13–39.

Shanahan, M. J., Hill, P. L., Roberts, B. W., Eccles, J., & Friedman, H. S. (2014). Conscientiousness, health, and aging: The life course of personality model. *Developmental Psychology, 50,* 1407–1425.

Yoo, J., Miyamoto, Y., Rigotti, A., & Ryff, C. D. (2017). Linking positive affect to blood lipids: A cultural perspective. *Psychological Science, 28,* 1468–1477.

Yoo, J., Miyamoto, Y., & Ryff, C. D. (2016). Positive affect, social connectedness, and health biomarkers in Japan and the US. *Emotion, 16*(8), 1137–1146.

Conclusion

Matthew T. Lee, Laura D. Kubzansky, and Tyler J. VanderWeele

The chapters in this volume affirm the value not only of specialized, discipline-specific research on the nature of well-being—its antecedents, and its consequences—but also of synthesizing interdisciplinary scholarship into a coherent body of research findings, theoretical explanations, and policy recommendations regarding well-being. Each of the 20 chapters makes a contribution to more than one scholarly discipline, and many bridge the social sciences and the humanities. In some cases, a disciplinary expert engaged with the methods or findings of an outside discipline. Other chapters were co-authored by scholars in the both humanities and social sciences. Still others were written by interdisciplinary experts. Beyond the individual chapters, the volume as a whole informs the meta-conversation about how scholars might draw on their specific expertise to transcend disciplinary boundaries and contribute to the collective work of conceptualizing and measuring well-being in ways that effectively advance our understanding of and ability to improve population health. In other words, we believe bringing together work from across often siloed disciplines will provide important insight regarding how individuals and social organizations can pursue the good life and build better societies. We hope that readers will appreciate each individual chapter on its own terms while also gaining a broader awareness of how the study of well-being might benefit from more sustained interdisciplinary dialogue. Ultimately, we hope our volume will encourage further efforts at synthesis by identifying and then building on areas of emerging consensus (see, for example, Chapter 17). The prospect of a "well-ordered" interdisciplinary science of well-being might continue to serve as guiding principle for work going forward (see Chapter 6).

Matthew T. Lee, Laura D. Kubzansky, and Tyler J. VanderWeele, *Conclusion* In: *Measuring Well-Being*. Edited by: Matthew T. Lee, Laura D. Kubzansky, and Tyler J. VanderWeele, Oxford University Press (2021). © Oxford University Press. DOI: 10.1093/oso/9780197512531.003.0022

Consensus and Disagreement in the Interdisciplinary Dialogue about Well-Being

Nearly everyone is in favor of promoting higher levels of well-being. But despite this bedrock consensus, many chapters in this volume—especially those describing the lively debate about measurement recommendations in Part 4—confirm that disagreements will invariably arise about how to go about measurement. How should well-being be defined? What are its essential domains? Are these domains in conflict with each other, such that tradeoffs are inevitable for the majority of people? How should the domains be measured? Which pathways to well-being or apparent effects of well-being involve causal relationships and which observed associations are actually spurious? Perhaps most fundamentally, philosophers have devoted substantial attention to the issue of whether a "radical kind of pluralism" (Chapter 7, p. 225) must eventually shipwreck interdisciplinary conversations because the term "well-being" refers to multiple incommensurate underlying constructs.

We expect that the "systematic cleavage" (Chapter 9, p. 278) between empirical measures of well-being and philosophical conceptualizations will continue to present difficulties. Across and within academic disciplines, different "interpretive communities" (Fish, 1980) understand well-being in ways that prioritize some domains, conceptualizations, and pathways over others based on the social standpoints and foundational assumptions that are shared by members of such communities. Conflicts are frequently generated by the presuppositional fault lines that separate such interpretive communities. Our introductory chapter reviewed some examples, including the focus on happiness and life satisfaction currently ascendant within social science disciplines compared to the primacy of more eschatologically "ultimate" concerns in some of the humanities, especially theology.

Our volume does not aim to resolve such tensions. Postmodern perspectives on human cultural variation would argue that a complete resolution is neither possible nor desirable. On the other hand, emerging post-postmodernist streams of thought contend that such relativistic views are not necessarily definitive and that coherent integration may in fact be possible. One conclusion is clear from the chorus of voices across the disciplines represented in our book: the interdisciplinary field of well-being will be enhanced when scholars more fully appreciate the cultural presuppositions that guide their conceptualization and measurement decisions (for explicit statements to this effect from theologians, see Chapters 10 and 11;

from psychologists, see Chapter 3; from philosophers, Chapters 7 and 9; from sociologists, Chapter 15; and from psychologists and a philosopher, see Chapter 13). Even the seemingly innocuous act of creating a composite measure of well-being implies a "philosophical commitment, to a kind of even-handed pluralism" (Chapter 13, p. 403). Margolis et al. (Chapter 13, p. 403) conclude: "There is no such thing as a value-free measure of human flourishing. We are all philosophers."

To affirm this point is not to suggest that synthesis is impossible or that we cannot make progress. Indeed, the overwhelming majority of participants in the Interdisciplinary Workshop on Happiness, Well-Being, and Measurement held at Harvard University that launched this volume were able to come to a consensus on a set of shared recommendations for selecting measures of well-being for various purposes (see VanderWeele et al., Chapter 17; but see also the dissenting viewpoint provided by Ryff, Boylan, and Kirsch in Part 4). As editors, we thought that it was fitting to conclude the volume with an active discussion and debate. After all, the free exchange of ideas has always enlivened the humanities and social sciences. We encourage the scholars among our readers to examine the arguments in Part 4, reflect on their own scholarship as well as on relevant debates in their fields of study, draw their own conclusions, and offer their own contributions to the ongoing dialogue. As Ryff, Boylan, and Kirsch (Chapter 18, p. 521) so eloquently put it, "the arbiters of such matters will not be the authors of the current volume, including ourselves, but rather members of the scientific community and government officials who must make difficult decisions in how to assess well-being."

We believe that such choices will be better informed if decision-makers follow the principles articulated by contributors to this volume. We have already mentioned the value of greater attention to presuppositions, and it is important enough that we reiterate it again. In addition, it will be helpful to adopt several other strategies when seeking to gain greater insight into population health and well-being, including giving greater weight to well-designed longitudinal studies rather than cross-sectional research (see Chapter 5), considering the thoughtful methodological advice provided by Tay, Jebb, and Scotney (Chapter 3), drawing on the extensive accumulated wisdom of those who have led large-scale investigations (Chapters 1 and 2), attending to important group differences with regard to the experience and expression of well-being (Chapters 4 and 16), and following the tried-and-true principles that guide well-ordered science (Chapter 6).

Even with these principles firmly in mind, reasonable people will disagree. To take just one example, the recommendations provided by VanderWeele and 18 co-authors (Chapter 17) accept the reality that some large surveys that guide policy decisions about well-being will have room for only a small number of questions about well-being itself. Ryff, Boyland, and Kirsch (Chapter 18) object to this approach. In their response, VanderWeele, Trudel-Fitzgerald, and Kubzansky (Chapter 19, p. 536) contend that "it is better to include one [well-being survey item] than none at all" (cf. VanderWeele et al., 2020). Ryff, Boyland, and Kirsch (Chapter 20, p. 547) dissent from this viewpoint and suggest that such a "stance perpetuates a simplistic view of well-being." This debate underscores two distinct types of risks. On the one hand, there is the risk that social policy will be determined in the absence of data about well-being. On the other, there is the risk that policy will be guided by overly simplistic data. In both cases, there is potential for inadequately informed decisions. We hope that decision-makers who find themselves on the horns of this genuine dilemma are able to benefit from the debate presented in this volume. With time, the right way forward—or some middle ground— may emerge although this, of course, may vary by context.

In addition to clarifying such dilemmas, contributors to our volume also offered examples of integrative thinking that underscore the complementary ways in which distinct disciplines and schools of thought might cross-pollinate to advance well-being. For example, a resourceful philosophical synthesis of the core ideas of Aristotle and Lacan—two thinkers who begin with radically different assumptions about human nature—contributes to an cohesive conception of well-being that supports a hybrid of objective list theories and desire theories (Chapter 8). And, despite significant differences, core philosophical and spiritual ideals from both East and West tend to support a unified view of inner peace that may be broadly applicable across cultures (Chapter 15). In addition, and contrary to concerns about epistemic crises across disciplines, traditional theological reflection on health and well-being supports a holistic view that views these outcomes as deeply interconnected with social, political, and economic forces, consistent with influential perspectives in social science and public health (Chapter 10; Link & Phelan, 1995; Subramanian, Kim, & Kawachi, 2005). Similarly, an integration of philosophy and psychology guided the creation of a more comprehensive measure of meaning in life (Chapter 12) and the use of a psychological measure to engage with the concept of friendship as understood by philosophers (Chapter 9). Also worth noting is that the development of a measure appropriate to one religious tradition can serve as a template for the subsequent elaboration of measures for other traditions (Chapter 16).

What Is Well-Being?

We conclude by returning to the question that motivated this volume: What is well-being? Our chapters demonstrate some of the substantial progress already made across disciplines, but we expect this question will continue to animate scholarly debate for many years to come. This is partly because people prioritize different aspects of well-being and quite often sacrifice one domain to enhance another (Adler, Dolanb, & Kavetsos, 2017). For example, theological virtues such as "poverty of spirit" or humility might be considered vices—"slave morality"—by philosophers such as Aristotle or Nietzsche (Chapter 10; Lee, 2014). Furthermore, "human life, as we experience it and investigate it in this world, is always already a complex mix of the good and the broken" (Chapter 10, p. 288). In other words, experiences cannot be neatly dichotomized into well-being or ill-being. Physical illness and its attendant suffering provide a good example. From a biomedical perspective, illness must be prevented or cured and pain must be eliminated. But from a spiritual perspective, illness and the suffering it causes may be viewed as a good rather than an evil when it awakens a person to their spiritual complacency and prompts the acquisition of virtue and spiritual growth. Illness is thus part of the "divine pedagogy" that purifies and refines the "spiritual intelligence" through suffering (Larchet, 2002, pp. 60–61). On this view, people who avoid serious physical illness may waste their lives by becoming content with hedonic happiness and unconcerned about deeper forms of meaning and purpose or spiritual well-being. Illness, rather than health, may be a gift.

Or consider physical safety, another apparently clear indication of well-being that becomes much more complicated once we adopt Messer's awareness of the world as an admixture of the good and the broken. When the first author of this concluding chapter was conducting interviews for a research project on the religious call to benevolent service (Lee, Poloma, & Post, 2013), one of the interviewees described the serious injuries he sustained from a violent assault that resulted from his ministry in a high-crime neighborhood. But the interviewee quickly turned the notion of safety on its head when he explained that, while growing up, his mother would frequently tell him that he was "not called to safety," that "the most dangerous place for Christians is to remain safe," and that Christians are "called to follow Christ, to suffer, to be with folks who are hurting." Within his interpretive community, an altruistic physical sacrifice was a small price to pay for the meaningful forms of well-being that he experienced through his benevolent work in a neighborhood that could well expose him to future assault and physical injury. Well-being, like altruism, is deeply interconnected with a group's moral code and ability to generate life-giving solidarity—in short, with culture (Lee, 2014).

We suggest that our starting question "what is well-being?" must eventually point beyond the individual to a deeper question: "What is well-being for?" Well-being is, of course, an end in itself, and it can often feel as if it is the sole responsibility of the individual to find ways to attain it. However, most philosophical and religious traditions connect the individual attainment of well-being with features of social organization, or even divine action, that promote or inhibit this outcome, with virtuous individual and group actions that benefit others rather than self, with healthy community and intergroup relations (Chapter 14), and, above all, with self-transcendent ends. Maslow (1970, p. 272), for example, argued that happiness and other conventional measures of individual well-being are not the proper aim of life; rather, the goal is to reach a higher level of human development, to become "a sound member of the human species." For Christian theologians, "at the core of the Christian ideal of the spiritual life stands the practice of neighbor love" (Chapter 11, p. 325). It would seem that happiness as a by-product of virtuous actions that benefit others is preferable, in most ethical systems, to just coping and/or selfish hedonism. Promoting good even in difficult situations and reliably doing what is right as a leader in a community is central to well-being.

Such virtuous awareness can extend beyond individuals to organizations and larger groups. For example, some business organizations have created a virtuous culture that socializes managers to take responsibility for the prevention of fatal worker "accidents," while organizations with nonvirtuous cultures may promote the belief that worker safety is beyond their control (Haines, 1997). The physical well-being of workers is therefore enhanced by the virtuousness of the culture and the organizational leaders, and the same may be true for psychological well-being. More generally, many contemporary organizations are rife with stifling practices, dehumanizing structures, unsatisfying relationships, and disengaged members, so it is no surprise that Gallup polls across a variety of economic sectors routinely find that only about one-third of members are "engaged" (Laloux, 2014; Miller, Latham, & Cahill, 2017). As complete well-being (VanderWeele, 2017) has attained more prominence among scholars, laypersons, and policy-makers, awareness among organizational leaders, members, and stakeholders is shifting toward understandings of well-being rooted in wholeness and virtue. More people are understanding their role as *stewards of the larger system* in which their organization is embedded, rather than attending only to duties required by their specific organizational role (Laloux, 2014; Scharmer & Kaufer, 2013). There is now a broad social movement developing around the goal of helping systems become more responsible for fostering complete well-being and equity for all, which is shifting the interdisciplinary dialogue about not only measuring well-being but also about determining who (and what) is responsible for promoting well-being (Well-Being in the Nation Network, 2019; see also Willett et al., 2019).

Conclusion

The chapters in this volume have made significant contributions to our knowledge of the interdisciplinary conceptualization and measurement of well-being. More work is needed, including the psychometric validation of many of the new measures that have been proposed, adding the voice of disciplines that were not as well-represented among our contributors (e.g., history and yet further engagement with economics and political science) and a more complete engagement with both concepts and data drawn from outside Western, educated, industrialized, rich, and democratic (WEIRD) societies (Henrich, Heine, & Norenzayan, 2010; Lambert et al., 2020).

As we write these final words, the social, political, and human costs of the COVID-19 pandemic continue to expand. Now, more than ever, we need clear thinking and effective policy-making to promote well-being for all. Scholars will not be the only voices in the debates to come about how to do this. But we believe that the tools of our trade—a commitment to learn from past wisdom, the application of logic and reason, the systematic search for empirical truths, an ability to make sense of patterns in the data—will continue to be of indispensable value. We hope that this volume inspires further work in these directions and provides some guidance about how to bring different disciplines into hospitable dialogue.

About the Authors

Matthew T. Lee is Director of Empirical Research at the Human Flourishing Program in the Institute for Quantitative Social Science at Harvard University and coauthor of *The Heart of Religion* (Oxford University Press, 2013). He is also Distinguished Visiting Scholar of Health, Flourishing, and Positive Psychology at Stony Brook University's Center for Medical Humanities, Compassionate Care, and Bioethics, and he previously served as Chair of the American Sociological Association's Section on Altruism, Morality, and Social Solidarity. His research explores pathways to human flourishing, benevolent service to others, and the integration of social science and the humanities.

Laura D. Kubzansky is Lee Kum Kee Professor of Social and Behavioral Sciences and co-Director of the Lee Kum Sheung Center for Health and Happiness at the Harvard T. H. Chan School of Public Health. Dr. Kubzansky has published extensively on the role of psychological and social factors in health. Ongoing research includes studying biobehavioral mechanisms linking emotions, social relationships, and health; defining, measuring, and modifying aspects of well-being; and workplace conditions in relation to well-being. She has served on the leadership team for multiple training programs for junior scholars and is primary investigator or co-investigator on numerous grants.

Tyler J. VanderWeele is the John L. Loeb and Frances Lehman Loeb Professor of Epidemiology in the Departments of Epidemiology and Biostatistics at the Harvard T. H. Chan School of Public Health, Director of the Human Flourishing Program, and Co-Director of the Initiative on Health, Religion, and Spirituality at Harvard University. His research concerns methodology for distinguishing between association and causation in observational studies, and his empirical research spans psychiatric, perinatal, and social epidemiology; the science of happiness and flourishing; and the study of religion and health, including both religion and population health and the role of religion and spirituality in end-of-life care. He has published more than 300 papers in peer-reviewed journals and is author of the book *Explanation in Causal Inference* (Oxford University Press, 2015).

Author Note

This work was supported in part by a grant from the John Templeton Foundation, by the Lee Kum Sheung Center for Health and Happiness, and by the Human Flourishing Program at Harvard University. The views expressed in this chapter represent the perspectives of the authors and do not reflect the opinions or endorsement of any organization. We have no known conflict of interest to disclose. Correspondence concerning this chapter should be directed to Matthew T. Lee, Human Flourishing Program, Harvard University, 129 Mt. Auburn St., Cambridge, MA, 02138 (matthew_lee@fas.harvard.edu).

References

Adler, M. D., Dolanb, P., & Kavetsos, G. (2017). Would you choose to be happy? Tradeoffs between happiness and the other dimensions of life in a large population survey. *Journal of Economic Behavior and Organization, 139*, 60–73.

Fish, S. F. (1980). *Is there a text in this class? The authority of interpretive communities.* Cambridge, MA: Harvard University Press.

Haines, F. (1997). *Corporate regulation: Beyond "punish or persuade."* New York: Oxford University Press.

Henrich, J., Heine, S. J., & Norenzayan, A. (2010). The weirdest people in the world?. *Behavioral and Brain Sciences, 33*(2-3), 61–83.

Laloux, F. (2014). *Reinventing organizations: A guide to creating organizations inspired by the next stage of human consciousness.* Brussels: Nelson Parker.

Lambert, L., Lomas, T., van de Weijer, M. P., Passmore, H. A., Joshanloo, M., Harter, J., . . . Diener, E. (2020). Towards a greater global understanding of wellbeing: A proposal for a more inclusive measure. *International Journal of Wellbeing, 10*(2), 1–18.

Larchet, J. (2002). *The theology of illness.* Crestwood, NY: St. Vladimir's Seminary.

Lee, M. T. (2014). The essential interconnections among altruism, morality, and social solidarity: The case of religious altruism. In V. Jeffries (Ed.), *The Palgrave handbook of altruism, morality, and social solidarity: Formulating a field of study* (pp. 311–331). New York: Palgrave Macmillan.

Lee, M. T., Poloma, M. M., & Post, S. G. (2013). *The heart of religion: Spiritual empowerment, benevolence, and the experience of God's love.* New York: Oxford University Press.

Link, B., & Phelan, J. (1995). Social conditions as fundamental causes of disease. *Journal of Health and Social Behavior, 35*, 80–94.

Maslow, A. H. (1970). *Motivation and personality* (2019 ed.). New Delhi: Prabhat Prakashan.

Miller, R., B. Latham, & Cahill, B. (2017). *Humanizing the education machine: How to create schools that turn disengaged kids into inspired learners.* Hoboken: Wiley.

Scharmer, O., & Kaufer, K. (2013). *Leading from the emerging future: From ego-system to eco-system economies.* San Francisco: Berrett-Koehler.

Subramanian, S. V., Kim, D., & Kawachi, I. (2005). Covariation in the socioeconomic determinants of self-rated health and happiness: A multivariate multilevel analysis of individuals and communities in the USA. *Journal of Epidemiology and Community Health, 59*(8), 664–669.

VanderWeele, T. J. (2017). On the promotion of human flourishing. *Proceedings of the National Academy of Sciences of the United States of America, 114*(31), 8148–8156.

VanderWeele, T. J., Trudel-Fitzgerald, C., Allin, P., Farrelly, C., Fletcher, G., Frederick, D. E., . . . Kubzansky, L. D. (2020). Brief well-being assessments, or nothing at all?. *Preventive Medicine* https://doi.org/10.1016/j.ypmed.2020.106095

Well-Being in the Nation Network. (2019). Theory of change and action plan: What does it take to secure legacies of intergenerational well-being for all? https://winnetwork. org/about/win-theory-of-change/

Willett W., Rockström J., Loken B., Springmann M., Lang T., Vermeulen S., . . . Jonell, M. (2019). Food in the Anthropocene: The EAT–Lancet Commission on healthy diets from sustainable food systems. *Lancet, 393*, 447–492.

Name Index

Subject Index

For the benefit of digital users, indexed terms that span two pages (e.g., 52–53) may, on occasion, appear on only one of those pages.

Boxes and figures are indicated by italic *b* and *f*, respectively.